OXFORD MEDICAL PUBLICATIONS

Epidemiology of the Rheumatic Diseases

Epidemiology of the Rheumatic Diseases

SECOND EDITION

Edited by

ALAN J. SILMAN

Professor of Rheumatic Diseases, ARC Epidemiology Unit,
Manchester University Medical School

and

MARC C. HOCHBERG

Professor of Medicine and Epidemiology and Preventive Medicine,
and Head of the
Division of Rheumatology and Clinical Immunology,
University of Maryland School of Medicine

with contributions from

CYRUS COOPER
MRC Environmental Epidemiology Unit,
University of Southampton

HEINER RASPE
Department of Social Medicine,
University Clinics Luebeck

ELAINE DENNISON
MRC Environmental Epidemiology Unit,
University of Southampton

VIOLETA RUS
Department of Medicine,
University of Maryland School of Medicine

ALI HAJEER
ARC Epidemiology Unit,
University of Manchester

DEBORAH P.M. SYMMONS
ARC Epidemiology Unit,
University of Manchester

GARY J. MACFARLANE
Unit of Chronic Disease Epidemiology,
University of Manchester

WENDY THOMSON
ARC Epidemiology Unit
University of Manchester

TERENCE W. O'NEILL
ARC Epidemiology Unit,
Manchester University

KAREN WALKER-BONE
MRC Environmental Epidemiology Unit,
University of Southampton

RA645
M85
E65
2001

OXFORD
UNIVERSITY PRESS

OXFORD

UNIVERSITY PRESS

Great Clarendon Street, Oxford OX2 6DP

Oxford University Press is a department of the University of Oxford.
It furthers the University's objective of excellence in research, scholarship,
and education by publishing worldwide in

Oxford New York

Athens Auckland Bangkok Bogota Bombay Buenos Aires Cape Town
Chennai Dar es Salaam Delhi Florence Hong Kong Istanbul Karachi
Kolkata Kuala Lumpur Madrid Melbourne Mexico City Mumbai Nairobi
Paris São Paulo Shanghai Singapore Taipei Tokyo Toronto Warsaw

and associated companies in
Berlin Ibadan

Oxford is a trade mark of Oxford University Press
in the UK and in certain other countries

Published in the United States
by Oxford University Press Inc., New York

© Oxford University Press, 2001

The moral rights of the author have been asserted

Database right Oxford University Press (maker)

First edition 1993
Second edition 2001

All rights reserved. No part of this publication may be reproduced,
stored in a retrieval system or transmitted, in any form or by any means,
without the prior permission in writing of Oxford University Press.
or as expressly permitted by law, or under terms agreed with the appropriate
reprographics rights organization. Enquiries concerning reproduction
outside the scope of the above should be sent to the Rights Department,
Oxford University Press, at the address above.

You must not circulate this book in any other binding or cover
and you must impose this same condition on any acquirer

A catalogue record for this title is available from the British Library

Library of Congress Cataloging in Publication Data

Silman, Alan J.
Epidemiology of the rheumatic diseases/Alan J. Silman and Marc C. Hochberg; with
contributions from Cyrus Cooper ... [et al.]–2nd ed.
(Oxford medical publications)
Includes bibliographical references and index.
1. Musculoskeletal system–Diseases–Epidemiology.   2. Rheumatism–Epidemiology
3. Connective tissues–Diseases–Epidemiology.   I. Hochberg, Marc.   II. Title.   III.
Series.
[DNLM: 1. Rheumatic Diseases–epidemiology. WE 544 S584e 2001]
RA645.M85 S55 2001   614.5′9723–dc21   2001036225

ISBN 0 19 263149 7 (Hbk)

10 9 8 7 6 5 4 3 2 1

Typeset by
EXPO Holdings, Malaysia
Printed in Great Britain
on acid-free paper by
Bookcraft (Bath) Ltd.
Midsomer Norton

Foreword

The revision of the 1993 Oxford University Press book *Epidemiology of the Rheumatic Diseases* by Alan Silman and Marc Hochberg is most welcome and timely at the start of the Bone and Joint Decade Initiative.

Despite the considerable impact of musculoskeletal diseases on the prevalence of disability and consumption of medical resources, rheumatic diseases are not mentioned in the WHO Burden of Disease list. This trend of looking only at fatal diseases is changing, but we have to provide the data on musculoskeletal diseases world-wide. This revised book will certainly be a guideline for WHO to fill the gap and change the trend.

Because of the ageing population all over the world, musculoskeletal disorders are forming an increasingly important contribution to the overall burden of disease. ILAR's (International League of Associations for Rheumatology) Standing Committee on Epidemiology, in which both authors of the book are leading members, has initiated the COPCORD study (Community Orientated Program for Control of Rheumatic Diseases) in Asia, South America, and Africa. These COPCORD studies have already shown that musculoskeletal problems are as common in developing countries as in the developed world. These data, together with the data reported in the revision of Epidemiology of the Rheumatic Diseases, are not only of primary importance for WHO Burden of Diseases records, but also for practising clinicians, researchers, educators, and leaders in the pharmaceutical industry.

The thing that matters is that the burden of chronic rheumatic diseases and its resulting disability will be reduced. This can only be achieved by a better knowledge of the epidemiology, improved education at the undergraduate and graduate level, and more research in basic and applied science, so that the patient will have appropriate medical and holistic therapy before disability sets in.

Rheumatology is a broad diagnostic specialty, akin to internal medicine, dealing with not only rheumatoid arthritis, systemic autoimmune diseases such as lupus, systemic sclerosis, vasculitis, spondyloarthropathies, and reactive arthritis, but also with osteoarthritis, osteoporosis, crystal arthropathies, back ache, and soft tissue rheumatism. The new edition of this book has additional chapters on Paget's disease, vasculitis, regional pain, and chronic widespread pain syndromes. For all of these diseases there are new pathophysiologic discoveries and therapeutic possibilities, and most importantly epidemiology is considerably changing due to the ageing of the population. This unique, updated epidemiology book will add to the globalization of rheumatology by giving better information on incidence and prevalence of rheumatic diseases and should support evidence-based strategies for future developments in the field of rheumatology.

The chapters do not just give incidence and prevalence of the different diseases but also definitions, criteria, risk factors, ethnic as well as geographical and genetic factors, morbidity and mortality.

The authors have to be congratulated with what they have achieved. It is more strenuous to revise and re-edit a book than to write the original one.

Professor Dr E.M. Jan Dequeker, MD, PhD, FRCP Edin.
President of ILAR

Acknowledgments

The authors would not have been able to complete the task without the considerable contribution of Dr Jacqui Pearson, our editorial assistant, responsible for undertaking much of the literature searching, citation checking, and reading of drafts. Cath Barrow, Margarita Cook, Cathy Morgan, Stephanie Crocker, and Mary Ingram from the ARC Unit in Manchester worked tirelessly helping to prepare the drafts, figures and the reference lists for publication. We are also grateful to a number of colleagues who reviewed earlier drafts of chapters. Particular thanks should be given to Dr Gonzalez-Gay for his comments on the chapter on polymyalgia rheumatica and giant cell arthritis and Professor David G. I. Scott for his considerable contribution to the chapter on vasculitis.

Contents

PART II: Connective tissue diseases

Contents

Introduction

Alan J. Silman and Marc C. Hochberg

Scope of epidemiology

In common usage the term epidemiology has two meanings. The first is the description of the occurrence of a disease and the risk factors—demographic, genetic, and environmental—for its development. The second covers a methodological approach to investigate not only disease occurrence and aetiology but also, and increasingly, to the development of criteria for disease classification, studies of natural history, intervention studies including clinical trials, and the evaluation of clinical tests. Thus textbooks of epidemiology are either reviews of data on disease occurrence and causation or are manuals for those wishing to apply epidemiological methods on a wider field.

The results of epidemiological studies should be capable of extrapolation to populations, the latter referring either in the demographic sense to a geographically defined denominator or to a theoretical population, for example all individuals with a disease or a risk factor. A common error is to apply the term 'epidemiological' to observations made on a personal series of perhaps a handful of cases. Thus reports of a 2:1 female excess in a clinical series of patients, case reports of disease concordant identical twins, or case series of disease developing after exposure to a specific environment agent are not epidemiological observations. They are, however, useful in generating hypotheses for formal study. The major problem, and this is particularly relevant to the rheumatic diseases, is the difficulty in undertaking sound epidemiological studies.

Problems in undertaking rheumatic disease epidemiology

A common theme that emerges in virtually all the conditions considered in this volume is the difficulty in deriving epidemiological data. The art of the epidemiologists is perhaps not in undertaking (the impossible)—the 'perfect' study—but in understanding the imperfections in studies, both self conducted and reported by others, and hence achieving a reasonable interpretation of the available data. Specific problems for the rheumatic diseases include:

1. The difficulty in defining a case. There are two issues, the first being the frequent occurrence of mild or indeterminate disease such as 'probable' rheumatoid arthritis (a term in regular use until 1988) and 'incomplete' SLE (see Chapter 7); the second being the occurrence of subclinical forms of disease whose significance is not well understood, for example asymptomatic radiographic osteoarthritis.

2. The lack of a clear distinction between the different disorders. One major problem in surveys is the difficulty in distinguishing mild rheumatoid arthritis from generalized osteoarthritis in its early stages. A second common example of confusion is the rare multisystem diseases for which a series of terms such as 'overlap syndrome' and 'mixed connective tissue disease' have been proposed which, in our opinion, hinder rather than enhance epidemiological understanding.

3. The difficulty in case ascertainment. Some chronic diseases such as cancer and insulin dependent diabetes will inevitably become clinically apparent both to the patient and his physician. Thus 'capture' of cases can be achieved by monitoring clinic facilities and, for some disorders, hospital inpatient statistics and even death certificates can be used. By contrast, the major rheumatic diseases such as rheumatoid arthritis and osteoarthritis, particularly in their early stage, are frequently not clinically obvious either to the patient or his

physician. The necessary alternative is therefore to undertake costly and time consuming population surveys.

4.   Verification of disease status typically necessitates radiographic examination, for example in osteoarthritis of the hip, which is not acceptable to many populations and regulatory bodies in the current climate of environment concern.

5.   Many of the rheumatic diseases are so rare that the size of population surveys required to determine prevalence are probably in excess of what is feasible. Furthermore, the optimal epidemiological approach to investigating disease causation, the prospective cohort study, is not applicable to the study of such rare disorders. As a consequence, most of the data on risk factors are derived from retrospective, clinic-based case-control studies. These are subject to several potential biases, which limit interpretation and extrapolation. Not surprisingly these methodological difficulties often produce conflicting results to the same question as illustrated in the subsequent chapters.

It would be wrong to assume, however, that epidemiology has been incapable of generating information about the rheumatic diseases. Indeed as this volume demonstrates there is a considerable amount of material available for interpretation.

Scope of this volume

The term rheumatic diseases does not have a clear boundary but perhaps could reasonably be taken as those diseases seen in rheumatological practice. We have concentrated on those disorders seen in the developed world and have not considered those conditions that are specific to very small geographical areas such as Kashin-Beck or Mseleni disease. The many forms of infectious arthritis, including acute rheumatic fever, have not been included as a specific topic, mainly because their epidemiological characteristics are those of the underlying infection and their detailed consideration are more appropriate to a text book of infectious diseases. By contrast we have included chapters on 'non-articular' or 'soft tissue' rheumatism including back pain. Although these disorders do not occur frequently in the pages of the major rheumatological journals or in the programmes of major rheumatological

meetings, they do affect large numbers in the population and form, for many, a large part of rheumatological practice. Osteoporosis has been included, though not strictly a rheumatic disease. Its study and indeed its management have recently become a major source of interest to rheumatologists.

It was our aim to have as unified a format as possible in discussing the epidemiological characteristics of the various disorders. The format has remained flexible to cope with the relevance of some of the headings used for the different disorders. In general, each chapter commences by discussing case definition and criteria. This is then followed by a review of data on occurrence—prevalence and incidence—and their demographic predictors, including trends over time, geographical, and racial variation. Risk factors are then assessed under three headings: genetic, host, and environmental. Under 'genetic' have been included data based both on classical genetic studies—familial aggregation and twin studies—followed by more recent studies of immunogenetic and other gene markers. The 'host' section refers to 'non-genetic' factors present in the host that might increase disease risk, including such items as body build, pregnancy history, and co-morbidity. There is a paucity of data on environmental risk factors for most of the rheumatic diseases. Exposure to infectious agents is a major theme of much research in inflammatory joint diseases but with little concrete data. Other environmental exposures such as diet, smoking and occupation are considered where the data warrants mention.

Since the first edition was published in 1993, there has been an enormous number of published studies in all aspects of the epidemiology of rheumatic diseases. Indeed there has probably been as much new material published in the past 7 years as there was in the previous 30 years. As a consequence, every chapter in the volume has been completely reworked and revised to exclude some of the historical and redundant material and to cover all the recent developments. Particular mention should be made of the recent advances in molecular genetics which has resulted in a considerable number of both hypothesis generating and hypothesis testing studies in all the major disorders.

We have included new chapters on the systemic vasculitides, including disorders such as Wegener's granulomatosis and Churg–Strauss syndrome, and on Paget's disease. The section on soft tissue rheumatism has been extensively rewritten and now presented in two separate chapters, the first on chronic widespread pain including fibromyalgia and the second covering the major regional pain syndromes affecting the cervical spine and upper limb. A further welcome addition is the introductory chapter reviewing data on the burden of rheumatic and musculoskeletal diseases as a whole based on population survey material. Changing concepts in disease classification as applied to chronic arthritis in childhood and the HLA-B27-related spondyloarthropathies have been incorporated into the text. In order to accommodate this new material without increasing the size of the book to an unmanageable proportion we have dropped the chapter in the first edition on the pharmaco-epidemiology. That chapter covered the epidemiology of adverse reactions to antirheumatic drugs. This is a field advancing to such an extent that it clearly merits a volume of its own. In addition we have also excluded, from this current volume, the contribution of epidemiology to understanding the natural history and outcome of rheumatic disorders and again these are important issues but the material currently available is so vast as to justify its publication elsewhere.

1 | *Population studies of musculoskeletal morbidity*

Deborah P. M. Symmons

Introduction

This chapter reviews the advantages and disadvantages of population-based studies of musculoskeletal morbidity and disability, and summarises the results available.

Epidemiological studies of occurrence should, ideally, be generalizable not only to the whole population in which they were conducted but also to other populations. This means that the cases included in the epidemiological study should be representative of all cases of that condition in the community. Indeed, this is the underlying assumption of many published papers—yet often it is not true. Cases of a condition in the community may be identified from a number of sources (Fig. 1.1). A number of factors determine whether people make their way up the pyramid. For example consider the situation where the researcher wishes to establish the prevalence of symptomatic osteoarthritis of the spine. He could conduct a population survey but this would be expensive. He could decide to base his study in primary care and include all individuals presenting with back pain. Whether or not individuals

with back pain seek medical attention will be determined by the severity of the pain, the degree to which it interferes with their everyday life, whether it prevents them from working, and whether they believe anything can be done to help. Some individuals with spinal osteoarthritis may present with referred pain to the leg which the primary care physician might incorrectly diagnose as intermittent claudication. Such an individual would not be included in the researcher's study. Even more factors come into play if the study is based on hospital ascertained cases. Whether an individual is referred to hospital depends not only on the characteristics (demographic, psychosocial, and condition) of the individual but also on the characteristics of the referring physician and of the hospital (distance away, facilities and skills available, and so on). Therefore, in order to avoid the issues of selection and referral bias, studies should, whenever possible, be conducted in the community.

Studies may be regarded as 'population-based' if they can be referred back to a general population defined by geopolitical boundaries (e.g. a country, county, or

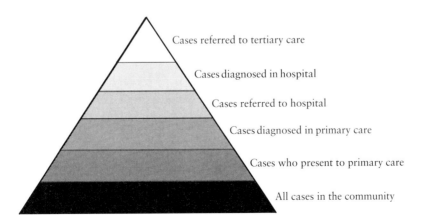

Fig. 1.1   The case ascertainment pyramid.

health authority area). This population will be either the denominator (if all cases have been identified) or the sampling frame.

Population-based studies—methodological issues

Advantages

The main advantage of a population-based study over a clinic-based study is that it is more likely to include representative cases and so to be generalizable. Thus studies whose aim is to identify the burden of illness within a community should be population rather than clinic based, except for conditions such as fractured neck of femur which lead more or less inevitably to hospital attendance. Studies which focus on symptoms rather than diagnoses can also address the issue of 'overlap' or 'double counting'. Many individuals have musculoskeletal pain at more than one site. Adding together the estimated number of individuals with knee pain, back pain, and shoulder pain using the results of different studies will give an inflated estimate of the overall burden of musculoskeletal pain. Studies which look at pain in a number of sites simultaneously offer a better estimate of overall morbidity and provide useful insights into patterns of pain. Similarly studies of locomotor disability are best conducted in the community since, in the individual, the aetiology of disability is often multi-factorial.

Studies of symptoms are not the same as studies of diagnoses. It is well recognized that many people with, for example, abnormal spinal radiographs do not have back pain and vice versa. Population surveys offer the opportunity to study in parallel the epidemiology of pathology (e.g. radiograph changes), specific diagnoses (where a clinical evaluation is included), musculoskeletal pain, and disability. The results are often intriguing!

Disadvantages

Cost

It is very expensive to conduct any type of community-based survey. This is especially so for musculoskeletal conditions where it is usually necessary to employ a minimum of two stages if any diagnostic label is to be applied. Few rheumatic conditions can be correctly classified on the basis of symptoms alone and it is usually necessary to conduct a physical examination and/or laboratory and radiological investigations before applying classification criteria. Community-based studies are especially expensive when investigating uncommon conditions. This is because the sample size has to be large in order to identify a reasonable number of cases. The US National Health and Examination Survey of 1970–1 included a clinical examination of 6913 subjects. Nevertheless, it was only possible to generate robust estimates of the prevalence of osteoarthritis (OA), rheumatoid arthritis (RA), bursitis and gout [1]. Studies of diseases which are less common have to use a different approach which may, nevertheless, be population-based [2].

Response bias

All the arguments about representativeness and generalizability of population-based studies are negated if a study has a low response rate. Whether or not an individual responds to a survey is seldom random. Generally, individuals are more likely to respond if they have the condition under investigation, are female, aged more than 45, and belong to a higher socio-economic grouping [3]. It is notoriously difficult to get young males to participate in population-based studies [4].

Wording of the question

Many population studies focus on symptoms. The results may be highly dependent on the wording of the questions. The question 'Have you had pain lasting for more than a day in the last week?' may yield an entirely different pattern from 'Have you had any pain in the last week?' and yet both are estimating the one-week period prevalence. Investigators seldom present data on the sensitivity, specificity, positive predictive value or repeatability of the questions and definitions which they have used and so it is difficult to choose the 'best' estimate of disease occurrence.

There is evidence that, even when the same question wording is used, higher prevalence estimates are produced by health interview surveys than by multi-purpose surveys [5]. Asking respondents whether they 'have' a particular illness will produce higher estimates than asking them if they 'suffer' from that illness.

The Mini-Finland Health Survey included a Health Interview and a Health Examination part, which were conducted independently of one another. The agreement between the two interviews conducted 4–6 months apart was only fair for musculoskeletal disorders (kappa = 0.44) although it was somewhat higher for inflammatory polyarthritis (kappa = 0.54) [6]. The interview data also showed poor agreement with the findings at examination (kappa = 0.38).

Self-reported diagnoses

Government-sponsored surveys tend to rely on self-reported symptoms and diagnoses. Individuals frequently do not know and cannot identify the specific musculoskeletal diseases that affect them. For this reason it is often necessary to use rather vague collective terms such as 'arthritis and rheumatism' when asking people to specify what is wrong with them. Methodology studies have shown that conditions which are severe and require treatment are more reliably reported than milder conditions [7].

Diagnostic uncertainty

Population-based studies inevitably include a greater proportion of mild cases than those based in a health-care setting. Definitions used in the clinic may be impractical in population studies. Even when classification criteria exist it can be surprising to find who does and who does not satisfy them. Many rheumatic conditions still have no standard definitions. In some situations, there may be competing definitions. For example a study which sets out to determine the overall prevalence of OA will have to wrestle with the fact that the standard classification criteria apply to OA of specific individual joints rather than the general condition. The lack of standard definitions for many conditions makes comparison between studies very difficult.

Some population-based studies (e.g. those from the Mayo clinic or based in primary care) have access to medical records. The accuracy of these studies is highly dependent on the quality of the record. For example, applying classification criteria for RA or systemic lupus erythematosus (SLE) requires that the attending physician (who may have had no prior knowledge that the epidemiological study was going to take place) has recorded regularly and accurately the pattern of joint involvement, and performed the relevant autoantibody tests and radiographs.

Comparability

Variations in the methodology, questionnaire design, and data collection instruments limit the comparability of studies. Since 1987 the European division of the World Health Organization (WHO) and the Central Bureau of Statistics of the Netherlands have been working together with the aim of developing common instruments and methodology for health interview surveys. The WHO is also developing a standardized interviewer administered questionnaire to be used in the assessment of disability—the WHO Disability Assessment Schedule (WHO-DAS).

Sources of data

Data sources for population-based studies fall into three broad categories:

(1)   routinely collected data;

(2)   government-sponsored surveys;

(3)   epidemiological surveys.

Routinely collected data

Death certificates

Mortality records are, with a few exceptions, of limited value in the study of rheumatic disease epidemiology because the rheumatological disorder is often not recorded on the death certificate. However, death certificate data may be useful, for example, for comparing the attributed causes of death of a cohort of patients known to have RA with those of the general population.

Morbidity registers

Some Scandinavian countries have registers of people who are disabled or who can reclaim the cost of medication for a particular condition. In Finland, since 1966, people with chronic inflammatory rheumatic diseases have been entitled to free or highly subsidised medication. The patient's physician has to complete a comprehensive medical certificate which has to be approved by an expert advisor on behalf of the sickness insurance scheme. The scheme covers the whole population. There are a number of caveats when interpreting epidemiological studies from this source. Only individuals requiring chronic medication are registered and so mild cases will be missed. Secondly, particularly for more severe diseases, there may be 'left censorship', that is patients who die early in the course of disease may not survive long enough to be registered. Thirdly, the physician's diagnosis may not conform to standard classification criteria, although there have been some validation exercises which suggest that, certainly for RA, there is reasonable agreement between the physician diagnosis and the American College of Rheumatology (ACR) (previously known as the American Rheumatism Association) criteria for RA [8].

In some countries morbidity registers have been established for cases of early arthritis presenting to primary care, for childhood rheumatic complaints or for vasculitis. In order to be useful for descriptive epidemiology such registers need to cover a large, well-defined population and to be able to ensure complete (or near complete) case ascertainment [9]. They also need to be able to check that people enrolled on the register do come from the population under study and do satisfy the definition of the disease being investigated. Because, in effect, they provide a system of ongoing population surveillance, they do permit the estimate and monitoring of disease incidence. Maintaining a registry of this type can be very costly. Published studies from single-disease morbidity registers are not considered in this chapter.

Primary care data

General practitioners (GPs) may contribute information to a computerized database or participate in surveys. In England and Wales, a General Practice Research database was set up in 1987. It covers over 500 practices and approximately three and a half million patients. It records on a common database the reason for every consultation. In the Netherlands, the Dutch Continuous Morbidity Registration Scheme uses records from GPs in the Nijmegen region. In both the UK and Holland, GPs also participate in surveys—the England and Wales GP morbidity surveys and the Dutch National Survey on Morbidity in General Practice.

In England and Wales, at the time of the 10-yearly censuses, a group of around 60 general practices participate in a morbidity survey. Thus the most recent, the 4th National Morbidity Survey, took place between 1st September 1991 and 31st August 1992. The study covered 1 per cent of the population (502 493 patients, 468 042 person years at risk). Using computer software developed specifically for the study, doctors and nurses recorded the reason for every consultation and whether this was the first consultation for this particular problem. They also recorded whether the condition was severe, intermediate, or minor. In addition, interviewers obtained socio-economic information on around 83 per cent of patients on the practice lists [10].

There are limitations to GP data. Although it does include diagnostic information, this represents the GP's opinion rather than conformity to specific diagnostic criteria. Comparison between countries is hindered by differences in the provision of primary care.

Hospital discharge data

In some countries information on the diagnosis at the time of hospital discharge is collated. This information is only of value epidemiologically for conditions which almost invariably lead to hospital admission, for example fractured neck of femur. Even then, people who die prior to or during hospital admission may be excluded and so the true incidence of the condition will be underestimated. A further limitation is that estimates of incidence require that a hospital admission can be identified as the first for that particular patient and that particular diagnosis. In some countries, such as the UK, hospital statistics are episode- rather than person-based.

Work absenteeism records

In some countries information on the reason for and duration of absence from work is collected. This can be used to examine the profile of rheumatological complaints in the workforce in general, and in specific occupations.

Studies in defined populations

The Rochester Epidemiology Program
Population-based studies are possible in Olmsted County, Minnesota because virtually all the health care is provided by the Mayo Clinic, the Olmsted Medical Group and their affiliated community hospitals, local nursing homes and a few private practitioners. Since 1910 all these institutions have used a common medical record system which includes inpatient and outpatient diagnoses, surgical procedures, and histology [11]. This information is all indexed centrally. Olmsted County comprises one city (Rochester—population in 1990 around 70 000) and 13 small towns and villages (population in 1990 around 35 700). The population is predominantly of Scandinavian origin, with less than 1 per cent being non-white. Although the population itself is relatively small, the fact that the centralized database has been in existence for almost 90 years means that it offers many million person-years of follow-up. The Rochester

Epidemiology Project is thus particularly suited to studying diseases with a stable incidence.

Elsewhere in the US, the databases of some large prepaid insurance programmes (for example the Kaiser Permanente Health Plan in the Western States) have been used to generate estimates of disease frequency. However, most cannot be regarded as truly 'population-based' since they do not include all the residents of a particular geopolitical area and there may be some selection bias as to who is accepted onto a particular programme.

Framingham

More than 40 years ago approximately 5000 people, randomly selected from the 30–60 year population of Framingham, Massachusetts, US who were free of overt cardiovascular disease, were enrolled in a longitudinal study [12]. It was estimated that the study population would yield about 1500 new cases of coronary heart disease during the planned 20 years of follow-up which would be sufficient to enable statistically reliable findings with respects to risk factors for the development of coronary artery disease. The subjects have been followed biennially with very low loss to follow-up. This framework of research has provided the opportunity to screen the subjects, for example for knee osteoarthritis [13] and for physical disability [14], and to use the baseline data and data recorded at previous reviews to examine risk factors for the development of OA.

Government-sponsored surveys

In many countries there are regular population surveys which examine social and demographic trends. These may, from time to time, include health related information such as the number of visits to a physician, and self-reported illness (acute and long-standing). Such studies are usually cross-sectional and can be used to estimate the prevalence of musculoskeletal symptoms and self-reported diagnoses. The sample size is usually too small to permit accurate estimates of incidence. They offer the opportunity of linking self-reported problems with sociodemographic data and for looking at health-related behaviour (such as smoking and alcohol consumption) and co-morbidity. They also capture cases that may not have sought medical help. In a number of countries there is the possibility of linking survey data with other sources of data, such as mortality and malignancy registers. For example in Sweden and Denmark residents have a personal identity number which enables data-linking. The following are examples of government-sponsored surveys.

United Kingdom

General Household Survey (GHS)

This is a continuous survey which has been running in Great Britain since 1971. It is based on a sample of the general, non-institutionalized population. For example in 1996/7, interviews were conducted with 17 043 people aged 16 or over from 9158 households [15]. The GHS includes questions on demography and fertility, family and household information, housing, health, employment, and education. Since 1972, the GHS has collected information on self-reported health. With regard to chronic conditions individuals are asked 'Do you have any long-standing illness, disability or infirmity—by long-standing I mean anything that has troubled you over a period of time?'. As a supplementary question, since 1988, they have been asked 'What was the matter with you?' and 'Did it limit your activities in any way?'

Health Survey for England (HSfE)

This annual survey has been running since 1991. Data are collected from a sample of individuals aged two or over living in private households in England. 60 postcode sectors are covered each month and 18 addresses are selected from each sector. Thus, the survey covers approximately 8860 households each year. The survey comprises a computer assisted interview (conducted by proxy for those aged 2–12) followed by a visit from a nurse. The survey focuses on cardiorespiratory health but in 1995 [5] it covered disability. It used a modification of the WHO's recommended sequence of questions about five areas of activities (loco-motion, personal care, seeing, hearing, and communication) [16].

United States

In the US the National Center for Health Statistics is responsible for a series of surveys which include

National Health Interview Survey (NHIS)

This is an ongoing household survey which includes around 111 000 people each year. It collects information through interviews and questionnaires on self-reported symptoms and diagnoses. The 1984 NHIS included a Supplement on Aging which was administered to 16 148 people aged over 55 years.

National Health and Nutrition Examination Survey (NHANES)

The first National Health Examination Survey (NHES) was conducted in 1960–62. This then evolved into the National Health and Nutrition Examination survey which is just completing its third programme:

I 1971–75. Included 20 749 people aged 1–74. A 'detailed' subsample of 6913 adults aged 25–74 had a general medical examination. They were examined for joint tenderness, swelling, range of movement and pain on movement. They also underwent X-rays of the knees and hips (except for women aged less than 50). The 2431 participants who responded positively to one of the questions on arthritis in the medical history interview completed the Arthritis Supplement. This supplement included questions about physical disability. Those people who underwent the medical examination were also included in the NHANES I Epidemiologic Follow-up Study which focused on mortality, disease, and disability occurring between 1982 and 84 [17]. This cohort has been used to study the impact of radiographic OA knee on subsequent symptoms and disability [18].

II 1976–79. Included osteoarthritis and disc degeneration as target conditions. It included radiographs of the lumbar and cervical spine.

III 1988–94. Divided into two 3-year national probability samples. Included questions on hand swelling and stiffness, osteoporosis, and hip fracture. All men and non-pregnant women aged 20 years and over were eligible for bone densitometry unless they had previously fractured both hips [19].

All these US surveys are based on probability samples of the US, civilian, non-institutionalized population.

Canada

Canadian Health Survey

This survey was conducted in 1978–9. It was based on interviews from a sample of households from all the Canadian provinces. It was based on the NHIS and included information on health problems and disability. 23 023 people participated of whom 17 492 were aged 16 or over.

Health and Activity Limitation Survey (HALS)

The HALS surveyed people, aged 16 and over, who were identified as having physical or psychological dis-

ability via the 1986 Canadian census. A total of 126 268 people participated. The HALS questionnaire included 12 activity specific questions and one non-specific activity question. Respondents were asked to attribute each limitation of activity to an underlying condition. It included individuals in private households and institutions.

Ontario Health Survey

This survey, conducted in 1990, was confined to the province of Ontario. It was a stratified cluster sample survey of private households. The main method of data collection was via an interview with one adult from the selected households who was asked to respond on behalf of all residents. In addition, all household members aged 12 and over were given a questionnaire to complete.

Finland

In Finland the Social Insurance Institution conducted national health interviews in 1964, 1968, 1976, and 1987. In addition, in 1966–72, 57 440 Finnish adults aged over 15 took part in the Mobile Clinic Health Examination Survey. This focused predominantly on cardiovascular risk factors [20] but, via record linkage, it has, for example, been used in epidemiological studies of risk factors for RA [21,22] . The Mini-Finland Health Survey conducted in 1978–80 included both health interview surveys and health examination surveys. The aim of the study was to establish the health status, morbidity, and health needs of Finns aged 30 and over. A sample of 8000 adults representative of the whole Finnish population was invited to participate and 7217 responded. The health examination survey focused on cardiovascular, respiratory, and musculoskeletal disorders, functional limitations, disabilities, and handicaps [6]. This group have also been involved in longitudinal studies via record linkage [23–25].

Other examples include the 1995 South Australia Health Omnibus Survey [26]. A recent publication of the European Commission [27] found that all 16 countries in Western Europe which it contacted had conducted at least one government-sponsored health survey in the previous 3 years. Such surveys often include information about musculoskeletal conditions, for example as part of a 'pick list' of chronic conditions. However, this is usually not the prime focus of the survey and, unless an investigator with a particular interest in musculoskeletal disorders conducts some secondary analysis on the data set, the full potential of the survey with regards to understanding the epidemiology of rheumatic disorders in that population will not be realized.

Epidemiological surveys

Epidemiological surveys to document the frequency and distribution of musculoskeletal disorders in populations were largely pioneered by the work of Kellgren and Lawrence in England in the 1950s [28]. The main purpose of these studies was to define the relative frequency of specific conditions and diagnoses. These surveys are reviewed in the relevant chapters of this book. This chapter focuses on studies of musculoskeletal symptoms and locomotor disability and studies which have attempted to measure the overall burden of musculoskeletal morbidity.

The COPCORD programme

During the period 1950–80 a variety of population studies of musculoskeletal disorders were conducted, mainly in Europe and North America. Very few studies were conducted in developing countries. In 1981, the International League Against Rheumatism (ILAR) and the WHO launched the Community Oriented Program for the Control of Rheumatic Diseases (COPCORD) [29]. COPCORD was to have three stages. In Stage I epidemiological data on the prevalence of rheumatic disease are collected. In Stage II primary health-care workers are educated about the management of the most common musculoskeletal disorders in their region. In Stage III improved health care is achieved and documented.

The original COPCORD stage I surveys had three phases and employed a minimum sample size of 1500. In the first phase volunteer primary health-care workers administered a simple questionnaire which asked about current pain (no minimum duration specified) and included a mannikin to indicate the site of pain. In the second phase, the district nurse interviewed positive responders. This questionnaire also included questions on pain and disability, as well as questions designed to identify people likely to be suffering from, for example, RA and gout. Individuals with significant complaints were invited to attend for the third phase, a medical examination [30].

More recently the questionnaire has been revised and validated [31]. The survey now comprises only two phases—an interviewer-administered questionnaire and a clinical examination of positive responders within 1–2 weeks. The questionnaire now covers seven domains: musculoskeletal pain (within the last 7 days and ever) plus a mannikin, other musculoskeletal symptoms, history of trauma, functional ability, coping, health seeking behaviour, and treatment. The Health Assessment Questionnaire (HAQ) [32] has been substituted for the original COPCORD disability questionnaire. Because of these changes, subtle variations in methodology and issues surrounding accurate translation the COPCORD studies are not directly comparable with one another but do provide a very valuable insight into the pattern of musculoskeletal symptoms and disability in otherwise unstudied populations.

Other epidemiological studies

There has been a renewed interest in community studies of musculoskeletal symptoms with the recognition that health-care systems should be based on an assessment of 'need'—i.e. the ability to benefit from health care. There are three steps in conducting an epidemiological health-care needs assessment: an understanding of the incidence and prevalence of musculoskeletal complaints; an appreciation of the availability and effectiveness of interventions; and an estimate of the proportion of people with a particular musculoskeletal disorder who would benefit from a particular intervention. This last step requires an understanding of the spectrum of severity within the cases of a particular disorder at a community level.

There have been few studies of the relative frequency of symptoms at different musculoskeletal sites and of the distribution of painful sites within the individual. In the 1986 Calderdale (West Yorkshire, UK) study, postal questionnaires were sent to one-third (25 168) of the local households. The questionnaire asked for demographic details of the household members, if any members suffered from any pain, swelling or stiffness in their joints, neck or back (and included a chart to indicate the site of the pain), and whether any members experienced disablement in six selected activities of daily living [33]. The 1996 Tameside (Greater Manchester, UK) study comprised a postal questionnaire sent to an age- and sex-stratified sample of 6000 adults from three general practices [34]. The questionnaire sought demographic details; asked about pain in the last month lasting for more than 1 week in a number of specified joint areas and included the modified HAQ [35]. The study was conducted in three phases. In the second phase, positive respondents were sent a questionnaire specific for their area of joint pain and in the third phase a sample of positive respondents for each joint area was invited to attend for a medical examination.

A recently published study used a question derived from NHANES I (Which of your joints have ever been painful, swollen, aching or tender on most days for at least 1 month?) in two groups of Japanese women aged 60 to 79—one in Japan and the other in Hawaii [36]. The total sample size was 860. The joint areas covered were shoulder, elbow, wrists, hands, hips, knees, ankles, feet, and spine.

Population studies of general musculoskeletal morbidity

Studies of musculoskeletal symptoms

Results of government-sponsored surveys

Tables 1.1 and 1.2 show the prevalence of self-reported musculoskeletal symptoms and conditions from NHANES I, II and III and the NHIS (US), the General Household Survey (UK) and two Canadian surveys. From these it is clear that musculoskeletal symptoms are extremely common in all three countries (usually the highest ranking category of symptoms). Overall, approximately one-quarter of the population has musculoskeletal symptoms with the back and the knee

being the most common sites of pain (Table 1.1). Back pain is more common in younger age groups and knee pain in older age groups. The phrasing of the questions in NHANES I, II, and III varies with regards to the duration of pain (see footnote Table 1.1) which means that the results from the three surveys are not directly comparable.

Generally, the prevalence of self-reported musculoskeletal conditions appears to be higher in the US than the UK but the results are not directly comparable because of differences in study methodology and condition definition (Table 1.2). The wording in the General Household Survey (UK) has remained constant. In the UK there appears to have been a secular increase in the age and gender-specific prevalence of self-reported musculoskeletal conditions. There is an approximately equal gender-specific prevalence of self-reported musculoskeletal conditions up to the age of 45. In older age-groups the prevalence is higher in women. In the US there has been no secular increase since 1980 in the proportion of people aged over 55 reporting physician-diagnosed arthritis (Table 1.3).

Results of epidemiological studies

The COPCORD studies
The majority of published COPCORD studies are from the Asia-Pacific basin (Tables 1.4 and 1.5). In addition

Table 1.1 The cumulative life time incidence of musculoskeletal symptoms, data from NHANES I, II and III (rate per 1000)

	NHANES I (1971–5)[a] Age (years)				NHANES II (1976–9)[b] Age (years)				NHANES III (1988–94)[c] Age (years)			
	25–44	45–64	67–74	All (25–74)	25–44	45–64	67–74	All (25–74)	18–44	45–64	65+	All (≥18)
All spinal and joint pain	205	364	396	241	158	384	401	201	199	341	496	283
Back pain				172	123	203	182	160	199	301	288	239
Neck pain				–	66	101	93	82	–	–	–	–
Other joint pain				–	123	251	281	190	–	–	–	–
knee				133				459				46
hip				82				228				31
hand				68				324				40
shoulder				67				346				
ankle				43				191				
elbow				42				244				
foot				32				156				
wrist				31				180				

Adapted from [37, 39, 43]
[a] Question: Have you ever had pain in your .... on most days for at least 1 month?
[b] Question: Have you ever had pain in your .... on most days for at least 2 weeks?
[c] Question: Have you ever had pain in your back for most days for 1 month or more?
     Have you ever had pain in your hand/knee/hip on most days for 1 month for 6 weeks or more?

Table 1.2 Prevalence of self-reported musculoskeletal conditions (per 1000)

United States (data from NHIS)

	1983–5 [1]					1989–90 [38]					1995 [39]			
	Age group (years)					Age group (years)					Age group (years)			
	18–44	45–64	65–74	75+	All	25–44	45–64	65–74	75+	All	18–44	45–64	65+	All
Arthritis	52	279	460	508	131	94	289	454	568	150	53	244	492	130
Male					95					117				97
Female					164					180				161
Back/spine											85	106	96	70
Male														59
Female														61

United Kingdom

	1988 [40]					1996–7 [15]				
	Age group (years)					Age group (years)				
	16–44	45–64	65–74	75+	All	16–44	45–64	65–74	75+	All
All musculoskeletal problems	80	189	267	377	124	105	254	307	402	198
Male	91	178	217	223	110	110	246	265	310	184
Female	71	199	307	399	137	100	262	342	470	211
Arthritis and rheumatism										
Male	12	81	131	141	42	16	97	148	188	88
Female	20	133	242	306	87	22	134	223	313	106
Back problems										
Male	42	72	39	26	38	50	89	60	30	62
Female	34	56	41	28	33	49	83	51	47	59
Other bone and joint problems										
Male	42	49	66	84	41	44	60	57	91	54
Female	20	22	47	96	27	29	45	67	110	46

Canada

	1978 [41]			1990 (Ontario only) [42]			
	Age group (years)			Age group (years)			
	15–64	65+	All	16–44	45–64	65–74	All (≥16)
All musculoskeletal problems	170	484	160	125	303	432	220
Arthritis and rheumatism							152
Back/neck disorders							81

Table 1.3 Proportion of people aged 55 and over who reported physician-diagnosed arthritis in the US (rate per 1000)

	1960–62	1976–80	1988–94
Total	372	443	398
Male	283	372	311
White male	281	373	305
Black male	302	364	355
Female	451	502	467
White female	451	492	460
Black female	450	597	572
Male			
55–59 years	244	300	189
60–64 years	288	334	290
65–69 years	321	351	337
70–74 years	284	357	372
75–79 years	297	–	411
80 years and over	–	–	388
Female			
55–59 years	437	397	317
60–64 years	451	471	461
65–69 years	390	506	473
70–74 years	533	528	512
75–79 years	498	–	548
80 years and over	–	–	554

Adapted from: [39,43].
Using data from: 1960–62 Health Examination survey; 1976–80 NHANES II; 1988–94 NHANES III.

to those shown in the tables a further study was conducted in Shanghai. Studies are also being conducted in Brazil, Chile, and Mexico [31]. The tables include other studies of similar design from the same region. It is clear that peripheral joint pain and back pain are common in all regions. Contrary to what might be expected, the prevalence of pain is higher in developed (e.g. Australia) than in developing countries, and higher in urban than rural parts of the same country. There are also intriguing differences in the pattern of knee pain between rural areas of Northern and Southern China (the two populations studied belong to the same ethnic group). Some attempts were made to estimate the relative frequency of OA, gout, and RA in these different settings but, apart from OA, the numbers of cases in each sample were small and the confidence intervals wide and overlapping.

Other epidemiological studies

As in the COPCORD studies, studies from Europe have shown that musculoskeletal pain is common, with the back and the knee being the most frequently affected sites (Table 1.6). In both the Tameside and the Calderdale studies, back pain was most common in the younger age groups (16–64) whereas knee pain became increasingly common with increasing age. In Tameside, knee pain was more common in men than women in the youngest age group (16–44 years), but for most other sites of pain and ages women had a higher prevalence of pain. Only knee pain and pain in multiple joints increased in frequency between the two oldest age bands in the Tameside study. Other studies have also suggested that the prevalence of certain musculoskeletal symptoms does not increase with age in the very elderly [48]. However, the majority of studies

Table 1.4 Prevalence of musculoskeletal symptoms in studies from the Asia-Pacific region (per cent of adult population)

Area	Reference	Sample size	Peripheral joint pain	Neck	Lower back	Shoulder	Elbow	Knee pain
Philippines[a]	[44]	950	18	7	7	2	3	5
Indonesia[a]	[30, 98]							
Rural		4683	18	5	15	11	10	12
Urban		1071	28	12	23	–	–	15
Malaysia[a]	[30]							
Malays		1267	9	7	7	4	3	11
Chinese		474	5	1	4	2	2	4
Indians		853	11	6	10	6	6	11
China (rural)	[30, 70]							
North		4192	33	5	28	5	4	27
South		5057	8	2	12	1	1	2
Thailand	[45]	2455	–	3	12	–	–	9
Tokelau								
Island	[46]	794	–	0.3	12	4	0.4	9[b]
Migrant	[47]	1333	–	2	10	3	–	8[b]
Australia[a]	[30]	1437	32	17	22	10	6	15

[a] COPCORD studies.
[b] Knee pain in association with clinical OA.

Table 1.5 Gender specific prevalence of musculoskeletal symptoms in studies from Asia Pacific region (per cent of adult population)

Area	Reference	Total sample size	Males						Females					
			Peripheral joint pain	Neck	Lower back	Shoulder	Elbow	Knee	Peripheral joint pain	Neck	Lower back	Shoulder	Elbow	Knee
Philippines[a]	[44]	950	–	8	7	2	8	5	–	6	8	3	17	5
Indonesia[a]	[30, 98]													
Rural		4683	17	4	17	14	5	–	19	5	13	15	6	–
Urban		1071	25	11	19	16	7	–	29	13	26	17	8	–
China	[30, 70]													
North		4192	33	5	28	–	–	–	47	8	43	–	–	–
South		5057	7	2	12	–	–	–	24	3	14	–	–	–
Tokelau														
Island	[46]	794	–	1	14	–	–	10	–	1	10	–	–	10
Migrant	[47]	1333	–	3	11	4	–	9	–	2	9	2	–	7

[a] COPCORD studies

Table 1.6   Distribution of pain by age and gender in two UK population surveys (per cent of respondents)

	Males age band				Females age band			
	16–44	45–64	65–74	75+	16–44	45–64	65–74	75+
Tameside, Greater Manchester [34][a]								
Neck	7	15	17	18	12	19	23	21
Lower back	20	24	20	17	20	27	32	30
Shoulder	9	19	16	20	12	19	26	24
Elbow	3	13	6	6	5	8	6	9
Hand	7	12	14	12	7	19	21	20
Hip	3	11	13	11	4	15	20	20
Knee	15	21	27	27	10	23	32	35
Most joints	2	7	8	11	2	9	16	19
Calderdale, West Yorkshire [33][b]								
Any joint symptoms	15	30	35	34	16	35	43	53

[a] Pain for > 1/52 in last month.
[b] Any pain, swelling or stiffness in joints, feet, or back.

(Tables 1.1, 1.2, and 1.3) suggest that while the prevalence of back pain does plateau or even fall after middle age, the prevalence of peripheral joint pain continues to rise even into extreme old age.

In the Tameside study, 47 per cent of the population reported having musculoskeletal pain lasting for at least 1 week in the previous month. In a population survey from Asturias, Spain, 45 per cent of responders had experienced musculoskeletal pain for at least 1 week in the previous year [49]. As with most other studies, back pain was the most frequent followed by neck, knee, and then shoulder pain. A Swedish study focused on rheumatic complaints of at least 6 weeks duration in 50–70 year olds [50]. The overall prevalence was 38 per cent. Back pain was the most frequent site of pain, followed by neck and then knee and shoulder pain.

Both the Tameside and Calderdale studies found that many people had pain at more than one site. Only 34 per cent of those with musculoskeletal pain had pain at only one site [34]. The most common combinations of pain were back and knee; neck and shoulder; and back and hip pain. Other studies have also shown that the more sites of pain that individuals have, the more likely they are to develop pain in previously unaffected areas [51,52]. There are a number possible explanations for this. One is that the pains have a common aetiology (e.g. heavy physical work) or pathology (e.g. osteoarthritis). Alternatively there may be psychosocial factors at play.

Table 1.7   Patient consultation rates and incidence and prevalence estimates based on attendance at primary care (4th National Morbidity Survey, England and Wales, 1991–2), rates per 10 000 person years at risk

	Age band					
	0–15	16–44	45–64	65–74	75+	Total
GP consultations for musculoskeletal conditions	381	1231	2354	2702	2915	1521
Rheumatoid arthritis						
Incidence	1	9	24	29	23	
Prevalence	2	16	71	111	94	38
Osteoarthritis						
Incidence	1	36	325	560	669	
Prevalence	1	52	559	1038	1386	315
Back pain						
Incidence	37	345	463	410	413	
Prevalence	42	394	556	495	509	591

Source: [53].

In contrast to the Indonesian COPCORD study which found a higher prevalence of musculoskeletal pain in an urban area, a study of two groups of Japanese women found a substantially higher cumulative prevalence of pain in a rural part of Japan than in an urban area of Hawaii (72.1 vs. 50.5 per cent) [36]. The differences were greatest for thoracic spine and knee pain. This suggests that the effect of environmental and occupation factors may vary in different settings and at different times of life.

Results from GP morbidity studies

As one might expect, the prevalence of symptoms as measured by attendance at primary care is lower than the prevalence of self-reported symptoms. In the 4th National Morbidity Survey in England and Wales (1991–2), 15 per cent of the total population (20 per cent of the adult population) consulted their GPs during the course of a year with musculoskeletal problems (Table 1.7) [53]. This was an increase from the previous survey in 1981–2 when 13 per cent of the population had consulted. A study from Sweden published in 1981 reported that 12 per cent of GP visits were for a musculoskeletal disorder [54]. Back pain was the most common musculoskeletal disorder among male consulters whereas back pain and soft tissue rheumatism each accounted for one third of consultations for musculoskeletal problems amongst women. Both this Swedish study and a study from Spain [49] reported that the consultation rates for rheumatic problems fell after the age of 65, but this pattern was not found in the 4th England and Wales morbidity survey [53]. It appears that the severity of pain is more important than the level of disability in determining when patients decide to consult a GP [49].

Studies of the relative frequency of specific rheumatic disorders

Results from routinely collected data

The Finland Register of Patients Entitled To Reimbursed Medication

The Finland register for the reimbursement of medication has been used to estimate the incidence of a variety of rheumatic disorders (Table 1.8). Since these studies were conducted concurrently in the same population, they provide a useful insight into the relative frequency of the different rheumatic disorders in the different age–sex groups. The figures for connective tissue disease are based on very small numbers and so are not robust. For example no new cases of SLE were registered during 1990 although, clearly, SLE does occur in the Finnish population. This register has also been used to demonstrate a changing peak in age of onset of RA in the Finnish population over the last 15 years [55] and for a variety of studies of mortality rates and cause of death in RA. These are reviewed in Chapter 2 on RA.

The Rochester Epidemiology Program

Table 1.9 shows the results from of a number of publications arising from the Rochester Epidemiology programme. They are not directly comparable because they cover different time periods and so are standardized to different populations. Nevertheless, they shed some light on the relative frequency of a variety of inflammatory conditions. It is of note, for example, that while the incidence of ankylosing spondylitis is higher than that of RA in men aged 25–44 the reverse is true for older men. The lower part of the table shows the tremendous burden of fractures related to bone fragility. The incidence of vertebral and proximal femur fracture continues to increase with age well into

Table 1.8 Incidence of specific rheumatic diseases in Finland[a] in 1990 (based on entitlement to subsidized medication)

Disease	Reference	Numberof cases	Incidence rate/100 000	95% CI
Rheumatoid arthritis	[55]	324	32.2	29.0–35.9
Ankylosing spondylitis	[56]	78	7.3	6.0–7.8
Psoriatic arthritis	[57]	65	6.1	4.6–7.6
Chronic reactive arthritis		22	2.0	1.3–3.1
Mixed connective tissue disease	[58]	9	0.8	0.4–1.7
Systemic sclerosis		4	0.4	0.1–1.0
Poly/dermatomyositis		4	0.4	0.1–10
Juvenile rheumatoid arthritis	[59]		14.0[b]	

[a] Based on 5/21 hospital districts (population 1 006 000 adults).
[b] 14/100 000 children.

Table 1.9   Incidence of specific rheumatic diseases in Rochester, Minnesota, US (rate per 100 000)

Disorder	Reference	Year of study	Males			Females		
			25–44	45–64	≥65	25–44	45–64	≥65
Rheumatoid arthritis	[60]	1955–85	17.0[a]	47.8	95.7	49.5[a]	113.9	118.9
SLE	[61]	1950–76	0.6	2.9	4.5	6.3	1.5	5.0
Ankylosing spondylitis	[62]	1935–89	23.0	8.1	3.8	6.3	2.7	1.4
Reiter's syndrome	[63]	1950–80	5.2	–	–	–	–	–
PMR	[64]	1970–91	–	18.7[b]	67.5	–	25.5[b]	116.7
Giant cell arthritis	[65]	1950–91	–	2.2[b]	14.8	–	6.4[b]	48.1
Osteoporotic-related fractures								
Distal forearm	[66]	1985–94	90.1[a]	114.5	137.0	131.0	415.0	769.4
Clinically diagnosed vertebral fracture	[67]	1985–89	18.3	53.8	241.7	22.6	164.3	850.0
Proximal femur	[68]	1983–92	3.0	30.8	516.0	2.8	57.9	1089.8

[a] Age 35–44.
[b] Age 50–64.

the ninth decade (Table 1.10) [69]. The Mayo clinic records have also shown a marked secular increase in the incidence of limb fractures over the last 20 years in the urban but not the rural community around Rochester [70].

Results from GP data

Estimates for incidence and prevalence were derived from the 4th National Morbidity survey based on attendance in primary care (Table 1.7) [53]. The highest incidence and prevalence figures were for back pain and osteoarthritis. These diagnoses are not based on any classification criteria and are substantially higher than those derived from other sources. For example, most rheumatologists would not expect to find such a high prevalence of osteoarthritis in children. Since the previous survey in 1981–2 the proportion of people consulting for osteoarthritis had risen by 55 per cent for men and 25 per cent for women; the proportion consulting for osteoporosis had doubled for

males and risen by 214 per cent for females. In contrast, the proportion consulting for rheumatoid arthritis had fallen by 15 per cent for men and 29 per cent for women. This might represent a true decline or might indicate that the diagnosis was being used more restrictively. The proportion consulting for back pain had, overall, remained fairly static.

Results from government-sponsored surveys

Estimates of the relative frequency of rheumatic disorders may be based on self report, or self report of physician diagnoses (Have you ever been told by a doctor that you have ...) from health surveys. The proportion of people aged 55 and over who reported physician-diagnosed arthritis (Table 1.3, cited in [37]) rose by 28 per cent in the 20 years between 1962 and 1980 but has since stabilized.

NHANES I included radiographs of the knees and hips in a subgroup of subjects. These radiographs were read independently by two rheumatologists (with arbi-

Table 1.10   Incidence of fractures in the elderly in Rochester, Minnesota, 1989–91(rate per 100 000 person years)

	Males						Females					
	60–64	65–69	70–74	75–79	80–84	85+	60–64	65–69	70–74	75–79	80–84	85+
Distal forearm	141	95	64	45	149	94	808	822	824	835	870	849
Proximal humerus	81	142	160	134	75	188	165	140	343	244	548	498
Vertebrae	81	497	415	668	1567	2533	349	682	1167	1566	2579	3132
Ribs	363	520	415	445	1045	1313	220	281	297	522	870	1581
Proximal femur	81	189	160	534	597	1501	165	221	275	861	1838	2488
All sites	1853	2815	2491	2716	4851	8443	3361	3849	4897	6524	9252	12031

Adapted from: [69].

Table 1.11 Prevalence of radiographic osteoarthritis (Grade 2–4) of the hip and knee from NHANES I (per cent)

	Men		Women	
	55–64	65–74	55–64	65–74
Radiographic OA hip	2.6	4.6	2.8	2.7
Radiographic OA knee	4.1	8.3	7.3	18.0
People with knee pain:				
Radiographic OA knee	20.2	29.6	14.4	32.3

Adapted from: [17].

tration by a third rheumatologist where necessary) using an ordinal scale (0–4) based on the Atlas of Standard Radiographs [71]. Osteoarthritis was defined as a radiograph grade of 2–4. Radiographic OA hip is a little more common in men than women whereas OA knee is substantially more common in women (Table 1.11) [17]. The prevalence of radiographic OA knee is considerably higher in those with knee pain, but nevertheless up to two-thirds of people with knee pain have no definite radiographic evidence of OA.

Population studies of locomotor disability

Issues of definition and measurement

Traditionally, medical research has concentrated on four aspects of disease: aetiology, pathology, manifestations, and prognosis. Following this model, epidemiological studies have focused on risk factors for disease, the incidence and prevalence of symptoms and diagnoses, and disease outcome (recovery or death). However, this does not reflect the severity of a disease or the impact on an individual's life. As summarized above, the prevalence of musculoskeletal symptoms is very high. However, many of these complaints may be trivial and of short duration. It is important to be able to assess whether these symptoms are having any impact on the individual's quality of life. From the patient's perspective the main consequences of musculoskeletal disorders are pain and disability which is likely to be predominantly in the locomotor and personal care domains.

The consequences of any disease process can be summarized using the concepts proposed by Philip Wood in the International Classification of Impairments,

Disabilities and Handicaps (ICIDH) [72]. The term impairment covers any loss or abnormality of anatomical, physiological, or psychological structure or function. Disability means any restriction in the ability to perform an activity in the manner or within the range considered normal. Handicap refers to the disadvantage conferred on an individual by an impairment or disability and depends on the individual's cultural and social setting. The ICIDH recognizes nine categories of disability (Table 1.12) [72]. The latest revision of the ICIDH turns the two rather negative terms of disability and handicap into more positive

Table 1.12 International Classification of Impairments, Disabilities, and Handicaps [72]

Classification of disabilities
1 Behaviour disabilities
1.1 Awareness disabilities
1.2 Disabilities in relationships
2 Communication disabilities
2.1 Speaking disabilities
2.2 Listening disabilities
2.3 Seeing disabilities
2.4 Other communication disabilities
3 Personal care disabilities
3.1 Excretion disabilities
3.2 Personal hygiene disabilities
3.3 Dressing disabilities
3.4 Feeding and other personal care disabilities
4 Locomotor disabilities
4.1 Ambulation disability
4.2 Confining disabilities (e.g. transfer)
4.3 Other locomotor disabilities (e.g. lifting)
5 Body disposition disabilities
5.1 Domestic disabilities
5.2 Body movement disabilities
5.3 Other body disposition disabilities
6 Dexterity disabilities
6.1 Daily activity disabilities
6.2 Manual activity disabilities
6.3 Other dexterity disabilities
7 Situational disabilities
7.1 Dependence, endurance disabilities
7.2 Environmental disabilities
7.3 Other situational disabilities
8 Particular skill disabilities
9 Other activity restrictions

attributes—activities and participation. Thus impairment measures the consequences of the disease at the level of the body, activities looks at the consequences of the disease for the person, and participation explores the consequences in the context of society. The WHO-DAS explores these concepts in six domains: understanding and communication with the world, getting around, self care, getting along with people, life activities (e.g. work, household tasks), and participation in society (e.g. involvement in family and community activities), in a series of 36 questions.

In fact, the ICIDH definition of disability is only one of many. Indeed, many government surveys regard a condition as disabling if it limits everyday activities. The Mini-Finland survey defined disability in three ways: reduced work capacity, requiring occasional assistance, and requiring regular assistance [73]. The Canadian Health Survey defined four levels of physical ability: no limitations; not limited in any major activity but some minor limitations; limited in at least one major activity; unable to do at least one major activity. Unfortunately, physical disability can claim almost as many measurement instruments as definitions. In clinical rheumatology a variety of tools have been developed over the last 50 years but few of these have been used in the population setting. The oldest measures are based on the clinical judgement of the observer. These include the Steinbrocker functional class assessment for RA [74]. The next generation of instruments were based on observed performance (e.g. the Keitel index [75]) but again these were impractical for population studies. Finally there came the self-report measures of which the most widely used are the HAQ [76] and the Arthritis Impact Measurement Scales (AIMS) [76]. Because the AIMS takes approximately 15–20 minutes to complete, only the HAQ has been used in population surveys.

Population studies using the Stanford Health Assessment Questionnaire

The HAQ is a tool which was originally developed for use in RA but which has proved of value in other settings. It comprises 20 questions covering eight domains of daily living (eating, dressing and grooming, reaching, arising, walking, hygiene, grip, and activities). Respondents rate their ability to perform each task from 0 (no difficulty) to 3 (unable to do). The scoring system uses the highest abnormal response from each domain with an adjustment for the use of aids or the need for assistance. The scores from the eight domains are then averaged to give an overall score from 0 (no disability) to 3 (severe disability). A summary of community surveys which have used either the HAQ or a modified version called the mHAQ [35], which uses only eight of the original 20 questions, is shown in (Table 1.13). A further study based in a UK general practice showed that the prevalence of a HAQ > 0 rose from around 13 per cent in men aged 55–59 to 62 per cent in men aged over 85; and from around 25 per cent in women aged 55–59 to around 85 per cent in women aged over 85 [78]. All showed an increasing level of disability with age and higher levels of disability in women than in men. In both the UK and the Netherlands 60 per cent of women aged over 75 reported some disability. As might be expected, the prevalence of disability increases with the number of areas of joint pain [33, 79].

The NHANES I Epidemiologic Follow-up study included 4428 people who were aged at least 50 years at the baseline assessment (in 1971–5) [80]. They were asked to complete a 26-item physical function questionnaire which was based on the HAQ (but included six additional questions). The questions were grouped in eight categories (as in the HAQ) and scored from

Table 1.13 Population based studies of physical disability using the HAQ

Country	Reference	Definition of disability	% of responders							
			Male				Female			
			16–44	45–64	65–74	75+	16–44	45–64	65–74	75+
UK	[34]	mHAQ > 0.5	6	16	13	22	7	14	19	36
Netherlands	[77]	HAQ ≥ 0.5	–	11[a]	20	41	–	18[a]	33	61
UK	[34]	mHAQ > 0	18	33	34	41	22	36	44	60

[a] Age 55–64.

Table 1.14 Prevalence of disabling (i.e. limiting activity) musculoskeletal conditions (rate per 1000)

United States

	1971–5 [37] Age group (years)				1989–90 [38] Age group (years)				
	25–44	45–64	65–74	All	25–44	45–64	65–74	75+	All
All musculoskeletal conditions	27	81	114	65					
Male				57					
Female				69					
Arthritis					10	51	99	146	28
Male									18
Female									36

United Kingdom

1995 [81]

	Age group (years)				
	16–44	45–64	65–74	75+	All ≥16
Arthritis and rheumatism	7	64	110	170	51
Back problems	13	28	25	31	22

Canada

1986–7 [82]

	Age group (years)				
	16–44	45–64	65–74	75+	All ≥15
All musculoskeletal conditions	25	75	126	192	50
Male			39		
Female			61		
Arthritis and rheumatism	6	39	86	151	27
Back problems	14	29	26	15	16
Other bone and joint problems	3	6	9	12	5

0–3 (as in the HAQ). The mean age at the baseline assessment was 62 years and approximately 10 years later 17 per cent had a disability score greater than one.

Studies using other measures of disability

Results from government-sponsored surveys

The results of a number of government surveys are shown in Table 1.14. These tend to use a definition of 'limiting everyday activity' for disability. Thus the sequence of questioning is 'Do you have any long-standing condition?' If the answer to this question is 'Yes' then the respondent is asked if this condition limits his activities. Methodological differences between studies make it difficult to draw any conclusions about the relative frequency of disability between countries and with time. All these studies show an increasing prevalence of disability related to musculoskeletal problems with age, and a higher prevalence in women than men. Co-morbidity is another important factor in determining whether or not a person with arthritis reports limitation of activity [73, 83]. In secondary analysis of the 1984–6 NHIS, Yelin and Felts estimated that 68 per cent of RA patients with no co-morbidity experienced limitation of activities of daily living, compared with 89 per cent of those with co-morbidity [83]. The equivalent figures for osteoarthritis were 59 per cent and 82 per cent. Data from the 1984 NHIS Supplement On Ageing show that people aged over 55 with arthritis have an average of 2.8 co-morbid conditions (in addition to their arthritis) compared to an average of 1.8 chronic conditions (in total) amongst those aged over 55 without arthritis [84].

The seven per cent of the US population with musculoskeletal problems account for approximately one-third of those with activity limitation [83]. In Canada musculoskeletal disorders also account for around 30 per cent of long-term disability [85] and in the UK musculoskeletal and connective disorders account for 34 per cent of all reported disability [5]. Inflammatory arthritis is more disabling than osteoarthritis, and osteoarthritis is more disabling than back pain [73, 84].

Rather surprisingly at least three countries (Canada, the Netherlands, and the UK) undertook national studies of the prevalence of disability in 1986–8 [86–88]. The Canadian Health and Activity Limitation Survey found that five per cent of the population were disabled due to musculoskeletal disorders [82]. The UK 1986 Disability Survey found that 6.2 per cent of adults living in private households were disabled due to musculoskeletal conditions [88].

More recently, the HSfE found that 18 per cent of people aged over 16 and living in private households reported having at least one disability out of the five covered; four per cent of men and five per cent of women had a serious disability. The prevalence rose sharply with age; 73 per cent of men and 75 per cent of women aged over 85 had at least one disability [5]. Among those with at least one disability the greatest proportion (34 per cent) attributed their disability to a musculoskeletal disorder (including 2 per cent due to RA and 2 per cent due to osteoarthritis).

Results from epidemiological surveys

The Calderdale study looked at six activities which often cause difficulties for people with arthritis: getting up and down stairs, gripping or holding objects, doing up buttons or zips, putting on shoes, socks or stockings, brushing or combing hair, and getting out of a low chair. The prevalence of disabling joint symptoms rose from 2.6 per cent in those aged 16–44 to 34.3 per cent in those aged over 75 years [33].

Results from the Framingham Study

The Framingham Disability Study was conducted in cycle 14 of the examinations of the Framingham population when the cohort members were aged between 55 and 84 years [14]; 2837 individuals took part. Disability was defined in three ways using validated instruments. The results showed a sharp gradient in disability across the three age groups 55–64, 65–74, 75–84. Whereas 96 per cent of 55–64 year olds could walk half a mile, only 77 per cent of 75–84 year olds were able to do so; 79 per cent of those aged 55–64 could perform heavy household work compared to 50 per cent of 75–84 year old. The most substantial gender differences were in the oldest age groups with women being more disabled than men. However, the authors emphasize the message that, even in the oldest age group, the majority of people are not significantly disabled and are leading independent lives.

Risk factors

Age and gender

Almost all the studies of musculoskeletal symptoms, different rheumatic disorders, and locomotor disability cited in this chapter have shown that the prevalence rises with age and is higher in women than in men. It is reasonably easy to explain the increase with age. The gender difference is more difficult to understand. The most common arthropathies OA and RA occur more frequently in women than men. The reasons for this are explored in the relevant chapters. It is not clear why women with these diseases should report more disability than men. This may be related to the tasks performed by women or may be because men overestimate (or women underestimate) what they are actually capable of doing. Alternatively the disease course may be more severe in women.

Ethnic origin

Despite the wealth of studies described in this chapter, it is difficult to be sure whether there are ethnic differences in the prevalence of pain and disability because of the differences in study design. The COPCORD studies (Tables 1.4 and 1.5) suggest that there may be. However, there may be just as marked differences within a single ethnic group in different environmental settings [36] as there are between ethnic groups in the same environmental setting. The US NHANES studies suggest that black men and women report a higher age- and gender-specific frequency of physician-diagnosed arthritis than their white counterparts [39]. Data from the 1989–91 NHIS suggest that Hispanics have a lower prevalence of all forms of arthritis than non-Hispanics [38]. The US NHANES studies also suggest that physical disability is more common in non-whites than whites [37] and that ethnic origin is the strongest predictor of disability.

Socio-economic factors

Data from a wide variety of sources and countries have shown that there is a relationship between socio-economic status, measured in a wide variety of ways, and the prevalence of musculoskeletal symptoms and disability (Table 1.15). In both the US [37, 38] and Canada [89], government-sponsored surveys have shown a link between the prevalence of self-reported symptoms, self-reported diagnoses, and self-reported locomotor disability and family income. While it can be argued that the musculoskeletal disorder may have lead to a drop in income, it is equally possible that the cause and effect operated in the reverse direction. Certainly the lower levels of education associated with musculoskeletal problems are likely to have preceded the onset of symptoms. The duration of formal education may be seen as a proxy for social class. In the UK, the GHS shows a link between the prevalence of self-reported musculoskeletal conditions and social class as measured by the occupation of the head of the household. Occupation, income, and level of formal education are strongly correlated. Leigh and Fries used four US national surveys, including NHANES I and NHIS 1986, to explore the independent effect of these three variables [90]. They found that the association between schooling and arthritis in employed men is largely accounted for by occupation and income. However, in women the relationship remained even when income and occupation were included. Badley and Ibaòez used data from the Canadian Health and Activity Limitation Survey (1986) and showed that increasing age, not being married, fewer years of schooling, lower income, and being unemployed were all independently associated with disability (whether or not the disability was related to musculoskeletal disorders) [89].

The Tameside study [34] also showed a link between the prevalence of pain at some (but not all) sites and the Carstairs index—a measure of social deprivation which is related to the individual's area of residence [91] (Table 1.16). There was a significant association between area of residence and the prevalence of back, hip, knee, and multiple joint pain. A relationship between area of residence and disability as measured by the mHAQ was noted in middle-aged men and women (45–64 years) but not in other age bands. It is possible that disability lead to financial disadvantage in those of working age so that they live in poorer areas.

There is also a well-recognized relationship between socio-economic factors and a variety of other chronic diseases. Using data from the US 1978 Social Security Survey of Disability and Work, Pincus *et al.* showed that 19 of the 23 health conditions reported by more than 1 per cent of the population differed significantly in reported frequency according to the level of formal education [92]. The 1983 Italian Health Survey [93], which included 58 462 individuals aged 25 and over, randomly selected to be representative of the whole population of Italy, found that the following chronic disorders were substantially less prevalent (reduced by 30 per cent or more) amongst those who were well educated (high school or university vs. primary school only): diabetes, myocardial infarction, other heart diseases, chronic bronchitis, asthma, peptic ulcer, liver cirrhosis, renal failure, and arthritis. The results were similar when occupation was used as an indicator of social class. The Mini-Finland Health Survey, which

Table 1.15 Relationship between socio-economic status and musculoskeletal problems

US

	NHANES I (age 25–74) 1971–5 [37]	NHIS (all ages) 1989–91 [38]	
	% with self-reported symptoms	% with self-reported arthritis	% with self-reported activity limit
Education			
< 12 years	36.7	13.6	4.8
12 years	27.6	18.6	3.1
> 12 years	24.6	16.1	2.5
Annual family income		Annual family income	
<$5,000	39.1	<$10,000 21.2	
$5,000–9,999	30.3	$10,000–19,999 19.1	
$10,000–14,999	27.5	$20,000–34,999 13.3	
≥$15,000	24.1	≥$35,000 11.4	

UK

Social class by occupation of head of household	GHS 1988 [40] Self-reported musculoskeletal condition	GHS 1996/7 [15] Self-reported musculoskeletal condition	HsfE [81] Self-reported musculoskeletal disability[a] Male	Female
V Unskilled	23.5	26.4	26	27
IV Semi-skilled	18.7	22.2	18	22
IIIM Skilled manual	16.3	21.5	19	20
IIIN Skilled non-manual	14.1	20.5	16	19
II Intermediate	13.2	16.0	14	15
I Professional	9.8	13.0	9	14

Canada

	Non-disabled [89]	Disabled with a musculoskeletal disorder [89]
Education		
≤ Grade 8	14.0	38.3
Secondary	40.3	32.5
> Secondary	45.7	29.2
Income		
<$10,000	9.1	21.4
$10,000–19,999	14.9	28.0
$20,000–29,999	17.3	16.9
$30,000–49,999	31.7	20.9
≥$50,000	26.9	12.8

[a] Any disability including sight, hearing, locomotor.

Table 1.16   Relationship between the prevalence of musculoskeletal symptoms (per cent) and a measure of social deprivation (from [34])

	Carstairs Index[a]					
	1/2	3	4	5	6/7	
Any musculoskeletal symptoms	48	50	53	57	56	[b]
Back	18	19	25	27	24	[b]
Neck	16	19	15	18	21	
Shoulder	16	18	19	18	20	
Elbow	6	6	7	7	8	
Hand	12	14	15	16	14	
Hip	9	11	13	14	11	[b]
Knee	19	23	25	25	27	[b]
Multiple joint pain	15	19	21	21	24	[b]

[a] The Carstairs Index is assigned to an individual based on their post ode. It is based on the proportion of people living in overcrowded accommodation, in social classes IV and V, unemployed men, and car ownership. There are 7 unequal categories: 1 is very affluent and 7 severely deprived.
[b] Significant trend.

included an independent interview and examination phase, suggested that there was some over-reporting of chronic morbidity in the less educated part of the population [6]. This study also found that the prevalence of disability (defined in three different ways) was highest in those with fewest years of formal education [73].

Previous pain experience

A number of population-based studies, particularly of low back pain and soft tissue syndromes have shown that the strongest risk factor for the development of a new episode of pain is having had an episode of pain in the past [51].

Psychological distress

There have been a number of longitudinal studies based in the general population or in industry which have shown that the level of psychological distress at baseline was a strong predictor of developing back pain or other musculoskeletal pain at a later time [94–96]. Magni *et al.*, using data from NHANES I, found that 18 per cent of the population with chronic pain had depression (using the depression scale of the Center for Epidemiologic Studies) compared to 8 per cent of the general population [97]. However, given that these data are cross-sectional, it is not possible to tell whether the pain caused the depression or vice versa. In the Mini-Finland survey, the prevalence of disability was higher in those who reported a lot of either physical or mental stress at work [73].

Summary

Studies from a wide variety of sources show that musculoskeletal symptoms and disability are extremely common in all parts of the globe. Back and knee pain are the most common sites of pain. Back pain is particularly common in people of working age with men and women being approximately equally affected. Knee pain is particularly common in the older age groups and the frequency continues to rise into extreme old age. Except in the youngest age groups, women have more knee pain than men (perhaps reflecting the epidemiology of the most common underlying diagnosis, osteoarthritis). The prevalence of physical disability rises sharply with age. Nevertheless, the majority of elderly people are not physically disabled. Musculoskeletal conditions are responsible for around one-third of physical disability in the community. There are many parts of the world for which there are no data on the prevalence of musculoskeletal disorders or physical disability.

References

1.   Lawrence RC, Hochberg MC, Kelsey JL *et al.* Estimates of the prevalence of selected arthritic and musculoskeletal diseases in the United States. *J Rheumatol* 1989; **16**: 427–441.
2.   Safavi KH, Heyse SP, Hochberg MC. Estimating the incidence and prevalence of rare rheumatologic diseases: a review of methodology and available data sources. *J Rheumatol* 1990; **17**: 990–993.

3. Criqui MH, Barrett-Connor E, Austin M. Differences between respondents and non-respondents in a population-based cardiovascular disease study. *Am J Epidemiol* 1978; **108**: 367–372.

4. Rönmark E, Lundqvist J, Lundbäck B, Nyström L. Non-responders to a postal questionnaire on respiratory symptoms and diseases. *Eur J Epidemiol* 1999; **15**: 293–299.

5. Department of Health. *Health Survey for England 1993*. London: The Stationery Office, Department of Health, 1995.

6. Heliövaara M, Aromaa A, Klaukka T, Knekt P, Joukamaa M, Impivaara O. Reliability and validity of interview data on chronic diseases. The Mini-Finland Health Survey. *J Clin Epidemiol* 1993; **46**: 181–191.

7. Jabine TB. Reporting chronic conditions in the National Health Interview Survey. A review of findings from evaluation studies and methodological test. *Vital Health Stat* 1987; **2**: 1–45.

8. Hakala M, Pöllänen R, Nieminen P. The ARA revised criteria select patients with clinical rheumatoid arthritis from a population based cohort of subjects with chronic rheumatic disease registered for drug reimbursement. *J Rheumatol* 1993; **20**: 1674–1678.

9. WHO working group. *The use of registers in the epidemiologic study of rheumatic diseases including planning*. Report of a WHO working group, Sweden 25–27 November 1985. *Scand J Rheumatol Suppl* 1988; **71**: 1–16.

10. McCormick A, Fleming D, and Charlton J. *Morbidity statistics from general practice 1991/2 (MSGP4)*. London: Office of Population Censuses and Surveys, 1994.

11. Kurland LT, Molgaard CA. The patient record in epidemiology. *Sci Am* 1981; **245**: 54–63.

12. Dawber TR, Meadors GF, Moore FE. Epidemiological approaches to heart disease: the Framingham study. *Am J Public Health* 1951; **41**: 279–286.

13. Felson DT, Hannan MT, Naimark A *et al*. Occupational physical demands, knee bending, and knee osteoarthritis: results from the Framingham Study. *J Rheumatol* 1991; **18**: 1587–1592.

14. Jette AM, Branch LG. The Framingham Disability Study: II. Physical disability among the aging. *Am J Public Health* 1981; **71**: 1211–1216.

15. Office for National Statistics: Social Survey Division. *Living in Britain: results from the 1996 general household survey*. London: The Stationery Office, 1998.

16. WHO and the Netherland Central Bureau of Statistics. *Third consultation to develop common methods and instruments for health interview surveys*. Voorburg: 1993.

17. Lawrence RC, Everett DF, Hochberg MC. Arthritis. In: Cornoni-Huntley JC, Huntley RR, Feldman JJ, eds. *Health status and well-being of the elderly: National Health and Nutrition Examination Survey I Epidemiologic followup study*. New York: Oxford University Press; 1990: 136–151.

18. Davis MA, Ettinger WH, Neuhaus JM, Mallon KP. Knee osteoarthritis and physical functioning: evidence from the NHANES I Epidemiologic Followup Study. *J Rheumatol* 1991; **18**: 591–598.

19. Looker AC, Orwoll ES, Johnston CCJr *et al*. Prevalence of low femoral bone density in older U.S. adults from NHANES III. *J Bone Miner Res* 1997; **12**: 1761–1768.

20. Reunanen A, Aromaa A, Pyörälä K, Punsar S, Maatela J, Knekt P. The Social Insurance Institution's coronary heart disease study. Baseline data and 5-year mortality experience. *Acta Med Scand Suppl* 1983; **673**: 1–120.

21. Heliövaara M, Aho K, Aromaa A, Knekt P, Reunanen A. Smoking and risk of rheumatoid arthritis. *J Rheumatol* 1993; **20**: 1830–1835.

22. Heliövaara M, Aho K, Knekt P, Reunanen A, Aromaa A. Serum cholesterol and risk of rheumatoid arthritis in a cohort of 52 800 men and women. *Br J Rheumatol* 1996; **35**: 255–257.

23. Heliövaara M, Mäkelä M, Aromaa A, Impivaara O, Knekt P, Reunanen A. Low back pain and subsequent cardiovascular mortality. *Spine* 1995; **20**: 2109–2111.

24. Heliövaara M, Aho K, Knekt P, Aromaa A, Maatela J, Reunanen A. Rheumatoid factor, chronic arthritis and mortality. *Ann Rheum Dis* 1995; **54**: 811–814.

25. Aho K, Heliövaara M, Maatela J, Tuomi T, Palosuo T. Rheumatoid factors antedating clinical rheumatoid arthritis. *J Rheumatol* 1991; **18**: 1282–1284.

26. Wilson D, Wakefield M, Taylor A. The South Australia health omnibus survey. *Health Promotion J Aust* 1992; **2**: 47–49.

27. Hupkens C. *Coverage of health topics by surveys in the European Union*. European Commission, 1997.

28. Lawrence JS. *Rheumatism in populations*. London: Heinemann, 1977.

29. Muirden KD. The origins, evolution and future of COPCORD. *APLAR J Rheum* 1997; **1**: 44–48.

30. Wigley RD. Rheumatic problems in the Asia-Pacific region. In: Wigley RD, ed. *The primary prevention of rheumatic diseases*. Carnforth: Parthenon Publishing, 1994: 21–25.

31. Bennett K, Cardiel MH, Ferraz MB, Riedemann P, Goldsmith CH, Tugwell P. Community screening for rheumatic disorder: Cross cultural adaptation and screening characteristics of the COPCORD core questionnaire in Brazil, Chile, and Mexico. *J Rheumatol* 1997; **24**: 160–168.

32. Fries JF, Spitz P, Kraines RG, Holman HR. Measurement of patient outcome in arthritis. *Arthritis Rheum* 1980; **23**: 137–145.

33. Badley EM, Tennant A. Changing profile of joint disorders with age: findings from a postal survey of the population of Calderdale, West Yorkshire, United Kingdom. *Ann Rheum Dis* 1992; **51**: 366–371.

34. Urwin M, Symmons D, Allison T *et al*. Estimating the burden of musculoskeletal disorders in the community: the comparative prevalence of symptoms at different anatomical sites, and the relation to social deprivation. *Ann Rheum Dis* 1998; **57**: 649–655.

35. Pincus T, Summey JA, Soraci SAJr, Wallston KA, Hummon NP. Assessment of patient satisfaction in activities of daily living using a modified Stanford Health Assessment Questionnaire. *Arthritis Rheum* 1983; **26**: 1346–1353.

36. Aoyagi K, Ross PD, Huang C, Wasnich RD, Hayashi T, Takemoto T. Prevalence of joint pain is higher among

women in rural Japan than urban Japanese-American women in Hawaii. *Ann Rheum Dis* 1999; **58**: 315–319.

37. Cunningham LS, Kelsey JL. Epidemiology of musculoskeletal impairments and associated disability. *Am J Public Health* 1984; **74**: 574–579.

38. National Arthritis Data Workgroup. Arthritis prevalence and activity limitation—United States, 1990. *Morb Mortal Wkly Rep* 1990; **43**: 433–438.

39. Praemer A, Furner S, Rice DP. *Musculoskeletal conditions in the United States*. American Academy of Orthopaedic Surgeons, 1999.

40. OPCS: Social survey division. *General household survey 1988*. London: HMSO, 1990.

41. Lee P, Helewa A, Smythe HA, Bombardier C, Goldsmith CH. Epidemiology of musculoskeletal disorders (complaints) and related disability in Canada. *J Rheumatol* 1985; **12**: 1169–1173.

42. Badley EM, Rasooly I, Webster GK. Relative importance of musculoskeletal disorders as a cause of chronic health problems, disability, and health care utilization: findings from the 1990 Ontario Health Survey. *J Rheumatol* 1994; **21**: 505–514.

43. Praemer A, Furner S, Rice DP. *Musculoskeletal conditions in the United States*. American Academy of Orthopaedic surgeons, 1992.

44. Manahan L, Caragay R, Muirden KD, Allander E, Valkenburg HA, Wigley RD. Rheumatic pain in a Philippine village. A WHO-ILAR COPCORD Study. *Rheumatol Int* 1985; **5**: 149–153.

45. Chaiamnuay P, Darmawan J, Muirden KD, Assawatanabodee P. Epidemiology of rheumatic disease in rural Thailand: a WHO-ILAR COPCORD study. Community Oriented Programme for the Control of Rheumatic Disease. *J Rheumatol* 1998; **25**: 1382–1387.

46. Wigley RD, Prior IA, Salmond C, Stanley D, Pinfold B. Rheumatic complaints in Tokelau. I. Migrants resident in New Zealand. The Tokelau Island migrant study. *Rheumatol Int* 1987; **7**: 53–59.

47. Wigley RD, Prior IA, Salmond C, Stanley D, Pinfold B. Rheumatic complaints in Tokelau. II. A comparison of migrants in New Zealand and non-migrants. The Tokelau Island migrant study. *Rheumatol Int* 1987; **7**: 61–65.

48. Bergstrom G, Bjelle A, Sundh V, Svanborg A. Joint disorders at ages 70, 75 and 79 years—a cross-sectional comparison. *Br J Rheumatol* 1986; **25**: 333–341.

49. Ballina-Garcia FJ, Hernandez-Mejia R, Martin-Lascuevas P, Fernandez-Santana J, Cueto-Espinar A. Epidemiology of musculoskeletal complaints and use of health services in Asturias, Spain. *Scand J Rheumatol* 1994; **23**: 137–141.

50. Jacobsson L, Lindgarde F, Manthorpe R. The commonest rheumatic complaints of over six weeks' duration in a twelve-month period in a defined Swedish population. Prevalences and relationships. *Scand J Rheumatol* 1989; **18**: 353–360.

51. Croft P. The epidemiology of pain: the more you have, the more you get. *Ann Rheum Dis* 1996; **55**: 859–860.

52. Papageorgiou AC, Croft PR, Thomas E, Ferry S, Jayson MIV, Silman AJ. Influence of previous pain experience on the episode incidence of low back pain: Results from the South Manchester Back Pain Study. *Pain* 1996; **66**: 181–185.

53. Office of Population Censuses And Surveys. *Morbidity statistics from general practice. Fourth national study 1991–2*. London: HMSO, 1995.

54. Bjelle A, Mägi M. Rheumatic disorders in primary care. A study of two primary care centres and a review of previous Swedish reports on primary care. *Scand J Rheumatol* 1981; **10**: 331–341.

55. Kaipiainen-Seppänen O, Aho K, Isomäki H, Laakso M. Shift in the incidence of rheumatoid arthritis toward elderly patients in Finland during 1975–1990. *Clin Exp Rheumatol* 1996; **14**: 537–542.

56. Kaipiainen-Seppänen O, Aho K, Heliövaara M. Incidence and prevalence of ankylosing spondylitis in Finland. *J Rheumatol* 1997; **24**: 496–499.

57. Kaipiainen-Seppänen O. Incidence of psoriatic arthritis in Finland. *Br J Rheumatol* 1996; **35**: 1289–1291.

58. Kaipiainen-Seppänen O, Aho K. Incidence of rare systemic rheumatic and connective tissue diseases in Finland. *J Intern Med* 1996; **240**: 81–84.

59. Kaipiainen-Seppänen O, Savolainen A. Incidence of chronic juvenile rheumatic diseases in Finland during 1980–1990. *Clin Exp Rheumatol* 1996; **14**: 441–444.

60. Gabriel SE, Crowson CS, O'Fallon WM. The epidemiology of rheumatoid arthritis in Rochester, Minnesota, 1955–1985. *Arthritis Rheum* 1999; **42**: 415–420.

61. Michet CJJ, McKenna CH, Elveback LR, Kaslow RA, Kurland LT. Epidemiology of systemic lupus erythematosus and other connective tissue diseases in Rochester, Minnesota, 1950 through 1979. *Mayo Clin Proc* 1985; **60**: 105–113.

62. Carbone LD, Cooper C, Michet CJ, Atkinson EJ, O'Fallon WM, Melton LJ. Ankylosing spondylitis in Rochester, Minnesota, 1935–1989. Is the epidemiology changing? *Arthritis Rheum* 1992; **35**: 1476–1482.

63. Michet CJ, Machado EB, Ballard DJ, McKenna CH. Epidemiology of Reiter's syndrome in Rochester, Minnesota: 1950–1980. *Arthritis Rheum* 1988; **31**: 428–431.

64. Salvarani C, Gabriel SE, O'Fallon WM, Hunder GG. Epidemiology of polymyalgia rheumatica in Olmsted County, Minnesota, 1970–1991. *Arthritis Rheum* 1995; **38**: 369–373.

65. Salvarani C, Gabriel SE, O'Fallon WM, Hunder GG. The incidence of giant cell arteritis in Olmsted County, Minnesota: apparent fluctuations in a cyclic pattern. *Ann Intern Med* 1995; **123**: 192–194.

66. Melton LJ, III, Amadio PC, Crowson CS, O'Fallon WM. Long-term trends in the incidence of distal forearm fractures. *Osteoporos Int* 1998; **8**: 341–348.

67. Cooper C, Atkinson EJ, O'Fallon WM, Melton LJ. Incidence of clinically diagnosed vertebral fractures: a population-based study in Rochester, Minnesota, 1985–1989. *J Bone Miner Res* 1992; **7**: 221–227.

68. Melton LJ, III, Therneau TM, Larson DR. Long-term trends in hip fracture prevalence: the influence of hip fracture incidence and survival. *Osteoporos Int* 1998; **8**: 68–74.

69. Melton LJ, III, Crowson CS, O'Fallon WM. Fracture incidence in Olmsted County, Minnesota: comparison

of urban with rural rates and changes in urban rates over time. *Osteoporos Int* 1999; **9**: 29–37.

70. Wigley RD, Zhang NZ, Hu DW *et al*. ILAR study of rheumatic diseases in China. IV Knee pain in Shiao Hong Men village. *APLAR Bull* 1990; **7**: 76–77.

71. Kellgren JM, Jeffrey MR and Ball J. *Atlas of standard radiographs. The epidemiology of chronic rheumatism.* Oxford: Blackwell Scientific Publications, 1963.

72. WHO. *International classification of impairments, disabilities and handicaps. A manual of classification relating to the consequences of disease.* Geneva: WHO, 1989.

73. Mäkelä M, Heliövaara M, Sievers K, Knekt P, Maatela J, Aromaa A. Musculoskeletal disorders as determinants of disability in Finns aged 30 years or more. *J Clin Epidemiol* 1993; **46**: 549–559.

74. Steinbroker O, Traeger CH, Batterman RC. Therapeutic criteria in rheumatoid arthritis. *JAMA* 1949; **140**: 659–662.

75. Keitel W, Hoffman H, Weber G. Ermittlung der prozentualen functsminderung der gelenke durch einen bewegungsfunktionstest in der rheumatologie. *Deut Gesundeheitwes* 1971; **26**: 1901–1903.

76. Meenan RF, Gertman PM, Mason JH. Measuring health status in arthritis. The arthritis impact measurement scales. *Arthritis Rheum* 1980; **23**: 146–152.

77. Odding E. *Locomotor disability in the elderly.* University of Rotterdam, 1994.

78. McAlindon TE, Cooper C, Kirwan JR, Dieppe PA. Knee pain and disability in the community. *Br J Rheumatol* 1992; **31**: 189–192.

79. Odding E, Valkenburg HA, Algra D, Vandenouweland FA, Grobbee DE, Hofman A. Association of locomotor complaints and disability in the Rotterdam study. *Ann Rheum Dis* 1995; **54**: 721–725.

80. Hubert HB, Bloch DA, Fries JF. Risk factors for physical disability in an aging cohort: The NHANES I epidemiologic followup study. *J Rheumatol* 1993; **20**: 480–488.

81. Department of Health. *Health Survey for England 1995.* London: The Stationery Office, 1997.

82. Reynolds DL, Chambers LW, Badley EM *et al*. Physical disability among Canadians reporting musculoskeletal diseases. *J Rheumatol* 1992; **19**: 1020–1030.

83. Yelin EH, Felts WR. A summary of the impact of musculoskeletal conditions in the United States. *Arthritis Rheum* 1990; **33**: 750–755.

84. Verbrugge LM, Lepkowski JM, Konkol LL. Levels of disability among U.S. adults with arthritis. *J Gerontol* 1991; **46**: S71-S83.

85. Badley E. The impact of musculoskeletal disorders on the Canadian population. *J Rheumatol* 1992; **19**: 337–340.

86. Statistics Canada, Department of the Secretary of State of Canada. *The health and activity limitation survey.* Ottawa: Statistics Canada, 1988.

87. Netherlands Central Bureau of Statistics. *Physical disability in the population of the Netherlands 1986/88.* The Hague: SDU Publishers, 1990.

88. Martin J, White A. *The prevalence of disability among adults. OPCS surveys of disability in Great Britain.* Report 1 OPCS. London: Social Survey Division, HMSO, 1988.

89. Badley EM, Ibañez D. Socioeconomic risk-factors and musculoskeletal disability. *J Rheumatol* 1994; **21**: 515–522.

90. Leigh JP, Fries JF. Occupation, income, and education as independent covariates of arthritis in four national probability samples. *Arthritis Rheum* 1991; **34**: 984–995.

91. Carstairs V, Morris R. *Deprivation and health in Scotland.* Aberdeen: Aberdeen University Press, 1991.

92. Pincus T, Callahan LF, Burkhauser RV. Most chronic diseases are reported more frequently by individuals with fewer than 12 years of formal education in the age 18–64 United States population. *J Chronic Dis* 1987; **40**: 865–874.

93. La Vecchia C, Negri E, Pagano R, Decarli A. Education, prevalence of disease, and frequency of health care utilisation. The 1983 Italian National Health Survey. *J Epidemiol Community Health* 1987; **41**: 161–165.

94. Bigos SJ, Battié MC, Spengler DM *et al*. A prospective study of work perceptions and psychosocial factors affecting the report of back injury. *Spine* 1991; **16**: 1–6.

95. Croft PR, Papageorgiou AC, Ferry S, Thomas E, Jayson MI, Silman AJ. Psychologic distress and low back pain. Evidence from a prospective study in the general population. *Spine* 1995; **20**: 2731–2737.

96. Leino PI, Hanninen V. Psychosocial factors at work in relation to back and limb disorders. *Scand J Work Environ Health* 1995; **21**: 134–142.

97. Magni G, Caldieron C, Rigatti-Luchini S, Merskey H. Chronic musculoskeletal pain and depressive symptoms in the general population. An analysis of the 1st National Health and Nutrition Examination Survey data. *Pain* 1990; **43**: 299–307.

98. Darmawan J, Valkenburg HA, Muirden KD, Wigley RD. Epidemiology of rheumatic diseases in rural and urban populations in Indonesia: a World Health Organisation International League Against Rheumatism COPCORD study, stage I, phase 2. *Ann Rheum Dis* 1992; **51**: 525–528.

PART I
Inflammatory joint disease

2 | *Rheumatoid arthritis*

Alan J. Silman

Criteria for diagnosis

Problems with criteria assignment in rheumatoid arthritis

The interpretation of epidemiological data, either in regard to the occurrence of, or risk factors for, rheumatoid arthritis (RA), is fundamentally dependent on the nature of the criteria used to define a case. Criteria that have been developed for use in the clinic, to ascertain cases for treatment trials, or studies of natural history, are likely to be inappropriate for epidemiological studies of the disorder. There are two main areas of concern. Firstly, RA, at the time of first onset, presents as with an inflammatory polyarthritis, which is often difficult to distinguish from other causes of inflammatory polyarthritis as well as from those individuals whose disease does not evolve into a specific diagnostic entity. There are no absolute tests that distinguish the nature of the arthritis at the time of onset. Indeed, it may be questioned whether it is appropriate to apply criteria for RA at disease onset given the concept that RA is a chronic, deforming, disabling disease and, by definition, can therefore not be ascertained at first presentation.

The second difficulty in relation to RA is in the use of criteria to ascertain cases in cross-sectional studies for the purposes of, for example, determining prevalence or, in genetic studies, classifying individual family members as case or non-case. In RA, a disease whose activity fluctuates, it is as important to be able to pick up inactive, or, indeed, totally remitted disease as it is to ascertain those with current evidence of disease. Older criteria sets were aware of this difficulty, for example [1], but more recent epidemiological studies do not seem to have taken account of the problem.

Available criteria sets

The first criteria to be developed for RA were those formulated by a consensus of experts and accepted by the American Rheumatism Association in 1956 [2]. These were subsequently revised in 1958 to make them more suitable for widespread use and are now commonly known as the 'Rome criteria' (Table 2.1) [3]. These criteria achieved widespread acceptability until the late 1980s and epidemiological studies up to this period predominantly used these criteria. An extension of these criteria (Table 2.2) [1] allowed for the inclusion of inactive disease. Subsequently, an alternative set of criteria were derived for epidemiological studies, the 'New York criteria' (Table 2.3) [4]. There were only four features for these criteria, but no rules were determined to define a case. In general, a cut-off of two or more positive features was found to be sensitive but

Table 2.1 Rome criteria for active RA

1. Morning stiffness
2. Pain on movement or tenderness in a joint[a]
3. Soft tissue swelling in a joint[a]
4. Soft tissue swelling of another joint[a]
5. Symmetrical soft tissue joint swelling simultaneously[a]
6. Subcutaneous nodules[a]
7. X-ray changes[b]
8. Positive rheumatoid factor

Probable RA—three or four criteria positive.
Definite RA—five or six criteria positive.
Classical RA—seven or eight criteria positive.
[a] Must be observed by a physician but does not include terminal interphalangeal joints.
[b] Can include juxta-articular osteoporosis.
Source: [4].

Table 2.2 Rome criteria for inactive RA

1. Past history polyarthritis
2. Symmetrical deformity of hand or feet joints
3. Radiological change
4. Positive rheumatoid factor

Probable RA—two criteria positive.
Definite RA—three or four criteria positive.

Table 2.3   New York criteria for RA

1. History of joint pain: ≥ 3 limb joints (PIP/MCP etc. on one side counts as a single joint)
2. Swelling, limitation of movement, subluxation or ankylosis of ≥ 3 limb joints PLUS symptoms of at least one joint pair; the involved joints must include at least one hand, wrist, or foot. There must also be symmetrical involvement of at least one joint pair
3. X-ray (grade 2 or more) erosive RA in hands, wrists, and feet
4. Positive serological reaction for RA

Positive: no rules, studies to indicate number and which criteria are satisfied.
Source: [4].

not specific, whereas using a cut-off of three features, the converse was the case.

These criteria sets were developed from consensus. By contrast, in 1987, the American Rheumatism Association (now the American College of Rheumatology) produced a revised version of their original criteria derived from an analytical approach comparing disease features in a series of patients attending specialist clinics, with an average disease duration of 7 years, from those with a number of other definitive diagnoses for example, osteoarthritis, fibromyalgia, and SLE. These criteria (Table 2.4) [5] have advantages over the original criteria in that the more precise definition of the individual features is used. They were also developed in two forms: a list system in which any individual with four of seven criteria could be classified as positive and a decision tree approach where five separate subsets could be used to define the disease (Table 2.4). This criteria set is now in widespread use, predominantly in the list (4/7) format. Initial evaluation showed very little difference between the original Rome criteria and the 1987 ARA criteria in clinic patients [6].

Problems in the 1987 ARA criteria for new onset disease

Early observations [7] showed the criteria only had a sensitivity of 74 per cent for recent onset disease. Indeed, in a more recent study of patients with disease

Table 2.4   The 1987 revised criteria for the classification of RA (traditional format)[a]. Modified from [5]

Criterion	Short title	Definition
1	Morning stiffness	Morning stiffness in and around the joints, lasting at least 1 h before maximal improvement. At least 3 joints.
2	Arthritis of 3 or more joint areas	Areas simultaneously have had soft tissue swelling or fluid (not bony overgrowth alone) observed by a physician. The 14 possible areas are right or left PIP, MCP, wrist, elbow, knee, ankle, and MTP joints.
3	Arthritis of hand joints	At least 1 area swollen (as defined above) in a wrist, MCP or PIP joint.
4	Symmetric arthritis	Simultaneous involvement of the same joint areas (as defined in (2)) on both sides of the body (bilateral movement of PIPs, MCPs, or MTPs is acceptable without absolute symmetry).
5	Rheumatoid nodules	Subcutaneous nodules, over bony prominences, or extensor in juxta-articular regions, observed by a physician.
6	Serum rheumatoid factor	Demonstration of abnormal amounts of serum rheumatoid factor by any method for which the result has been positive in <5% of normal control subjects.
7	Radiographic changes	Radiographic changes typical of RA on posteroanterior hand and wrist radiographs, which must include erosions or unequivocal bony decalcification localized in or most marked adjacent to the involved joints (osteoarthritis changes alone do not qualify).

[a] For classification purposes, a patient shall be said to have RA if he/she has satisfied at least four of the seven criteria. Criteria 1 to 4 must have been present for at least 6 weeks. Patients with two clinical diagnoses are not excluded. Designation as classic, definite, or probable RA is not to be made.

Alternative classification based on fulfilling the following subsets:
1. Criteria 2 and 3
2. Criteria 2 and 6
3. Criteria 2 and 7
4. Criteria 4 and 6
5. Criteria 3 and 6.
Criteria for this classification excludes PIP.

Table 2.5 Performance of 1987 ARA criteria in ascertaining new incident cases of RA, reproduced with permission of the *Journal of Rheumatology* from [10]

Format	Sensitivity %	Specificity %
4/7	62	50
Decision tree	78	35

onset of less than 6 months [8], the criteria had 84 per cent sensitivity even in patients where virtually 100 per cent were seropositive and erosive. Other recent reports suggest a sensitivity of 90 per cent for early synovitis [9]. The most robust analysis of the performance of the criteria in early disease came from a population-based incident cohort of individuals presenting with joint inflammation in the peripheral joints. The value of the 1987 criteria in relation to both hospital physician opinion and predicting disease course over the subsequent 3 years was evaluated. The criteria had relatively low sensitivity and even lower specificity against physician's opinion (Table 2.5). Furthermore, the likelihood ratio (that is the improvement in odds in predicting specific outcomes of random chance) for those who were ARA criteria positive was only between 1.1 and 1.7, in predicting those individuals who 3 years later would either be severely disabled, have persistent

disease, or have radiographic erosions. Given the fact that individuals continued to accumulate the individual criteria features during the progression of disease, allowing a cumulative approach to criteria satisfaction over the course of disease does improve the sensitivity [10].

Problems in using 1987 ARA criteria detecting current disease

A population study amongst the Pima Indians [11] showed that the use of the 1987 criteria, which essentially detect currently active disease only, had a sensitivity of 28 per cent for detecting presumed cases of ever having RA. This was much lower than the use of the combined Rome criteria for both active and inactive disease. A similar problem emerged in relation to a twin study where the aim was to ascertain the lifetime disease status of both pairs of a twinship [12]. To account for the remitting nature of the disease and the possibility that cases might be missed, a proposed modification of the 1987 criteria [12], allowing such individuals to be included, has been made (Table 2.6).

The impact of applying these modifications was considerable (Table 2.7), with an improvement in sensitivity of about 30 per cent without any appreciable loss of

Table 2.6 Modification to 1987 ARA criteria to improve ascertainment of inactive cases. Reproduced with permission of the *Journal of Rheumatology* from [12]

	Criterion	Current	Ever
1.	Morning stiffness in and around the joints lasting at least 1 h before maximal improvement	Reported in the 6 weeks prior to interview	At any time in the disease course
2.	Arthritis of 3 or more joint areas	With soft tissue swelling or fluid at current examination	With swelling at current examination or deformity and a documented history of swelling
3.	Arthritis of hand joints: Involvement of at least one area in a wrist MCP or PIP joint	With soft tissue swelling or fluid at current examination	With swelling at current examination or deformity and a documented history of swelling
4.	Symmetrical arthritis: Simultaneous involvement of the same joint areas on both sides of the body	With soft tissue swelling or fluid at current examination	With swelling at current examination or deformity and a documented history of swelling
5.	Rheumatoid nodules: Subcutaneous nodules	Present or current examination	Present at current examination or documented in the past
6.	Serum rheumatoid factor	Detected at current examination	Present at current examination or documented in the past to have been positive in the past by any assay method
7.	Radiographic changes	Erosive changes typical of RA on posteroanterior hand and wrist radiographs	Erosive changes typical of RA on posteroanterior hand and wrist radiographs

An individual satisfying four or more criteria was classified as having RA.

Table 2.7 Comparison of the performance of different criteria sets of the *Journal of Rheumatology* for ascertaining cases of RA, reproduced with permission from [12]

Criteria set	Sensitivity %	Specificity %
New York (≥2)	95	65
New York (≥3)	84	87
Rome (definite)	62	78
1987 ARA (4/7)	57	87
Modified 1987 ARA (4/7)	88	87
1987 ARA (decision tree)	58	83
Modified 1987 ARA (decision tree)	89	78

specificity. There is no doubt that without the use of such a process, either implicitly or explicitly, prevalence based studies will severely under-estimate the occurrence of the disease. The other problem in relation to the criteria is that individual features may not be unambiguously ascertained and, in practice, a number of borderline cases emerge. The application of 'fuzzy' criteria to allow for different levels of confidence also substantially improve the discrimination of these criteria [13].

Occurrence

Problems in defining occurrence

The problems in defining occurrence are not unique to RA but the latter provides a useful model. Incidence rate, defined as the rate of new cases arising in the population at risk over a given time period, is obviously appropriate for RA. The number of cases arising in a population under study over a period of time is ascertained and expressed as incidence per 1000 person years of observation which is conventionally referred to as annual incidence per 1000 population. There are two approaches used for assessing incidence, both of which have problems in relation to RA. The first is to undertake duplicate surveys in the same population and to estimate the number of new cases occurring in the interval between surveys. The problem with such an approach is that to ascertain the rate with any statistical precision, in a disease as relatively rare as RA, requires very large population surveys that are both expensive and difficult logistically. Further, cases that develop and either die or fully recover between surveys will be missed by the second survey. An alternative and much cheaper approach is to constantly monitor, either retrospectively or prospectively, the clinical facilities where all patients from the target population with RA are likely to attend, with a view to ascertaining all clinically diagnosed new cases. Assumptions about the use of medical care facilities by the target population may, however, be erroneous: some individuals with the disease may not attend or may not be diagnosed. Additionally, the retrospective approach relies on accurate contemporary medical records and standardization of diagnosis is more difficult to achieve. The problem of the alternative, prospective approach is that compliance by the participating physicians in recording accurate data may wane over time. Computerized diagnostic indices are useful but unless they apply to all possible physicians seeing patients from a fixed denominator population then under-ascertainment is likely to occur. The rarity of the disease is a problem for all approaches and to derive robust estimates of occurrence in individual age sex groups requires prolonged observation of a large population over many years. Therefore only recently have reliable data on the population incidence of RA become available.

The concept of prevalence representing all existing cases with RA is also deceptively simple and methodologically simpler. Thus a cross-sectional survey of a population sample will yield all cases whether diagnosed or not. Further, the occurrence of existing cases is not as rare as the rate of new cases developing, and a cross-sectional study may give reliable estimates from a relatively modest sample size (around 2000). The problem comes from deciding on the inclusion criteria. In most series, the number of active cases who would satisfy any criteria set are small and many of the cases will be either be in remission because of drug therapy or due to natural history. Further, there may be no objective evidence at the time of survey of disease presence such as joint deformity or radiological evidence of joint destruction. In reality, most apparent point prevalence estimates include a variable and unstated proportion of past cases. Thus such studies are ascertaining both currently active cases and an unknown proportion of cases at any time in the past. Thus it is the measurement of cumulative or life time prevalence that is being attempted, though cases that remitted totally many years prior to the study will be ignored by both subject and investigator. Some studies have included all ever-diagnosed cases alive at a notional prevalence day, for example [14], though the interpretation of such a figure is unclear. The problem in interpreting the data that follow is that published studies have not clearly distinguished whether they are adopting a point or cumulative prevalence approach and comparisons between data have to be made with caution [15].

Occurrence in populations of European origin

Incidence

The major studies reporting the incidence of RA in populations of European origin are summarized in Table 2.8. A number of the earlier studies are difficult to interpret given the methodological problems discussed above. The data recorded from the United Kingdom Royal College of General Practitioners [18,19] suggest incidence rates which are so much higher than other recorded rates that they almost certainly reflect diagnostic inaccuracy. Similarly, the original data from surveys in the North of England in the 1950s and 1960s [17] almost certainly ascertain cases that were not RA.

The most recent studies have been remarkably consistent. In brief, studies based on ascertained cases in the North East and mid-West of the United States [14,30] have suggested age-adjusted incidence rates of

Table 2.8   Incidence studies of RA: populations of European origin

Reference	Population/period	Case ascertainment	Incidence (95% CI) per 1000 person years		
			Males	Females	Both
[16]	Massachusetts, US 1968	Hospital referrals			0.29
[17]	Leigh and Wensleydale, England 1959–68	New cases between duplicate surveys	8	12	10
[18]	UK 1970–72	Primary care diagnosed attenders	1.63	4.20	2.99
[19]	UK 1981–82	Primary care diagnosed attendes	1.50	3.34	2.47
[20]	Olmsted County, US 1950–74	Computerized register of diagnosed cases	0.22	0.48	0.37
[21]	Norway 1969–84	Hospital registers	0.10	0.26	0.21
[22]	Finland 1979–84	National drug reimbursement register	–	–	0.70
[23]	US (nurses) 1976–84	Biennial questionnaires	–	0.12	–
[24]	Seattle, US (women) 1987–89	Prospective ascertainment from local hospitals	–	0.24	–
[25]	Norfolk, UK 1990	Prospective follow-up of primary care attenders	0.16 (0.11–0.23)	0.43 (0.35–0.53)	
[26]	Lorraine, France 1986–89	Diagnosed cases	0.05	0.12	0.09
[27]	Finland 1980–1990	National drug reimbursement register	–	–	0.27 (0.24–0.30)
[28]	Joannina, Greece 1987–95	Referrals to local rheumatologists	0.12 (0.04–0.20)	0.36 (0.21–0.51)	0.24 (0.15–0.33)
[29][a][b]	Oslo, Norway 1988–93	Register from all local clinical sources cases only	0.14 (0.12–0.16)	0.37 (0.33–0.41)	0.26 (0.24–0.28)
[14]	Olmsted County, US 1975–85	Computerized register of diagnosed cases	0.47 (0.32–0.61)	0.88 (0.71–1.05)	0.68 (0.57–0.80)
[30]	Massachusetts, US 1987–90	Computerized register of diagnosed cases	0.22 (0.13–0.32)	0.60 (0.46–0.75)	0.42 (0.23–0.60)
[31]	Finland 1995	National drug reimbursement register	0.24	0.43	0.33

[a] RF positive.
[b] Similar data recently also published from northern Norway [355]

between 0.7 and 0.4 per 1000 person years at risk. Data from European studies based on ascertained cases have shown rates lower than this with an incidence of approximately 0.25 per 1000 person years [27–29]. In all studies, the female rate is between two to three times higher than the male rate. There do appear to be suggestions of geographical variation even within Europe. Thus a study from France [26] showed an incidence of approximately 0.1 per 1000 person years. Recent data from Finland suggest regional differences even within a country [356].

Data from the Norfolk Arthritis Register (NOAR) in the UK [25] adopted a different approach insofar as that study attempted to ascertain all cases of joint inflammation based on their attendance in primary care. After a structured, standardized follow-up to determine whether such individuals satisfied criteria for RA or not, there was a very strong similarity between these data and the other studies from Europe as shown in Table 2.8. As discussed earlier, with an increasing period of observation, the likelihood of satisfying the criteria for RA increases. Thus in NOAR, after 5 years of observation, the incidence increased from 0.13 to 0.25/1000 person years (pyr) in males and from 0.3 to 0.54 in females [32].

Influences of age and gender

A number of recent studies have been able to provide relatively robust estimates of the influence of age and gender on the incidence of RA, both in Europe (Tables 2.9 and 2.10) [25,29] and in the US (Table 2.11) [14]. All the studies are consistent in showing the considerable rarity of RA in young males, i.e. under the age of 35. Although the absolute female excess is greater with increasing age, the relative excess in females is greatest in those under the age of 50 in all studies. There is evidence, particularly from the Norfolk studies but also from the other studies, that the gender difference narrows. Indeed in the Norfolk study, in the very oldest age group, men had a higher incidence.

The influence of age is also remarkably constant in these studies. In contrast to widespread belief, in both males and females the incidence of the disease increases with increasing age and does not peak in the fifth or sixth decades. There is a suggestion that there is a decline in incidence in the very elderly (i.e. those over 75), but this is likely to be due to a reduction in susceptibility. Thus the conclusion has to be that RA is a disease of increasing age. However, the possibility of a birth cohort influence that could explain this is discussed below.

Prevalence

There have been more surveys on the prevalence of RA in populations of European origin than any other

Table 2.9 Age specific incidence rates for RA, Norfolk, UK, 1990[a], reproduced with permission of Oxford University Press from [25]

Age	Incidence/100 000	
	Males	Females
15–24	3	12
25–34	6	15
35–44	6	45
45–54	12	67
55–64	27	77
65–74	38	80
75–84	77	40
All 15+	16 (11–23)	43 (35–53)

[a] Age-adjusted to England and Wales population.

Table 2.10 Age specific incidence rates for RA Oslo, Norway, 1988–1993, reproduced with permission of the *Journal of Rheumatology* from [29]

Age	Incidence/100 000		
	Males	Females	All
20–29	3	12	8
30–39	4	18	11
40–49	6	29	17
50–59	22	57	40
60–69	40	73	58
70–79	43	72	61
All (20–79)	14 (95% CI 12–16)	37 (95% CI 33–41)	26 (95% CI 24–28)

Table 2.11 Age and sex specific incidence rates for RA in Rochester, Minnesota, 1955–1985, modified from [14]

Age	Incidence/100 000		
	Males	Females	All
35–44	17	50	34
45–54	39	103	73
55–64	59	126	97
65–74	89	130	115
75–84	110	123	119
85+	0	44	33
All 15+[a]	50	98	75
	(95% CI 41–59)	(95% CI 87–109)	(95% CI 68–83)

[a] Age adjusted to US population.

Table 2. 12 Prevalence of RA in European populations

Reference	Population	Age	N	Prevalence definite RA %		
				Males	Females	Both
[33][a]	Rhonda, Wales	15+	19 722	0.7	0.6	
	Glamorgan, Wales	15+	4621	1.0	1.1	
[34]	Leigh and Wensleydale, England	15+	2234	0.5	1.6	1.1
[35]	Sofia, Bulgaria	15+	4318	0.3	1.2	0.9
[36]	Piestany, Czechoslovakia	15+	1420	0.3	0.5	0.4
[37][b]	Rotterdam, Netherlands	15+	19647	0.5	1.2	0.9
[38]	National sample, Sweden	15+	39 418			0.7
[39]	Oberhorlen, Germany (1963)	15+	421	2.6	0.6	1.2
	Oberhorlen, Germany (1968)	15+	415	0.6	0.4	0.5
[40][c]	National sample, Denmark	15+	19 100	0.3	1.2	0.8
	Samso, Denmark	15+	4557	0.5	1.2	0.8
[41][d]	Jondal, Norway	≥16–75	803	0.5	1.2	0.7
[42]	Sjobo, Sweden	40–70	5262			0.7
[43]	Heinola, Finland	≥30	8000	1.0	2.7	1.9
[44]	Hanover, Germany	25–74	11 534			0.5
[45]	Manchester, England	16+	1045	0.2	1.4	0.8
[46][e]	Oslo, Norway	20–79	5886	0.2	0.7	0.4
[47]	Chiawani, Italy	16+	3294	0.1	0.5	0.3
[48]	Belgrade, Serbia	20+	2184	0.1	0.3	0.2
[49][f]	Siberia, Russia	15+	974			0.7
[50]	Dublin, Ireland	18+	1227			0.5
[51][a]	Brittany, France	18+	2740	0.3	0.9	0.6
[52]	Halland, Sweden	20–74	3928			0.5

[a] Based on a number of diagnosed cases attending local hospitals.
[b] Not ARA criteria, including some 'probable cases'.
[c] Based on a screening study for hand function.
[d] Supplemented population register data.
[e] Similar data recently published from northern Norway [355].
[f] Prevalence is very high in some Russian populations in recent reports [357]

Table 2.13 Prevalence of RA in North American populations

Reference	Population	Age	N	Prevalence definite RA %		
				Males	Females	Both
[53]	Pittsburgh, US	15+	798	0.4	1.0	0.7
[54]	Puerto Rico	15+	3883	0.2	0.4	–
[55]	Michigan, US	6+	7207	0.2	0.6	0.4
[56]	US adults	18–79	6672	0.5	1.7	1.0
[57]	US whites	15+	4552	–	–	0.9

rheumatic disease, although few have been sufficiently large to produce robust estimates of the occurrence by different age groups. Studies in populations of European origin in Europe are shown in Table 2.12 and those of North American origin in Table 2.13. Probably the most remarkable feature is the consistency in the results obtained despite the different approaches to study. As shown in Table 2.12, studies in the 1970s and 1980s suggested a prevalence in the population overall of approximately 1 per cent, although more recent studies from Norway [46–48] have shown much lower prevalences of less than 0.5 per cent. A possibility for this is a decline in incidence as discussed below. There have been a number of older population surveys of prevalence of RA in populations of European origin in the United States (Table 2.13). However, interestingly, there have been no such studies recently and estimates of prevalence have been derived from ascertained cases alive on prevalence day (e.g. [14]). It is of interest to note that in that population, even allowing for the fact that many of these cases might be totally limited and inactive, the overall prevalence was approximately 1 per cent.

Occurrence in Native American populations

There have been a large number of studies, predominantly the prevalence but also the incidence, of RA in a number of Native American Indian populations and, in brief, many of these populations have shown the highest recorded occurrence of any population in the world (Table 2.14). The Pima Indians in particular from Arizona [67] have a very high occurrence. This population has been subjected to regular biennial examination and from the interval cases it has been possible to ascertain the incidence of disease. The

Table 2.14 Prevalence of RA in Native American populations

Reference	Population	Age	N	Prevalence definite RA %		
				Males	Females	Both
[58]	Haida Indians, Queen Charlotte Island	15+	209	–	–	1.0
[59]	Pima Indians, US	30+	–	0.6	2.5	1.3
	Blackfeet Indians, US	30+	–	1.3	1.4	1.4
[60]	Alaskan Eskimos	15+	1443	0.5	1.0	0.8
[61]	Yakima Indians, US	18–79	501	–	3.4	–
[62]	Chippewa Indians, US	18+	205	4.8	8.2	6.8
[63]	Inuit Eskimos, Canada	15+	2055	0	1.8	–
[64]	Yupik Eskimos	18+	4600	0.2	1.0	0.6
[65]	Pima Indians, US	20+	1449	3.2	7.0	5.3
[66]	Southeast Alaskan Indians	19+	5169	1.3	3.5	2.4
[67]	Pima Indians, US	15+	2894	1.0	3.1	
[68]	Inupiat Indians, Alaska, US	20+	1651	0.6	2.3	1.4
	Yupik Eskimos, Alaska, US	20+	2135	0.1	1.0	0.6

Table 2.15 Prevalence of RA in populations of African origin

Reference	Population	Age	N	Prevalence definite RA %		
				Males	Females	Both
[69]	Kingston, Jamaica	35–64	530	1.5	2.2	1.9
[70][a]	Igbo-ora, Ishera, Nigeria; and Cavalia, Liberia	5+	1027	0.8	1.2	1.0
[71]	Rural, Tswana tribe Phokeng, South Africa	15+	801	–	–	0.1
[72]	Soweto, South Africa	15+	964	Nil	1.4	0.9
[73]	Xhosa, Tribe Transkei, South Africa	18+	577	–	–	0.7
[74]	Lesotho	15+	1070	Nil	0.4	0.3
[75]	Rural, Venda, South Africa	18+	543	Nil	Nil	Nil [b]
[76]	Igbo-ora, Nigeria	18+	2000	Nil	Nil	Nil
[45][c]	Manchester, England	16+	1163	Nil	0.5	0.3

[a] Includes 'mild disease'.
[b] Prevalence of 0.03% in larger population based on cases attending local hospitals.
[c] Subjects of Afro-Caribbean origin.

most recent data suggested an overall incidence of 3.8 per 1000 person years (95% CI 1.7–5.9) with, again, a significant excess in females (OR 4.9, 95% CI 2.2–7.6) per 1000 pyr compared to males (OR 2.7, 95% CI 0–6.2) per 1000 pyr. Other Native American populations with very high incidence include the Chippewa Indians [62] and the Inupiat Indians from Alaska [66,68] .

Occurrence in populations of African origin

By contrast to the Native American populations, studies in African populations have shown remarkably low prevalences (Table 2.15). In one study in the rural Venda [75], no case was found in 543 subjects. In another study in a rural population from Nigeria [76], no case was found in over 2000 individuals participating in a population survey. Interestingly, in that survey, which was derived from a population of some 40 000, not a single case of RA was revealed by monitoring the clinic facilities set up to provide health care for the villagers. Whether these differences are due to genetic background or to environmental effects is unknown. There have been few population surveys in populations of African origin outside the African continent. In a study of Afro-Caribbeans in Manchester, UK, a prevalence of 0.3 per cent was observed. A figure lower than that observed in the European population living in the same area [45]. These data therefore suggest the difference is more likely to be related to genetic and constitutional factors than environmental ones. However, by contrast, a study from Soweto in South Africa

[72] showed a prevalence similar to white South Africans and was much higher than prevalence figures observed for rural African populations.

Occurrence in Asian and Australasian populations

A number of studies of prevalence of RA have also been conducted in South East Asian and Australasian populations (Table 2.16). In general, these data show prevalence figures that are lower than those from European populations, although there are some interesting differences. Populations from the Indian subcontinent [80,88,358] showed prevalence figures similar to European groups, whereas populations from South East Asia showed figures very similar to African populations. There does appear to be some environmental effect insofar as in the Pakistani population, the prevalence in affluent areas was twice that in the poor area [88]. Not entirely consistent with this are the results from a large multi-centre studies in Taiwan [89] where the prevalence in an urban area was three times that in a rural area.

Occurrence in Middle Eastern populations

Finally, a few surveys have been undertaken of populations from the Middle East, the data is shown in Table 2.17. There are no consistent findings, but the results are broadly similar to the average figures seen in Europe and other Asian populations.

Table 2.16   Prevalence of RA in Asian and Australasia population surveys

Reference	Population	Age	N	Prevalence definite %		
				Males	Females	Both
[77]	Kinmet, China	15+	5629	0.2	0.4	0.3
[78]	Beijing, North China	20+	4192			0.3
	Shanton, South China	20+	5057			0.3
[79]	Hong Kong	15+	2002			0.3
[80]	Delhi, India	16+	39 826			0.8
[81]	Rural, Indonesia	15+	4683			0.2
	Urban, Indonesia	15+	1071			0.3
[82] Quoted in [83]	Shizuoka, Japan	All ages	2802	0.5	1.1	0.8
[84]	Osaka, Japan	All ages	3318	0	0.3	0.17
[83]	Japan	15+				
	Hiroshima		11 306	0.2	0.5	0.4
	Nagasaki		4963	0.1	0.4	0.3
[85]	Kinki, Japan	All ages	7364			0.3
[86]	Hiroshima and Nagasaki, Japan	15+	11 393	0.4	0.7	
[87]	Kamitonda, Japan	All ages	2276			0.3
[88]	Karachi, Pakistan:	15+				
	Poor area		2220			0.9
	Affluent area		2012			2.0
[89]	Taiwan, Rural	20+	3000	0.2	0.4	0.3
	Taiwan, Urban		6000	0.6	1.2	0.9
[90]	Europeans, New Zealand	20+	432	0.5	2.2	–
[91]	Maoris, New Zealand	20+	175	3.8[a]	4.0[a]	
[92]	Philippines, Manila	15+	3006			0.2
[93]	Shantou, China	16+	22 049			0.2
[94][b]	Kamitonda, Wakayama, Japan	All ages	~3000			
	1975			0.11	0.57	0.34
	1985			0.2	0.44	0.32
	1996			0.11	0.24	0.17

[a] Definite and probable.
[b] Point prevalence for 1996.

Table 2.17   Prevalence of RA in Middle Eastern populations

Reference	Population	Age	N	Prevalence definite %		
				Males	Females	Both
[95]	Jerusalem, Israel	20+	6760	Nil	0.4	
[96]	National sample, Iraq	16+	6999			1.0
[97]	Oman	16+	1925			0.8
[98]	Saudi Arabia	16+	5891	6.18	0.25	0.22

Summary of geographical data on occurrence

The most striking observation is not the variability in occurrence, but the similarity with little evidence of 'orders of magnitude' differences in the occurrence between the different populations. In fact, it is indeed remarkable that, some Native American populations apart, all recent studies have been consistent in finding prevalence proportions between 2 and 10 per 1000 population. It is difficult to get a consistent pattern as to whether the differences that do emerge can be explained by environmental or constitutional/genetic factors. One hypothesis is that RA is a disease of urbanization and that rural populations, particularly in the developed world, have a very low occurrence. Although this is broadly true, the low occurrence of the disease in Hong Kong [79] and the low occurrence in Afro-Caribbeans compared to their European neighbours in inner-city Manchester in the UK, would perhaps argue that in these populations at least, one should search for genetic factors to explain their infrequent occurrence.

Time trends

Mortality

Mortality data can be used as a proxy for the combined effects of both incidence and case survival and hence an observation of declining population mortality for RA would be consistent either with a fall in incidence or a reduction in the severity of diagnosed cases. The problem, of course, is the frequent failure to mention RA on death certificates and there are a

number of studies confirming the high rate of under-recording of this disease as a contributor to death [99]. Multi-cause coding may not solve this problem [100]. A study of trends in mortality from Australia covering the period 1950–1981 [101] did not clearly state whether it included all mentions of RA on death certificates or only those with RA as the underlying cause of death. In brief, however, there was no significant trend apparent overall in age adjusted death rates during this period, although there was evidence of a recent decline in mortality rate in women, particularly those in the older age groups (Fig. 2.1) [101]. What was interesting from this data was the observation that there was no improvement in the survival of men with RA as judged by age at death, particularly against a background of generally falling mortality in the population.

RA is not a new disease and has been described in historical writings and portrayed in paintings for at least 200–300 years although, for example, compared to osteoarthritis, evidence from skeletal remains of its early existence is difficult to obtain.

Incidence or severity

Trends in RA can be considered both in terms of disease incidence and severity of those who develop the disease. There is an inherent circularity in this distinction as all the diagnostic criteria include recognized indices of severity, positive rheumatoid factor and radiological erosions, and thus failure to satisfy the criteria might reflect absence of disease or a less severe form. Changes in severity over time could also reflect both the underlying aggressiveness of the disorder or advances in therapy despite evidence from formal clinical trials that current therapeutic options are not significantly more effective than 'older' options. One problem in examining trends in severity is that such studies are frequently based on samples of patients attending specialist hospital units and could therefore reflect changes in referral or attendance patterns.

Trends in incidence

The examination of trends necessitates the continual monitoring of a fixed population with access to contemporary medical records; the latter permitting retrospective correct diagnostic assignment. Such a system can only work if the monitoring system can detect all the cases in a defined population. Such a system exists in the Rochester Epidemiology Program based at the

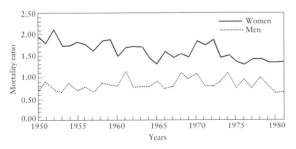

Fig. 2.1 Trends in age-adjusted population mortality rates from RA for Australia 1950–85. 1950 = 100 both sexes. Reproduced from Wicks IP, Moore J, Fleming A. *Ann Rheum Dis* 1988; **47**: 563–569 [101] with permission from the BMJ Publishing Group.

Table 2.18   Recent trends in incidence of RA results from three population monitoring studies

Reference	Population	Case Ascertainment	Year(s)	Incidence/1000 pyr	(95% CI)
[67]	Pima Indians US	Biennial examination	1966–73 1974–82 1983–90	8.9 6.2 3.8	(5.9–11.9) (3.8–8.6) (1.7–5.9)
[27]	Finland (National)	Register for drug reimbursement	1980 1985 1990	0.40 0.39 0.32	(0.35–0.45) (0.34–0.44) (0.27–0.36)
[14]	Olmsted County, Minnesota, US	Computerized register of all patient diagnosis	1955–64 1965–74 1975–85	0.90 0.72 0.68	(0.75–1.05) (0.60–0.85) (0.57–0.80)

Mayo Clinic. This institution, together with the Olmsted Medical Practice, provide the only source of medical care for the population of Olmsted County in Minnesota. Although retrospective examination of medical records will omit those who never seek medical attention for their symptoms and standardization of diagnosis is difficult, the utility of such a system in documenting trends in new cases over long periods of time is clear. The data analysed from 1955–1985 [14] (Table 2.18) show a generalized decrease in incidence during this period. This decline was greater in females: 120 to 88/100 000 pyr between 1955–1964 and 1975–1985, than in males: 564 to 47/100 000 pyr. However, possibly due to small numbers, there was considerable random fluctuation over this period.

The most striking evidence of a decline in incidence in North America comes from the results of the biennial examination of the Pima Indians [67]. These data (Table 2.18) showed a startling decline between 1996–1973 and 1983–1990. However, in this population, the fall in incidence was similar in males (5.9–2.7/1000 pyr) and females (11.5–4.9/1000 pyr) between 1963–1973 and 1983–1990 respectively.

Long-term trends in European populations are less easily available. UK data are available from an ongoing survey of all patients attending one of 30 participating general practitioners who send back to the 'Central' unit a 'weekly return' of the numbers attending with a list of specific diagnoses, which include RA. Data from this source [102] showed a statistically significant decline of approximately 7.5 per 100 000 per year between 1976 and 1987, equivalent to a halving in the incidence rate. Although most of the participating doctors remained the same during the period of observation, the possibility cannot be excluded that there was a decline in completeness of recording during that period. Another source of data from UK primary care comes from the morbidity surveys conducted by a larger group of general practitioners who were 'forced' to make a diagnosis about every patient consultation. These surveys in 1970–72 [18] and 1981–82 [19] all relied on the recorded diagnosis from the general practitioner and were not standardized. Results comparing these reveal that there was a small but statistically significant decline in incidence between these surveys.

Whole population data are also available from those countries that have population morbidity register for specific disorders. Interpretation of trends from such sources is difficult as in addition to the persistent problem of changes in registration completeness, there may be selective changes in the severity of cases recorded. Such registers are extensively available in Scandinavia. Data from Finland [103] have recently been published. This source demonstrated an annual incidence of registered seropositive RA that showed a small decline between 1980 and 1990 (Table 2.18) which, on further investigation, was proportionately due to a greater decline in rheumatoid factor negative disease. Data from Wakayama, Japan based on a small number of incident cases suggested a significant decreased incidence from 0.43 to 0 between 1965 and 1996, this decrease was restricted to females [94].

Period of onset or period of birth

Trends in incidence by calendar year of presentation or diagnosis may not reflect true temporal patterns of disease. As discussed above, most studies of the incidence of RA carried out over a short period of time demonstrate a marked increase in risk with increasing age. Although this might represent a true age effect, an alternative explanation is that the oldest groups in those populations were at highest risk based on their year of birth and that follow-up over a long period would confirm that the age-specific incidence rates would fall. Indeed, in the Finnish Register study, there was evidence of a shift towards an older age at onset with a decline in incidence in the youngest age groups [103]. A similar result was found in a Japanese study with an increase in mean age of onset from 38 to 47 years between 1960–1965 and 1985–1990 [104].

If the presumed environmental exposure which triggers RA occurs early in life it might be more appropriate, therefore, to examine trends in disease in successive generations defined by their cohort of birth. Lawrence was the first to suggest the possibility that the risk of RA could be related to the period in which an individual was born for the reasons stated above [17]. In a prospective study in Oberhörlen, West Germany in the 1960s, the maximal incidence was found to be in those aged 65 and over. This was compared to the maximal prevalence of existing cases in the cross-sectional survey in the same population was found in the decade below that age [39]. Gabriel attempted to examine the influence of birth cohorts on incidence rates between 1955 and 1985 [14]. Small numbers limit the conclusions, but there are some suggestions in that data that individuals born between 1880 and 1895 had the highest age-specific rates. Further, a shift towards an increasing age at onset in Japanese patients between 1960 and 1990 was thought to be due, at least in part, to a birth cohort effect [104]. Analyses of the Finnish data suggest fairly convincing evidence of a decline in age-specific incidence in more recent birth cohorts (Fig. 2.2) [103].

Using data from the Leigh and Wensleydale population surveys on the prevalence of rheumatoid factor positivity (using the SCAT test) in relation to period of birth, Lawrence [17], revealed: (i) in urban populations, rheumatoid factor positivity increases with age in cross-sectional studies, (ii) in a 10-year follow-up period in an urban population, there was a tendency for individuals to have a fall in titre, (iii) on an analysis by year of birth, the rate of positivity fell in successive cohorts from those born in 1885/94; indicating perhaps that latter group had a peculiarly high risk. Lawrence hypothesized that the reduction in titre in the older age groups was consistent with an effect of improvement in atmospheric pollution resulting from the Clean Air Act in 1956.

Trends in severity

RA may become a less severe disease over time, possibly related to changes in treatment [105,106]. Data on

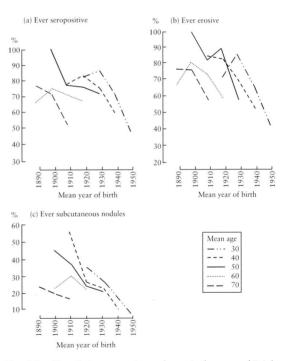

Fig. 2.3 Trends in proportions of certain features of RA by birth cohorts of patients with established disease. (a) Ever seropositive, (b) ever erosive, (c) ever subcutaneous nodules. Reprinted from Silman AJ, Davies P, Currey HLF, Evans SJW, Is rheumatoid arthritis becoming less severe? *Journal of Clinical Epidemiology*, **36**, 891–897. Copyright (1983), with permission from Elsevier Science [107].

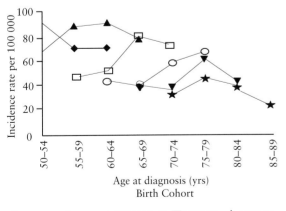

◆ 1925–29   ▲ 1920–24   □ 1915–19   ▼ 1905–09   ★ 1900–04

Fig. 2.2 Incidence of RA in women according to their birth cohort and age at diagnosis. Reproduced with permission from [103].

disease severity were analysed on a birth cohort basis using three indicators of disease severity, these were ever seropositive, ever erosive, and ever having subcutaneous nodules. The results from all three analyses were similar (Fig. 2.3) [107]. These figures show that successively more recent generations were less likely to be positive for any of the above features. Further examination showed that the trends were not linear and that there was a severity peak in patients presenting in around 1960 with the majority of the birth cohorts displaying their maximum severity around that year [107].

Population data from Finland has also shown a decline in the proportion of registered disabled as a result of musculoskeletal conditions being due to RA [22] and that the average level of disability declined between 1978 and 1989 [108].

Trends in mortality

There has also been evidence, in population terms, of a reduction in mortality due to RA, also consistent with a decline in severity [109].

Genetic factors

Familial clustering

An increased rate of occurrence of RA in first degree relatives (FDR) of RA probands could obviously be compatible both with a greater shared environment or a greater shared genetic constitution. There have been a number of studies comparing the occurrence in FDR of probands with a matched control group (Table 2.19). Lawrence [17] clearly pointed out the potential for bias in such studies in that the FDR of affected individuals are more likely to recall or respond positively to questionnaires or interviews on joint symptoms than random population controls. In one recent study, false negative rates were found to be negligible, but 60 per cent of proband recalled cases in their FDR were false positives [125]. Indeed, logistically, it is difficult to achieve a high response rate in control families, the affected families being more motivated to participate. There is a considerable variation in the reported risk in FDR though those studies that used standard criteria for diagnosis based on the results of clinical examination found that the increased rate in all FDR was small, at around two (Table 2.19). Most of these studies did not adjust for age and sex differences between the probands' and the controls' FDR. In addition, the

majority of the probands were derived from hospital series and it is likely that such patients have more severe disease and perhaps are more likely to be ascertained because they have a family history. In the only community-based study [123], a non-significant increased risk of 1.6 was observed (Table 2.19). A meta-analysis of available studies with population controls suggested that the overall increased risk was approximately two. An alternative approach is to undertake, in the same population, a comparative study of the prevalence of RA in FDR of affected probands and in the general population. In the one such study from Utah, the increased familial risk might be as high as 10-fold [126].

Certain subgroups of relatives do appear to be at greater risk. Younger age at onset increases the risk [127], but the effect of gender is inconsistent. In one survey, siblings of affected female cases were three times more likely to have RA than siblings of male cases [128]. By contrast, using a survival analysis approach suggested that the FDR of male cases were at greater risk [127]. Disease risk is also greater in those with severe disease [129]. Certainly there is a substantially increased risk in the previously unaffected FDR of families already demonstrated to have multiple affected cases. For example in one follow-up survey of unaffected first-degree relatives in multiply affected families, an incidence of 8/1000 pyr (95% CI 4.2–13.6) was found. This is substantially in excess of all quoted rates for the incidence of the disease [130].

The data on familial risk has been used to determine what genetic model of inheritance might be appropriate for this disease. Using existing data, one analysis suggested that a two-locus, multiplicative model would be appropriate in explaining the occurrence of the disease, with HLA being one of the major loci involved [131]. However, in an analysis of the data from 247 families [127], a recessive major gene model was proposed. One intriguing suggestion is that genetic anticipation might occur in relation to RA. This term describes the phenomenon that successive generations experience disease onset earlier in life in a more severe form. This is possibly due to an expansion in the tandemly repeated trinucleotide sequences close to the presumed disease susceptibility genes. Such a phenomenon have been observed in studies of two family sets [132,133] with the suggestion that in successive generations the disease is occurring 10 years earlier. One problem, however, with such an approach is the left censorship bias due to the fact that it is only those older mothers who can be captured in surveys of this type.

Table 2.19 Familial aggregation of RA

Reference	Probands Source	Criteria	N	Controls Source	N	Source RA Information in Relatives	Criteria	Relative risk RA FDR	
[110]	Clinic	Clinical	532	Relatives of hospital and normal population	532	Interview from proband	Clinical	2.1 siblings	1.8 parents
[111]	Clinic	Clinical	333		343			2.8 siblings	1.8 parents
[112]	Hospital	Clinical	224	Relatives of non-RA clinical attenders and normals	488	Interview	Clinical	5.9	
[113]	Clinic	Clinical	192	Relatives	192	Interview of matched hospital controls	Clinical	15.8	
[114]	Clinic	Clinical	293	Relatives	293	Interview of hospital patients and employees	Clinical	2.3	
[115]	Population	ARA definite	67	Household sample	183	Examination	ARA definite	2.0	
[116]	Hospital	Clinical	28	Relatives of sero-positive negative RA	35	Examination	Various	0.8	
[117]	Hospital	ARA	31	Relatives of sero-negative RA	31	Examination	ARA definite	4.3	
[118]	Clinic	Rome active	140	Spouses	102	Examination	Rome active	2.7	
[119]	Hospital Clinical	N/S		N/S		Examination	N/S	1.4	
[120]	Population	ARA	N/S	Relatives of matched population controls	N/S	Examination	ARA	1.5 siblings	4.0 parents
[121]	Populations	ARA	76	Same		Examination	ARA	1.2	
[122]	Clinic	New York	201	Spouses[a]		Proband interview plus medical records	New York	1.7	
[123]	Community	1987 ARA	207	Local population	180	Interview and examination	1987 ARA	1.6 (0.3–8.7)	
[124]	Clinic	1987 ARA	126		94	Self report from proband	N/A	4.4 (1.7–11.1)	

[a] Controls were spouses of proband, and spouses of proband's children, siblings, uncles, aunts, nephews and nieces. Prevalence in controls based on prevalence survey in same population [34].

One interesting observation found in two studies of affected sibling pairs [134,135] is that there is no greater similarity either in age of onset or calendar year of onset between pairs of cases than within pairs. The hypothesis for these analyses is that a closer age of onset would be expected if genetic factors were important in explaining concordance and a closer calendar year of onset if environmental factors were of relevance. The fact that neither observation was found would be compatible with the hypothesis that these families arise by chance based on the random distribution of RA in the population.

Twin studies

Studies of twins can provide useful information on the aetiology of RA. Firstly, the widest use of twin studies is to compare the concordance for disease in monozygotic (MZ) and dizygotic (DZ) twin pairs. The theory is that there should be no greater similarity in environmental exposure between MZ and (same sexed) DZ twins and that any excess in disease concordance in the former proves a genetic contribution to disease. Secondly, the concordance rates in MZ and DZ twins gives an upper limit on the penetrance of the presumed disease susceptibility gene or genes and can be used to infer the proportionate genetic contribution. Finally, a comparison of the affected and unaffected twin in MZ pairs might be of value in suggesting clues to putative environmental factors.

There are some major sources for error in RA twin studies. Firstly, cross-sectional studies may underestimate the true concordance as follow-up over time of initially unaffected twin pairs may reveal the subsequent development of disease [136]. Secondly, there is an undoubted publication bias towards reporting con-

cordant twins [137] and analyses based on the pooled experience from published studies [121] is impossible to interpret. Thirdly, it is likely that MZ twins share environment to a greater extent even than same sexed DZ twins, perhaps due to a greater psychological affinity, and differences in concordance between MZ and DZ twins might not reflect the operation of genetic factors.

There have been a large number of twin studies in RA, though most are too small to provide useful data (Table 2.20). The earlier reports are either only available in published proceedings or reported by 'personal communication' in later publications. It is also difficult to interpret the results of studies undertaken before 1950, given the lack of discrimination between the different types of inflammatory joint disease before that time. The results from the Danish twin register [137] have been criticized as the diagnosis was based only on questionnaire and the completion rate was less than 50 per cent [121]. The first UK study [121] relied on notification by rheumatologists from both the UK and the Netherlands and only includes hospital attendees. There was a very high rate of seronegative arthritis in the twins examined that might reflect other diagnostic entities. In addition, the results of that study, which have never been published in full, are based only on 162 twin sets despite the fact that 382 twin sets were examined [121]. The results from the Finnish nation-

Table 2.20   Concordance in twins

Reference	Source of twins	Monozygotic		Dizygotic	
		N	Concordance (%)	N	Concordance (%)
a	N/A	N/A	22.0	N/A	17.5
b	N/A	17	35.3	16	12.5
c	N/A	5	60.0	9	11.1
[138]	Media	6	50.0	6	16.7
	Twin register	8	0	9	0
[139]	Patients attending one centre	8	0		
[140]	Danish twin register	47	34.0	141	7.1
[119]	Clinic attenders: Seropositive	20	30.0	73	4.0
	Seronegative	18	0	51	0
[141]	Questionnaire to population twin register	73	12.3	173	3.5
[142]	Survey of clinic attenders and media campaign	91	15.4	112	3.6
[143]	Australian twin register	14	21 (6–44)	9	0 (0–25)
[144]	Danish national register	13	0	36	8.3

a Kaufmann and Scheerer (1928) quoted in [145].
b Claussen and Steiner (1938) quoted in [119].
c Edstrom (1941) quoted in [146].

wide twin register [141] are based on ascertainment of cases resulting from notification to statutory authority for free medicines and thus there may be considerable under-ascertainment of mild cases. The results from this study showed much lower concordance rates: MZ, 12 per cent; DZ, 4 per cent. A large study from the United Kingdom which examined all twins and verified zygosity using DNA fingerprinting yielded results remarkably similar to the Finnish data: MZ, 15 per cent; DZ, 4 per cent [142].

It is possible to use twin concordance data from MZ and DZ pairs to infer something about the heritability of the disease, that is the proportionate role of genetic factors in explaining disease susceptibility. The concordance figures are not useful in this respect as they are dependent on prevalence; the higher the prevalence the higher the twin concordance. A recent analysis of the heritability of the two largest studies [119,141,142,147] showed a remarkable consistency in that heritable factors accounted for 60 per cent of cases [148]. Nonetheless, these estimates are still based on the assumption that the degree of shared environment is the same between same sex DZ and MZ pairs.

One problem with the twin studies that have been undertaken is that they are capturing the disease status in the second twin at an arbitrary point in time. On further follow-up more twins would develop the disease and it is perhaps more appropriate to use a life-table approach to compare the 'disease free survival' in the initially unaffected co-twins of both the MZ and DZ probands. When this was done [142], the incidence rates were 12.0 and 2.4/1000 pyr in the MZ and DZ pairs respectively, equivalent to an age and sex adjusted rate ratio of 4.2 (95% CI 1.3–13.7).

The Finnish study [141] showed a greater similarity in age of onset between the concordant MZ (mean difference 4.7 years) than the concordant DZ pairs (mean difference 11.0). Interestingly, in that study the concordant MZ twins tended to have severe disease [149]. There was no influence of sex on concordance in any of the major studies. In the recent UK series, there was no evidence of greater disease similarity within the concordant MZ pairs [150].

Disease discordant MZ pairs are often taken as an indication of environmental factors, although there are some factors associated with the biology of twinning, including X-chromosome inactivation and genetic imprinting, which might explain why presumably genetically identical individuals are discordant for disease [151]. However, in the UK series of twins no abnormal evidence of X inactivation was demonstrated [152].

Discordant twin pairs have been subject to a number of investigations of putative environmental agents and these are discussed elsewhere (see below, for example in relation to smoking and hormonal influences).

Genetic susceptibility markers: HLA-DRB1

The strongest evidence in support of the genetic contribution to RA disease susceptibility comes from the consistent association observed between alleles in the highly polymorphic HLA-DRB1 gene of HLA class II and RA. The initial discovery of the association between HLA-DR4 and RA [153] has been replicated in many populations (Table 2.21). High-resolution DNA methods of HLA typing have identified a number of different alleles within the HLA-DRB1 which are associated with RA. The key discovery was that all of the DRB1 alleles that are associated with RA share a very similar amino-acid sequence (glutamine-lysine/arginine-arginine-alanine-alanine) in positions 70–74 in the third hypervariable region in that gene. This shared sequence is commonly referred to as the RA shared epitope (SE) [172]. As shown in Table 2.22, the specific SE bearing allele does vary considerably between population. In part, this represents the predominant SE bearing allele in that population. For example the Native American groups have a very high population frequency of *1402 whereas other *04 alleles are rare in these populations. Conversely, *0405 alleles are predominant in some Asian and European populations, but rare in Northern Europe populations (Table 2.22).

What is unclear is why, within a population, there is variability in the strength of the association between different variants of the shared epitope. The results of two studies [192,193] from populations of Northern European origin (Tables 2.23 and 2.24) show a clear gradient of risk with *0101 showing only a very weak relationship, with *0404 showing a much stronger relationship. If the shared epitope sequence was the disease susceptibility sequence *per se* this difference in relationship would be unexpected. There does appear to be consistent evidence from studies that those individuals that are 'homozygous' for the SE are at greater risk than those individuals carrying a single copy. There is also a variable association even with individuals homozygous for SE. The most striking observation (Table 2.23 and 2.24) is that the greatest risk is for those individuals that carry two different variants of the SE, specifically those individuals who have the genotype *0401/*0404. This was initially referred to as a compound heterozygote [192]. The strong

Table 2.21   HLA DR4 and DRI antigen associations in different populations

Reference	Population	Source RA Cases	Criteria	N	Controls	DR4 (%)		DR1 (%)	
						RA	Controls	RA	Controls
[153]	US whites	Clinic	ARA	80	Healthy	70	28	–	–
[154]	US blacks	Clinic	ARA	35	Healthy	45.7	14.3	28.6	28.6
[155]	US blacks	Clinic	ARA	98	Healthy	22.2	7.4	15.9	11.7
[156]	UK	Clinic							
	Caucasians		N/S	100	Healthy	74	38	28	20
	Asians (Indian subcontinent)		N/S	35	Healthy	17.1	14.3	60	16.7
[157]	Japan	Clinic	ARA	63	Healthy	71.4	41.8		
[158]	Mexicans	Clinic	ARA	20	Healthy	50	6		
[159]	Italians	Clinic	ARA	54	Healthy	18.5	12.3	25.9	12.8
[160]	Japan	Clinic	ARA	88	N/S	70.5	46.1	13.6	9.6
[161]	North India	Clinic	ARA	62	Healthy	67.7	12.5	17.7	15
[162]	Thais	Clinic	ARA	30	N/S	23.3	16.3	3.3	0
[163]	US Yakima Indians	N/S	ARA	29	Healthy	41	38	7	10
[62]	US Chippewa Indians	Population survey	ARA	12	From survey	100	68		
[164]	Netherlands	Population survey	ARA	53	Healthy	32	24.4		
[165]	French	Clinic seropositive	ARA	77	Healthy	66.2	16.3	16.9	13.6
[166]	Greeks	Clinic	ARA	118	Healthy	34.5	31	20.3	12.1
[167]	Israel Jews								
	Ashkenazi	Clinic	ARA	44	Healthy	54.4	40	22.7	16.7
	Non-Ashkenazi	Clinic	ARA	29	Healthy	38	36.7	6.9	15
[168]	Switzerland	Clinic	ARA	132	Unrelated and	43.9 ⎫		30.5 ⎫	
				143	non-selective	44.0 ⎬ 19.9		33.6 ⎬ 17.3	
				Both	blood donors	44.0 ⎭		32.2 ⎭	
[169]	South African blacks	Clinic	ARA	100	Zulu blood donors	44	9.6	4	4.7
[170]	Chile	Clinic	ARA	64	Healthy	48	32	27	16
[171]	Kuwait Arabs	Clinic	ARA	85	N/S	29.4	15	9.4	16.1

Seropositive only increase in DRW10 gene frequencies.
N/S = not stated.
[a] Two studies compared.

relationship between this genotype and disease is clear, though why this should be so is unknown.

Association between HLA and RA: severity or susceptibility

There are a number of lines of evidence suggesting that HLA alleles are possibly of greater influence on disease severity rather than on disease susceptibility *per se*. An early study on subjects ascertained from a community survey showed only a very weak relationship between HLA-DR4 and RA [164]. A more recent study, based on the NOAR incident-based cohort, also shows a very modest relationship between HLA and RA [194]. These observations would suggest that the previously described strong associations might be explained by the relationship with disease severity. Two large studies examining the influence of SE on one indicator of

Table 2.22 HLA DRB1 alleles carrying presumed RA susceptibility epitope in third hypervariable region

Allele	Reference	Associated with RA in populations
*0101	[173]	Non-Greeks
	[175]	Japanese
	[176]	Japanese
*0102	[177]	Israeli Jews
*0401	[178]	Norway
	[179]	Greeks
	[180]	Indians
	[181]	US Whites
	[182]	New Zealand Caucasians
	[183]	Korea
	[174]	Europe/ North America
*0404	[178]	Norway
	[184]	Chinese
	[185]	Siberia
	[174]	Europe/ North America
*0405	[182]	New Zealand Polynesians
	[186]	Spanish
	[184]	Chinese
	[180]	Indians
	[176]	Japanese
*0408	[177]	Israeli Jews
	[187]	Chile
	[185]	Siberia
*1001	[173]	Greeks
	[188]	Tamils
	[189]	Basques
	[177]	Israeli Jews
*1402	[190]	Yakima Indians
	[191]	Tinglit Indians

Table 2.23 Differential HLA DRB1[a] and genotype risk and RA: I, modified from [192]

Genotype	Risk ratio
DRX/DRX[b]	1
DR1/DRX	3
DR1/DR1	5
DR4 (0401)/X	6
DR14 (0404)/X	4
DR1/DR14	9
DR1/DR4	21
DR4/DR14	49

[a] Based on serological typing.
[b] i.e. not DR1/DR4.

Table 2.24 Differential HLA DRB1[a] and genotype risk and RA: II, reproduced with permission of the Journal of Rheumatology [193]

Genotype	Odds ratio (95% CI)
SE –/–	1 (reference)
*0101/SE–	2.9 (1.4–6.2)
*0401/SE–	3.6 (1.9–6.6)
*0404/SE–	3.7 (1.3–10.5)
SE+ (any)/SE–	3.5 (2.1–5.9)
*0101/*0101	1.1 (0.3–4.8)
*0401/*0401	4.6 (1.7–12.7)
*0101/*0401	7.3 (2.3–23.3)
*0401/*0404	25.6 (3.3–202)
SE+ (any)/SE+ (any)	7.8 (4.0–15.1)

[a] Based on serological typing

severity (radiographic erosions) are shown in Table 2.25. The study in the Norfolk arthritis patients showed only weak relationships compared with the prevalent-derived cases by MacGregor *et al.* [193].

Contribution of HLA-DRB1 to genetic susceptibility

The current issue is what proportion of the likely genetic susceptibility to RA can be explained by genes within the HLA region and what proportion might be explained by genes yet to be revealed. A mathematical approach to understanding this question can be derived from considering the sibling recurrence risk and the observed absence of HLA haplotype sharing, identical by dissent, in RA-affected sibling pairs [131,195]. If the sibling recurrence risk is as low as two then the proportion of susceptibility encoded by HLA may be as high as 80 per cent. However, in disease subgroups where recurrence risk may be as high as five then perhaps two-thirds of the genetic encoded susceptibility remains to be revealed.

Contribution of non-HLA-DRB1 genes in the MHC region

The MHC region on the short arm of chromosome six is an area rich in genes with effects on the immune

Table 2.25 Relationship between HLA DRB1 and erosion risk

Reference	Case source	SE –/–	SE +/–	SE +/+
[194]	Community incident cases	1	1.8 (1.3–2.4)	2.5 (1.8–3.6)
[193]	Prevalent cases	1	4.3 (2.4–7.6)	9.7 (4.8–19.6)

system and immune response. Thus despite the strong evidence of association with HLA DRB1, there have been several studies examining the role of other loci within the MHC region. There is very strong linkage disequilibrium between loci and it is virtually impossible using genetic epidemiology to separate out, for example, influences of DRB1 from DQA1. Some have suggested that the DQA locus could be the primary susceptibility site [196]. Tumour necrosis factor (TNF) genes are also found in this region with evidence of strong TNF HLA-DRB haplotype effects on RA [197]. The story is not so simple as, for example, TNFα-1 appeSars to be a susceptibility gene for RA independent of HLA-DRB1 [198].

Contribution of genes outside the MHC region

The recognition that non-HLA genes are likely to be involved in RA susceptibility has lead to a considerable number of investigations using a variety of approaches. As the overall contribution of any one gene might be small, studies are frequently underpowered to detect effects. Similarly, study designs such as whole genome scans (see below) that are performing large numbers of significance tests simultaneously are subject to a high likelihood of type 1 errors. Thus, it is important that the positive results of such studies are replicated in other patient populations. Three approaches are being used:

1. Sibling pair whole genome scans—this approach has the possibility of identifying areas of potential linkage based on a greater than expected 'identity by descent'—i.e. affected sibling pairs are genetically more similar at a given locus than random expectations. A European study of 261 families (97 test sample and 164 validation sample) was highly suggestive of a susceptibility locus on chromosome 3 with a large number of other areas that were worthy of follow-up [199]. A Japanese study of only 41 families found evidence of linkage with loci on chromosomes 1, 8, and X [200]. These and other areas are being tested in whole genome screens on sibling pair collections from the UK [201] and the USA [172].

2. Candidate gene studies—given the complexity of RA pathogenesis it is possible to produce a very long list of genes that might be implicated [202]. Studies have been undertaken using: traditional case–control study design; family based control

methods to avoid population stratification effects (with the most widely analytical approach being the transmission disequilibrium test); and linkage within sibling pairs. Such studies have highlighted possible roles for a variety of cytokine genes [203,204], hormonal influence on immune response [205,206], and other immune-associated molecules [207,208]. Such studies are limited by the need to have an *a priori* candidate.

3. Whole genome scans association studies—the ideal study design would be one that could screen an infinite number of markers using the more powerful association approach. Such studies, involving perhaps the screening of up to 100 000 markers (compared to the 3–400 used in the sibling pair screens discussed above) could be feasible using single nucleotide polymorphisms [126]. The technology is rapidly becoming available for the high throughput automated genotyping and it is likely that this approach will be increasingly used.

Non-genetic host factors

Influence of pregnancy and sex hormones

The striking female excess in incidence with the maximal relative increase being during the reproductive period has resulted in many investigators considering the role of pregnancy and hormonal factors in disease susceptibility. The well-described pregnancy-induced remission of active disease and the anecdotal comments of the relationship of disease activity to different phases in the menstrual cycle have all contributed to the concept that there are important hormonal influences on disease susceptibility. These have been investigated in a number of ways.

Nulliparity and infertility

It was suggested 35 years ago [209] that subfertility was a risk factor for the subsequent development of RA. There have been a large number of case–control studies (Table 2.26), which typically have suggested that women who are nulliporous have a subsequent increased risk of developing RA. However, not all studies have been consistent in this regard, as shown in the table. Furthermore, in a large prospective study linking pregnancy history with death certificate

Table 2.26 Pregnancy history and RA

Reference	Cases	Controls			Odds Ratio (95% Confidence Intervals)		
	N	Source	N	Nulliparity	Abortions	Stillbirths	
[209]	54[a]	Community	54	2.7 (1.1–6.7)			
	172[b]		235		0.7 (0.4–1.4)	0.7 (0.2–2.7)	
[210]	102	OA	122	0.8 (0.3–2.3)	3.7 (2.0–6.7)		
[211][a]	40	Female relatives	67	0.5 (0.1–5.4)	1.2 (0.5–2.9)	12.5 (1.6–19.1)	
[212]	324	Community	324	3.2[c]			
[213]	270	OA	292	1.8 (1.1–3.0)			
		Community	245	1.8 (1.0–3.1)			
[214]	195	OA			0.4 (0.3–0.7)	1.0 (0.4–2.6)	
		Community	233		0.9 (0.5–1.6)	1.8 (0.5–6.9)	
[215]	135	Soft tissue					
		OA	378	1.4 (0.9–2.2)			
[216]	144	Community	605		0.9 (0.6–1.4)	0.9 (0.3–2.7)	
[217]	60	Community	160	0.4 (0.15–1.3)	0.16 (0–14)		
[218]	269[d]	Population	15 000	1.1 (0.8–1.5)			

[a] Married pre-RA onset.
[b] Pregnancies pre-RA onset.
[c] Not stated.
[d] Cohort study.

mention of RA [219], no relationship was found with parity and subsequent mortality. In addition, however, to women who are nulliporous, there is additional evidence to suggest that conception is more difficult in women with RA. In one case–control study [216], women with RA had a 40 per cent greater likelihood of having delayed conception for more than a year compared to controls. In a further case–control study, a four-fold increase was observed in self-reported fertility problems compared to population controls [220]. In that study, the cases were affected twins with non-affected co-twins. A further analysis comparing the risk of infertility in the unaffected co-twins with the affected sibling showed that the latter also had a two-fold increased risk of infertility. A large study from Finland [218] compared the subsequent development of RA in over 15 000 women recruited between 1966 and 1972 and followed-up to 1989 using national registers. In these data there was no relationship at all between parity and the development of RA. There is certainly no evidence that voluntary refraining from becoming pregnant is associated with the increased incidence of RA. As an example, a review of data of marital status showed that the risk of RA was the same in married to that in single women [221]. It does appear that it is not the lack of pregnancy *per se* but rather the reason for problems in pregnancy that might

be associated with disease risk. This is discussed further below.

Others have investigated the possibility of an increased risk of fetal loss prior to disease onset. Again, the data on this topic are inconsistent (Table 2.26) and probably the overall conclusion is that there is no increase rate of prior fetal loss.

Timing of pregnancy

There are some very interesting data in relation to the timing of pregnancy and onset of RA. There is very convincing data [222–224] that the pregnancy period itself is associated with 40 to 80 per cent reduction in onset of RA. By contrast, in the post-partum period, there is a substantial increased risk. Thus in the first 3 months post-partum in one case-control study, an increase of 5.6 was found (95% CI 1.8–17.6) and this increase was magnified when restricted to onsets after the first pregnancy (OR 10.8, 95% CI 1.3–91) [222].

Breast feeding

One hypothesis raised by the increase in incidence in the post-partum period is the potential role of breast feeding. In a case–control study [225], breast-feeding after the first pregnancy was associated with a 5.4-fold increased risk of developing RA (2.5–11.4). A two-fold increased after a second pregnancy presumably related to attraction in susceptible women, the increases were greater in women whose RA were severe (seropositive and erosive) and in that group there was an eight-fold increase. The increase was also maximal in those women who had developed their disease after the age of 30. In a further case–control study a two-fold increased risk was associated with breast feeding when women with RA were compared with their unaffected co-twin. Given that it was expected that there would be over-matching in relation to breast-feeding from these groups. These data also support this hypothesis. Support for the breast-feeding theory comes from other studies showing an increased risk of severe disease in relation to breast-feeding [226]. However, in one study from a national

survey [219], women who breast fed had, on long-term follow-up, a decreased mortality in RA. The significance of these findings is unclear. One possible explanation for the association with breast feeding is its relationship with prolactin that might be proinflammatory. Indeed, the genes coding for prolactin production are based on the shorter arm of chromosome 6 and both women who breast feed [217] and women who are nulliporous [227] have, in part, an explanation for their disease occurrence in relation to carrying HLA-DR4.

A possible protector effect of oral contraceptive hormones

The first suggestion that oral contraceptive (OC) use has a protective effect against RA came from a pro-

Table 2.27   Case–control studies of oral contraceptive use and RA

Reference	Source of		Number of		Source of OC Data
	Cases	Controls	Cases	Controls	
[230]	Hospital	Soft tissue rheumatism	228	302	Postal questionnaire
[231]	Hospital	Non-arthritic attenders same clinic	229	458	Medical records
[232]	Hospital inpatients	Community	76	152	Postal questionnaire
[233]	Married, hospital	Sampling from 90% local population	182	182	Medical records
[234]	Hospital	Osteoarthritis or soft tissue rheumatism	148	186	Postal questionnaire
[235]	Hospital		100	100	Interview
[236]	Incident cases	Community	359	1357	Interview
[213]	Hospital	Osteoarthritis	150	157	Postal Questionnaire
		Community	150	180	
[237]	Group health co-operative	Random sample of pharmacy users	71	280	Pharmacy records
[215]	Incident cases	Osteoarthritis	135	378	Interview
[238]	Family study	Sisters of cases	86	118	Questionnaire
[220]	Affected twin in family study	General population	60	160	Questionnaire
[226]	Hospital	Community	176	145	Questionnaire
[239]	Incident	Community	167	178	Questionnaire/ interview

spective study of 23 000 UK women who, on follow-up, had a 50 per cent reduction in subsequent incidence of RA compared with women who had never used the OC [228]. Interestingly, subsequent follow-up of the same cohort of women showed that the gap in incidence narrowed suggesting that OC use postpones the development of RA rather than prevents [229]. Nevertheless, there have been a substantial number of further studies, both case–control and cohort, to address the same question. The details of these studies are summarized in Tables 2.27 to 2.30. There is a considerable disparity in the results between these studies and an attempt has been made to resolve this by undertaking statistical meta-analyses [23,241,242] with the overall conclusion that all OC use, either ever used or currently used, is associated with an approximately 50 per cent reduction in incidence. Given the variability in the constituent of oral contraceptive pills both between countries (and hence between studies) and over time, it is difficult to come up with a consistent or hormonal explanation. The alternative is that it is the postponement of pregnancy resulting from OC use rather than OC use *per se* that is responsible for the reduction in disease.

Table 2.28   Results from case–control studies of oral contraceptive use and RA

Reference	Odds ratio (95% CI) for reduction in risk versus		
	Ever users	Current users	Ex-users
[232]	0.70 (0.40–1.24)	1.21 (0.58–2.52)	0.37 (0.16–0.86)
[230]	0.42 (0.27–0.65)	0.45 (0.28–0.75)	0.40 (0.22–0.72)
[231]	1.7 (0.8–3.5)		
[233]	1.1 (0.7–1.7)	1.3 (0.7–2.4)	1.0 (0.6–1.7)
[234]	0.57 (0.32–1.00)		
[235]	1.29 (0.64–2.58)		
[237]	2.0 (0.97–4.2)	1.0 (0.4–2.2)	
[215]	0.39 (0.24–0.63)	0.58 (0.32–1.08)	
[238]	0.37 (0.11–1.24)		
[213]	0.56 (0.29–1.12)[a] 0.60 (0.30–1.17)[b]		
[226]	6.71 (0.41–1.23)[c] 6.76 (0.5–1.14)[d]		
[220]	0.43 (0.2–1.1)		
[239]	0.88 (0.5–1.6)	0.22 (0.06–0.9)	

[a] versus hospital controls.
[b] versus population controls.
[c] < 5 years use.
[d] >5 years use.

Table 2.29   Prospective studies of OC use and RA

Reference	Population	Source of OC data	Exposed	Non-exposed	Follow-up (years)	Data
[228]	General practice	Medical records	23 000	23 000	4	Reports from general practitioner
[240]	Family planning clinics	Interview	9 600	7 300	12–15	Questionnaire
[229]	General practice	Medical records	23 000	23 000	20	As above
[23]	Married nurses	Questionnaire	55 000	62 000	7.5	Questionnaire

Table 2.30　Results of prospective studies of OC use and RA

Reference	Relative risk (95% CI) for:		
	Ever users	Current users	Ex users
[228]	0.68 (0.45–1.03)	0.49 (N/S)	0.84 (N/S)
[240][a]	1.12 (0.79–1.79)	1.33 (N/S)	1.00 (N/S)
[229]	–	0.82 (0.59–1.15)	0.94 (0.72–1.22)
[23]	1.0 (0.6–1.4)	1.3 (0.3–6.5)	1.0 (0.6–1.4)

[a] Calculated.

Postmenopausal oestrogen use

One of the problems in relation to the hypothesis linking OC use to RA onset is that OC use is predominantly restricted to women under the age of 40 whereas the vast majority of RA onset is after this age. It is therefore reasonable to consider whether oestrogens taken for non-contraceptive reasons have the same preventive role. In brief, there is no consistent evidence that post-menopausal hormone use is associated with any change in occurrence of disease. An initial case–control study [234] showed a halving in RA risk to those who ever took hormone therapy, but further case–control studies [243], a retrospective cohort study [244], and an incidence-based case–control study [245] have shown no evidence of protection from such therapy.

Sex hormones

There have been a number of epidemiological studies examining the hypothesis that, independent of origin, the sex hormones level as determined in the serum may be a marker for disease risk. Although there have been a number of case–control studies in males (Table 2.31) suggesting that low testosterone level is associated with

RA, the problem is that as disease activity itself might suppress testosterone level, this low hormone level may be the effect rather than cause. Indeed, in the one major prospective study published to date [250] of over 19 000 men who were followed-up from 1973 to 1989, in a nested case–control study, there was no difference in the testosterone or dihydroepiandrosterone (DHEAS) level at baseline between those men that developed RA compared to those men that did not. Similarly, no change was noted for women. Indeed, in further studies [251], it was suggested that the reduction in DHEAS level in RA was related to disease activity by studying hormone levels between affected individuals and their non-affected siblings. There is also no consistent data of sex hormones in women (Table 2.32). Similarly, in studies of serum prolactin levels, these have not revealed, in general terms, any influence of serum hormone levels. Such 'static' studies do not reflect the true hormonal environment of an individual and more dynamic tests are indicated. In one such study, thyrotrophin (TRH) stimulation showed an exaggerated prolactin response in RA women compared to controls who also had increased basal levels of prolactin. Interestingly in that study, this effect was maximal in those women who were HLA-DR4 positive [258].

Table 2.31　Sex steroid levels in males with RA

Reference	Cases	Controls		Result
	N	Source	N	
[246]	7	Normal	6	Androgens ↓
[247]	31	Normal	95	Serum testosterone ↓
		Ankylosing spondylitis	33	Derived free testosterone ↓
[248]	25	Osteoarthritis	25	Derived free testosterone ↓
[249]	87	Normal	141	Free testosterone ↓
		Ankylosing spondylitis	48	Serum testosterone ↓

Table 2.32 Sex steroid levels in females with RA

Reference	Cases	Controls		Results
	N	Source	N	
[252]	8	Normals	8	Adrenal adrogenic anabolic metabolite excretion ↓
[253]	21	Osteoarthritis	19	No difference In premenopausal women Testosterone and DHEAS[a] in postmenopause ↑
[254]	10	Disease	11	No difference testosterone or DHEAS
		Normals	13	
[255]	77	Normals	44	Testosterone ↓ DHEAS ↓
[256]	31	Osteoarthritis	32	No difference testosterone or DHEAS
[257]	49	Normals Postmenopausal	49	Testosterone ↓ DHEAS ↓

[a] Dihydroepiandrosterone.

Co-morbidity

There have been a number of reports of other pathologies associated (positively or negatively) with the development of RA. Some of the more sustained ideas are considered below.

Hypercholesterolaemia

Many studies have suggested an increased likelihood of cardiovascular death in RA patients [259,260]. The relationship may not be simply as a consequence of the disease and its treatment, as an elevated serum cholesterol predicts the future development of RA [261]. This report is in contrast to previous unpublished findings of a prospective study in Pima Indians suggest that low cholesterol level was associated with a subsequent increased risk [262].

Prior tonsillectomy and appendectomy

Circumstantial support for an infective aetiology came from the observation, 10 years ago, of an increased risk of tonsillectomy and appendectomy for the development of RA [263] with the suggestion that such surgery reduced host defence mechanisms. Despite a further study confirming this association [264], three other studies failed to reproduce this result [265–267] and there have been criticisms of the methodology of the first study [268]. A recent population-based, case–control study also showed no evidence of an effect.

Thyroid disease

There is an increased risk of autoimmune thyroid disease, and indeed other autoimmune conditions such as insulin-dependent diabetes mellitus, in both RA cases and their relatives [269]. The reason for this is unclear though the link is not apparently HLA linked (see above).

Schizophrenia

It had been suggested in many studies that schizophrenia and RA are negatively associated [270,271]. A recent survey comparing the incidence of schizophrenia in patients with appendicitis to that in those with RA found a higher incidence in the latter [272]. In a major national survey linking a psychiatric care register with a hospital inpatient register, subjects with schizophrenia had 44 per cent of the risk of subjects with affective disorder of being hospitalized for RA [273].

Atopy

RA is considered a Th1 cytokine driven disorder with Th1 cytokines predominating over Th2. By contrast, atopy is a Th2 disease. It might be hypothesised that atopy, and its clinical correlates of asthma, hay fever, and eczema, would be less frequent in RA. In a case–control study a reduced frequency of atopy was observed based on clinical history (OR 0.4, 95% CI 0.2–0.8) [274] and a study of hayfever [275]. These findings were replicated in a recent large case control study [359].

Environmental factors: non-infectious

As mentioned above, the geographical variation in the occurrence of RA, particularly in the developed world, is relatively low. Furthermore, such variation that does exist might be explained by genetic factors and it thus appears that perhaps environmental influences might only be relatively limited. From a pathological point of view, it seems likely that an abnormally sustained response to infection might be the most likely environmental trigger for the disease, but a number of other environmental triggers have been investigated and these are reviewed briefly.

Education and social class

Variations in the incidence in relation to either social class or level of education might act as a pointer to influences of lifestyle. However, such data that do exist show virtually no influence of either of these two variables on susceptibility to arthritis. Some earlier studies had suggested that RA risk was inversely related to income and occupational status [56,276]. A number of subsequent reports in the 1960s and early 1970s, however, showed no relationship with occupational class for example [86,277,278]. Within the 500 000 adult population covered by NOAR, there was no evidence of a trend of increasing incidence of RA with declining social class [279]. A further analysis of that data set showed no correlation at postcode level between the incidence of disease and a variety of indicators of deprivation such as poor housing derived from census indicators. Two recent studies on education [280,281] found no association between the number of years in full-time education and the risk of RA. A recent, but small, study in Pakistan also showed no evidence of increase in occurrence of disease in a poor area compared to an affluent area in that country [88].

Obesity

Somewhat surprisingly, there have been a number of recent studies suggesting obesity to be a risk factor in the development of RA. In a case–control study of women with recent onset of RA, those in the highest quintile of body weight, had a 40 per cent increased risk compared to the rest of the population. In an incident-based case–control study covering both sexes, those with severe obesity (body mass index ≥30) had a substantially increased risk of 3.7 (95% CI 1.1–12.3) which was observed in both sexes, although in women it was particularly marked premenopausally [282]. Another recent case–control study [281] also observed an increased risk for those with a body mass index ≥0 of 1.8 (95% CI 1.2–2.8), although after adjusting for age, smoking, and marital status, this increase became non-significant. There is no obvious reason why obesity should be a risk factor, although it is possible it is related to the increased circulating oestrogen present in individuals who have high levels of adipose tissue.

Diet

The role of diet in susceptibility to RA and influencing its ultimate outcome has traditionally been a major concern of sufferers and there is an enormous scientific literature on the role of a large number of nutrients on the disease. Evaluating the role of specific nutrients in susceptibility to RA is, however, very difficult. It is obviously necessary to determine premorbid diet, but recall for this, even in recent onset cases, is subject to considerable error. It is also very difficult to isolate single nutrients for analysis given the confounding present within most typical diets. Prospective studies have yet to be completed and the existing data relies entirely on retrospective case–control studies either of long-standing (prevalent) or recent (incident) cases. Two groups of nutrients have been investigated in detail: (i) omega-3 fatty acids and (ii) trace minerals and other elements.

There is a theoretical basis for investigating the possible role of omega-3 fatty acids, which are predominantly derived from fish oils, as being protective in the development of RA insofar as they would compete with arachiedonic acids and hence lead to reduction in inflammation. Randomized clinical trials [283,284] were suggestive that diets high in eicosapentaenoic acid (EPA) and docosahexaenoic acid (DHA) both had a favourable effect on the outcome of RA. In addition, olive oil (whose main constituent is oleic acid and omega-9 fatty acid) may also be beneficial in controlling disease [284]. In a case–control study in Greek patients [285] consumption of olive oil, at least 30 times per month, was associated with a four-fold reduction in the incidence of RA compared to those with the lowest frequency of intake. Similar findings were observed for those individuals who had a strict adherence to the festival of lent, which in Greece is typically associated with abstinence from meat. In that same study, individuals who ate at least 12 portions of fish per month had a two-thirds reduction in risk of disease compared to those only consuming fish once or twice per month. A much larger case–control study was reported comparing 324 cases with 1245 controls [286] which suggested that those whose fish intake was predominantly from oily fish such as salmon or trout and who were in the top quartile of consumption had half of the risk of developing RA compared to those below the bottom quartile. Similar results were obtained and an estimate of total omega-3 fatty acid consumption was evaluated. Interestingly, the result was much clearer (and statistically significant) when the cases were restricted to only those who were rheumatoid factor positive. A more recent study from Greece suggested that both frequency of olive oil and independently of cooked vegetables consumption, were inversely related to RA risk [287].

The other area of interest has been in relation to vitamins, trace elements, and minerals in a diet. RA has been linked both to increased copper [288] and copper deficiency [289]. Serum selenium has also been reported to be lower in RA [290,291] although this could be a result of disease activity, it is possible of aetiological importance [292]. Selenium probably does have antiviral and anti-inflammatory effects. In the large case–control study above, no influence was found of calcium, phosphorous, or iron intake and indeed there was no evidence for association in relation to vitamin A, C, or E intake. These latter data are in contrast to the results from a Finnish case–control study [293] which showed that those in the lowest tertile for α-tocopherol had almost a doubling in risk of RA, similarly those in the lowest tertile for β-carotene also had a doubling in risk. However, this was a small study and neither of these risks were statistically significant.

Cigarette smoking

A possible link between cigarette smoking and susceptibility to RA has only recently been investigated. However, over 25 years ago, in a population study, it was shown that rheumatoid factor production was

Table 2.33 Epidemiological studies of cigarette smoking and RA

Reference	Cases (N)	Controls (N)	Odds ratio[a] (95% CI) for never smoking			Comments
[296,354]	7697	370 000	Current		1.2 (1.1–1.3)	Women's Health Cohort Study; modest influence of duration and number of cigarettes smoked
			Ex		1.0 (0.95–1.1)	
[297]	113	116 666	Current		1.3 (0.9–2.1)	Cohort study with questionnaire diagnosis of female nurses
			Ex		1.5 (0.9–2.3)	
[298]	135	178	Current		0.5 (0.4–0.8)	Smoking history after disease onset
[240]	78				2.4	Cohort study of females only
[299]	349	1 457	Current		1.3 (0.9–1.8)	Results are from women only; stronger association with increasing pack years
			Ex		1.2 (0.8–1.7)	
[300]	150	150	Current		3.7 (1.6–10.1)	Controls were unaffected twins; risks higher in monozygotic twins
			Ever		3.9 (1.6–10.5)	
[301]	512	53 000	Males	Current	4.0 (2.1–7.7)	Cohort study; cases determined by record linkage; results are for seropositive disease; no increase in seronegative group; small number of female cases
				Ex	2.8 (1.4–5.6)	
			Females	Current	1.1 (0.4–2.6)	
				Ex	0.8 (0.4–1.7)	
[282]	165	178	Current		0.95 (0.6–1.6)	Results similar for both sexes
			Ex		1.7 (0.95–3.1)	
[281]	361	5 851	Current	Males	2.4 (1.5–3.9)	Cases from population register; seropositive cases have almost five-fold increase
				Females	1.1 (0.8–1.6)	

[a] Relative risk for cohort studies.

associated with smoking, particularly in males [294]. This finding was replicated in a prospective study from Finland, again showing that men who smoked were at greater risk of developing rheumatoid factor positivity [295]. Interestingly, in that survey, the association was with rheumatoid factor production in the absence of RA. A summary of nine epidemiological studies of cigarette smoking with RA is shown in Table 2.33. There is only a single study that has shown no evidence of a risk, indeed that study showed smoking was protective in the development of RA. However, in that study smoking history was determined after the onset of the disease [215] and it is entirely likely that after the development of RA that there is an increased tendency to give up smoking. The remaining studies shown in the table are all suggestive of an increased risk from cigarette smoking although the magnitude of the risk does vary. A very recent study showed a 13-fold increase risk for those with over 40 pack years of smoking [360]. There is no consistent finding in studies that the risk is maximal in males. Similarly, any increased risk is not restricted to those who are current smokers at the time of disease onset, but, if anything, seems greater in those who are exsmokers. In support of the rela-tionship between rheumatoid factor and cigarette smoking, are those studies [281,282,301] which showed that the risk of developing RA was virtually restricted to those with rheumatoid-factor-positive disease.

Alcohol consumption

There is a very modest, but unsubstantiated, assumption that regular consumption of alcohol may protect against the development of RA. In one case–control study of recent onset cases, women who consumed at least two alcoholic drinks a day, had a 50 per cent reduction in risk of RA (OR 0.5, 95% CI 0.2–1.7) compared with all other alcohol groups. This reduction was limited to postmenopausal women and was not substantiated when lifetime alcohol consumption was considered. A study examining alcohol consumption at the time of first presentation [298] showed that women who consumed one to two alcoholic drinks a day had a 60 per cent of RA compared to those with no regular alcohol consumption, and those with more than three drinks a day had a 30 per cent risk. However, one major limitation to this study is that this refers to the alcohol consumption at the time of first presentation and it is entirely plausible that women had ceased alcohol drinking following the onset of disease. A recent analysis showed a lower alcohol-related mortality in subjects with RA [302]. This may reflect either a decreased risk of RA or changing habits after arthritis onset.

Occupation-related exposures

The first specific occupational hazard suggested as related to RA followed the observation of an increased rate of RA in coal miners who had massive pulmonary fibrosis in south Wales [303]. However, formal epidemiological studies showed that, in that region, coal miners did not have a higher prevalence of RA compared to non-miners. Association of RA with silicosis was also demonstrated in a study of Pyrite miners in Italy, but that study was uncontrolled and most of the cases probably did not have RA [304]. A more recent study of 1026 granite workers, working in the industry between 1940 and 1971 and followed up to 1981, showed the incidence of RA was 1.7/1000 person years compared to a general population risk in that population of a fifth of that. Interestingly, most of the affected miners in that population did not have silicosis [305]. In a recent US study, a two-fold increased RA risk was observed in individuals registered as suffering from occupation-induced silicosis [306]. There have been few detailed studies undertaken involving careful ascertainment of occupational exposure across a whole range of occupational groups. In the largest study undertaken so far in 13 Swedish counties covering half a million individuals, linkage was undertaken between census data and hospital admission databases for RA. A job exposure matrix approach was used to examine the relationship between both specific occupational titles and exposures. The overall summary of results found there was very little evidence of occupational links to RA. There was a statistically significant, but very modest, increase in risk, in men who had used organic solvents, but no relation to any other chemical exposures. The relationship between silicone and RA has also been investigated. Though the interest in this exposure has come predominantly from its use in surgical implants, such as breast implants, rather than occupational exposure. The major interest from exposure to silicone implants has been in the development of connective tissue diseases such as scleroderma, but in recent reports [298,307,308] there was not an increased risk of RA in women who had a silicone breast implant. A recent meta-analysis of all available data also failed to find evidence of an increased risk [309].

Environmental factors: infectious agents

General considerations

The most favoured aetiological model for RA is an infection with a micro-organism in a genetically susceptible host [310]. The nature of possible viral or other agents has been the subject of considerable investigation with only limited success. From an epidemiological prospect, few infectious agents show the same geographical ubiquity as RA though, as discussed below, Epstein-Barr virus (EBV) is an interesting exception. This is not to rule out the likely possibility of aetiological heterogeneity, i.e. RA could result from a number of viral insults. A number of epidemiological studies have used the retrospective interview approach to determine the likelihood of increased prior infection in cases compared to controls. Such an approach is subject to considerable misclassification. However, these studies have shown no evidence of differences in exposure to a long list of possible infectious agents [282,311].

Disease clustering in time

Some epidemiological support for an infectious aetiology comes from the observation, as mentioned above, of a birth cohort effect in regard to rheumatoid factor positivity both in the general population [17] and in patients with RA [107]. Such an effect may represent early life exposure to an infectious agent. A formal analysis for clustering in the NOAR failed to reveal any evidence of important clustering in time or time/place which would be expected if RA occurred as a consequence of epidemic infection [312].

Detailed investigation of aetiological factors within family clusters has failed to provide evidence to support an infectious cause. Thus both for affected sibling pairs [134,135] and spouse couples [313] there was a considerable median delay between the onset of disease in both the affected members.

Blood transfusion

The intriguing possibility was raised that blood transfusion was associated with subsequent increased risk of RA in a case–control study which showed an odds ratio of 3.6 (95% CI 1.5–8.8) in relation to blood transfusion occurring at least 10 years prior to the onset of RA. This was based on studies of incident cases interviewed within a short time after disease onset [282]. Such an observation was more common in females than in males and more common in those who were rheumatoid factor positive. If this association is true, one likely explanation is clearly that blood transfusion carries an infectious agent that over the long term increases the likely development of RA. Recently, an alternative explanation has been put forward insofar as the donor cells in the transfused blood may persist in the recipient's bone marrow. Such a phenomenon has been used to explain the likelihood of scleroderma, a kind of graft versus host reaction (e.g. see [314]). Whether such a relationship holds for RA is unknown.

Other epidemiological evidence supporting the role of an infectious agent comes from work suggesting that ownership of pets, particularly cat ownership, is associated with an increased risk of RA [315,316]. In these studies, it was cat ownership rather than any other pet that was particularly associated with disease onset, both in the 5-year period predisease and also pre pubertally.

Immunization

Immunization has been long considered as a possible trigger for the development of RA. Cases have been described following a number of immunizations, for example hepatitis B [317]. The interesting possibility was that non-live vaccines, for example tetanus toxoid, may be associated with an increased risk of onset. In NOAR, 3 per cent of the first 600 patients reported having a tetanus immunization in the 6 weeks prior to RA development [282]. Although this exposure occurred two and a half times more frequently in patients with RA than controls, owing to small numbers, confidence intervals around this estimate were wide and no robust conclusions could be drawn. It has been known for several years, however, that immunization itself can be associated with a rise in rheumatoid factor production [318]. This hypothesis remains to be investigated further.

Epstein–Barr virus

The most widely investigated virus has been EBV following the first report in 1975 [319] of an antibody to EBV in the sera of patients with RA. A number of sero-epidemiological studies comparing antibody frequencies to a number of different EBV associated antigens between case and control patients have confirmed the high titres of antibodies against a variety of EBV-related antigens: viral capsid antigen, early antigen, EB nuclear antigen and nuclear antigen (RANA); for example see [320–323]. However, not all studies have been positive, for example see [324], and the differences from a control population have not always been either biologically or statistically significant. Around the time of RA onset, there is evidence of increased production of anti-E3 and anti-E11 antibodies [325]. PCR-based studies have demonstrated an increase in EBV viral DNA in probands compared with their unaffected relatives [326] and at the synovial cell level, there is increasing evidence of EBV infection [327]. Thus EBV-DNA was found more frequently in the synovial tissue of 84 RA patients compared with 81 controls [328]. By contrast, synovial membrane biopsies in 37 RA patients failed to reveal substantive evidence of EBV infection [329].

Epidemiologically, the geographical distribution of infectious mononucleosis and RA are similar and the former is apparently unknown in countries with a low prevalence of RA [330]. These separate observations perhaps can be reconciled by considering the effect of age. In countries with a low prevalence of RA, infection with EBV is virtually universal by the age of three and the infection is clinically silent; whereas in high prevalence countries infection occurs at a later age and is more likely to be clinically apparent with, for example, infectious mononucleosis. However, the increased rate of RANA is seen in most populations, including Mexican and American Indians and Afghans [331]. The evidence for EBV infection as a cause of RA is also constrained by the lack of clinical evidence that acute EBV is arthritogenic, unlike, for example, rubella, hepatitis, and mumps [332].

Human parvovirus

Human parvovirus (HPV) has been another candidate following the first description of infection with this agent leading to erythema infectiosum [333]. HPV probably has little relevance for RA, despite two early reports from the UK: the first showing that 19/153 patients with early synovitis had evidence of HPV infection [334] and the second describing joint problems in 17 patients following an HPV outbreak [335]. Neither study had appropriate control groups nor were there any patients with a persistent arthritis. One interesting observation came from HLA analysis [336] of the patients from one of these series [334] which

showed that the HLA-DR4 positive rate was similar to that found in RA, although HLA-DR4 is probably a marker for the persistence of HPV-related arthritis rather than RA [337].

In a further serological study comparing patients with non-specific inflammatory arthritis (possible early RA) to normal controls, two of the patients had evidence of recent HPV infection (IgM positive) and there was a higher rate of IgG positivity to HPV in the patients (92 per cent) than in the other two groups (68 and 61 per cent respectively). Two large studies of recent-onset RA suggested that HPV could, at best, have only a very limited role in RA [338,339]. A study of discordant MZ twins also showed no evidence that HPV infection explained the disease discordance [340].

Proteus

It has been suggested that RA is a reactive arthritis to *Proteus mirabilis* infection in the urinary tract. *Proteus* can be isolated from the urine of RA patients more often than from controls [341] and antibodies to *Proteus* are raised during active disease [342]. This is not a consistent finding [343] and thus the aetiological significance of the association has been questioned [344].

Other infectious agents

Retroviruses have also been studied based on the similarity between RA and the arthritis produced by lentevirus in animals, for example caprine arthritis encephalitis in goats. However, attempts in humans to show evidence of retrovirus infection have been unsuccessful [345–347]. There appears to be no strong evidence that HTLV-1 or -11 are linked to human RA [310]. Although polyarthritis can occur in HTLV-1 carriers, which may in some individuals be indistinguishable from RA [348]. There are also very good mycoplasma-induced animal models of RA and in these models chronicity and severity, like in humans, are related to genetic factors [349]. Clinical and epidemiological studies in humans have, however, failed to support a mycoplasma source, although a recent report demonstrated the isolation of mycoplasma antigens from the synovial fluid of six patients with RA [350]. It is also likely that the response to mycobacterial antigen, as with HPV, is enhanced in HLA-DR4 positive individuals [351]. Statistically significant increases were found, using PCR techniques, of infection with various mycoplasma species in 28 RA patients compared to controls [352].

There have been studies on numerous other microorganisms, not only viruses and bacteria but also protozoa [353], with no overall conclusion.

References

1. Kellgren JH. Diagnostic criteria for population studies. *Bull Rheum Dis* 1962; **13**: 291–292.
2. Ropes MW, Bennett GA, Cobb S, Jacox R, Jessar RA. Proposed diagnostic criteria for rheumatoid arthritis. *Bull Rheum Dis* 1956; **7**: 121–124.
3. Ropes MW, Bennett GA, Cobb S, Jacox R, Jessar RA. Revision of diagnostic criteria for rheumatoid arthritis. *Bull Rheum Dis* 1958; **9**: 175–176.
4. Bennett PH, Wood PHN. *Population studies of the rheumatic diseases: Proceedings of the third international symposium*. Amsterdam: Excerpta Medica, 1968.
5. Arnett FC, Edworthy SM, Bloch DA *et al.* The American Rheumatism Association 1987 revised criteria for the classification of rheumatoid arthritis. *Arthritis Rheum* 1988; **31**: 315–324.
6. Bernelot-Moens HJ, van de Laar MA, van der Korst JK. Comparison of the sensitivity and specificity of the 1958 and 1987 criteria for rheumatoid arthritis. *J Rheumatol* 1992; **19**: 198–203.
7. Dugowson CE. Incidence of rheumatoid arthritis in women. *Arthritis Rheum* 1989; **32**: B80.
8. Kaarela K, Kauppi MJ, Lehtinen KE. The value of the ACR 1987 criteria in very early rheumatoid arthritis. *Scand J Rheumatol* 1995; **24**: 279–281.
9. Hulsemann JL, Zeidler H. Diagnostic evaluation of classification criteria for rheumatoid arthritis and reactive arthritis in an early synovitis outpatient clinic. *Ann Rheum Dis* 1999; **58**: 278–280.
10. Harrison BJ, Symmons DP, Barrett EM, Silman AJ. The performance of the 1987 ARA classification criteria for rheumatoid arthritis in a population based cohort of patients with early inflammatory polyarthritis. *J Rheumatol* 1998; **25**: 2324–2330.
11. Jacobsson LT, Knowler WC, Pillemer S *et al.* A cross-sectional and longitudinal comparison of the Rome criteria for active rheumatoid arthritis (equivalent to the American College of Rheumatology 1958 criteria) and the American College of Rheumatology 1987 criteria for rheumatoid arthritis. *Arthritis Rheum* 1994; **37**: 1479–1486.
12. MacGregor AJ, Bamber S, Silman AJ. A comparison of the performance of different methods of disease classification for rheumatoid arthritis. Results of an analysis from a nationwide twin study. *J Rheumatol* 1994; **21**: 1420–1426.
13. Leitich H, Adlassnig KP, Kolarz G. Development and evaluation of fuzzy criteria for the diagnosis of rheumatoid arthritis. *Methods Inf Med* 1996; **35**: 334–342.
14. Gabriel SE, Crowson CS, O'Fallon WM. The epidemiology of rheumatoid arthritis in Rochester, Minnesota, 1955–1985. *Arthritis Rheum* 1999; **42**: 415–420.
15. MacGregor AJ, Silman AJ. A reappraisal of the measurement of disease occurrence in rheumatoid arthritis. *Br J Rheumatol* 1992; **19**: 1163–1165.
16. O'Sullivan JB, Cathcart ES. The prevalence of rheumatoid arthritis. Follow-up evaluation of the effect of criteria on rates in Sudbury, Massachusetts. *Ann Intern Med* 1972; **76**: 573–577.
17. Lawrence JS. *Rheumatism in populations*. London: William Heinemann Medical Books, 1977.
18. Royal College of General Practitioners. Office of populations, censuses and surveys, Department of health and social security. *Morbidity statistics from general practice 1971–2. Second national morbidity study*. London: HMSO, 1979.
19. Royal College of General Practitioners. Office of populations, censuses and surveys, Department of health and social security. *Morbidity statistics from general practice 1981–2. Third national morbidity study*. London: HMSO, 1986.
20. Linos A, Worthington JW, O'Fallon WM, Kurland LT. The epidemiology of rheumatoid arthritis in Rochester, Minnesota: a study of incidence, prevalence, and mortality. *Am J Epidemiol* 1980; **111**: 87–98.
21. Gran JT, Magnus J, Mikkelsen K, Nygaard H, Brath HK. The incidence of classical and definite rheumatoid arthritis in Lillehammer, Norway. *Scand J Rheumatol* 1986; **59**: A11.
22. Isomaki HA. Rheumatoid arthritis as seen from official data registers. Experience in Finland. *Scand J Rheumatol* 1989; **18**: 21–24.
23. Hernandez-Avila M, Liang MH, Willett WC *et al.* Exogenous sex hormones and the risk of rheumatoid arthritis. *Arthritis Rheum* 1990; **33**: 947–953.
24. Dugowson CE, Koepsell TD, Voigt LF, Bley L, Nelson JL, Daling JR. Rheumatoid arthritis in women: incidence rates in group health cooperative, Seattle, Washington, 1987–1989. *Arthritis Rheum* 1991; **34**: 1502–1507.
25. Symmons DP, Barrett EM, Bankhead CR, Scott DG, Silman AJ. The incidence of rheumatoid arthritis in the United Kingdom: results from the Norfolk Arthritis Register. *Br J Rheumatol* 1994; **33**: 735–739.
26. Guillemin F, Briancon S, Klein JM, Sauleau E, Pourel J. Low incidence of rheumatoid arthritis in France. *Scand J Rheumatol* 1994; **23**: 264–268.
27. Kaipianen-Seppänen O, Aho K, Isomaki H, Laakso M. Incidence of rheumatoid arthritis in Finland during 1980–1990. *Ann Rheum Dis* 1996; **55**: 608–611.
28. Drosos AA, Alamanos I, Voulgari PV *et al.* Epidemiology of adult rheumatoid arthritis in northwest Greece 1987–1995. *J Rheumatol* 1997; **24**: 2129–2133.
29. Uhlig T, Kvien T, Glennas A, Smedstad LM, Forre O. The incidence and severity of rheumatoid arthritis, results from a county register in Oslo, Norway. *J Rheumatol* 1998; **25**: 1078–1084.
30. Chan KWA, Felson DT, Yood RA, Walker AM. Incidence of rheumatoid arthritis in central Massachusetts. *Arthritis Rheum* 1993; **36**: 1691–1696.

31. Kaipianen-Seppänen O, Aho K. Incidence of chronic inflammatory joint diseases in Finland in 1995. *J Rheumatol* 2000; **27**: 94–100.

32. Wiles N, Symmons DP, Harrison B *et al*. Estimating the incidence of rheumatoid arthritis: trying to hit a moving target? *Arthritis Rheum* 1999; **42**: 1339–1346.

33. Miall WE, Ball J, Kellgren JH. Prevalence of rheumatoid arthritis in urban and rural populations in south Wales. *Ann Rheum Dis* 1958; **17**: 263–272.

34. Lawrence JS. Prevalence of rheumatoid arthritis. *Ann Rheum Dis* 1961; **20**: 11–17.

35. Tzonchev VT, Pilossoff T, Kanev K. Prevalence of inflammatory arthritis in Bulgaria. In: Bennett PH, ed. *Population studies of the rheumatic diseases: Proceedings of the third international symposium.* Amsterdam: Excerpta Medica, 1968: 60–63.

36. Sit'aj S, Sebo M. Rheumatoid arthritis and ankylosing spondylitis in Czechoslovakia. In: Bennett PH, ed. *Population studies of the rheumatic diseases.* Amsterdam: Excerpta Medica, 1968: 64–66.

37. den Oudsten SA, Planten O, Posthuma EPS. Longitudinal survey of RA in an urban district of Rotterdam. In: Bennett PH, ed. *Population studies of the rheumatic diseases: Proceedings of the third international symposium.* Amsterdam: Excerpta Medica, 1968: 99–105.

38. Hellgren L. The prevalence of rheumatoid arthritis in different geographical areas in Sweden. *Acta Rheumatol Scand* 1970; **16**: 293–303.

39. Behrend T, Lawrence JS, Behrend H, Fischer K. Prevalence of rheumatoid arthritis in rural Germany. *Int J Epidemiol* 1972; **1**: 153–156.

40. Sorensen K. Rheumatoid arthritis in Denmark. Two population studies. *Dan Med Bull* 1973; **20**: 86–93.

41. Haavik TK. Rheumatoid arthritis in a Norwegian community (Jondal). A study based on the local doctor's file. *Scand J Rheumatol* 1979; **8**: 184–186.

42. Recht L, Brattstrom M, Lithman T. Chronic arthritis: Prevalence, severity and distribution between primary care and referral centres in a defined rural population. *Scand J Rheumatol* 1989; **18**: 205–212.

43. Aho K, Heliövaara M, Sievers K, Maatela J, Isomaki H. Clinical arthritis associated with positive radiological and serological findings in Finnish adults. *Rheumatol Int* 1989; **9**: 7–11.

44. Mau W, Raspe HH, Wasmus A, Zeidler H. Prevalence and course of rheumatoid arthritis according to the ARA 1987 criteria in caucasians. *Arthritis Rheum* 1991; **34**: D106.

45. MacGregor AJ, Riste LK, Hazes JMW, Silman AJ. Low prevalence of rheumatoid arthritis in black-Caribbeans compared with whites in inner city Manchester. *Ann Rheum Dis* 1994; **53**: 293–297.

46. Kvien TK, Glennas A, Knudsrod OG, Smedstad LM, Mowinckel P, Forre O. The prevalence and severity of rheumatoid arthritis in Oslo: results form a county register and a population survey. *Scand J Rheumatol* 1997; **26**: 412–418.

47. Cimmino MA, Parisi M, Moggiana G, Mela GS, Accardo S. Prevalence of rheumatoid arthritis in Italy: the Chiavari study. *Ann Rheum Dis* 1998; **57**: 315–318.

48. Stojanovic R, Vlajinac H, Palic-Obradovic D, Janosevic S, Adanja B. Prevalence of rheumatoid arthritis in Belgrade, Yugoslavia. *Br J Rheumatol* 1998; **37**: 729–732.

49. Erdes S, Alekseeva LI, Krylov MI, Kariakin AN, Benevolenskaia LI. Rasprostranennost' revmatoidnogo artrita i revmatoidnogo faktora u korennykh zhitelei Severo-Vostochnoi Sibiri. *Ter Arkh* 1999; **71**: 9–12.

50. Power D, Codd M, Ivers L, Sant S, Barry M. Prevalence of rheumatoid arthritis in Dublin, Ireland: a population based survey. *Ir J Med Sci* 1999; **168**: 197–200.

51. Saraux A, Guedes C, Allain J *et al*. Prevalence of rheumatoid arthritis and spondyloarthropathy in Brittany, France. *J Rheumatol* 1999; **26**: 2622–2627.

52. Simonsson M, Bergman S, Jacobsson LT, Petersson IF, Svensson B. The prevalence of rheumatoid arthritis in Sweden. *Scand J Rheumatol* 1999; **28**: 340–343.

53. Cobb S, Warren JE, Merchant WR, Thompson DJ. An estimate of the prevalence of rheumatoid arthritis. *J Chronic Dis* 1957; **5**: 636–643.

54. Mendez-Bryan R, Gonzalez-Alcover R, Roger L. Rheumatoid arthritis: prevalence in a tropical area. *Arthritis Rheum* 1964; **7**: 171–176.

55. Mikkelsen WM, Dodge HJ, Duff IF, Kato H. Estimates of the prevalence of rheumatic diseases in the population of Tecumseh, Michigan, 1959–60. *J Chronic Dis* 1967; **20**: 351–369.

56. Engel A. Rheumatoid arthritis in US adults 1960–62. In: Bennett PH, ed. *Population studies of the rheumatic diseases.* Amsterdam: Excerpta Medica, 1968: 83–89.

57. Cathcart ES, O'Sullivan JB. Rheumatoid arthritis in a New England town. A prevalence study in Sudbury, Massachusetts. *N Engl J Med* 1970; **282**: 421–424.

58. Gofton JP, Robinson HS, Price GE. A study of rheumatic disease in a Canadian Indian population. II rheumatoid arthritis in the Haida Indians. *Ann Rheum Dis* 1964; **23**: 364–371.

59. O'Brien WM, Bennett PH, Burch TA, Bunim JJ. A genetic study of rheumatoid arthritis and rheumatoid factor in Blackfeet and Pima Indians. *Arthritis Rheum* 1967; **10**: 163–179.

60. Beasley RP, Retailliau H, Healey LA. Prevalence of rheumatoid arthritis in Alaskan Eskimos. *Arthritis Rheum* 1973; **16**: 737–742.

61. Beasley RP, Willkens RF, Bennett PH. High prevalence of rheumatoid arthritis in Yakima Indians. *Arthritis Rheum* 1973; **16**: 743–748.

62. Harvey J, Lotze M, Stevens MB, Lambert G, Jacobson D. Rheumatoid arthritis in a Chippewa band. I. Pilot screening study of disease prevalence. *Arthritis Rheum* 1981; **24**: 717–721.

63. Oen K, Postl B, Chalmers IM *et al*. Rheumatoid diseases in an Inuit population. *Arthritis Rheum* 1986; **29**: 65–74.

64. Boyer GS, Lanier AP, Templin DW. Prevalence rates of spondyloarthropathies, rheumatoid arthritis, and other rheumatic disorders in an Alaskan Inupiat Eskimo population. *J Rheumatol* 1988; **15**: 678–683.

65. del Puente A, Knowler WC, Pettit DJ, Bennett PH. High incidence and prevalence of rheumatoid arthritis in Pima Indians. *Am J Epidemiol* 1989; **129**: 1170–1178.

66. Boyer GS, Templin DW, Lanier AP. Rheumatic diseases in Alaskan Indians of the southeast coast: high pre-

valence of rheumatoid arthritis and systemic lupus erythematosus. *J Rheumatol* 1991; **18**: 1477–1484.

67. Jacobsson LT, Hanson RL, Knowler WC *et al*. Decreasing incidence and prevalence of rheumatoid arthritis in Pima Indians over a twenty-five-year period. *Arthritis Rheum* 1994; **37**: 1158–1165.

68. Boyer GS, Benevolenskaya LI, Templin DW *et al*. Prevalence of rheumatoid arthritis in circumpolar native populations. *J Rheumatol* 1998; **25**: 23–29.

69. Lawrence JS, Bremner JM, Ball J, Burch TA. Rheumatoid arthritis in a subtropical population. *Ann Rheum Dis* 1966; **25**: 59–66.

70. Muller AS, Valkenburg HA, Greenwood BM. Rheumatoid arthritis in three west African populations. *East Afr Med J* 1972; **49**: 75–83.

71. Beighton P, Solomon L, Valkenburg HA. Rheumatoid arthritis in a rural South African Negro population. *Ann Rheum Dis* 1975; **34**: 136–141.

72. Solomon L, Robin G, Valkenburg HA. Rheumatoid arthritis in an urban South African Negro population. *Ann Rheum Dis* 1975; **34**: 128–135.

73. Meyers OL, Daynes G, Beighton P. Rheumatoid arthritis in a tribal Xhosa population in the Transkei, South Africa. *Ann Rheum Dis* 1977; **36**: 62–65.

74. Moolenburgh JD, Valkenburg HA, Fourie PB. A population study on rheumatoid arthritis in Lesotho, Southern Africa. *Ann Rheum Dis* 1986; **45**: 691–695.

75. Brighton SW, de la Harpe AL, van Staden DJ, Badenhorst JH, Myers OL. The prevalence of rheumatoid arthritis in a rural African population. *J Rheumatol* 1988; **15**: 405–408.

76. Silman AJ, Holligan S, Birrell F *et al*. Low prevalence of rheumatoid arthritis in a rural Nigerian population. *Arthritis Rheum* 1991; **34**: D107.

77. Beasley RP, Bennett PH, Lin CC. Low prevalence of rheumatoid arthritis in Chinese. Prevalence survey in a rural community. *J Rheumatol Suppl* 1983; **10**: 11–15.

78. Wigley RD, Zhang NZ, Zeng QY *et al*. Rheumatic diseases in China: ILAR-China study comparing the prevalence of rheumatic symptoms in northern and southern rural populations. *J Rheumatol* 1994; **21**: 1484–1490.

79. Lau E, Symmons D, Bankhead C, MacGregor A, Donnan S, Silman A. Low prevalence of rheumatoid arthritis in the urbanized Chinese of Hong Kong. *J Rheumatol* 1993; **20**: 1133–1137.

80. Malaviya AN, Kapoor SK, Singh RR, Kumar A, Pande I. Prevalence of rheumatoid arthritis in the adult Indian population. *Rheumatol Int* 1993; **13**: 131–134.

81. Darmawan J, Muirden KD, Valkenburg HA, Wigley RD. The epidemiology of rheumatoid arthritis in Indonesia. *Br J Rheumatol* 1993; **32**: 537–540.

82. Oshima Y. Clinical findings of collagen disease. V. Rheumatism. *J Jap Soc Intern Med* 1960; **50**: 774–780.

83. Wood JW, Kato H, Johnson KG, Uda Y, Russell WJ, Duff IF. Rheumatoid arthritis in Hiroshima and Nagasaki, Japan. Prevalence, incidence, and clinical characterisation. *Arthritis Rheum* 1967; **10**: 21–31.

84. Shichikawa K. Epidemiology of rheumatoid arthritis. *Jap J Clin Med* 1963; **21**: 1034–1042.

85. Shichikawa K. Prevalence of rheumatic disease in Japan. In: Bennett PH, ed. *Population studies of the rheumatic diseases: Proceedings of the third international symposium*. Amsterdam: Excerpta Medica, 1968: 55–59.

86. Kato H, Duff IF, Russell WJ *et al*. Rheumatoid arthritis and gout in Hiroshima and Nagasaki, Japan. A prevalence and incidence study. *J Chronic Dis* 1971; **23**: 659–679.

87. Shichikawa K, Takenaka Y, Maeda A, Yoshino R, Tsujimoto M, Ota H. A longitudinal population survey of rheumatoid arthritis in a rural district in Wakayama. *Ryumachi* 1981; **21** (Suppl.): 35–43.

88. Hameed KT, Gibson T, Kadir M, Sultana S, Fatima Z, Syed A. The prevalence of rheumatoid arthritis in affluent and poor urban communities of Pakistan. *Br J Rheumatol* 1995; **34**: 252–256.

89. Chou CT, Pei L, Chang DM, Lee CF, Schumacher R, Liang MH. Prevalence of rheumatic diseases in Taiwan: a population study of urban, surburban, rural differences. *J Rheumatol* 1994; **21**: 302–306.

90. Prior IAM, Evans JG, Morrison RBI, Rose BS. The Carterton study: 6 patterns of vascular, respiratory, rheumatic and related abnormalities in a sample of New Zealand European adults. *N Z Med J* 1970; **72**: 169–177.

91. Rose BS, Prior IAM. A survey of rheumatism in a rural New Zealand Maori community. *Ann Rheum Dis* 1963; **22**: 410–415.

92. Dans LF, Tankeh-Torres S, Amante CM *et al*. The prevalence of rheumatic diseases in a Filipino urban population: a WHO-ILAR COPCORD Study. World Health Organization. International League of Assciations for Rheumatology. Community Oriented Programme for the Control of the Rheumatic Diseases. *Lupus* 1997; **6**: 399–403.

93. Zeng Q, Huang S, Chen R. 10-year epidemiological study on rheumatic diseases in Shantou area. *Chung Hua Nei Ko Tsa Chih* 1997; **36**: 193–197.

94. Shichikawa K, Inoue K, Hirota S *et al*. Changes in the incidence and prevalence of rheumatoid arthritis in Kamitonda, Wakayama, Japan, 1965–1996. *Ann Rheum Dis* 1999; **58**: 751–756.

95. Adler E, Abramson JH, Elkan Z, Hador SB, Goldberg R. Rheumatoid arthritis in a Jerusalem population. Epidemiology of the disease. *Am J Epidemiol* 1967; **85**: 365–377.

96. Al Rawi ZS, Alazzawi AJ, Alajili FM, Alwakil R. Rheumatoid arthritis in population samples in Iraq. *Ann Rheum Dis* 1978; **37**: 73–75.

97. Pountain G. The prevalence of rheumatoid arthritis in the Sultanate of Oman. *Br J Rheumatol* 1991; **30**: 24–28.

98. Al Dalaan A, Al Ballaa S, Bahabri S, Biyari T, Al Sukait M. The prevalence of rheumatoid arthritis in the Qassim region of Saudi Arabia. *Ann Saudi Med* 1998; **18**: 396–397.

99. Lindahl B. In what sense is rheumatoid arthritis the principal cause of death? A study of the National Statistics Office's way of reasoning based on 1224 death certificates. *J Chronic Dis* 1985; **38**: 963–972.

100. Lindahl BI, Johansson LA. Multiple cause-of-death data as a tool for detecting artificial trends in the underlying cause statistics: a methodological study. *Scand J Soc Med* 1994; **22**: 145–158.

101. Wicks IP, Moore J, Fleming A. Australian mortality statistics for rheumatoid arthritis 1950–81: analysis of death certificate data. *Ann Rheum Dis* 1988; **47**: 563–569.

102. Silman AJ. Has the incidence of rheumatoid arthritis declined in the United Kingdom? *Br J Rheumatol* 1988; **27**: 77–79.

103. Kaipianen-Seppänen O, Aho K, Isomaki H, Laakso M. Shift in the incidence of rheumatoid arthritis toward elderly patients in Finland during 1975–1990. *Clin Exp Rheumatol* 1996; **14**: 537–542.

104. Imanaka T, Shichikawa K, Inoue K, Shimoaka Y, Takenaka Y, Wakitani S. Increase in age at onset of rheumatoid arthritis in Japan over a 30 year period. *Ann Rheum Dis* 1997; **56**: 313–316.

105. Porter DR, Capell HA, McInnes I *et al*. Is rheumatoid arthritis becoming a milder disease? Or are we starting second-line therapy in patients with milder disease? *Br J Rheumatol* 1996; **35**: 1305–1308.

106. Ward M, Fries J. Trends in antirheumatic medication use among patients with rheumatoid arthritis, 1981–1996. *J Rheumatol* 1998; **25**: 408–416.

107. Silman AJ, Davies P, Currey HLF, Evans SJW. Is rheumatoid arthritis becoming less severe? *J Chronic Dis* 1983; **36**: 891–897.

108. Aho K, Kaipianen-Seppänen O, Heliövaara M, Klaukka T. Epidemiology of rheumatoid arthritis in Finland. *Semin Arthritis Rheum* 1998; **27**: 325–334.

109. Coste J, Jougla E. Mortality from rheumatoid arthritis in France, 1970–1990. *Int J Epidemiol* 1994; **23**: 545–552.

110. Lewis-Fanning E. Report of enquiry into the aetiological factors associated with RA. *Ann Rheum Dis* 1950; **9**: 1–94.

111. Barter RW. Familial incidence of rheumatoid arthritis and acute rheumatism in 100 rheumatoid arthritics. *Ann Rheum Dis* 1952; **11**: 39–44.

112. Stecher RM, Hersh AH, Solomon WM, Wolpaw R. The genetics of rheumatoid arthritis. Analysis of 224 families. *Am J Hum Genet* 1953; **5**: 118–138.

113. Neri Serneri GG, Bartoli L. Cosidetto malattie del collageno. II sulla eredopatalogia delle megenchimopatie realtive. *Acta Genet Med (Rome)* 1965; **5**: 502–511.

114. Short CL, Bauer W, Reynolds WE. Rheumatoid arthritis. Cambridge, Mass: Harvard University Press; 1957.

115. Lawrence JS, Ball J. Genetic studies on rheumatoid arthritis. *Ann Rheum Dis* 1958; **17**: 160–168.

116. Bremner JM, Alexander WRM, Duthie JJR. Familial incidence of rheumatoid arthritis. *Ann Rheum Dis* 1959; **18**: 279–284.

117. de Blecourt JJ, Boerma FW, Vorenkamp EO. Rheumatoid arthritis (RA) factor in near relatives of sero-positive and sero-negative patients with rheumatoid arthritis. *Ann Rheum Dis* 1962; **21**: 339–341.

118. Veenhof-Garmann AM, Steiner FJF, Westendorp-Boerma Jea. The prevalence of rheumatoid arthritis and rheumatoid factor in relatives and spouses of sero-positive and seronegative patients suffering from definite or classical rheumatoid arthritis. In: Bennett PH, ed. *Population studies of the rheumatic diseases:*

Proceedings of the third international symposium . Amsterdam: Excerpta Medica, 1968: 123–127.

119. Lawrence JS. The epidemiology and genetics of rheumatoid arthritis. *Rheumatology* 1969; **2**: 1–36.

120. Hellgren L. Inheritance of rheumatoid arthritis. *Acta Rheumatol Scand* 1970; **16**: 211–216.

121. Lawrence JS. Heberden oration, 1969. Rheumatoid arthritis—nature or nurture? *Ann Rheum Dis* 1970; **29**: 357–379.

122. Wasmuth AG, Veale AMO, Palmer DG, Highton TC. Prevalence of rheumatoid arthritis in families. *Ann Rheum Dis* 1972; **31**: 85–91.

123. Jones MA, Silman AJ, Whiting S, Barrett EM, Symmons DPM. Occurrence of rheumatoid arthritis is not increased in the first degree relatives of a population based inception cohort of inflammatory polyarthritis. *Ann Rheum Dis* 1996; **55**: 89–93.

124. Koumantaki Y, Giziaki E, Linos A *et al*. Family history as a risk factor for rheumatoid arthritis: a case-control study. *J Rheumatol* 1997; **24**: 1522–1526.

125. Kwoh CH, Whiteley DM, Venglish CM. Accuracy of patients' report of rheumatoid arthritis among first-degree relatives. *Am J Epidemiol* 1992; **136**: 1017.

126. Seldin MF, Amos CI, Ward R, Gregersen PK. The genetics revolution and the assault on rheumatoid arthritis. *Arthritis Rheum* 1999; **42**: 1071–1079.

127. Lynn AH, Kwoh CK, Venglish CM, Aston CE, Chakravarti A. Genetic epidemiology of rheumatoid arthritis. *Am J Hum Genet* 1995; **57**: 150–159.

128. Deighton CM, Wentzel J, Cavanagh G, Roberts DF, Walker DJ. Contribution of inherited factors to rheumatoid arthritis. *Ann Rheum Dis* 1992; **51**: 182–185.

129. Deighton CM, Roberts DF, Walker DJ. Effect of disease severity on rheumatoid arthritis concordance in same sexed siblings. *Ann Rheum Dis* 1992; **51**: 943–945.

130. Silman AJ, Hennessy E, Ollier B. Incidence of rheumatoid arthritis in a genetically predisposed population. *Br J Rheumatol* 1992; **31**: 365–368.

131. Rigby AS, Voelm L, Silman AJ. Epistatic modelling in rheumatoid arthritis: an application of the Risch theory. *Genet Epidemiol* 1993; **10**: 311–320.

132. Deighton C, Heslop P, McDonagh J, Walker D, Thomson G. Does genetic anticipation occur in familial rheumatoid arthritis? *Ann Rheum Dis* 1994; **53**: 833–835.

133. McDermott E, Khan MA, Deighton C. Further evidence for genetic anticipation in familial rheumatoid arthritis. *Ann Rheum Dis* 1996; **55**: 475–477.

134. Silman AJ, Ollier WER, Currey HLF. Failure to find disease similarity in sibling pairs with rheumatoid arthritis. *Ann Rheum Dis* 1987; **46**: 135–138.

135. Sanders PA, Grennan DM. Age and year of onset differences in siblings with rheumatoid arthritis. *Br J Rheumatol* 1990; **29**: 128–130.

136. Tarp U, Graudal HK. Seropositive rheumatoid arthritis in monozygotic twin sisters carrying HLA-DR4 or DR4 associated with B27. *J Rheumatol* 1989; **16**: 1530–1532.

137. O'Brien WM. Twin studies in rheumatic diseases. *Arthritis Rheum* 1968; **11**: 81–86.

138. Thymann G. Polyarthritis in twins. *Acta Genet* 1957; **7**: 148–150.

139. Meyerowitz S, Jacox RF, Hess DW. Monozygotic twins discordant for rheumatoid arthritis: a genetic, clinical and psychological study of 8 sets. *Arthritis Rheum* 1968; **11**: 1–21.

140. Harvald B, Hague M. Hereditary factors elucidated by twin studies. In: *Genetics and the epidemiology of chronic diseases*. Washington: US Public Health Services; 1965: 61.

141. Aho K, Koskenvuo M, Tuominen J, Kaprio J. Occurrence of rheumatoid arthritis in a nationwide series of twins. *J Rheumatol* 1986; **13**: 899–902.

142. Silman AJ, MacGregor AJ, Thomson W *et al*. Twin concordance rates for rheumatoid arthritis: results from a nationwide study. *Br J Rheumatol* 1993; **32**: 903–907.

143. Bellamy N, Duffy D, Martin N, Mathews J. Rheumatoid arthritis in twins: a study of aetiopathogenesis based on the Australian twin registry. *Ann Rheum Dis* 1992; **51**: 588–593.

144. Svendsen AJ, Holm NV, Petersen PH, Junker P. Prominance of environmental factors in the etiopathogenesis of rheumatoid arthritis. A nation-wide population based twin study. *Arthritis Rheum* 1998; **41**: 191 Suppl.

145. Falls HF. Skeletal system, including joints. In: Sorsby A, ed. *Clinical genetics*. London: Butterworth, 1953: 282.

146. Grossman AJ, Leifer P, Batterman RC. The occurrence of rheumatoid arthritis in twins. *Acta Rheumatol Scand* 1956; **2**: 161–169.

147. Aho K, Tuomi T, Palosuo T, Kaarela K, Essen RV, Isomaki H. Is seropositive rheumatoid arthritis becoming less severe? *Clin Exp Rheumatol* 1989; **7**: 287–290.

148. MacGregor AJ, Snieder H, Rigby AS *et al*. Characterizing the quantitative genetic contribution to rheumatoid arthritis using data from twins. *Arthritis Rheum* 2000; **43**: 30–37.

149. Jarvinen P, Koskenvuo M, Koskimies S, Kotaniemi K, Aho K. Rheumatoid arthritis in identical twins: a clinical and immunogenetic study of eight concordant pairs derived from a nationwide twin panel. *Scand J Rheumatol* 1991; **20**: 159–164.

150. MacGregor AJ, Bamber S, Carthy D *et al*. Heterogeneity of disease phenotype in monozygotic twins concordant for rheumatoid arthritis. *Br J Rheumatol* 1995; **34**: 215–220.

151. Gregersen PK. Discordance for autoimmunity in monozygotic twins. Are 'identical' twins really identical? *Arthritis Rheum* 1993; **36**: 1185–1192.

152. Trejo V, Derom C, Vlietinck R *et al*. X chromosome inactivation patterns correlate with fetal-placental anatomy in monozygotic twin pairs: implications for immune relatedness and concordance for autoimmunity. *Mol Med* 1994; **1**: 62–70.

153. Stastny P. Association of the B cell alloantigen DRw4 with rheumatoid arthritis. *N Engl J Med* 1978; **298**: 869–871.

154. Karr RW, Rodey GE, Lee T, Schwartz BD. Association of HLA-DRw4 with rheumatoid arthritis in black and white patients. *Arthritis Rheum* 1980; **23**: 1241–1245.

155. Alarcon GS, Koopman WJ, Acton RT, Barger BO. DR antigen distribution in blacks with rheumatoid arthritis. *J Rheumatol* 1983; **10**: 579–583.

156. Woodrow JC, Nichol FE, Zaphiropoulos G. DR antigens and rheumatoid arthritis: a study of two populations. *BMJ* 1981; **283**: 1287–1288.

157. Nakai Y, Wakisaka A, Aizawa M, Itakura K, Nakai H, Ohashi A. HLA and rheumatoid arthritis in the Japanese. *Arthritis Rheum* 1981; **24**: 722–725.

158. Gorodezky C, Lavalle C, Castro-Escobar LE, Miranda-Limon JM, Escobar-Gutierrez A. HLA antigens in Mexican patients with adult rheumatoid arthritis. *Arthritis Rheum* 1981; **24**: 976–977.

159. Ferraccioli G, Peri F, Nervetti A, Ambanelli U, Savi M. Toxicity due to remission inducing drugs in rheumatoid arthritis. Association with HLA-B35 and Cw4 antigens. *J Rheumatol* 1986; **13**: 65–68.

160. Maeda H, Juji T, Mitsui H, Sonozaki H, Okitsu K. HLA DR4 and rheumatoid arthritis in Japanese people. *Ann Rheum Dis* 1981; **40**: 299–302.

161. Mehra NK, Kaul R, Taneja V, Chaudhuri TK, Jhinghan B, Malaviya AN. HLA-Linked susceptibility to rheumatoid arthritis in North India. *Tissue Antigens* 1987; **31**: 220–223.

162. Parivisutt L, Chandanayingyong D, Nilganuwong S. Rheumatoid arthritis in Thais. In: Dawkins RL, Christiansen FT, Zilko PJ, eds. *Immunogenetics in rheumatology*. Amsterdam: Excerpta Medica, 1982: 98–100.

163. Willkens RF, Hansen JA, Malmgren JA, Nisperos B, Mickelson EM, Watson MA. HLA antigens in Yakima Indians with rheumatoid arthritis. Lack of association with HLA-Dw4 and HLA-DR4. *Arthritis Rheum* 1982; **25**: 1435–1439.

164. de Jongh BM, van Romunde LK, Valkenburg HA, de Lange GG, van Rood JJ. Epidemiological study of HLA and GM in rheumatoid arthritis and related symptoms in an open Dutch population. *Ann Rheum Dis* 1984; **43**: 613–619.

165. Bardin T, Legrand L, Naveau B *et al*. HLA antigens and seronegative rheumatoid arthritis. *Ann Rheum Dis* 1985; **44**: 50–53.

166. Papasteriades CA, Kappou ID, Skopouli FN, Barla MN, Fostiropoulos GA, Moutsopoulos HM. Lack of HLA-antigen association in Greek rheumatoid arthritis patients. *Rheumatol Int* 1985; **5**: 201–203.

167. Brautbar C, Naparstek Y, Yaron M *et al*. Immunogenetics of rheumatoid arthritis in Israel. *Tissue Antigens* 1986; **28**: 8–14.

168. Swiss Federal Commission for the Rheumatic Diseases SfR. HLA-DR antigens in rheumatoid arthritis. A Swiss collaborative study; final report. *Rheumatol Int* 1986; **6**: 89–92.

169. Mody GM, Meyers OL. Rheumatoid arthritis in blacks in South Africa. *Ann Rheum Dis* 1989; **48**: 69–72.

170. Massardo L, Jacobelli S, Rodriguez L, Rivero S, Gonzalez A, Marchetti R. Weak association between HLA-DR4 and rheumatoid arthritis in Chilean patients. *Ann Rheum Dis* 1990; **49**: 290–292.

171. Sattar MA, Al Saffar M, Guindi RT, Sugathan TN, Behbehani K. Association between HLA-DR antigens and rheumatoid arthritis in Arabs. *Ann Rheum Dis* 1990; **49**: 147–149.

172. Gregersen PK. The North American Rheumatoid Arthritis Consortium—bringing genetic analysis to

bear on disease susceptibility, severity, and outcome. *Arthritis Care Res* 1998; **11**: 1–2.

173. Carthy D, Ollier W, Papasteriades C, Pappas H, Thomson W. A shared HLA-DRB1 sequence confers RA susceptibility in Greeks. *Eur J Immunogen* 1993; **20**: 391–398.

174. Ollier W, Thomson W. Population genetics of rheumatoid arthritis. *Rheum Dis Clin N Am* 1992; **18**: 741–759.

175. Yukioka M, Wakitani S, Murata N *et al.* Elderly-onset rheumatoid arthritis and its association with HLA-DRB1 alleles in Japanese. *Br J Rheumatol* 1998; **37**: 98–101.

176. Wakitani S, Murata N, Toda Y *et al.* The relationship between HLA-DRB1 alleles and disease subjects of Rheumatoid arthritis in Japanese. *Br J Rheumatol* 1997; **36**: 630–636.

177. Gao X, Gazit E, Livneh A, Stastny P. Rheumatoid arthritis in Israeli Jews: shared sequences in the third hypervariable region of DRB1 alleles are associated with susceptibility. *J Rheumatol* 1991; **18**: 801–803.

178. Rønningen KS, Spurkland A, Egeland T *et al.* Rheumatoid arthritis may be primarily associated with HLA-DR4 molecules sharing a particular sequence at residues 67–74. *Tissue Antigens* 1990; **36**: 235–240.

179. Stavropoulos C, Spyropoulou M, Koumantaki Y *et al.* HLA-DRB1 alleles in Greek rheumatoid arthritis patients and their associations with clinical characteristics. *Eur J Immunogen* 1997; **24**: 265–274.

180. Taneja V, Giphart MJ, Verduijn W, Naipal A, Malaviya AN, Mehra NK. Polymorphism of HLA-DRB, -DQA1, and -DQB1 in rheumatoid arthritis in Asian Indians. Associations with DRB1*0405 and DRB1*1001. *Hum Immunol* 1996; **46**: 35–41.

181. Mu M, King M, Criswell L. Relative predispositional effects and mode of inheritance of HLA-DRB1 alleles among community-based caucasian females with rheumatoid arthritis. *Genet Epidemiol* 1998; **15**: 123–134.

182. Tan PLJ, Farmiloe S, Roberts M, Geursen A, Skinner MA. HLA-DR4 subtypes in New Zealand Polynesians. *Arthritis Rheum* 1993; **36**: 15–19.

183. Hong GH, Park MH, Takeuchi F, Oh MD, Song YW. Association of specific amino acid sequence of HLA-DR with rheumatoid arthritis in Koreans and its diagnostic value. *J Rheumatol* 1996; **23**: 1699–1703.

184. Seglias J, Li EK, Cohen MG, Wong RWS, Potter PK, So AK. Linkage between rheumatoid arthritis susceptibility and the presence of HLA-DR4 and Dr*gb allelic third hypervariable region sequences in southern Chinese persons. *Arthritis Rheum* 1992; **35**: 163–167.

185. Konenkov V, Sartakova M, Kimura A. Oligonucleotide genotyping of HLA-DRB1 04 and HLA-DQB1 03 among Russians in west Siberia suffering from rheumatoid arthritis. *Exp Clin Immunogenet* 1994; **11**: 187–191.

186. Yelamos J, Garcia-Lozano JR, Moreno I *et al.* Association of HLA-DR4-Dw15 (DRB1*0405) and DR10 with rheumatoid arthritis in a Spanish population. *Arthritis Rheum* 1993; **21**: 811–814.

187. Gonzalez A, Nicovani S, Massardo L *et al.* Influence of the HLA-DRB shared epitope on susceptibility to and clinical expression of RA in Chilean patients. *Ann Rheum Dis* 1997; **56**: 191–193.

188. Mody GM, Hammond MG. Differences in HLA-DR association with rheumatoid arthritis among migrant Indian communities in South Africa. *Br J Rheumatol* 1994; **33**: 425–427.

189. de Juan MD, Belmonte J, Barado J *et al.* Differential associations of HLA-DR antigens with rheumatoid arthritis (RA) in Basques: high frequency of DR1 and DR10 and lack of association with HLA-DR4 or any of its subtypes. *Tissue Antigens* 1994; **43**: 320–323.

190. Willkens RF, Nepom GT, Marks CR, Nettles JW, Nepom BS. Association of HLA-Dw16 with rheumatoid arthritis in Yakima Indians. Further evidence for the 'shared epitope' hypothesis. *Arthritis Rheum* 1991; **34**: 43–47.

191. Templin DW, Boyer GS, Lanier AP *et al.* Rheumatoid arthritis in Tlingit Indians: clinical characterization and HLA associations. *J Rheumatol* 1994; **21**: 1238–1244.

192. Wordsworth P, Pile KD, Buckely JD *et al.* HLA heterozygosity contributes to susceptibility to rheumatoid arthritis. *Am J Hum Genet* 1992; **51**: 585–591.

193. MacGregor A, Ollier W, Thomson W, Jawaheer D, Silman AJ. HLA-DRB1*0401/0404 genotype and rheumatoid arthritis: Increased association in men, young age at onset, and disease severity. *J Rheumatol* 1995; **22**: 1032–1036.

194. Thomson W, Harrison B, Ollier B *et al.* Quantifying the exact role of HLA-DRB1 alleles in susceptibility to inflammatory polyarthritis: results from a large, population-based study. *Arthritis Rheum* 1999; **42**: 757–762.

195. Rigby AS, Silman AJ, Voelm L *et al.* Investigating the HLA component in rheumatoid arthritis: an additive (dominant) mode of inheritance is rejected, a recessive mode is preferred. *Genet Epidemiol* 1991; **8**: 153–175.

196. Seidl C, Korbitzer J, Badenhoop K *et al.* Protection against severe disease is conferred by DERAA- bearing HLA-DRBI alleles among HLA-DQ3 and HLA-DQ5 positive rheumatoid arthritis patients. *Hum Immunol* 2001; **62**: 523–9.

197. Hajeer AH, Worthington J, Silman AJ, Ollier WE. Association of tumor necrosis factor microsatellite polymorphisms with HLA-DRB1*04-bearing haplotypes in rheumatoid arthritis patients. *Arthritis Rheum* 1996; **39**: 1109–1114.

198. Mulcahy B, Waldron LF, McDermott MF *et al.* Genetic variability in the tumor necrosis factor-lymphotoxin region influences susceptibility to rheumatoid arthritis. *Am J Hum Genet* 1996; **59**: 676–683.

199. Cornelis F, Faure S, Martinez M *et al.* New susceptibility locus for rheumatoid arthritis suggested by a genome-wide linkage study. *Proc Natl Acad Sci U S A* 1998; **95**: 10746–10750.

200. Shiozawa S, Hayashi S, Tsukamoto Y *et al.* Identification of the gene loci that predispose to rheumatoid arthritis. *Int Immunol* 1998; **10**: 1891–1895.

201. Worthington J, Ollier WE, Leach MK *et al.* The Arthritis and Rheumatism Council's National Repository of Family Material: pedigrees from the first 100 rheumatoid arthritis families containing affected sibling pairs. *Br J Rheumatol* 1994; **33**: 970–976.

202. John S, Hajeer A, Marlow A *et al*. Investigation of candidate disease susceptibility genes in rheumatoid arthritis: principles and strategies. *J Rheumatol* 1997; 24: 199–201.

203. Cox A, Camp NJ, Cannings C *et al*. Combined sib-TDT and TDT provide evidence for linkage of the inter-leukin-1 gene cluster to erosive rheumatoid arthritis. *Hum Mol Genet* 1999; 8: 1707–1713.

204. John S, Myerscough A, Marlow A *et al*. Linkage of cytokine genes to rheumatoid arthritis. Evidence of genetic heterogeneity. *Ann Rheum Dis* 1998; 57: 361–365.

205. Fife M, Fisher S, John S *et al*. Multipoint linkage analysis of a candidate gene in rheumatoid arthritis: suggestive evidence of linkage of linkage to the CRH genomic region. *Arthritis Rheum* 1999; 42: S232.

206. John S, Myerscough A, Eyre S *et al*. Linkage of a marker in intron D of the estrogen synthase locus to rheumatoid arthritis. *Arthritis Rheum* 1999; 42: 1617–1620.

207. John S, Marlow A, Hajeer A, Ollier W, Silman A, Worthington J. Linkage and association studies of the natural resistance associated macrophage protein 1 (NRAMP1) locus in rheumatoid arthritis. *J Rheumatol* 1997; 24: 452–457.

208. McDermott M, Kastner DL, Holloman JD *et al*. The role of T-cell receptor beta chain genes in the susceptibility to rheumatoid arthritis. *Ann N Y Acad Sci* 1995; 756: 173–175.

209. Kay A, Bach F. Subfertility before and after the development of rheumatoid arthritis in women. *Ann Rheum Dis* 1965; 24: 169–173.

210. Kaplan D. Fetal wastage in patients with rheumatoid arthritis. *J Rheumatol* 1986; 13: 875–877.

211. Silman AJ, Roman E, Beral V, Brown A. Adverse reproductive outcomes in women who subsequently develop rheumatoid arthritis. *Ann Rheum Dis* 1988; 47: 979–981.

212. del Junco DJ, Annegers JF, Coulam CB, Luthra HS. The relationship between rheumatoid arthritis and reproductive function. *Br J Rheumatol* 1989; 28 (Suppl. I): 33.

213. Spector TD, Roman E, Silman AJ. The pill, parity, and rheumatoid arthritis. *Arthritis Rheum* 1990; 33: 782–789.

214. Spector TD, Silman AJ. Is poor pregnancy outcome a risk factor in rheumatoid arthritis? *Ann Rheum Dis* 1990; 49: 12–14.

215. Hazes JM, Dijkmans BC, Van den Broucke JP, de Vries RR, Cats A. Reduction of the risk of rheumatoid arthritis among women who take oral contraceptives. *Arthritis Rheum* 1990; 33: 173–179.

216. Nelson JL, Voigt LF, Koepsell TD, Dugowson CE, Daling JR. Pregnancy outcome in women with rheumatoid arthritis before disease onset. *J Rheumatol* 1992; 19: 18–21.

217. Brennan P, Ollier B, Worthington J, Hajeer A, Silman AJ. Are both genetic and reproductive associations with rheumatoid arthritis linked to prolactin? *Lancet* 1996; 1: 106–109.

218. Heliövaara M, Aho K, Beunanen A, Knekt P, Aromaa A. Parity and risk of rheumatoid arthritis in Finnish women. *Br J Rheumatol* 1995; 34: 625–628.

219. Brun JG, Nilssen S, Kvale G. Breast feeding, other reproductive factors and rheumatoid arthritis. A prospective study. *Br J Rheumatol* 1995; 34: 542–546.

220. Brennan P, Silman AJ. An investigation of gene-environmental interaction in the etiology of rheumatoid arthritis. *Am J Epidemiol* 1994; 140: 453–460.

221. Silman AJ. Epidemiology of rheumatoid arthritis. *APMIS* 1994; 102: 721–728.

222. Silman AJ, Kay A, Brennan P. Timing of pregnancy in relation to the onset of rheumatoid arthritis. *Arthritis Rheum* 1992; 35: 152–155.

223. Koepsell T, Dugowson C, Voigt L, Lee J, Nelson L, Daling J. Reduced incidence of rheumatoid arthritis during pregnancy. *Arthritis Rheum* 1990; S29: 117.

224. Lansink M, de Boer A, Dijkmans BA, Van den Broucke JP, Hazes JM. The onset of rheumatoid arthritis in relation to pregnancy and childbirth. *Clin Exp Rheumatol* 1993; 11: 171–174.

225. Brennan P, Silman A. Breast-feeding and the onset of rheumatoid arthritis. *Arthritis Rheum* 1994; 37: 808–813.

226. Jorgensen C, Picot MC, Bologna C, Sany J. Oral contraception, parity, breast feeding, and severity of rheumatoid arthritis. *Ann Rheum Dis* 1996; 55: 94–98.

227. Nelson JL, Dugowson C, Richards M, Koepsell T, Gooley T, Hansen JA. Risk of rheumatoid arthritis, parity and the DRB1 'shared epitope' sequence. *Arthritis Rheum* 1995; 38: S232.

228. Wingrave SJ, Kay CR. Reduction in incidence of rheumatoid arthritis associated with oral contraceptives. *Lancet* 1978; 1: 569–571.

229. Hannaford PC, Kay CR, Hirsch S. Oral contraceptives and rheumatoid arthritis: new data from the Royal College of General Practitioners' oral contraception study. *Ann Rheum Dis* 1990; 49: 744–746.

230. Van den Broucke JP, Valkenburg HA, Boersma JW *et al*. Oral contraceptives and rheumatoid arthritis: further evidence for a preventive effect. *Lancet* 1982; 2: 839–842.

231. Linos A, Worthington JW, O'Fallon WM, Kurland LT. Case-control study of rheumatoid arthritis and prior use of oral contraceptive. *Lancet* 1983; 1: 1299–1300.

232. Allebeck P, Ahlbom A, Ljungstrom K, Allander E. Do oral contraceptives reduce the incidence of rheumatoid arthritis? A pilot study using Stockholm county medical information system. *Scand J Rheumatol* 1984; 13: 140–146.

233. del Junco DJ, Annegers JF, Luthra HS, Coulam CB, Kurland LT. Do oral contraceptives prevent rheumatoid arthritis? *JAMA* 1985; 254: 1938–1941.

234. Van den Broucke JP, Witteman JC, Valkenburg HA *et al*. Non-contraceptive hormones and rheumatoid arthritis in perimenopausal and postmenopausal women. *JAMA* 1986; 255: 1299–1303.

235. Darwish MJ, Armenian HK. A case-control study of rheumatoid arthritis in Lebanon. *Int J Epidemiol* 1987; 16: 420–424.

236. Koepsell T, Dugowson C, Nelson JL, Voigt L, Daling JR. Rheumatoid arthritis in women in relation to oral contraceptive use. *Am J Epidemiol* 1992; 136: 996.

237. Moskowitz MA, Jick SS, Burnside S *et al*. The relation-ship of oral contraceptive use to rheumatoid arthritis. *Epidemiology* 1990; **1**: 153–156.

238. Hazes JMW. Influence of oral contraception on the occurrence of rheumatoid arthritis in female sibs. *Scand J Rheumatol* 1990; **19**: 306–310.

239. Brennan P, Bankhead C, Silman A, Symmons D. Oral contraceptives and rheumatoid arthritis: results from primary care-based incident case-control study. *Semin Arthritis Rheum* 1997; **26**: 817–823.

240. Vessey MP, Villard-Mackintosh L, Yeates D. Oral con-traceptives, cigarette smoking and other factors in relation to arthritis. *Contraception* 1987; **35**: 457–465.

241. Spector TD, Hochberg MC. The protective effect of the oral contraceptive pill on rheumatoid arthritis: an overview of the analytic epidemiological studies using meta-analysis. *J Clin Epidemiol* 1990; **43**: 1221–1230.

242. Pladevall-Vila M, Delclos G, Varas C, Guyer H, Brugues-Tarradellas J, Anglada-Arisa A. Controversy of oral contraceptives and risk of rheumatoid arthritis: meta-analysis of conflicting studies and review of conflicting meta-analyses with special emphasis on analysis heterogeneity. *Am J Epidemiol* 1996; **144**: 1–14.

243. Carette S, Marcoux S, Gingras S. Post menopausal hor-mones and the incidence of rheumatoid arthritis. *J Rheumatol* 1989; **16**: 911–913.

244. Spector TD, Brennan P, Harris P, Studd JWW, Silman AJ. Does estrogen replacement therapy protect against rheumatoid arthritis? *J Rheumatol* 1991; **18**: 1473–1476.

245. Koepsell TD, Dugowson CE, Nelson JL, Voigt LF, Daling JR. Non-contraceptive hormones and the risk of rheumatoid arthritis in menopausal women. *Int J Epidemiol* 1994; **23**: 1248–1255.

246. Cutolo M, Belleari E, Accardo S *et al*. Preliminary results of serum androgen level testing in men with rheumatoid arthritis. *Arthritis Rheum* 1984; **27**: 958–959.

247. Gordon D, Beastall GH, Thomson JA, Sturrock RD. Androgenic status and sexual function in males with rheumatoid arthritis and ankylosing spondylitis. *Q J Med* 1986; **60**: 671–679.

248. Spector TD, Perry LA, Tubb G, Silman AJ, Huskisson EC. Low free testosterone levels in males with rheu-matoid arthritis. *Ann Rheum Dis* 1988; **47**: 65–68.

249. Spector TD, Ollier WER, Perry LA, Edwards A, Silman AJ. Testosterone levels in males: a comparative study of rheumatoid arthritis. *Clin Rheumatol* 1989; **8**: 37–41.

250. Heikkila R, Aho K, Heliövaara M *et al*. Serum andro-gen-anabolic hormones and the risk of rheumatoid arthritis. *Ann Rheum Dis* 1998; **57**: 281–285.

251. Deighton CM, Watson MJ, Walker DJ. Sex hormones in postmenopausal HLA-identical rheumatoid arthritis discordant sibling pairs. *J Rheumatol* 1992; **19**: 1663–1667.

252. Masi AT, Josipovic DB, Jefferson WE. Low adrenal androgenic-anabolic steroids in women with rheuma-toid arthritis (RA): gas liquid chromatographic studies of RA patients and matched normal control women indicating decreased 11-deoxy-17-ketosteroid excretion. *Sem Rheum Arth* 1984; **14**: 1–23.

253. Cutolo M, Balleari E, Giusti M, Monachesi M, Accerdo S. Sex hormone status in women suffering from rheu-matoid arthritis. *J Rheumatol* 1986; **13**: 1019–1023.

254. Dougados M, Nahoul K, Benhamou L, Amor B. Androgen plasma levels in female rheumatoid arthritis patients. *Arthritis Rheum* 1983; **26**: 935–936.

255. Feher KG, Feher T, Merety K. Interrelationship between the immunological and steroid hormone parameters in rheumatoid arthritis. *Exp Clin Endocrinol* 1986; **87**: 38–42.

256. Spector TD, Silman AJ. Oral contraceptives and rheumatoid arthritis. Bias in observational studies of cause—effect relationships. *J Chronic Dis* 1987; **40**: 1063–1064.

257. Sambrook PN, Eisman JA, Champion GD, Pocock NA. Sex hormone status and osteoporosis in post-menopausal women with rheumatoid arthritis. *Arthritis Rheum* 1988; **31**: 973–978.

258. Jorgensen C, Maziad H, Bologna C, Sany J. Kinetics of prolactin release in rheumatoid arthritis. *Clin Exp Rheumatol* 1995; **13**: 705–709.

259. Myllykangas-Luosujarvi R, Aho K, Kautiainen H, Isomaki H. Cardiovascular mortality in women with rheumatoid arthritis. *J Rheumatol* 1995; **22**: 1065–1067.

260. Wallberg-Jonsson S, Ohman M, Dahlqvist S. Cardio-vascular morbidity and mortality in patients with rheumatoid arthritis in Northern Sweden. *J Rheumatol* 1997; **24**: 445–451.

261. Heliövaara M, Aho K, Knekt P, Reunanen A, Aromaa A. Serum cholesterol and risk of rheumatoid arthritis in a cohort of 52 800 men and women. *Br J Rheumatol* 1996; **35**: 255–257.

262. del Puente A. Personal communication.

263. Gottlieb NL, Page WF, Appelrouth DJ, Palmer R, Kiem IM. Antecedent tonsillectomy and appendectomy in rheumatoid arthritis. *J Rheumatol* 1979; **6**: 316–323.

264. Fernandez-Madrid F, Reed AH, Karvonen RL, Granda JL. Influence of antecedent lymphoid surgery on the odds of acquiring rheumatoid arthritis. *J Rheumatol* 1985; **12**: 43–48.

265. Wolfe F, Young DY. Rheumatoid arthritis and antecedent tonsillectomy. *J Rheumatol* 1983; **10**: 309–312.

266. Patel SB, Eastmond CJ. Preceding tonsillectomy and appendicectomy in rheumatoid and degenerative arthri-tis. *J Rheumatol* 1983; **10**: 313–315.

267. Linos AD, O'Fallon WM, Worthington JW, Kurland LT. The effect of tonsillectomy and appendectomy on the development of rheumatoid arthritis. *J Rheumatol* 1986; **13**: 707–709.

268. Bombardier C. Some pitfalls of the case-control approach to the investigation of rheumatoid disease. *J Rheumatol* 1979; **6**: 247–250.

269. Silman AJ, Ollier WER, Bubel MA. Autoimmune thyroid disease and thyroid autoantibodies in rheuma-toid arthritis patients and their families. *Br J Rheumatol* 1989; **28**: 18–21.

270. Spector TD, Silman AJ. Does the negative association between rheumatoid arthritis and schizophrenia pro-vide clues to the aetiology of rheumatoid arthritis? *Br J Rheumatol* 1987; **26**: 307–310.

271. Eaton WW, Hayward C, Ram R. Schizophrenia and rheumatoid arthritis: a review. *Schizophr Res* 1992; **6**: 181–192.

272. Lauerma H, Lehtinen V, Jourkamaa M, Jarvelin MR, Helenius H, Isohanni M. Schizophrenia among patients treated for rheumatoid arthritis and appendicitis. *Schizophr Res* 1998; **29**: 255–261.

273. Mors O, Mortensen PB, Ewald H. A population-based register study of the association between schizophrenia and rheumatoid arthritis. *Schizophr Res* 1999; **40**: 67–74.

274. Allanore Y, Hilliquin P, Coste J, Renoux M, Menkes C. Decreased prevalence of atopy in rheumatoid arthritis. *Lancet* 1998; **351**: 497.

275. Verhoef CM, van Roon JA, Vianen ME, Bruijnzeel-Koomen CA, Lafeber FP, Bijlsma JW. Mutual antagonism of rheumatoid arthritis and hay fever; a role for type 1/type 2 T cell balance. *Ann Rheum Dis* 1998; **57**: 275–280.

276. King SH, Cobb S. Psychosocial factors in the epidemiology of rheumatoid arthritis. *J Chronic Dis* 1958; **7**: 466–475.

277. Marcolongo R, Spaziani L. Analisi computerizzata su alcuni fattori condizionanti la prevalenza e la distribuzione dell'artrite reumatoide. *Reumatismo* 1971; **23**: 185–210.

278. Jacob DL, Robinson H, Masai AT. A controlled home interview study of factors associated with early rheumatoid arthritis. *Am J Public Health* 1972; **62**: 1532–1537.

279. Bankhead C, Silman A, Barrett B, Scott D, Symmons D. Incidence of rheumatoid arthritis is not related to indicators of socioeconomic deprivation. *J Rheumatol* 1996; **23**: 2039–2042.

280. Masi AT, Fecht T, Aldaq JC. History of smoking cigarettes, but not years of education correlated with the subsequent development of rheumatoid arthritis: preliminary findings from a community-wide, prospective, nested, case-control study. *Arthritis Rheum* 1996; **39**: S301.

281. Uhlig T, Hagen KB, Kvien TK. Current tobacco smoking, formal education, and the risk of rheumatoid arthritis. *J Rheumatol* 1999; **26**: 47–54.

282. Symmons DPM, Bankhead CR, Harrison BJ *et al.* Blood transfusion, smoking, and obesity as risk factors for the development of rheumatoid arthritis: results from a primary care-based incident case-control study in Norfolk, England. *Arthritis Rheum* 1997; **40**: 1955–1961.

283. Kremer JM, Bigauoette J, Michalek AV, Timchalk MA, Lininger L. Effects of manipulation of dietary fatty acids on clinical manifestation. *Lancet* 1985; **1**: 184–187.

284. Kremer JM, Lawrence DA, Jubiz W, Digiacomo R, Rynes R. Dietary fish oil and olive oil supplementation in patients with rheumatoid arthritis. Clinical and immunologic effects. *Arthritis Rheum* 1990; **33**: 810–820.

285. Linos A, Kaklamanis E, Kontomerkos A *et al.* The effect of olive oil and fish consumption on rheumatoid arthritis—a case control study. *Scand J Rheumatol* 1991; **20**: 419–426.

286. Shapiro JA, Koepsell TD, Voigt LF, Dugowson CE, Kestin M, Nelson L. Diet and rheumatoid arthritis in women: a possible protective effect of fish consumption. *Epidemiology* 1996; **7**: 256–263.

287. Linos A, Kaklamani VG, Kaklamani E *et al.* Dietary factors in relation to rheumatoid arthritis: A role for olive oil and cooked vegetables? *Am J Clin Nutr* 1999; **70**: 1077–1082.

288. Scudder PR, Al Timimi D, McMurray W, White AG, Zoob BC, Dormandy TL. Serum copper and related variables in rheumatoid arthritis. *Ann Rheum Dis* 1978; **37**: 67–70.

289. Rainsford KD. Environmental metal ion perturbations, especially as they affect copper status, and are factors in the etiology of arthritis conditions: an hypothesis. In: Sorenson JRJ, ed. *Inflammatory disease and copper*. Clifton: Humana Press, 1982: 137–142.

290. Mottonen T, Hannonen P, Seppala O, Alfthan G, Oka M. Glutathione and selenium in rheumatoid arthritis. *Clin Rheumatol* 1984; **1**: 195–200.

291. O'Dell JR, Lemley-Gillespie S, Palmer WR, Weaver AL, Moore GF, Klassen LW. Serum selenium concentrations in rheumatoid arthritis. *Ann Rheum Dis* 1991; **50**: 376–378.

292. Peretz A, Neve J, Vertongen F, Famaeyu JP, Molle L. Selenium status in relation to clinical variables and corticosteroid treatment in rheumatoid arthritis. *J Rheumatol* 1987; **14**: 1104–1107.

293. Heliövaara M, Knekt P, Aho K, Aaran RK, Alfthan G, Aromaa A. Serum antioxidants and risk of rheumatoid arthritis. *Ann Rheum Dis* 1994; **53**: 51–53.

294. Mathews JD, Whittingham S, Hooper BM, Mackay IR, Stenhouse NS. Association of autoantibodies with smoking, cardiovascular morbidity, and death in the Busselton population. *Lancet* 1973; **2**: 754–758.

295. Tuomi T, Heliövaara M, Palosuo T, Aho K. Smoking, lung function, and rheumatoid factors. *Ann Rheum Dis* 1990; **49**: 753–756.

296. Karlson EW, Min Lee I, Cook NR, Manson JE, Buring JE, Hennekens CH. A retrospective cohort study of cigarette smoking and risk of rheumatoid arthritis in female health professionals. *Arthritis Rheum* 1999; **42**: 910–917.

297. Hernandez-Avila M, Liang MH, Willett WC *et al.* Reproductive factors, smoking, and the risk for rheumatoid arthritis. *Epidemiology* 1990; **1**: 285–291.

298. Hazes JMW, Dijkmans BAC, Van den Broucke JP, de Vries RRP, Cats A. Lifestyle and the risk of rheumatoid arthritis: cigarette smoking and alcohol consumption. *Ann Rheum Dis* 1990; **49**: 980–982.

299. Voight LF, Koepsell TD, Nelson L, Dugowson CE, Daling JR. Smoking, obesity, alcohol consumption and the risk of rheumatoid arthritis. *Epidemiology* 1994; **5**: 525–532.

300. Silman AJ, Newman J, MacGregor AJ. Cigarette smoking increases the risk of rheumatoid arthritis: results from a nationwide study of disease-discordant twins. *Arthritis Rheum* 1996; **39**: 732–735.

301. Heliövaara M, Aho K, Aromaa A, Knekt P, Reunanen A. Smoking and risk of rheumatoid arthritis. *J Rheumatol* 1993; **20**: 1830–1835.

302. Myllykangas-Luosujarvi R, Aho K, Kautiainen H, Hakala M. Reduced incidence of alcohol related deaths in subjects with rheumatoid arthritis. *Ann Rheum Dis* 2000; **59**: 75–76.

303. Miall WE, Caplan A, Cochrane AL, Kilpatrick GS. An epidemiological study of rheumatoid arthritis associated with characteristic chest x-ray appearances in coalworkers. *BMJ* 1953; **4**: 1231–1236.

304. Franzinelli A, Marcolongo R. Epidemiologia dell'artrite, reumatoide e del fattore reumatoide. *Reumatismo* 1971; **23**: 222–235.

305. Klockars M, Koskela RS, Jarvinen E, Kolari PJ, Rossi A. Silica exposure and rheumatoid arthritis: a follow up study of granite workers 1940–81. *Br Med J Clin Res Ed* 1987; **294**: 997–1000.

306. Rosenman KD, Moore FM, Reilly MJ. Connective tissue disease and silicosis. *Am J Ind Med* 1999; **35**: 375–381.

307. Edworthy SM, Martin L, Barr SG, Birdsell DC, Brant RF, Fritzler MJ. A clinical study of the relationship between silicone breast implants and connective tissue disease. *J Rheumatol* 1998; **25**: 254–260.

308. Wolfe F, Anderson J. Silicone filled breast implants and the risk of fibromyalgia and rheumatoid arthritis. *J Rheumatol* 1999; **26**: 2025–2028.

309. Janowsky EC, Kupper LL, Hulka BS. Meta-analyses of the relation between silicone breast implants and the risk of connective-tissue diseases. *N Engl J Med* 2000; **342**: 781–790.

310. Krause A, Kamradt T, Burmester GR. Potential infectious agents in the induction of arthritides. *Curr Opin Rheumatol* 1996; **8**: 203–209.

311. Walker DJ, Griffiths ID, Madeley D. Autoantibodies and antibodies to microorganisms in rheumatoid arthritis: comparison of histocompatible siblings. *J Rheumatol* 1987; **14**: 426–428.

312. Silman AJ, Bankhead C, Rowlingson B, Brennan P, Symmons D, Gatrell A. Do new cases of rheumatoid arthritis cluster in time or in space? *Int J Epidemiol* 1997; **26**: 628–634.

313. Schweiger F, Bell DA, Little AH. Coexistence of rheumatoid arthritis in married couples: a search for etiological factors. *J Rheumatol* 1981; **8**: 416–422.

314. Nelson J, Furst D, Maloney S et al. Microchimerism and HLA-compatible relationships of pregnancy in scleroderma. *Lancet* 1998; **351**: 559–562.

315. Gottlieb NL, Ditchek N, Poiley J, Kiem IM. Pets and rheumatoid arthritis. An epidemiologic survey. *Arthritis Rheum* 1974; **17**: 229–234.

316. Bond C, Cleland LG. Rheumatoid arthritis: are pets implicated in its etiology? *Semin Arthritis Rheum* 1996; **25**: 308–317.

317. Gross K, Combe C, Kruger K, Schattenkirchner M. Arthritis after hepatitis B vaccination. Report of three cases. *Scand J Rheumatol* 1995; **24**: 50–52.

318. Levine PR, Axelrod DA. Rheumatoid factor isotypes following immunization. *Clin Exp Rheumatol* 1985; **3**: 147–149.

319. Alspaugh MA, Tan EM. Antibodies to cellular antigens in Sjogren's syndrome. *J Clin Invest* 1975; **55**: 1067–1073.

320. Alspaugh MA, Henle G, Lennette ET, Henle W. Elevated levels of antibodies to Epstein-Barr virus antigens in sera and synovial fluids of patients with rheumatoid arthritis. *J Clin Invest* 1981; **67**: 1134–1140.

321. Ng KC, Brown KA, Perry JD, Holborow EJ. Anti-RANA antibody: a marker for seronegative and seropositive rheumatoid arthritis. *Lancet* 1980; **1**: 447–479.

322. Catalano MA, Carson DA, Slovin SF, Richman DD, Vaughan H. Antibodies to Epstein-Barr virus-determined antigens in normal subjects and in patients with seropositive rheumatoid arthritis. *Proc Natl Acad Sci USA* 1979; **76**: 5825–5828.

323. Ferrell PB, Aitcheson CT, Pearson GR, Tan EM. Seroepidemiological study of relationships between Epstein-Barr virus and rheumatoid arthritis. *J Clin Invest* 1981; **67**: 681–687.

324. Venables PJ, Ross MG, Charles PJ, Melsom RD, Griffiths PD, Maini RN. A seroepidemiological study of cytomegalovirus and Epstein-Barr virus in rheumatoid arthritis and sicca syndrome. *Ann Rheum Dis* 1985; **44**: 742–746.

325. Kouri T, Petersen J, Rhodes G et al. Antibodies to synthetic peptides from Epstein Barr nuclear antigen-1 in sera of patients with early rheumatoid arthritis and in preillness sera. *J Rheumatol* 1990; **17**: 1442–1449.

326. Newkirk MM, Duffy KN, Paleckova A et al. Herpes viruses in multicase families with rheumatoid arthritis. *J Rheumatol* 1995; **22**: 2055–2061.

327. Scotet E, David-Ameline J, Peyrat M et al. T cell response to Epstein-Barr virus transactivators in chronic rheumatoid arthritis. *J Exp Med* 1996; **184**: 1791–1800.

328. Saal JG, Krimmel M, Steidle M et al. Synovial Epstein-Barr virus infection increases the risk of rheumatoid arthritis in individuals with the shared HLA-DR4 epitope. *Arthritis Rheum* 1999; **42**: 1485–1496.

329. Niedobitek G, Lisner R, Swoboda B et al. Lack of evidence for an involvement of Epstein-Barr virus infection of synovial membranes in the pathogenesis of rheumatoid arthritis. *Arthritis Rheum* 2000; **43**: 151–154.

330. Aho K, Raunio V. EB-virus and rheumatoid arthritis: new insights into their interrelation. *Medical Biology* 1982; **60**: 49–52.

331. Vaughan JH, Carson DA, Fox RI. The Epstein-Barr virus and rheumatoid arthritis. *Clin Exp Rheumatol* 1983; **1**: 265–272.

332. Depper JM, Zvaifler NJ. Epstein-Barr virus—its relationship to the pathogenesis of rheumatoid arthritis. *Arthritis Rheum* 1981; **24**: 755–761.

333. Anderson MJ, Jones SE, Fisher-Hoch SP et al. Human parvovirus, the cause of erythema infectiosum (fifth disease)? *Lancet* 1983; **1**: 1378.

334. White DG, Woolf AD, Mortimer PP, Cohen BJ, Blake DR, Bacon PA. Human parvovirus arthropathy. *Lancet* 1985; **1**: 419–421.

335. Reid DM, Reid TMS, Brown T, Rennie JAN, Eastmond CJ. Human parvovirus-associated arthritis: a clinical and laboratory description. *Lancet* 1985; **1**: 422–425.

336. Klouda PT, Corbin SA, Bradley BA, Cohen BJ, Woolf AD. HLA and acute arthritis following human parvovirus infection. *Tissue Antigens* 1986; **28**: 318–319.

337. Gendi NS, Gibson K, Wordsworth BP. Effect of HLA type and hypocomplementaemia on the expression of parvovirus arthritis: one year follow up of an outbreak. *Ann Rheum Dis* 1996; **55**: 63–65.

338. Nikkari S, Luukkainen R, Mottonen T *et al*. Does parvovirus B19 have a role in rheumatoid arthritis? *Ann Rheum Dis* 1994; **53**: 106–111.

339. Harrison B, Silman A, Barrett E, Symmons D. Low frequency of parvovirus infection in a population-based cohort of patients with early inflammatory polyarthritis. *Ann Rheum Dis* 1998; **57**: 375–377.

340. Hajeer AH, MacGregor AJ, Rigby AS, Ollier WER, Carthy D, Silman AJ. Influence of previous exposure to human parvovirus B19 infection in explaining susceptibility to rheumatoid arthritis: an analysis of disease discordant twin pairs. *Ann Rheum Dis* 1994; **53**: 137–139.

341. Wilson C, Corbett M, Ebringer A. Increased isolation of Proteus mirablis species from rheumatoid arthritis patients compared to osteoarthritis patients and healthy controls. *Br J Rheumatol* 1990; **29**: 99.

342. Ebringer A, Ptaszynska T, Corbett M *et al*. Antibodies to proteus in rheumatoid arthritis. *Lancet* 1985; **2**: 305–307.

343. Deighton CM, Gray JW, Bint AJ, Walker DJ. Anti-proteus antibodies in rheumatoid arthritis same-sexed sibships. *Br J Rheumatol* 1992; **31**: 241–245.

344. Gaston H. Proteus—is it a likely aetiological factor in chronic polyarthritis? *Ann Rheum Dis* 1995; **54**: 157–158.

345. Pelton BK, North M, Palmer RG *et al*. A search for retrovirus infection in systemic lupus erythematosus and rheumatoid arthritis. *Ann Rheum Dis* 1988; **47**: 206–209.

346. Panayi G, Dalgleish AG. Retroviruses in rheumatoid arthritis. *Ann Rheum Dis* 1986; **45**: 439.

347. Galeazzi M, Tuzi T, Amici C, Benedetto A. Rheumatoid arthritis and human T cell lymphotropic retrovirus. *Arthritis Rheum* 1986; **29**: 1533–1534.

348. Hasunuma T, Sumida T, Nishioka K. Human T cell leukemia virus type-I and rheumatoid arthritis. *Int Rev Immunol* 1998; **17**: 291–307.

349. Cassell GH, Davis JK, Lindsey JR, Cole BC, Hartley MW. Arthritis of rats and mice: implications for man. *Isr J Med Sci* 1981; **17**: 608–615.

350. Clark HW, Coker-Vann MR, Bailey JS, Brown TM. Detection of mycoplasmal antigens in immune complexes from rheumatoid arthritis synovial fluid. *Ann Allergy* 1988; **60**: 394–398.

351. Ottenhoff THM, Torres P, las Aguas J *et al*. Evidence for an HLA-DR4-associated immune-response gene for Mycobacterium tuberculosis. A clue to the pathogenesis of rheumatoid arthritis? *Lancet* 1986; **2**: 310–313.

352. Haier J, Nasralla M, Franco AR, Nicolson GL. Detection of mycoplasmal infections in blood of patients with rheumatoid arthritis. *Rheumatology* 1999; **38**: 504–509.

353. Wyburn-Mason R. The naeglerial causation of rheumatoid disease and many human cancers. A new concept in medicine. *Med Hypotheses* 1979; **5**: 1237–1249.

354. Karlson EW, Lee IM, Cook NR, Manson JE, Buring JE, Hennekens CH. A retrospective cohort study of cigarette smoking and risk of rheumatoid arthritis in female health professionals. *Arthritis Rheum* 1999; **42**: 910–917.

355. Riise T, Jacobsen BK, Gran JT. Incidence and prevalence of rheumatoid arthritis in the county of Troms, northern Norway. *J Rheumatol* 2000; **27**: 1386–1389.

356. Kaipiainen-Seppanen O, Aho K, Nikkarinen M. Regional differences in the incidence of rheumatoid arthritis in Finland in 1995. *Ann Rheum Dis* 2001; **60**: 128–132.

357. Erdes S, Alekseeva LI, Titov AV, Ryazantseva TA, Benevolenskaya LI. Spondylarthropathies and rheumatoid arthritis in some Finno-Ugrian populations in Russia. *Ter Arkh* 2000; **72**: 50–52.

358. Chopra A, Patil J, Billempelly V *et al*. Prevalence of rheumatic diseases in a rural population in western India: a WHO-ILAR COPCORD Study. *J Assoc Physicians India* 2001; **49**: 240–246.

359. Hilliquin P, Allanore Y, Coste J, Renoux M, Kahan A, Menkes CJ. Reduced incidence and prevalence of atopy in rheumatoid arthritis. Results of a case-control study. *Rheumatology* 2000; **39**: 1020–1026.

360. Hutchinson D, Shepstone L, Moots R, Lear JT, Lynch MP. Heavy cigarette smoking is strongly associated with rheumatoid arthritis (RA), particularly in patients without a family history of RA. *Ann Rheum Dis* 2001; **60**: 223–227.

3 | *Juvenile idiopathic arthritis*

Wendy Thomson and Alan J. Silman

Introduction

Juvenile idiopathic arthritis (JIA) is now the accepted term for the constellation of clinical syndromes characterized by childhood inflammatory arthritis, not explained by causes such as trauma, infection, haemophilia, and connective tissue disorders. The epidemiology of childhood connective tissue disorders, such as SLE, scleroderma, and polymyositis, are considered elsewhere in this volume, as part of the discussion of their epidemiology in adults. Some robust studies (for example [1]) have provided useful estimates of the relative incidence rates of the various connective tissue diseases in childhood.

Although in theory, children can satisfy criteria for adult inflammatory rheumatic disorders such as rheumatoid arthritis, psoriatic arthritis (PSA) and various of the spondylarthropathies such as anklosing spondylitis (AS), it is more usual to combine their childhood onsets with other non-specific inflammatory joint disorders under a single umbrella term such as JIA. This is beneficial as, firstly, childhood presentations are frequently atypical and, secondly, there is considerable overlap. As a consequence, the broad syndrome of JIA is frequently subdivided by its clinical pattern, particularly at onset, in order to define homogeneous subgroups which may be better suited for epidemiological study. The classifications are described in the next section.

Studies undertaken to date have not used consistent schemes, making it difficult to compare studies. European studies have predominantly used the term juvenile chronic arthritis (JCA) with North American studies adopting the term juvenile rheumatoid arthritis (JRA), reflecting the use of EULAR and ARA criteria respectively. As in Oen and Cheang [2], this may have implications for explaining the variation in results. As a shorthand, this chapter will use the term JIA highlighting, where relevant, the criteria used. Whatever the preferred term, however, this chapter describes the epidemiology of a fairly broad group of ill-defined disorders.

Classification

Classification of the chronic arthritides of childhood has been problematic since its first description in the late 1890s. Diament-Berger [3] and Still [4] led the way by recognizing the clinical heterogeneity within the childhood arthritides, proposing that they were at least three distinct subtypes. Ansell and Bywaters [5] first proposed that classification of childhood arthritides should be based on the characteristics of the disease at onset and, although since then classification has evolved substantially, this basic premise still remains. In fact, this led to the development of two classification systems, one within the US, the other in Europe. In 1972, the American Rheumatism Association (later the American Congress of Rheumatology) proposed a set of criteria for what they called juvenile rheumatoid arthritis (JRA) [6]. Modifications to the criteria were made in 1977 [7] and the revised criteria are still in widespread use today. In Europe, the original Taplow criteria [5,8] were modified and, in 1978, the proposed criteria of EULAR were published for the classification of juvenile chronic arthritis (JCA). These criteria have been widely used throughout Europe.

The main features of the two classification systems are given in Table 3.1. The major differences are the disease duration and the fact that the EULAR criteria are inclusive of other forms of juvenile arthritis such as AS, whereas the ARA criteria are exclusive.

Both sets of criteria have also undergone modification. The age at onset is often used to divide pauciarticiular patients, in particular, into those with an early or late onset, although the cut-off between these two groups has never been agreed. Antinuclear anti-

Table 3.1 Classification systems for JCA and JRA

EULAR/WHO critiera—juvenile *chronic* arthritis defined as:

1. Age of onset less than 16
2. Duration of arthritis for a minimum of 3 months
3. Classification by onset: pauci-articular, polyarticular, systemic
4. Exclusion of other diseases, as far as possible, up to one year from the onset of symptoms

ARA criteria—juvenile *rheumatoid* arthritis defined as:

1. Age at onset less than 16 years
2. Arthritis in one or more joint
3. Duration of disease for at least 6 weeks
4. Exclusion of other forms of juvenile arthritis

body positivity and/or the presence of chronic anterior uveitis has also been used to subdivide pauciarticular patients. Within EULAR, children who have polyarticular disease and are rheumatoid factor (RF) positive are termed 'juvenile rheumatoid arthritis'. Patients classified according to the ARA criteria are often divided into RF positive and negative. A further problem is that there are no universally accepted criteria for juvenile-onset spondylarthropathies, psoriatic arthritis, arthritis associated with inflammatory bowel disease or reactive arthritis. Despite these problems, both classification systems have gained widespread use and are often used inter-changeably, despite the fact that they do not identify comparable groups of patients.

In 1994, a task force was set up by the International League of Associations for Rheumatology (ILAR) to develop a new classification for the arthritides of childhood which it was hoped would supersede both the EULAR and ARA classification systems and provide a universally accepted and biologically relevant set of criteria. The ILAR classification system was first published in 1995 [9] and contained seven disease subtypes. These criteria were modified in 1997 [10]. Modifications included:

(1) systemic patients, previously subdivided into definite and probable were grouped together;

(2) patients with oligoarthritis were subdivided into those with persistent oligoarticular disease and those which extended to polyarticular disease;

(3) the addition of an eighth subtype, 'other arthritis, for those patients who fulfilled criteria for none of the categories or fulfilled criteria for more than two of the other categories.

Further minor modifications have recently been proposed [116,117] and the criteria are still not considered perfect [118].

The term juvenile idiopathic arthritis (JIA) was adopted to replace both JRA and JCA. JIA indicates disease of childhood (i.e. less than 16 years of age) of no known aetiology, characterized primarily by arthritis persistent for at least 6 weeks. Classification is made 6 months after disease onset into one of eight categories (Table 3.2)

Table 3.2 ILAR classification system for juvenile idiopathic arthritis

1. Systemic onset JIA—arthritis with or preceded by daily fever of at least 2 weeks' duration, that is documented to be quotidian for at least 3 days and accompanied by one or more of: tansient evanescent rash, lymphadenopathy, hepatomegaly, or serositis.
2. Persistent oligoarthritis—arthritis affecting 1–4 joints during first 6 months of disease which continues to affect no more than 4 joints throughout the disease course.
3. Extended oligoarthritis—arthritis affecting 1–4 joints during first 6 months of disease which affects a cumulative total of 5 joints or more after the first 6 months of disease.
4. Polyarthritis (RF negative)—arthritis affecting 5 or more joints during first 6 months of disease, tests for RF are negative.
5. Polyarthritis (RF positive)—arthritis affecting 5 or more joints during first 6 months of disease, tests for RF are positive (2 tests at least 3 months apart).
6. Psoriatic arthritis—arthritis and psoriasis or arthritis and at least 2 of dactylitis, nail abnormalities, or family history of psoriasis in at least 1 first-degree relative.
7. Enthesitis related arthritis—arthritis with enthesitis or arthritis or enthesitis with at least 2 of sacroiliac joint tenderness and/or inflammatory spinal pain, presence of HLA-B27, or family history of associated disease.
8. Other arthritis—does not fulfil criteria for any of the other categories or fulfills criteria for more than 1 category.

Each category has its own set of specific characteristics, exclusions, and descriptors.

Validation studies are now underway [11,12] and the ILAR classification is still open to further modifications. All previous classifications have been based on the clinicians' perceptions of clinical disease patterns. More recently, Thomas *et al.* [13] used a statistical approach, latent class analysis, to try to define underlying subtypes of JIA that best explained the observed relationship between laboratory and clinical variables. This type of approach may provide additional insights into how the ILAR criteria could be modified.

Incidence

The incidence of JIA and its subtypes is derived typically from a retrospective review of all medical records of children from a defined catchment population, attending referral centres. Some studies have included a survey of all relevant physicians in an attempt to ascertain missed cases, but poor response rates and difficulties in recall and case verification due to lack of contemporary records increase the difficulty. As an example is a major Belgian study aimed at all relevant clinicians; a response rate of 15 per cent emerged [14] which gives little confidence in the results obtained.

In a very detailed analysis, Oen and Cheang [2] showed that the use of physician surveys was likely to give an incidence twice that of studies based on clinic-derived cases alone. Criteria used also have an influence with studies based on the ACR criteria also

revealing a high incidence. It is impossible to determine if these differences reflect true underlying differences in occurrence or the methodological variations described.

There have been a very large number of incidence studies undertaken over the past 40 years from several countries. The data are presented separately for European (Table 3.3) and North American populations (Table 3.4). The results are perhaps surprisingly consistent given the differences in approach. Recent European studies [15–17] suggest an incidence of around 1–2 per 10 000 children years, although a study from East Berlin [18] revealed a much lower rate. Rates in North American populations of European origin are similar to these [19], although data from Canada are more similar to the Berlin data [20,21]. The assumption must be that those countries with the lower rates may be under-ascertaining cases.

Prevalence

Data on prevalence are difficult to interpret, as studies use this term to describe two distinct phenomena: the first is based either on a population survey to identify individuals with current evidence of disease or on ascertaining current attenders over (say) a 1-year period, and the second is to identify any child with an 'ever' diagnosis and count them as a case if alive on prevalence day. It is thus not surprising that these, as well as the other methodological differences discussed above for the incidence studies, have an important

Table 3.3 Incidence of juvenile idiopathic arthritis: European populations

Reference	Country	Region	Period	Criteria	Incidence/100 000 (95% CI)
[99]	Finland	Helsinki	1982	ARA	18.2 (10.8–28.7)
[100]	Denmark	North Jutland	1970–77	ARA	6
			1981–82		8
[101]	France	Paris	1981–82	ARA	19
		Brittany			13
[102]	Sweden	South-uzt	1984–88	EULAR	10.9 (9.4–12.4)
[15]	Finland	3 regions	1980	ARA	13.8
			1985	ARA	15.1
			1990	ARA	13.5
[16]	UK	Liverpool	1990–94	EULAR	10 (7–13)
		Canterbury			10 (6–14)
[18]	Germany	East Berlin	1980–88	EULAR	3.5 (2.8–4.4)
[17]	Norway	Tromso	1985–94	EULAR	22.6
[14]	Belgium	National	1973–88	EULAR	11.7

Table 3.4 Incidence of juvenile idiopathic arthritis: American populations

Reference	Country	Population	Period	Criteria	Incidence/ 100 000 (95% CI)
[24]	Canada	British Columbia – Europeans – Haida	1966–75	ARA	2.6 7.2
[103]	US	Michigan	1960–70		9.2
[104]	US	Rochester	1960–70	ARA	13.9 (9.9–18.8)
[32]	US	Baltimore Blacks	1979–80	ARA	6.1 (0.8–23.8)
[31]	Costa Rica	Hispanic	1993–95	EULAR	6.8 (4.1–9.6)
[20]	Canada	Countrywide	1991–93	ARA	3.1 (2.7–3.7)
[21]	Canada	Manitoba	1975–92	ARA	5.3
[22]	US	Inupiats	1970–82	ARA	28 (10.3–61.0)
[27]	US	Yupik Alaska	1970–82	ARA	42.5 (27.2–63.3)
[19]	US	Rochester	1960–93	ARA	11.7 (8.7–14.5)
[52]	Canada	Sakatoon	1981–89	ARA	8.0
[28]	US	SE Africa Tlingitis	1970–84	ARA	38.6 (23.2–66.2)

Table 3.5 Prevalence of juvenile idiopathic arthritis in different populations: European

Reference	Country	Case ascertainment	Criteria	Number of cases	Prevalence/100 000
[105]	Poland	Diagnosed cases	?	775	7
[106]	Slovakia	Diagnosed cases	?	95	8
[107]	Czech Rep	Diagnosed cases	?	595	23
[101]	France:				
	Paris	Diagnosed cases	EULAR	74	8
	Brittany			62	10
[108]	Sweden	Diagnosed cases	EULAR	223	56
[109]	Belgium	Diagnosed cases	EULAR	N/S	2.0
[39]	Sweden	Diagnosed cases	EULAR	248	64
[110]	Belgium	Population survey	EULAR	3	100
[18]	Germany	Diagnosed cases	EULAR	105	20
[17]	Norway	Diagnosed cases	EULAR	109	148
[29]	Turkey	Population survey	EULAR	30	64
[111]	UK	Diagnosed cases	?	14	200

impact on the results obtained [2]. The results from several prevalence studies undertaken in the past 20 years are shown for European, North American, and other populations (Tables 3.5, 3.6, and 3.7). The prevalences vary considerably and are very difficult to interpret. Given that death is exceptionally rare, it is possible to do some simple calculations. As shown in Table 3.8, the average age of onset is around 7–8 years, thus in childhood, if the disease is persistent, the duration (to age 16) is around 8 years. Thus, if the incidence is between 5 and 20 per 100 000 person years

(Tables 3.4 and 3.5) then the prevalence should be between 40 and 160. Figures outside these boundaries from the earlier European studies quoted probably represent serious underestimates.

Age and gender

JIA and its subtypes are defined by having an onset during childhood and, therefore, cannot occur after the age of 16. Clearly childhood onset of 'adult' disorders such as rheumatoid arthritis and ankylosing spondylitis

Table 3.6   Prevalence of juvenile idiopathic arthritis in different populations: North American

Reference	Country	Case ascertainment	Criteria	Number of cases	Prevalence/100 000
[112]	US	Population survey	?	249	220
[113]	US	Diagnosed cases	ACR	55	27
[104]	US	Diagnosed cases	ACR	15	113
[114]	US	Population survey	ACR	109	121
[32]	US	Diagnosed cases	ACR	4	26
[2]	Canada	Diagnosed cases	ACR	15	45
[52]	Canada	Diagnosed cases	ACR	115	40
[19]	US				
	– 1980	Diagnosed cases	ACR	65	94.3
	– 1990				86.1

Table 3.7   Prevalence of juvenile idiopathic arthritis in different populations: others

Reference	Country	Case ascertainment	Criteria	Number of cases	Prevalence/100 000
[30]	Kuwait	Diagnosed cases	ARA	41	22
[115]	Australia	Population survey	EULAR	9	400

Table 3.8   Incidence of juvenile idiopathic arthritis by age and gender

Age	Incidence/100 000		
	Males	Females	Both
0–3	12.4	41.1	26.3
4–7	5.2	29.0	16.8
8–11	27.4	19.9	23.8
12–15	19.5	27.0	23.2
ALL	16.1	29.4	22.6

Source: [17].

Table 3.9   Influence of age and gender on subtype

Subtype	N	Female:male	Mean age (range)
Pauciarticular	305	2.4:1	5.6 (0.3–16.5)
Polyarticular	154	5.1:1	1.3 (1.2–16.8)
Systemic	62	1.1:1	5.2(0.4–16.3)

Source: [20]

do occur, although the correct classification may only become apparent in adult life. The age and gender influence on occurrence will depend on the distribution of specific subtypes prevalent in any population. In some native North American populations, the predominant subtype is a spondylarthropathy, and hence there is a strong male preponderance [22]. In population studies, the occurrence of all subtypes is typically 1.5–2 times as high in females as in males (for example [18]). The gender difference varies by type, being greatest for polyarticular disease and least for systemic [23]. Age is the other major influence on gender, though this is partly explained by subtype. Recent data from Norway (Table 3.8) [17] show that the female excess is most marked under the age of 8. In adolescent onset, there was little different between the genders. The data for the genders combined (Table 3.8) show a fairly con-

stant incidence with age but, as indicated above, this conceals the influence of age on subtype. These differences may not be as great as once considered. In a large Canadian study of 521 children, the age at onset in the polyarticular group was only moderately higher than either the pauciarticular or systemic onset groups (Table 3.9) [20].

Race and geography

The data on incidence and prevalence can be used to examine influences of race (ethnicity) and geography—though these two cannot be easily separated. The British Columbia study suggested a very low occurrence in Chinese [24]. There do not appear to have been any formal epidemiological studies in South East Asian populations. In Japanese [25] and Thai [26] children, polyarticular disease is relatively more common than pauciarticular disease. Native American groups have very high incidence rates. In Manitoba, native populations had four times the incidence as Europeans [21]. Native Eskimo [22,27] and North American Indian [24,28] have much higher incidence rates than other populations. Some of these differences can be explained by the occurrence of specific subtypes. Thus, in the Yupik [27], the large majority are spondylarthopathic in type. By contrast, in the Tlinglit Indians, a broad spectrum of subtypes was observed [28].

Occurrence is similar in Turkish [29] and Arab [30] populations as in Europeans. Data from other population groups is sparse. An incidence study from Costa Rica, a hispanic population, revealed a similar incidence to other American groups [31].

African groups may have a low occurrence. The disease had a low prevalence in Baltimore blacks [32] and the proportion of black children in a Los Angeles series was only about a quarter of what might have been expected from their proportion in the population as a whole [33]. In general, African groups show a relatively higher proportion of pauciarticular disease [34].

Within countries, there are differences in prevalence, for example Canada [20], but it is difficult to know whether these represent real differences or the consequences of both random variation and differences in ascertainment. Even within an individual province, such as Manitoba, there is wide regional variation [21]. In the one study reporting such an analysis, there was no statistical evidence of non-random distribution (clustering) [35].

Time trends

There has been considerable interest in examining the influence of time on the onset of JIA. The underlying hypothesis is that the disease in some children may be initiated by an infectious agent which might occur in epidemics. Time trends have been examined over short periods looking for clustering or seasonality of onset, as well as charting incidence over longer periods of time to determine any underlying secular trends.

Clusters based on year of birth have been reported [36] which might be related to epidemics of influenza A. In that study, it was hypothesized that patients may have been sensitized to influenza *in utero* and 'challenged' by a different strain occurring later in life. There is an inconsistency in the literature relating to seasonality and onset. Some studies suggested a seasonal influence [37,38] with the latter study ascertaining no onsets between November and March compared to 17 between April and July. By contrast, a formal cluster

Table 3.10 Time trends in incidence of juvenile idiopathic arthritis

Period	Incidence (95% CI)/100 000		
	All	Pauciarticular	Systemic
1960–69	15.0 (8.7–14.8)	11.3 (5.7–16.9)	1.2 (0–2.3)
1970–79	14.1 (8.0–20.1)	9.0 (4.1–14.0)	3.3 (0.4–6.7)
1980–93	7.8 (3.9–11.7)	5.8 (2.5–9.1)	0

Source: [19].

analysis of time difference in onset between all pairs in a national survey in Denmark was negative [35]. In Canada also, no seasonal trend was apparent [21].

There are stronger data supportive of year-to-year variation. Data from Rochester [19] (Table 3.10) have shown a consistent decline since 1960, with the greatest decline being in pauciarticular disease. Finnish national data [15] showed no change between 1980 and 1990, though in both studies the number of systemic cases was too small to make useful comment. There was also no change in incidence in diagnosed cases in Berlin over the period 1980–88 [18].

The possibility has been raised [21] of a cyclical pattern in incidence, with peaks possibly occurring every 5 years. Thus in data from Manitoba (Fig. 3.1), there were peaks in 1986 and 1991 and troughs in intervening years. Though the authors (see below) postulated a relationship with infection, random fluctuation due to small numbers, needs to be considered. This may be the explanation for other reported year-to-year changes in incidence [39].

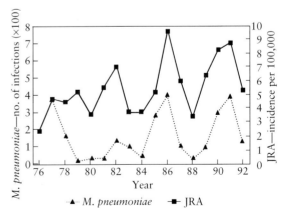

Fig. 3.1 Comparison of trends in JRA incidence and *M. pneumoniae* infection. Reproduced with the permission of the *Journal of Rheumatology* from [21].

Genetics

Familial clustering

JIA is a heterogeneous group of disorders, generally considered to be a complex genetic trait [40]. Evidence for this comes from a variety of sources such as twin studies, family studies, and disease association studies. The degree of disease concordance in monozygotic twins gives an indication of the level of involvement of genetic factors within given disease. Reports of twins concordant for JIA are very rare. Meyerowitz *et al.* [41] reported on eight sets of twins disconcordant for RA, three of which had juvenile onset, one seropositive the other two pauciarticular. Ansell *et al.* reported 11 twin pairs (five monozygotic (MZ) and six dizygotic (DZ)) [42]. Two pairs, both MZ, were concordant for disease. This study was later extended to include a total of 24 twin pairs (12 MZ and 12 DZ) in which six MZ pairs, but no DZ pairs, were concordant for disease [43]. Baum and Fink reported on a set of female MZ twins concordant for seronegative erosive arthritis [44]. Kapusta *et al.* reported on JIA which occurred in a mother and her identical twin sons and Husby *et al.* described a set of twins concordant for clinical features, including iritis, but discordant for amyloidsis and monoconal gammopathy [45,46]. The largest and most recent study comes from the National Institute of Arthritis and Musculoskeletal and Skin Diseases sponsored Research Registry for JRA affected sibling pair (ASP) [47]. Of 118 ASPs on the register, there are 14 pairs of twins. One pair comprises a girl with polyarticular onset and a boy with pauciarticular onset and disease course. The other 13 pairs wereconcordant for gender (nine female, four male), disease onset (10 pauciarticular, three polyarticular), and disease course (eight pauciarticular, five polyarticular).

Studies of familial clustering outside twins of JIA are also rare [42,48–53]. In the most recent study, Moroldo *et al.* studied 71 ASPs from the National Institute of Arthritis and Musculoskeletal and Skin Diseases sponsored Research Registry for JRA ASP, of which 63 per cent were concordant for gender and 76 per cent for onset type [77]. This study fully demonstrated a higher than expected degree of concordance for JIA onset type. The estimated λs for JIA is 15, although data from the Registry suggests that this may vary between different JIA subtypes [40].

Immunogenetics

Further evidence that genetic as well as environmental factors play a role in JIA originate from association-based studies. There have been many studies aimed at identifying the genes involved in JIA; the majority of these have focused on genes within the MHC. The earliest reports for HLA Class I were of an association between HLA-B27 and older children with pauciarticular onset disease [54] and of an increase in HLA-A2 in pauciarticular patients with an early disease onset [55]. The first studies looking at HLA Class II in juvenile arthritis demonstrated an increase in HLA-DR5 and DR8, and also in early onset pauciarticular patients [56,57]. Since then, there have been numerous studies of both Class I and Class II associations in JIA, with the Class I associations being consistently more limited than those for Class II. Many of the early studies were reviewed by Donn and Ollier [58].

The most recent, and one of the largest studies, used both serological and molecular-based methods to look for Class I and Class II associations in 680 children with JRA [59]. A summary of their results is given in Table 3.11. In general, their data support that of previous studies.

Systemic onset disease shows the weakest and most limited HLA associations. Some studies have reported an association with HLA-DR8 [60,61] and HLA-DR5 [62,60]. However, the most consistent finding is that of an increase in HLA-DR4 [57,63–66], although this was not confirmed in a study of 108 French children with systemic onset disease [67].

Children with polyarticular disease are often subdivided into seropositive and seronegative. Seropositive polyarticular children are generally considered to be immunogenetically similar to adult RA. Early studies of children with RF-positive polyarticular disease demonstrated an increase in HLA-DR4 [68]. This similarity with adult RA has been confirmed in many further studies [69–71]. In a Japanese population, it was shown to be HLA-DRB1*0405 which was increased in both RF-positive polyarticular JRA cases and RF-positive adult RA cases [25]. In contrast to previous studies, a recent examination of a small number of children with RF-positive polyarticular JRA in the regions of Cree and Ojibway (n = 18) found no association with any RA shared epitope positive allele, but did find an increase in HLA-DRB1*0901 [72].

Seronegative polyarticular JIA has been associated with HLA-DR8 [60,70,71,73] and HLA-DQ4 (DQA1*0401/DQB1*0402) [71,73]. An increase in

Table 3.11 HLA associations with JIA: stratified by major subgroup

Subgroup by onset	HLA allele	No. cases	% positive	No. controls	% positive	p value	OR (95%CI)
All							
	A2	680	62	254	52	0.001	1.5 (1.2–1.8)
	B27	680	14	254	8	0.05	1.8 (1.3–2.6)
	DR5(11)	680	29	254	14	0.05	1.8 (1.4–2.4)
	DRB1*1104	319	10	203	5	0.05	2.0 (1.2–3.3)
	DR8	680	19	254	7	0.001	3.0 (2.1–4.3)
	DRB1*0101	319	20	203	13	0.05	1.7 (1.2–2.4)
	DQA1*0101/4	452	32	86	24	0.05	1.4 (1.1–1.8)
	DQA1*0103	452	11	186	17	<0.001	0.6 (0.4–0.8)
	DQA1*03	452	24	186	35	<0.001	0.6 (0.4–0.8)
	DQA1*0401	452	6	186	21	<0.001	0.3 (0.2–0.4)
	DPB1*0201	464	34	210	24	0.001	1.6 (1.2–2.1)
Pauciarticular							
	A2	377	68	254	52	0.001	2.0 (1.6–2.5)
	B27	377	19	254	8	0.001	2.6 (1.8–3.4)
	DR4	377	16	254	31	<0.001	0.4 (0.3–0.6)
	DRB1*0401	206	4	203	11	<0.001	0.4 (0.2–0.6)
	DR5(11)	206	32	254	14	0.001	2.8 (2.1–3.9)
	DRB1*1104	206	12	203	5	0.001	2.5 (1.5–4.1)
	DR6(13)	377	29	254	22	0.05	1.4 (1.1–1.9)
	DR7	377	12	254	23	<0.001	0.5 (0.3–0.6)
	DR8	377	25	254	7	0.001	4.3 (2.9–6.2)
	DQA1*03	264	15	186	35	<0.001	0.3 (0.2–0.5)
	DPB1*0201	268	43	210	24	0.001	2.4 (1.8–3.1)
Polyarticular							
	DR1	184	25	254	18	0.001	1.5 (1.1–2.1)
	DRB1*0101	80	23	203	13	0.05	2.0 (1.2–3.1)
	DR5(11)	184	23	254	14	0.05	1.8 (1.3–2.5)
	DR7	184	16	254	23	<0.001	0.6 (0.4–0.9)
	DR8	184	13	254	7	0.001	2.0 (1.2–3.0)
	DRB1*1301	80	2	203	23	0.05	0.08 (0.03–0.2)
	DQA1*0101/4	121	40	186	24	0.001	2.1 (1.5–3.0)
	DQA1*0103	121	10	186	17	<0.001	0.5 (0.3–0.8)
	DQA1*0401	121	12	186	21	<0.001	0.5 (0.3–0.8)
Systemic							
	DR4	119	40	254	31	0.05	1.5 (1.1–2.0)
	DRB1*1301	70	24	203	10	0.05	2.8 (1.7–4.6)
	DQA1*0401	67	7	186	21	<0.001	1.0 (0.5–2.0)

Source: data derived from [69].

HLA-DP3 (DPB1*0301) has also been found in some studies [71,73]. The largest number of studies have looked at HLA associations with pauciarticular disease, particularly in children with an early age of disease onset. The finding of an increased HLA-A2 in pauciarticular patients with an early disease onset [55], has been confirmed in many studies [58,74,75], molecular methods indicating that it is the HLA-A*0201 sub-type that is increased [56]. In keeping with many previous studies, Murray *et al.* [59] reported an increase in DR5 [11], DR8, DR6 [13], and DPB1*0201 [58,76].

Murray *et al.* [59] also confirmed the decrease in HLA-DR4 and DR7 which are consistently reported to be reduced in all JIA subgroups other than RF-positive polyarticular JIA. Why there should be multiple HLA associations, particularly with pauciarticular disease, has not yet been fully established. Some possible mechanisms are reviewed in Albert and Scholz [76].

A subdivision of JIA patients according to age at disease onset is common practise, but varies between studies; under 5, under 6, and under 8 all having been used to define early onset disease. This makes comparisons between studies difficult. Murray *et al.*

[59] also aimed to define more precisely the age limits of HLA-associated risks in JRA. They show that there are HLA-specific windows of susceptibility which are unique to each JIA subtype.

There is always a worry with population-based studies in that any associations found are due to population stratification rather than linkage. However, Moroldo *et al.* [77], using transmission disequilibrium test in 101 caucasian North American families, established linkage between the MHC and pauciarticular onset JRA and Prahalad *et al.* confirmed this using allele sharing in affected sib pairs [78]. The affected sib pair study also established evidence of linkage between polyarticular JRA and the HLA-DR region. In this study of 80 ASPs, 10 per cent of sibpairs shared zero alleles compared with the 25 per cent expected, giving an estimated λs for HLA-DR of 2.5. Given that the λs for JIA is estimated as 15, then the proportional λs for HLA-DR is 17 per cent, leaving a further 83 per cent of the genetic risk unaccounted for. Some of the additional risk may come from other genes within the MHC but it is likely that other non-MHC genes will also be involved. Identification of non-HLA, JIA susceptibility genes is the focus of many current studies.

Non-genetic factors

There have been very few investigations of possible environmental and related risk factors. The major aetiological hypothesis is that the disease results from an infectious trigger in a genetically susceptible host. There is no evidence that socioeconomic factors are associated. Thus parental occupation, maternal education, and over-crowding are not found to be risk factors [35,79]. Indeed, inexplicably, it is high parental income that was associated with an increased risk [35].

Environmental factors around birth may be important [36,79] with the latter study showing that breast-fed children had 40 per cent of the risk of never-breast-fed, with evidence of a duration–protection effect: those breast-fed for more than 3 months having half the risk of those fed for less than that period [79].

Infectious agents

The cyclical pattern in onset of JIA has been shown to mirror the occurrence in the same population of epidemics of *Mycobacterium pneumoniae* and respiratory syncitial virus (Fig. 3.1) [21]. Thus the peak years of

onset (1985, 1991) mirrored epidemics with these agents. Case-control studies have been performed to determine the possible role of viral infection(s) as either a trigger or direct pathogen in JIA. Numerous viruses, including wild-type rubella, influenza A, mumps, varicella, hepatitis B, parvovirus, Coxsackie virus, Epstein–Barr virus, and Ross River virus are associated with arthritic complications [80]. To test the hypothesis that viral infection causes JIA (i.e. chronic arthritis), several groups have determined virus-specific antibody levels in serum from patients and control subjects for indirect evidence of previous or ongoing infection [36,81–87].

A comparison of sera from 42 children with JIA and 46 age- and sex-matched healthy controls for antibodies to mumps, measles, and poliovirus showed similar antibody levels. By contrast, JIA patients had a significantly higher geometric mean rubella antibody titre than that of controls. JIA suggests a possible role of rubella virus infection in the aetiology or pathogenesis of JIA [83]. Similar findings have been reported by others [81,82], although with differences in their interpretation. Linnemann *et al.* [82]) studied sera from 85 patients with well-documented JIA and age- and sex-matched controls for rubella antibody and serum immunoglobulin levels and noted a significant direct correlation between serum IgA and rubella antibody titres. The raised rubella antibody levels seen in JIA patients could most probably reflect a general increase in serum immunoglobulins. Indeed, the work by Phillips [84] on JIA support this interpretation and suggest that small-to-moderate elevations of viral antibody titres result from a generalized hyper-responsiveness in humoral immunity in these patients which is reflected in hyperglobulinaemia. Other work [86], however, supports a direct role for rubella virus in some cases of JIA. Rubella virus from either peripheral blood or synovial fluid mononuclear cells was isolated in seven of 19 patients (one of five cases with systemic onset, two of two cases with polyarthritis, and four of 12 cases with pauciarthritis) compared to none of 16 health controls. Thus, antecedent rubella infection, or even immunization with wild-type rubella vaccine [88], could lead to JIA. Recently there has been a case report linking *Bartonella* infection with systemic JIA [119].

Lyme disease

One infectious condition which can produce an arthritis that mimics JIA is Lyme disease. The arthritis is typically episodic involving only one or a few large joints [89–91]; thus, its clinical similarity to pauciarticular JIA. Lyme disease was originally described in a geographic cluster of cases of JIA in a rural Connecticut community in 1977 [92]; it is now recognized as the most commonly reported vector-transmitted disease in the US [93] and is known to occur in a world-wide distribution with cases reported in Canada [90], the UK [94], Europe, Scandinavia, Japan, China, Australia, and the Soviet Union [95,96]. Lyme disease is caused by a spirochete, *Borrelia burgdorferi*, which is transmitted via a bite from a tick of the *Ixodes ricinus* family. In the US, *I. dammini* is the responsible vector in the east and midwest, while *I. pacificus* occurs in the far west. In Europe, the vector is *I. racinun*, while in Japan, the vector is *I. persulcatus* [95]. The vector ecology of Lyme disease is felt to explain its geographic and seasonal distribution; this topic has been recently reviewed elsewhere [97]. The case definition for epidemiological studies, developed by the Centres for Disease Control, emphasizes the central role of erythema migrans, the pathognomonic skin lesion, and the need for laboratory confirmation of infection with measurement of IgG or IgM antibodies against *B. burgdorferi* in subjects with arthritis alone [96]. Studies of seroprevalence of *Borrelia* in 'sporadic' JIA patients showed higher levels in controls suggesting that outside Lyme disease this organism is unimportant in explaining disease susceptibility [98].

References

1. Pelkonen PM, Jalanko HJ, Lantto RK, Makela AL, Pietikainen MA, Savolainen HA et al. Incidence of systemic connective tissue diseases in children: a nation-wide prospective study in Finland. *J Rheumatol* 1994; 21: 2143–2146.
2. Oen KG, Cheang M. Epidemiology of chronic arthritis in childhood. *Semin Arthritis Rheum* 1996; 26: 575–591.
3. Diament-Berger MS. *Du rhumatisme noueux (polyarthrite déformante) chez les enfants*. Paris: Lecrosnier et Babé, 1891.
4. Still GF. On a form of chronic joint disease in children. *Med Chir Trans* 1897; 80: 47–59.
5. Ansell BM, Bywaters EGL. Prognosis in Still's disease. *Bull Rheum Dis* 1959; 9: 189–192.
6. Brewer Jr EJ, Bass JC, Cassidy JT, Duran BS, Fink CW, Jacobs JC et al. Criteria for the classification of juvenile rheumatoid arthritis. *Bull Rheum Dis* 1972; 23: 712–719.
7. Brewer Jr EJ, Bass J, Baum J, Cassidy JT, Fink C, Jacobs J et al. Current proposed revision of JRA Criteria. JRA Criteria Subcommittee of the Diagnostic and Thera-

peutic Criteria Committee of the American Rheumatism Section of The Arthritis Foundation. *Arthritis Rheum* 1977; 20 (2 Suppl.): 195–199.
8. Bywaters EGL. Report from the subcommittee on diagnostic criteria for juvenile rheumatoid arthritis (Still's disease). In: Bennett PH, Wood PHN, eds. *Population studies of the rheumatic diseases: proceedings of the Third International Symposium, New York, June 5th–10th, 1966*. Amsterdam: Excerpta Medica Foundation, 1968: 241.
9. Fink CW. Proposal for the development of classification criteria for idiopathic arthritides of childhood [see comments] [published erratum appears in *J Rheumatol* 1995; 22: 2195]. *J Rheumatol* 1995; 22: 1566–1569.
10. Petty RE. Viruses and childhood arthritis. *Ann Med* 1997; 29: 149–152.
11. Foeldvari I, Bidde M. Validation of the proposed ILAR classification criteria for juvenile idiopathic arthritis. International League of Associations for Rheumatology. *J Rheumatol* 2000; 27: 1069–1072.
12. Ramsey SE, Bolaria RK, Cabral DA, Malleson PN, Petty RE. Comparison of criteria for the classification of childhood arthritis. *J Rheumatol* 2000; 27: 1283–1286.
13. Thomas E, Barrett JH, Donn RP, Thomson W, Southwood TR. Subtyping of juvenile idiopathic arthritis using latent class analysis. British Paediatric Rheumatology Group. *Arthritis Rheum* 2000; 43: 1496–1503.
14. De Clercq L, Joos R, Veys EM, Mielants H, Castro S, Ackerman C et al. Epidemiologic survey of juvenile chronic arthritis in Belgium. *Arthritis Rheum* 1992; 35: S191.
15. Kaipiainen-Seppanen O, Savolainen A. Incidence of chronic juvenile rheumatic diseases in Finland during 1980–1990. *Clin Exp Rheumatol* 1996; 14: 441–444.
16. Symmons DP, Jones M, Osborne J, Sills J, Southwood TR, Woo P. Pediatric rheumatology in the United Kingdom: data from the British Pediatric Rheumatology Group National Diagnostic Register. *J Rheumatol* 1996; 23: 1975–1980.
17. Moe N, Rygg M. Epidemiology of juvenile chronic arthritis in northern Norway: a ten-year retrospective study. *Clin Exp Rheumatol* 1998; 16: 99–101.
18. Kiessling U, Doring E, Listing J, Meincke J, Schontube M, Strangfeld A et al. Incidence and prevalence of juvenile chronic arthritis in East Berlin 1980–88. *J Rheumatol* 1998; 25: 1837–1843.
19. Peterson LS, Mason T, Nelson AM, O'Fallon WM, Gabriel SE. Juvenile rheumatoid arthritis in Rochester, Minnesota 1960–1993. Is the epidemiology changing? *Arthritis Rheum* 1996; 39: 1385–1390.
20. Malleson PN, Fung MY, Rosenberg AM. The incidence of pediatric rheumatic diseases: results from the Canadian Pediatric Rheumatology Association disease registry. *J Rheumatol* 1996; 23: 1981–1987.
21. Oen K, Fast M, Postl B. Epidemiology of juvenile rheumatoid arthritis in Manitoba, Canada, 1975–92: cycles in incidence. *J Rheumatol* 1995; 22: 745–750.
22. Boyer GS, Lanier AP, Templin DW. Prevalence rates of spondyloarthropathies, rheumatoid arthritis, and other rheumatic disorders in an Alaskan Inupiat Eskimo population. *J Rheumatol* 1988; 15: 678–683.

23. Bowyer S, Roettcher P. Pediatric rheumatology clinic populations in the United States: results of a 3 year survey. Pediatric Rheumatology Database Research Group. *J Rheumatol* 1996; **23**: 1968–1974.

24. Hill R. Juvenile arthritis in various racial groups in British Columbia. *Arthritis Rheum* 1977; **20** (2 Suppl.): 162.

25. Okubo H, Itou K, Tanaka S, Watanabe N, Kashiwagi N, Obata F. Analysis of the HLA-DR gene frequencies in Japanese cases of juveniles rheumatoid arthritis and rheumatoid arthritis by oligonucleotide DNA typing. *Rheumatol Int* 1993; **13**: 65–69.

26. Pongpanich B, Daengroongroj P. Juvenile rheumatoid arthritis: clinical characteristics in 100 Thai patients. *Clin Rheumatol* 1988; **7**: 257–261.

27. Boyer GS, Lanier AP, Templin DW, Bulkow L. Spondyloarthropathy and rheumatoid arthritis in Alaskan Yupik Eskimos. *J Rheumatol* 1990; **17**: 489–496.

28. Boyer GS, Templin DW, Lanier AP. Rheumatic diseases in Alaskan Indians of the southeast coast: high prevalence of rheumatoid arthritis and systemic lupus erythematosus. *J Rheumatol* 1991; **18**: 1477–1484.

29. Ozen S, Karaaslan Y, Ozdemir O, Saatci U, Bakkaloglu A, Koroglu E *et al*. Prevalence of juvenile chronic arthritis and familial Mediterranean fever in Turkey: a field study. *J Rheumatol* 1998; **25**: 2445–2449.

30. Khuffash FA, Majeed HA. Juvenile rheumatoid arthritis among Arab children. *Scand J Rheumatol* 1988; **17**: 393–395.

31. Arguedas O, Porras O, Fasth A. Juvenile chronic arthritis in Costa Rica. A pilot referral study. *Clin Exp Rheumatol* 1995; **13**: 119–123.

32. Hochberg MC, Linet MS, Sills EM. The prevalence and incidence of juvenile rheumatoid arthritis in an urban Black population. *Am J Public Health* 1983; **73**: 1202–1203.

33. Hanson V, Kornreich H, Bernstein B, King KK, Singsen B. Prognosis of juvenile rheumatoid arthritis. *Arthritis Rheum* 1977; **20** (2 Suppl.): 279–284.

34. Pagan TM, Arroyo IL. Juvenile rheumatoid arthritis in Caribbean children: a clinical characterization. *Bol Asoc Med P R* 1991; **83**: 527–529.

35. Nielsen HE, Dorup J, Herlin T, Larsen K, Nielsen S, Pedersen FK. Epidemiology of juvenile chronic arthritis: risk dependent on sibship, parental income, and housing. *J Rheumatol* 1999; **26**: 1600–1605.

36. Pritchard MH, Matthews N, Munro J. Antibodies to influenza A in a cluster of children with juvenile chronic arthritis. *Br J Rheumatol* 1988; **27**: 176–180.

37. Feldman BM, Birdi N, Boone JE, Dent PB, Duffy CM, Ellsworth JE *et al*. Seasonal onset of systemic-onset juvenile rheumatoid arthritis. *J Pediatr* 1996; **129**: 513–518.

38. Lindsley CB. Seasonal variation in systemic onset juvenile rheumatoid arthritis. *Arthritis Rheum* 1987; **30**: 838–839.

39. Andersson Gäre B, Fasth A. Epidemiology of juvenile chronic arthritis in southwestern Sweden: a 5-year prospective population study. *Pediatrics* 1992; **90**: 950–958.

40. Glass DN, Giannini EH. Juvenile rheumatoid arthritis as a complex genetic trait. *Arthritis Rheum* 1999; **42**: 2261–2268.

41. Meyerowitz S, Jacox RF, Hess DW. Monozygotic twins discordant for rheumatoid arthritis: a genetic, clinical and psychological study of 8 sets. *Arthritis Rheum* 1968; **11**: 1–21.

42. Ansell BM, Bywaters EGL, Lawrence JS. Familial aggregation and twin studies in Still's disease: juvenile chronic polyarthritis. *Rheumatology* 1969; **2**: 37–61.

43. Ansell BM. Chronic arthritis in childhood. *Ann Rheum Dis* 1978; **37**: 107–120.

44. Baum J, Fink C. Juvenile rheumatoid arthritis in monozygotic twins: a case report and review of the literature. *Arthritis Rheum* 1968; **11**: 33–36.

45. Kapusta MA, Metrakos JD, Pinsky L, Shugar JL, Naimark AP. Juvenile rheumatoid arthritis in a mother and her identical twin sons. *Arthritis Rheum* 1969; **12**: 411–413.

46. Husby G, Williams-RC J, Tung KS, Smith FE, Cronin RJ, Sletten K *et al*. Immunologic studies in identical twins concordant for juvenile rheumatoid arthritis but discordant for monoclonal gammopathy and amyloidosis. *J Lab Clin Med* 1988; **111**: 307–314.

47. Prahalad S, Ryan MH, Shear ES, Thompson SD, Glass DN, Giannini EH. Twins concordant for juvenile rheumatoid arthritis. *Arthritis Rheum* 2000; **43**: 2611–2612.

48. Ansell BM, Bywaters EGL, Lawrence JS. A family study in Still's disease. *Ann Rheum Dis* 1962; **21**: 243–252.

49. Yodfat Y, Yossipovitch Z, Cohen I, Shapira E. A family with a high incidence of juvenile rheumatoid arthritis. *Ann Rheum Dis* 1972; **31**: 92–94.

50. Omenn GS. Genetics of rheumatic diseases. *Arthritis Rheum* 1977; **20** (2 Suppl.): 473–483.

51. Hochberg MC, Bias WB, Arnett Jr FC. Family studies in HLA-B27 associated arthritis. *Medicine* (Baltimore) 1978; **57**: 463–475.

52. Rosenberg AM, Petty RE. Similar patterns of juvenile rheumatoid arthritis within families. *Arthritis Rheum* 1980; **23**: 951–953.

53. Clemens LE, Albert E, Ansell BM. Sibling pairs affected by chronic arthritis of childhood: evidence for a genetic predisposition. *J Rheumatol* 1985; **12**: 108–113.

54. Rachelefsky GS, Terasaki PI, Katz R, Stiehm ER. Increased prevalence of W27 in juvenile rheumatoid arthritis. *N Engl J Med* 1974; **290**: 892–893.

55. Oen K, Petty RE, Schroeder ML. An association between HLA-A2 and juvenile rheumatoid arthritis in girls. *J Rheumatol* 1982; **9**: 916–920.

56. Fernandez-Vina MA, Falco M, Sun Y, Stastny P. DNA typing for HLA class I alleles: I. Subsets of HLA-A2 and of -A28. *Hum Immunol* 1992; **33**: 163–173.

57. Glass DN, Litvin DA. Heterogeneity of HLA associations in systemic onset juvenile rheumatoid arthritis. *Arthritis Rheum* 1980; **23**: 796–799.

58. Donn RP, Ollier WER. Juvenile chronic arthritis: a time for change. *Eur J Immunogen* 1996; **23**: 245–260.

59. Murray KJ, Moroldo MB, Donnelly P, Prahalad S, Passo MH, Giannini EH *et al*. Age-specific effects of juvenile rheumatoid arthritis-associated HLA alleles. *Arthritis Rheum* 1999; **42**: 1843–1853.

60. Morling N, Friis J, Heilmann C, Hellesen C, Jakobsen BK, Jorgensen B et al. HLA antigen frequencies in juvenile chronic arthritis. *Scand J Rheumatol* 1985; **14**: 209–216.

61. Fantini F, Gerloni V, Murelli M, Gattinara M, Negro A, Sciascia T et al. HLA phenotypes in subsets of pauciarticular onset juvenile chronic arthritis (JCA). *Eur J Pediatr* 1987; **146**: 338–338.

62. Forre O, Dobloug JH, Hoyeraal HM, Thorsby E. HLA antigens in juvenile arthritis: genetic basis for the different subtypes. *Arthritis Rheum* 1983; **26**: 35–38.

63. Miller ML, Aaron S, Jackson J, Fraser P, Cairns L, Hoch S et al. HLA gene frequencies in children and adults with systemic onset juvenile rheumatoid arthritis. *Arthritis Rheum* 1985; **28**: 146–150.

64. Singh G, Mehra NK, Taneja V, Seth V, Malaviya AN, Ghai OP. Histocompatibility antigens in systemic-onset juvenile rheumatoid arthritis. *Arthritis Rheum* 1989; **32**: 1492–1493.

65. Bedford PA, Ansell BM, Hall PJ, Woo P. Increased frequency of DR4 in systemic onset juvenile chronic arthritis. *Clin Exp Rheumatol* 1992; **10**: 189–193.

66. Date Y, Seki N, Kamizono S, Higuchi T, Hirata T, Miyata K et al. Identification of a genetic risk factor for systemic juvenile rheumatoid arthritis in the 5'-flanking region of the TNFalpha gene and HLA genes. *Arthritis Rheum* 1999; **42**: 2577–2582.

67. Desaymard C, Kaplan C, Fournier C, Manigne P, Hayem F, Kahn M-F et al. Étude des marqueurs du système majeur d'histocompatibilité et de l'hétérogénéité clinique de la forme systémique d'arthrite chronique juvénile: a propos de 108 patients. *Rev Rhum Ed Fr* 1996; **63**: 11–18.

68. Stastny P, Fink CW. Different HLA-D associations in adult and juvenile rheumatoid arthritis. *J Clin Invest* 1979; **63**: 124–130.

69. Vehe RK, Begovich AB, Nepom BS. HLA susceptibility genes in rheumatoid factor positive juvenile rheumatoid arthritis. *J Rheumatol* 1990; **26** (Suppl): 11–15.

70. Fernandez-Vina MA, Fink CW, Stastny P. HLA antigens in juvenile arthritis: pauciarticular and polyarticular juvenile arthritis are immunogenetically distinct. *Arthritis Rheum* 1990; **33**: 1787–1794.

71. Ploski R, Vinje O, Ronningen KS, Spurkland A, Sorskaar D, Vartdal F et al. HLA class II alleles and heterogeneity of juvenile rheumatoid arthritis: DRB1*0101 may define a novel subset of the disease. *Arthritis Rheum* 1993; **36**: 465–472.

72. Oen K, El Gabalawy HS, Canvin JM, Hitchon C, Chalmers IM, Schroeder M et al. HLA associations of seropositive rheumatoid arthritis in a Cree and Ojibway population. *J Rheumatol* 1998; **25**: 2319–2323.

73. Barron KS, Silverman ED, Gonzales JC, Owerbach D, Reveille JD. DNA analysis of HLA-DR, DQ, and DP alleles in children with polyarticular juvenile rheumatoid arthritis. *J Rheumatol* 1992; **19**: 1611–1616.

74. Hall PJ, Burman SJ, Laurent MR, Briggs DC, Venning HE, Leak AM et al. Genetic susceptibility to early onset pauciarticular juvenile chronic arthritis: a study of HLA and complement markers in 158 British patients. *Ann Rheum Dis* 1986; **45**: 464–474.

75. Brunner HI, Ivaskova E, Haas JP, Andreas A, Keller E, Hoza J et al. Class I associations and frequencies of class II HLA-DRB alleles by RFLP analysis in children with rheumatoid-factor-negative juvenile chronic arthritis. *Rheumatol Int* 1993; **13**: 83–88.

76. Albert ED, Scholz S. Juvenile arthritis: genetic update. *Baillieres Clin Rheumatol* 1998; **12**: 209–218.

77. Moroldo MB, Donnelly P, Saunders J, Glass DN, Giannini EH. Transmission disequilibrium as a test of linkage and association between HLA alleles and pauciarticular-onset juvenile rheumatoid arthritis. *Arthritis Rheum* 1998; **41**: 1620–1624.

78. Prahalad S, Ryan MH, Shear ES, Thompson SD, Giannini EH, Glass DN. Juvenile rheumatoid arthritis: linkage to HLA demonstrated by allele sharing in affected sibpairs. *Arthritis Rheum* 2000; **43**: 2335–2338.

79. Mason T, Rabinovich CE, Fredrickson DD, Amoroso K, Reed AM, Stein LD et al. Breast feeding and the development of juvenile rheumatoid arthritis. *J Rheumatol* 1995; **22**: 1166–1170.

80. Steere AC, Malawista SE. Viral arthritis. In: McCarty Jr DJ, ed. *Arthritis and allied conditions*. Philadelphia: Lea and Febiger, 1985: 1697–1712.

81. Cassidy JT, Shillis JL, Brandon FB, Sullivan DB, Brackett RG. Viral antibody titers to rubella and rubeola in juvenile rheumatoid arthritis. *Pediatrics* 1974; **54**: 239–244.

82. Linnemann Jr CC, Levinson JE, Buncher CR, Schiff GM. Rubella antibody levels in juvenile rheumatoid arthritis. *Ann Rheum Dis* 1975; **34**: 354–358.

83. Ogra PL, Chiba Y, Ogra SS, Dzierba JL, Herd JK. Rubella-virus infection in juvenile rheumatoid arthritis. *Lancet* 1975; **1**: 1157–1161.

84. Phillips PE. Infection and chronic rheumatic disease in children. *Semin Arthritis Rheum* 1980; **10**: 92–99.

85. De Vere-Tyndall A, Bacon T, Parry R, Tyrrell DA, Denman AM, Ansell BM. Infection and interferon production in systemic juvenile chronic arthritis: a prospective study. *Ann Rheum Dis* 1984; **43**: 1–7.

86. Chantler JK, Tingle AJ, Petty RE. Persistent rubella virus infection associated with chronic arthritis in children. *N Engl J Med* 1985; **313**: 1117–1123.

87. Denman AM. A viral aetiology for juvenile chronic arthritis? *Br J Rheumatol* 1988; **27**: 169–170.

88. Chantler JK, Ford DK, Tingle AJ. Persistent rubella infection and rubella associated arthritis. *Lancet* 1982; **1**: 1323–1325.

89. Steere AC, Schoen RT, Taylor E. The clinical evolution of Lyme arthritis. *Ann Intern Med* 1987; **107**: 725–731.

90. Bollegraaf E. Lyme disease in Canada. *Can Med Assoc J* 1988; **139**: 233–234.

91. Steere AC. Lyme disease. *N Engl J Med* 1989; **321**: 586–596.

92. Steere AC, Malawista SE, Snydman DR, Shope RE, Andiman WA, Ross MR et al. Lyme arthritis: an epidemic of oligoarticular arthritis in children and adults in three Connecticut communities. *Arthritis Rheum* 1977; **20**: 7–17.

93. Ciesielski CA, Markowitz LE, Horsley R, Hightwoer AW, Russell H, Broome CV. The geographic distribution of Lyme disease in the United States. *Ann N Y Acad Sci* 1988; **539**: 283–288.

94. Muhlemann MF, Wright DJ. Emerging pattern of Lyme disease in the United Kingdom and Irish Republic. *Lancet* 1987; **1**: 260–262.

95. Rahn DW. Lyme disease: clinical manifestations, diagnosis, and treatment. *Semin Arthritis Rheum* 1991; **20**: 201–218.

96. Rahn DW, Craft J. Lyme disease. *Rheum Dis Clin North Am* 1990; **16**: 601–615.

97. Burgdorfer W. Vector / host relationships of the Lyme disease spirochete, Borrelia burgdorferi. *Rheum Dis Clin North Am* 1989; **15**: 775–787.

98. Banerjee S, Banerjee M, Cimolai N, Malleson P, Proctor E. Seroprevalence survey of borreliosis in children with chronic arthritis in British Columbia, Canada. *J Rheumatol* 1992; **19**: 1620–1624.

99. Kunnamo I, Kallio P, Pelkonen P. Incidence of arthritis in urban Finnish children. A prospective study. *Arthritis Rheum* 1986; **29**: 1232–1238.

100. Ostergaard PA, Lillquist K, Rosthoj S, Urfe P. [Occurrence and types of juvenile rheumatoid arthritis in the County of Jutland 1970–1977 and 1978–1986] Incidens og typer af juvenil reumatoid arthritis i Nordjyllands Amt i perioden 1970–1977 og 1978–1986. *Ugeskr Laeger* 1988; **150**: 342–346.

101. Prieur AM, Le Gall E, Karman F, Edan C, Lasserre O, Goujard J. Epidemiologic survey of juvenile chronic arthritis in France. Comparison of data obtained from two different regions. *Clin Exp Rheumatol* 1987; **5**: 217–223.

102. Andersson Gäre B. Juvenile arthritis–who gets it, where and when? A review of current data on incidence and prevalence. *Clin Exp Rheumatol* 1999; **17**: 367–374.

103. Cassidy JT, Petty RE, Sullivan DB. Occurrence of selective IgA deficiency in children with juvenile rheumatoid arthritis. *Arthritis Rheum* 1977; **20** (2 Suppl.): 181–183.

104. Towner SR, Michet Jr CJ, O'Fallon WM, Nelson AM. The epidemiology of juvenile arthritis in Rochester, Minnesota 1960–1979. *Arthritis Rheum* 1983; **26**: 1208–1213.

105. Arendarczyk Z. [Rheumatoid arthritis in children up to the age of 15 in Poland]Wystepowanie reumatoidalnego zapalenia stawow u dzieci do lat 15 na terenie Polski. *Pediatr Pol* 1977; **52**: 73–78.

106. Cernay J, Jakubcova I, Vrsanska A, Michalko J, Mozolova D. [Juvenile rheumatoid arthritis, incidence and most frequent symptoms (author's transl)]Juvenilna reumatoidna artritida. Incidencia a najcastejsie priznaky. *Cas Lek Cesk* 1977; **116**: 331–335.

107. Havelka S, Hoza J, Kamenicka E. [Epidemiology of juvenile chronic arthritis in Czechoslovakia]K epidemiologii juvenilni chronicke artritidy v Ceske socialisticke republice. *Cesk Pediatr* 1986; **41**: 531–534.

108. Andersson Gäre B, Fasth A, Andersson J, Berglund G, Ekstrom H, Eriksson M et al. Incidence and prevalence of juvenile chronic arthritis: a population survey. *Ann Rheum Dis* 1987; **46**: 277–281.

109. Joos R, Veys EM, De Clercq L, Mielants H, Castro S, Ackerman C et al. Epidemiologic survey of juvenile chronic arthritis in Belgium. I. Incidence and prevalence. *J Rheumatol* 1993; **20** (Suppl. 37): 61.

110. Mielants H, Veys EM, Maertens M, Goemaere S, De Clercq L, Castro S et al. Prevalence of inflammatory rheumatic diseases in an adolescent urban student population, age 12 to 18, in Belgium. *Clin Exp Rheumatol* 1993; **11**: 563–567.

111. Steven MM. Prevalence of chronic arthritis in four geographical areas of the Scottish Highlands. *Ann Rheum Dis* 1992; **51**: 186–194.

112. Bonham GS. Prevalence of chronic skin and musculoskeletal conditions. United States -1976. *Vital Health Stat* 1978; **124**: 1–57.

113. Gewanter HL, Roghmann KJ, Baum J. The prevalence of juvenile arthritis. *Arthritis Rheum* 1983; **26**: 599–603.

114. Newacheck PW, Halfon N, Budetti PP. Prevalence of activity limiting chronic conditions among children based on household interviews. *J Chron Dis* 1986; **39**: 63–71.

115. Manners PJ, Diepeveen DA. Prevalence of juvenile chronic arthritis in a population of 12-year-old children in urban Australia. *Pediatrics* 1996; **98**: 84–90.

116. Fantini F. Classification of chronic arthritis of childhood (juvenile idiopathic arthritis): Criticisms and suggestions to improve the efficiency of the Santiago-Durban criteria. *J Rheumatol* 2001; **28**: 456–459.

117. Hofer ME, Mony R, Prieur AM. Juvenile idiopathic arthritides evaluated prospectively in a single center according to the Durban criteria. *J Rheumatol* 2001; **32**: 1083–1090.

118. Petty RE. Growing pains: The ILAR Classification of juvenile idiopathic arthritis. *J Rheumatol* 2001; **28**: 927–928.

119. Tsukahara M, Tsuneoka H, Tateishi H, Fujita K, Uchida M. *Bartonella* infection associated with systemic juvenile rheumatoid arthritis. *Clin Infect Dis* 2001; **32**: E22–E23.

4 | *Psoriatic arthropathy*

Alan J. Silman

Introduction

Epidemiologically, the concept of psoriatic arthritis is a complex one. Initially described over 150 years ago as the association of arthritis in a patient with psoriasis [1], the concept has been considerably refined as the understanding of different clinical and pathological entities of arthritis has increased. The dilemma seems superficially simple: if all the cases observed can be explained by the chance co-occurrence of two groups of relatively common disorders, psoriasis and specific types of inflammatory arthritis such as rheumatoid arthritis and ankylosing spondylitis, then the syndrome is not appropriate for consideration in an epidemiological sense. Alternatively, if either there is a distinct clinical or pathological type of arthritis restricted to psoriasis, or the presence of psoriasis increases the susceptibility to certain specific types of arthritis, then it is relevant to consider this disorder as a separate entity and investigate its epidemiology. There is also a middle ground and that is the possibility that the presence of psoriasis modifies the clinical and other features of any concurrent arthritis although the latter's occurrence is no different from that observed in the non-psoriatic population.

Is there a distinct entity of psoriatic arthritis?

In a population-based study in the Netherlands on 3659 individuals, there was no significantly increased risk of arthritis in the 41 individuals detected with psoriasis compared with the rest of the population [2] and the authors concluded that psoriatic arthritis did not exist. In reality, the sample size was too small to exclude the possibility of an increased risk. Furthermore, the cross sectional approach used was insensitive at picking up all the potential cases of the syndrome given the considerable interval reported by others between the development of psoriasis and the subsequent development of arthritis [3].

Undoubtedly, cases of rheumatoid and other forms of arthritis will occur by chance in psoriasis patients but there are two lines of evidence suggesting that psoriatic arthritis is not rheumatoid. Firstly, approximately 75 per cent of those patients with psoriasis who develop an arthritis typical of rheumatoid arthritis are rheumatoid factor negative [4]. It is this seronegativity that is taken as one of the hallmarks of the disease. However, the frequency of rheumatoid factor positivity in a general psoriatic population is low and it may be that psoriasis inhibits the production of rheumatoid factor [5]. Secondly, there are certain clinically distinctive features of psoriatic arthritis, including nail involvement (pitting etc.) and the predilection for the arthritis to involve the distal interphalangeal (DIP) joints, that have been proposed as evidence of a distinct syndrome. Support for this comes from a comparison of rheumatoid factor negative arthritis patients with and without psoriasis: the former having a greater rate of DIP involvement [6]. The strongest epidemiological study to address this question was the Norfolk Arthritis Register—a total population register of incident inflammatory polyarthritis [7]. The clinical, serological, and radiographic characteristics were compared between the 51 consecutive subjects with psoriasis and the 915 with inflammatory arthritis alone included on the register. The results showed that the subjects with psoriasis were significantly less likely to be rheumatoid factor positive erosive at 1 year and to be in remission at 1 year and were more likely to have DIP involvement at presentation [8] (Table 4.1).

Classification of psoriatic arthritis

In an attempt to clarify these issues, there have been many attempts at classifying the arthritis seen in

Table 4.1 Comparison of disease features in subjects with inflammatory polyarthritis between those with and without psoriasis; reproduced with permission of *Journal of Rheumatology* from [8]

Feature	Prevalence (%) in those		Difference (95% CI)
	With psoriasis n = 51	Without psoriasis n = 915	
DIP swelling	10 (20)	114 (13)	7 (−4,18)
Symmetry	32 (63)	571 (63)	0 (−13,14)
Rheumatoid nodules	2 (4)	57 (6)	−2 (−8,3)
Satisfy RA criteria	29 (57)	582 (64)	−7 (−21,7)
PIP swelling	35 (69)	561 (61)	8 (−6,20)
MCP swelling	32 (63)	602 (66)	−3 (−17,11)
Remission at 1 year	3 (6)	114 (13)	−7 (−13,0)
Erosions at 1 year	7/32 (22)	204/520 (39)	−17 (−32,−2)

psoriasis patients. Most would accept four basic categories: oligoarticular, polyarticular, spondylitic, and DIP joint arthritis. There are indeed considerable overlaps. Firstly, the oligoarticular group with a few large joints involved that frequently have clinical or radiological evidence of a 'central' arthritis (spondylitis or sacroiliitis). Similarly the spondylitic group frequently presented with an oligoarthritis. The polyarticular group may be restricted to those who are rheumatoid factor negative but frequently they may also develop features of a central arthritis. Furthermore, although the DIP group may express arthritis in this joint group alone, DIP joint involvement not infrequently occurs in

the presence of involvement of other joint groups [9]. Most experts would suggest that isolated peripheral enthesitis should be considered a subset of psoriatic arthritis. There is also increasing interest in the SAPHO syndrome [10] but its relationship to psoriatic arthritis is unclear.

In an attempt to convey these concepts and to clarify what will be considered in this chapter, the contribution of psoriatic arthritis to the 'universe' of inflammatory arthritis is shown in Fig. 4.1. The size of the circles is not meant to illustrate the relative size of the groups.

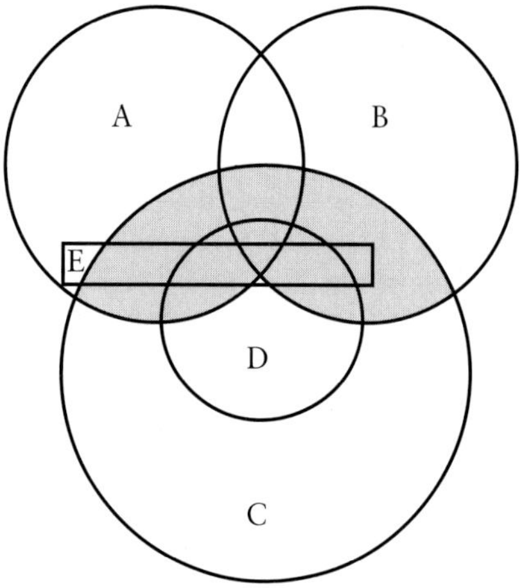

Criteria for psoriatic arthritis

Given what has been stated above, it is not surprising that psoriatic arthritis has proved a difficult disorder to define as an entity for study. It is also necessary to have criteria for both the skin and the joint components. Baker [11] listed the criteria (Table 4.2a) to be used in

Fig. 4.1 Diagrammatic representation of inter-relationships between psoriasis and the various components of psoriatic arthritis. A – peripheral inflammatory joint disease, B – central inflammatory joint disease, C – psoriasis, D – nail involvement, E – DIP joint involvement, hatched area – 'psoriatic arthritis'.

Table 4.2a Criteria for borderline psoriasis

1. Palpable scalp lesions

2. Scalp involvement is patchy (i.e. distinguishing it from dandruff)

3. Classical plaques required if eczema or related condition also present

4. Toe nail lesions alone insufficient

5. In the absence of unequivocal skin involvement nail changes of pitting and onycholysis are acceptable

6. Flexural lesions in the absence of psoriasis elsewhere are only acceptable if fungal infection excluded and margins clearly defined

7. Pustular lesions on palms and soles not acceptable alone

Source: [11].

Table 4.2b Criteria for psoriatic arthritis in presence of psoriasis

---

1. Joint pain in 3 or more limb joints (joint groups); no duration stipulated

2. Soft tissue swelling, limitation subluxation of ankylosis of 3 or more limb joints, including at least involvement of one joint in hands, wrists or feet, excluding first CMC, first MTP, and hips

OR

Satisfying New York criteria for ankylosing spondylitis

Source: [4].

Table 4.3 Comparison of performance of existing classification criteria sets for arthritis patients with psoriasis; reproduced with permission of *Journal of Rheumatology* from [16]

Criteria set	Sensitivity[a] (n=92)	Specificity[a] (n = 130)
Moll and Wright	61	100
ESSG	65	100
Amor	65	99
Any	84	100

[a]Based on clinician's judgement on presence/ absence arthritis.

cases of borderline psoriasis, the clear case needing no comment. Moll and Wright [4] suggested that the existing, internationally agreed criteria for the presence of rheumatoid arthritis and ankylosing spondylitis could be applied to the diagnosis of psoriatic arthritis as the emphasis was on ensuring inflammation at the relevant joint sites. However, one problem is that the 1987 revised ARA criteria for rheumatoid arthritis [12] are positive in over 70 per cent of cases of psoriatic arthritis [13]. There are three criteria sets for inflammatory polyarthritis suggested for use in patients with psoriasis: Moll and Wright, 1973 (Table 4.2b) [4], European Spondyloarthritis Study Group (ESSG) 1991 (Table 4.2c) [14], and French [15]. Undoubtedly they ascertain different individuals and, in use, have a lower sensitivity compared to expert clinical opinion (Table 4.3) [16]. An optimal case definition appropriate for epidemiological surveys is lacking.

Table 4.2c The European Spondyloarthropathy Study Group preliminary criteria for the classification of spondyloarthropathy

---

1. Inflammatory spinal pain

OR

2. Synovitis—asymmetric or predominantly in the lower limbs

And one or more of:

1. Positive family history

2. Psoriasis

3. Inflammatory bowel disease

4. Urithritis, cervicitis, or acute diarrhoea within 1 month before arthritis

5. Buttock pain alternating between right and left gluteal areas

6. Enthesopathy

7. Sacroiliitis

Source: [14]

Occurrence

The prevalence of psoriatic arthritis has been described using a number of approaches. Firstly, there have been a few population surveys describing the point prevalence based on the co-occurrence, at the time of the survey, of both psoriasis and a 'relevant' arthritis. Secondly, the prevalence of clinically ascertained cases alive at an arbitrary point describes the prevalence of 'ever diagnosed'. Thirdly, and more frequently, there have been surveys of patients with psoriasis to determine the cumulative prevalence of arthritis up to the point of the survey. Finally, the point prevalence estimates of psoriasis in series of patients with arthritis have been described. The latter two approaches are hampered in their interpretation by a lack of knowledge of the selection factors involved in determining entry to the survey. Thus patients with psoriasis attending a dermatologist are not a random cross-section of all psoriasis patients and almost certainly represent a more severely affected group, and possibly also a group with an increased rate of co-morbidity including arthritis. Despite the different potential approaches to estimating the occurrence of psoriatic arthritis, the occurrence of psoriatic arthritis is influenced considerably by the occurrence of psoriasis and it is useful to briefly review this.

Prevalence of psoriasis

A questionnaire survey of 14 000 individuals aged 20–54 in Finland obtained a cumulative prevalence of 5 per cent, which was the same in both sexes [17]. The concern with such data, based on self-reports, is in overestimating the true occurrence.

More stringent approaches have suggested lower but similar proportions. Large population studies of over 100 000 individuals in the Faroes [18] and over

20 000 individuals in different regions of Sweden [19] were consistent in suggesting a point prevalence of around 2.5 per cent of the adult population. The Health Interview Survey in 1980 in the US (quoted by Lawrence *et al.* [20]), suggested a point prevalence of 0.7 per cent with equal rates in men and women. This was based on diagnosis made by a physician which could be an under ascertainment. A survey of 738 general surgical patients in the UK by a trained dermatologist, observed a prevalence of 1.5 per cent [21]. The most recent survey of Lapps [22] yielded a prevalence of 1.4 per cent based on the review of medical records. One problem in interpreting these data is the difference between surveys of current disease, which are likely to be less subject to error but would miss remitted problems, and surveys of 'ever affected' which are almost impossible to validate.

Effect of age

Psoriasis is obviously a disorder that can occur at any age and has a variable duration. It would appear that the first attack occurs early in life and onset in the elderly is rare. Psoriasis itself is not infrequent in childhood: cumulative frequency 0.3 per cent [23], yet psoriatic arthritis is rare. The age-specific cumulative incidence rates based on the questionnaire survey in Finland mentioned above (Table 4.4) [17] are of interest in demonstrating the lack of an age effect on pre-

valence. The most obvious deduction is that onset is confined to early adult life or childhood with few new cases emerging subsequently. As discussed below, this pattern is reflected in the modest influence of age on the occurrence of psoriatic arthritis in contrast to other forms of inflammatory arthritis.

Population surveys of psoriatic arthritis

Data on the prevalence of psoriatic arthritis derived from population surveys are very few in number given the rarity of the disorder. In the first reported study in 1969 of 39 418 individuals aged 7 and over [24], the prevalence of inflammatory arthritis of the 'rheumatoid type', in association with psoriasis, was 2.2/10 000 in females and only slightly higher in males. The results of this survey showed that 3 per cent of individuals detected with rheumatoid arthritis had psoriasis and similarly 3.1 per cent of psoriasis patients had definite rheumatoid arthritis. Both these proportions were higher than matched non-arthritic (1.8 per cent) and non-psoriatic controls (0.6 per cent). Hellgren refined his arthritis group into those he considered to have psoriatic arthritis. As a consequence 27 per cent of males and 18 per cent of females with 'rheumatoid arthritis' and psoriasis were considered to have psoriatic arthritis. Overall, of the 2 per cent in that population with psoriasis, 1.15 per cent of males and 1.1 per cent of females had psoriatic arthritis equivalent to a prevalence of two per 10 000. More recent surveys (Table 4.5) suggest that the estimate was out by a factor of 10.

In the major population survey in the Netherlands [6], the population surveyed was smaller and the estimates less robust. In all, 41 individuals were discovered with psoriasis and eight had various forms of inflammatory arthritis both central and peripheral. Restricting analysis to those individuals who were rheumatoid factor negative and had nail lesions, yielded the estimate of 1.1/1000 shown (Table 4.5). It would be appropriate to point out that the Dutch study was more rigorous in the methods used to detect arthri-

Table 4.4 Population prevalence of psoriasis

| Age | Prevalence (%) | |
	Males	Females
20–24	4.0	5.3
25–29	4.9	5.8
30–34	4.8	5.0
35–39	5.3	4.5
40–44	5.0	4.2
45–49	4.5	3.3
50–54	4.7	Not studied

Source: [17].

Table 4.5 Population prevalence estimates of psoriatic arthritis

Reference	Population/ Country	Prevalence per 1000	
[6]	Netherlands	All inflammatory arthritis	2.2
		Rheumatoid factor negative plus nail involvement	1.1
[22]	Norway: Lapps		2.0
[25]	US		1.0 (0.8–1.2)

tis, including radiology and serology to all, and thus case ascertainment was likely to be higher. A study of 2508 Norwegian Lapps based on medical records revealed five cases of psoriatic arthritis in 35 psoriasis patients [22]. A study of 6047 psoriasis sufferers in Moscow also estimated that the population prevalence of psoriatic arthritis to be around 1/1000 [26].

Prevalence estimates based on the ascertainment of ever diagnosed cases in Olmsted County, Minnesota [25], was a similar order of magnitude though such an approach would miss underdiagnosed cases but over include those with totally remitted disease.

Surveys of arthritis in psoriasis patients

The results from surveys of psoriasis patients in hospital and other clinical series have shown much higher rates of arthritis (Table 4.6). The table describes the data from a number of differently derived psoriasis populations and there are wildly differing estimates of the frequency of arthritis. The obvious explanations for the observed differences are: (i) different levels of stringency in ascertaining cases; (ii) use of different criteria in making the diagnosis; and probably most importantly, (iii) differences in the psoriasis population studied and the possibility that in many studies the psoriasis individuals investigated were selectively more likely to have arthritis.

The different approaches used to ascertain cases are illustrated. Thus the largest survey of the Finnish Psoriatic Society [33] used a questionnaire to obtain data on arthritis whereas other studies used detailed clinical and radiographic assessment. It is also likely that individuals with psoriasis are more likely to join such a self-help group if additionally they have another problem such as arthritis. Indeed, radiographic sacroiliitis is very common in psoriatic arthritis [36], and failure to undertake pelvic X-rays could under-estimate the true occurrence of arthritis. The criteria used to define a case are rarely adequately considered. Only in the recent Italian study [16] was the influence of the different criteria available on prevalence considered. Selection factors, however, are the greatest barrier to interpreting these data. Clinic attendees with psoriasis may be selectively more likely to be referred if they have joint problems. This hypothesis is supported from the Dutch population study [2,6] in that patients with psoriasis are more likely to complain to a physician of joint pains, in the absence of obvious arthritis, than a comparable non-psoriatic population.

Surveys of psoriasis in arthritis patients

The same methodological constraints that apply to the interpretation of the occurrence of arthritis in psoriasis patients apply to the reverse. Baker [21] reviewed the

Table 4.6 Cumulative prevalence of inflammatory arthritis in patient series with psoriasis

Reference	Source of psoriasis patients	N	Source of arthritis data				Prevalence (%)		
			Patient self-report	Clinical history and examination	X-ray pelvis joints	X-ray peripheral	Males	Females	Both
[27]	Inpatients	543		✔			5.8	7.9	
[28]	Clinic attenders	1346		✔					7
[24]	Population survey	534		(Medical record review)	✔	✔	1.2	1.1	
[29]	Inpatients	500		✔	✔	✔	20	19	
[30]	Clinic attenders	100		✔	✔				12
[31]	Clinic attenders	61		✔	✔	✔			42
[6]	Population survey	41		✔	✔	✔			20
[32]	Clinic attenders	1285		✔					21
[33]	Members of Psoriatic Society	1517	✔						26
[34]	Clinic attenders	459	✔						17
[35]	Clinic attenders	555	✔						7
[16]	Clinic attenders	205		✔	✔				36[a] 22[b]

[a] Based on clinician opinion.
[b] Based on Moll and Wright criteria.

available data at that time and surprisingly found a consistent rate of psoriasis of between 2.5 and 7 per cent in patient series with arthritis. Many of these surveys were undertaken before the separate identification of specific inflammatory arthritis subgroups was considered but it provides a useful insight into the 'hospital prevalence' of the disorder. Recent population data from the Norfolk Arthritis Register discussed above showed a prevalence of approximately 5 per cent in new patients with peripheral inflammatory polyarthritis [8].

Incidence

There are a number of sources of incident data of psoriatic arthritis which in European and North American populations generate very similar estimates of between 3 and 6 per 100 000 person years (pyr). The Olmsted County Study, relying on all diagnosed cases, suggested an average incidence between 1980 and 1991 of 6.7 (95% CI 5.1–8.4)/100 000 pyr [25]. Data from Finland relying on registration to receive free medication and hence will selectively exclude those with mild disease as well as lacking diagnostic validation, generated an almost identical incidence of 6.1 (95% CI 4.6–7.6)/100 000 pyr in 1990 [37]. Data from the Norfolk Arthritis Register on the incidence of peripheral inflammatory polyarthritis with co-existent psoriasis generated a lower incidence of 3.5 (95% CI 2.3–5.1)/100 000 pyr in males and 3.4 (95% CI 2.3–4.9)/100 000 pyr in females, possibly reflecting a more stringent approach to case definition [8].

Age and gender

The influence of age and gender on these incidence estimates is shown for both the Finnish (Table 4.7) and the UK data (Table 4.8). The UK data show very little difference between the genders and a remarkable similar incidence in all age groups. The Finnish data suggest a unimodal distribution by age, with a peak in the 45–54 year age group.

The equality in prevalence between the sexes has already been referred to and this reflects, in part, the lack of a sex difference in the occurrence of psoriasis. This equality probably hides sex differences in the different clinical subgroups. Thus the peripheral arthritis type is associated with a 2:1 female excess whilst the spondylitic type, perhaps not surprisingly, is associated with a 2:1 male excess [38]. Unlike the incidence data there are no population data on the prevalence rates of

Table 4.7 Incidence of psoriatic arthritis: Finland patients on national register eligible for drug reimbursement; reproduced with permission of Oxford University Press from [37]

Age	Incidence
16–24	0.7
25–34	2.4
35–44	6.2
45–54	11.8
55–64	7.7
65–74	3.6
75–84	3.1
Total	6.1 (95% CI 4.6–7.6)

Table 4.8 Incidence of psoriatic arthritis: Norfolk, UK—patients presenting to primary care with peripheral inflammatory arthritis; reproduced with permission of *Journal of Rheumatology* from [8]

Age	Incidence/100 000 (95% CI)	
	Males	Females
15–24	0 (0–2.8)	0.8 (0.02–4.3)
25–34	4.9 (2.0–10)	4.3 (1.6–9.5)
35–44	5.3 (2.1–11)	4.5 (1.6–9.7)
45–54	4.7 (1.2–10)	3.2 (0.9–8.1)
55–64	4.8 (1.6–11)	5.5 (2.0–12)
65–74	3.1 (0.3–7.5)	5.5 (2.0–12)
75+	1.6 (0.04–8.8)	0 (0–3.4)
Total	3.5 (2.3–5.1)	3.4 (2.3–4.9)

Table 4.9 Age and sex frequency distribution of arthritis in psoriatic patients

Age	Percentage frequency distribution in (n = 227)	
	Males	Females
<16	1	6
16–25	10	17
26–35	18	20
36–45	27	23
46–55	21	22
56–65	16	12
66–75	6	1
75+	0	0

Source: [3].

psoriatic arthritis by age, and the age data are collected from the age distribution of clinical series of patients. Such data can only give an estimate of the relative occurrence at different ages rather than the absolute age risk. The results from one large series of 227 patients are shown in Table 4.9 [3]. There are no clear differences in the age trends between the sexes. Forty percent of female and 30 per cent of male cases have presented prior to the age of 35 and only a handful present after the age of 65. These are obviously different from the patterns observed in rheumatoid arthritis (see Chapter 2) and would support the concept that psoriatic arthritis is a distinct syndrome. However, in children, girls develop the disease at a much younger age than boys (4.5 versus 10 years) [39], perhaps reflecting the greater occurrence of sacroiliitis in boys.

The large majority of cases occur after the onset of the psoriasis as would be expected from the age trends [40,41], though in approximately 10 per cent of instances the arthritis predates the psoriasis and perhaps in a further 10 per cent the onset is simultaneous [3]. There are no consistent differences in the pattern of arthritis observed in relation to the timing of onset.

Race and geography

There are very few data on the geographical distribution of psoriatic arthritis either between different areas or different ethnic groups. Psoriasis itself is apparently rare in Indonesia, Kenya, and Uganda [28] and absent in Eskimos both in Alaska and Siberia [42]. By contrast, however, it has increased in occurrence in Ashkenazi Jews, this latter group in clinical series also having a relatively high incidence of psoriatic arthritis. Psoriatic arthritis is well described in African populations [31] and there are no apparent differences between South African blacks and whites. A study comparing the occurrence in different ethnic groups in Singapore suggested that Indians had twice the expected frequency compared to Chinese or Malays, in the same environment [43].

Genetics

There have been a number of family studies examining the rate of various clinical features in the first degree relatives (FDR) of probands with psoriatic arthritis. Few have compared their findings to a control series of FDR but the existence of clustering in families seems reasonable. Baker *et al.* [44] discovered one definite and four 'probable' psoriatic arthritis cases in 47 FDR examined from 53 probands. Kammer *et al.* [45] dis-

covered 3 per cent of 213 FDR who had psoriatic arthritis. The occurrence of inflammatory polyarthritis of all types was twice that expected in FDR of psoriatic arthritis [41]. In one controlled study, the prevalence of psoriatic arthritis in FDR was compared between probands with psoriatic arthritis and those with psoriasis and another form of arthritis. Ten cases were found in the FDR of the former and none in 20 probands with the latter, confirming that the increased risk is confined to those with clear-cut psoriatic arthritis [46]. Some 'super' families have also been reported, in many of which psoriatic arthritis occurs in some individuals with spondyloarthritic disorders in the absence of psoriasis occurring in other relatives [47]. In one pedigree, 11 out of 15 individuals examined had either psoriasis or arthritis [48]. Compared to the expected population rates, the FDRs of psoriatic arthritis probands would appear to have a 40-fold increase of psoriatic arthritis, a 20-fold increase of psoriasis, a three-fold increase in psoriasis-negative and seronegative arthritis, and a six-fold increase in sacroiliitis [46]. Psoriasis itself is not surprisingly increased in frequency, being found in 17 per cent of 213 FDR in one series [45]. Lawrence [5] reported a difference in the prevalence of psoriasis in siblings of probands with psoriasis alone (26 per cent) and psoriasis with arthritis (8 per cent). There is evidence of differential parental transmission with psoriatic arthritis in an offspring more likely if the father, rather than the mother, is affected. Similarly offspring of an affected father are twice as likely to be affected as those of an affected mother [49]. These observations are suggestive of maternal imprinting, i.e., genetic suppression of a maternal derived gene in favour of a paternal one. Interestingly this phenomenon is also seen in psoriasis [50].

There have been no studies of series of twins and only isolated case reports. In one set of monozygotic twins, the affected twin had widespread destructive arthritis with psoriasis whilst, by the age of 67, the co-twin was unaffected both by psoriasis and arthritis [51]. By contrast, in an interesting report of triplets consisting of a pair of monozygotic twins and a fraternal co-twin, the monozygotic twins both had psoriasis, the one with a peripheral arthritis and the other with a spondylitic arthritis, by contrast the fraternal co-twin was completely normal [52]. Such reports, whilst of interest individually, do not provide a coherent message. Finally, the significance of an isolated case report of the disease in an individual with Down's syndrome is unclear but may represent another avenue to genetic research [53].

As psoriatic arthritis represents the clinical co-occurrence of both psoriasis and inflammatory arthritis then the key question is: are there specific genetic susceptibility factors for psoriatic arthritis over and above those linked (i) to psoriasis alone and (ii) to the different forms of arthritis? It would therefore be expected that, compared to population controls, subjects with psoriatic arthritis would be more likely to carry susceptibility alleles for psoriasis, for example HLA-Cw*0602, and for certain forms of spondyloarthritis, for example HLA-B*27. It may be likely that specific psoriatic arthritis susceptibility alleles exist.

Susceptibility to psoriasis

There are long-standing, consistently reported associations between psoriasis and the serologically determined class I antigens B13, B17, and Cw6 [45,54,55]. Molecular typing methods have suggested that the primary and quantitatively most important association is with HLA-Cw*0602 [56]. The existence of a major psoriasis susceptibility locus on chromosome 6p has been confirmed by a number of whole genome scans of affected sibling pairs with the strongest linkage being with marker 6p21.3 [50,57,58]. Further investigation of this area identified a susceptibility haplotype which was telomeric to HLA-C but likely to be in the region carrying the disease susceptibility allele [59]. In addition, such whole genome scans have identified a number of non-HLA linked susceptibility loci including 17q and 4q [58–62].

Psoriatic arthritis versus population controls

There have been a large number of studies comparing HLA class I alleles between psoriatic arthritis patients with population controls (Table 4.10). As expected from the association discussed above in relation to psoriasis *per se*, consistently, HLA-B13, B17, and Cw6 have been increased, in many cases substantially, with large relative risks. As with psoriasis, molecular typing has shown that it is the Cw*0602 allele where the greatest risk lies [80] which is also associated with a younger age of onset. In addition to an association in European groups, HLA-B17 is also raised in African blacks with psoriatic arthritis [31]. In addition to these class I associations, the class II allele DR7 is also raised, although these alleles are in linkage disequilibrium with each other: the fact that one is raised would be expected from the rise in the others. Statistically the primary association was suggested to be with DR7 [74]. Studies have also found a strong and consistent association with B38 [69,70,76,79,81]. The association with HLA-B27 observed in some series reflects the occurrence in their subjects of a spondylitic arthropathy. Interestingly, the HLA-DRB1 alleles, such as *0401 raised in rheumatoid arthritis, are not increased in either the peripheral or central forms of psoriatic arthritis. HLA-DQ2 is also associated, which is probably not primary [82]. However, other MHC loci such as LMP2 and LMP7, which might have been relevant in relation to the role of CD8 +ve cells in the pathogenesis of psoriatic arthritis, are not related to disease risk [83].

Psoriatic arthritis versus psoriasis controls

The results from these studies (Table 4.11) are of potentially greater interest. The previously described association with HLA class I alleles B13 and B17 no longer hold, and indeed there is evidence to suggest from many of the studies a weaker association of psoriatic arthritis with these. A similar observation holds for HLA-Cw6. There is also no consistent pattern with HLA-DR7 [70,74]. By contrast, the association with HLA-B38 is only seen in the psoriatic arthritis patients: individuals with psoriasis alone having the frequencies seen in the normal population. HLA-B27, as might be expected, is increased in those psoriasis patients with arthritis.

Comparison between clinical subtypes

A few studies have had sufficient patients to compare the HLA linked susceptibility between the different clinical subtypes of the disease (Table 4.12). Broadly there are no consistent differences in the psoriasis associated alleles (B13, B17, Cw6, and DR7) between peripheral and central joint involvement. Similarly, HLA-B38 which did appear to be selectively associated with psoriatic arthritis, does not differentiate between these clinical types. HLA-B27 is seen much less frequently in psoriatic spondylitis than in ankylosing spondylitis (see Chapter 5) although it is increased compared to the background population rate of around 8 per cent in Western groups (Tables 4.10 to 4.12). In most series, HLA-B27 does differentiate between peripheral and central arthritis although the discrimination is not absolute.

In summary, in addition to the expected susceptibility to psoriatic arthritis from those alleles conferring

Table 4.10 HLA antigen associations with psoriatic arthritis (I) comparison with population controls

Reference	N		Gene/allele frequency (%)													
			B7		B13		B17		B27		B38		CW6		DR7	
	Cases	Controls	Cases	Controls	Cases	Controls	Cases	Controls	Cases	Controls	Cases	Controls	Cases	Controls	Cases	Controls
[63]	44	89			27	3			14	10						
[64]	156	386			15	5			9	6						
[65]	60	–							38	NA						
[66]	23	–			13	NA	30	NA	10	NA						
[67]	40	254			7	10	22	9	28	6						
[68]	82	100			7	4	20	6	28	9						
[69]	28	160	11	25	7	8	21	11	21	9	36	7				
[45]	100	346	10	31	9	5	13	10	32	6						
[70]	52	60			12	4	17	8	19	0	23	4	34	14	42	24
[31]	21[a]	300[a]			19	5	33	6								
[31]	26[b]	251[b]					42	25								
[71]	100	322			7	5	20	6	12	9			20	7	36	19
[72]	30	153			8	2	29	7	38	12			71	21	50	27
[73]	92	5000			17	5	17	8	21	8						
[74]	50	550			18	5	32	9	26	9			50	24	34	29
[75]	158	242	23	18	10	5	17	6	25	7	10	5	19	7	34	30
[76]	101	147			8	3	12	7	4	2	19	3	6	3	28	27
[77]	28	276	25	22			32	8	11	8					50	31
[78]	104	109					19	5	22	4	24	7	20	4		
[79]	193	2706					5	3	17	8			32	18		
[80]	94	100											32	18		

[a] White South Africans.
[b] Black South Africans.

Table 4.11 HLA antigen associations with psoriatic arthritis (II) comparison with psoriasis

| Reference | N | | Gene/allele frequency (%) | | | | | | | | | | | | | |
| | | | B7 | | B13 | | B17 | | B27 | | B38 | | CW6 | | DR7 | |
	Cases	Controls	Cases	Controls	Cases	Controls	Cases	Controls	Cases	Controls	Cases	Controls	Cases	Controls	Cases	Controls
[84]	108	83			14	13	21	27	15	7	10	0				
[85]	74	125				13	22	50	42	12						
[69]	28	32					21	28	21	13	36					
[70]	52	60	10	8	7	15	17	38			23	7	34	50	42	58
[71]	100	80	22	8	7	17	20	36	12	6			20	46	36	5
[72]	24	30			8	17	29	37	38	7			71	84	50	30
[74]	50	50			18	14	32	42	26	8			50	72	34	62
[75,86]	158	101	18	8	10	15	17	34	25	7	10	10	19	33	34	49

Table 4.12 HLA antigen associations with psoriatic arthritis (III) comparison between peripheral and axial (spondylo) arthritis types

| Reference | N | | B13 | | B17 | | B27 | | B38 | | CW6 | | DR7 | |
	Peripheral[a]	Axial[a]	Axial	Peripheral	Axial	Peripheral	Axial	Peripheral	Axial	Peripheral	Axial	Peripheral	Axial	Peripheral
[84]	68	40	16	10	26	13	7	28	6	15				
[67]	17	23	6	9	35	13	18	35						
[68]	54	28	11	0	11	14	11	60						
[85]	40	28		11	30	7	33	64						
[75,86]	65	35	6		21	4	15	28	12	14	15	19	37	31
[87]	33	27	6	11	11	7	18	48	0	11	52	35		
[76]	38	30	5	10			14	0	19	17	5	0	32	28
[78]	30	28			–	25	10	54			17			

[a] Groups not strictly comparable as patients with evidence of both patterns of joint involvement have been allocated in different studies to either or neither of these categories.

susceptibility to psoriasis, HLA-B38 does carry a susceptibility confined to the development of arthritis, independent of the type of arthritis. The final test, however, is whether this allele is also increased in rheumatoid factor negative arthritis individuals in the absence of psoriasis. There are few studies addressing this issue but in one study there was no difference [73]. Therefore, there is no single HLA allele that uniquely confers a combined risk of both psoriasis and arthritis in the same individual.

Non-MHC markers

Loci on chromosomes other than the sixth (the site of the HLA region) have also been investigated on the hypothesis that psoriatic arthritis is polygenic. There were no associations between specific Gm allotypes (markers for immunoglobulin heavy chain genes) and psoriatic arthritis [88]. Other studies using DNA probes for the switch region of immunoglobulin heavy chain genes on chromosome 14 showed a particular polymorphic pattern in 61 per cent of psoriatic arthritis probands compared to only 12 per cent of psoriasis individuals [89] though this has not been replicated. It would seem likely therefore that genes in the immunoglobulin region, despite the absence of rheumatoid factor, increase the susceptibility to arthritis in patients with psoriasis. By contrast there appears to be no association with the T cell receptor gene [90].

Environmental factors

There have been relatively few studies of potential environmental factors in the aetiology of psoriatic arthritis. The most interesting data have concerned the roles of viral infection and preceding trauma.

Role of micro-organisms

Most interest has centered on the role of hepatitis C and human immunodeficiency virus (HIV) infection. Hepatitis C infection was linked to disease development in one patient who was treated with interferon-α (IFN) [91]. It may be that IFN treatment may be of relevance. A case of arthritis has been reported in a psoriatic patient treated with IFNγ [92]. Hepatitis C antibodies, detected using a recombinant immunoblot assay, were recently found twice as frequently in psoriatic arthritic patients as in psoriasis (12 per cent

versus 6 per cent), the latter being double the expected population frequency [93].

Both psoriasis [94] and psoriatic arthritis [95–97] have been described following HIV infection and this subject has been extensively reviewed [98,99]. It is likely that up to 2 per cent of HIV infected men may develop psoriatic arthritis. Studies in African populations, where HIV infection is epidemic, showed HIV infection rates of 94 per cent in subjects with psoriatic arthritis compared to a local frequency of around 30 per cent [100]. Similar findings were observed in Zimbabwean patients [101].

Support for a possible viral aetiology for psoriatic arthritis comes from studies showing high blood levels of an adenylic acid polymer (2–5A) synthesized in the presence of double stranded DNA, which is thought to be a marker for viral replication. Increased levels of this polymer were found in patients with psoriatic arthritis but not in rheumatoid arthritis and non-arthritis controls [102]. A cross reacting antibody to the antigen pso p27 was found in the scales of patients with psoriasis and in the serum and synovial fluid of patients with arthritis [103]. Pso p27 is a virus like particle associated with retrovirus and might suggest a common viral link between the two disorders.

A bacterial aetiology was also suggested from controlled studies comparing antibody levels to the group A streptococcal endotoxin and antideoxyribonuclease β [104]. Increased levels were found in 50 per cent of sera from psoriatic arthritis patients compared to 23 per cent, 23 per cent, and 10 per cent in psoriasis, rheumatoid arthritis, and normal controls respectively.

Trauma

The concept that arthritis can develop after trauma is not a new one and there have been reports of inflammatory, but rheumatoid factor negative, arthritis developing after trauma [105,106]. Furthermore, the development of psoriasis at the site of skin trauma, the so called Koebner phenomenon, is well recognized and some have argued that the development of psoriatic arthritis may reflect a deep Koebner phenomenon [107]. Many cases have been described. The first report of arthritis developing 6 years after trauma, at the site of trauma, was over 30 years ago [108]. Since then there have been several case reports [109–113]. In the last two reports, of two and three cases respectively, the suggestive nature of the link was enhanced by the first affected joint being at the site of the trauma. There have been two epidemiological studies. In the first there was a six-fold greater reporting of immediately prior trauma, including surgery and accidents, in 138 patients with psoriatic arthritis compared to controls [114]. In the most recent study [115] 8 per cent of 300 patients reported some trauma in the 3 months preceding onset compared to less than 2 per cent of RA patients. Interestingly, of the 25 post-traumatic cases, one-third developed their first signs of their psoriatic arthritis immediately after the trauma [116]. Psoriatic arthritis has been reported after tattooing [117] but whether this was a consequence of trauma *per se* or of an associated infection is not clear.

Other environmental factors

There are limited studies of other environmental factors: subjects with psoriasis have lower serum levels of selenium, copper, and some unsaturated fatty acids compared to controls, but whether this represents a possible dietary cause of the disease or its effects is unknown [118]. There are no studies on education, social class, or similar variables, though the 30-year-old Swedish prevalence study [24] showed no significance in occurrence between urban and rural areas.

References

1. Alibert JL. *Précis théorique et pratique sur les maladies de la peau*. Paris: Caille and Ravier; 1822.
2. van Romunde LK, Valkenburg HA, Swart Bruinsma W, Cats A, Hermans J. Psoriasis and arthritis. I. A population study. *Rheumatol Int* 1984; 4: 55–60.
3. Roberts MET, Wright V, Hill AGS, Mehra AC. Psoriatic arthritis: Follow up study. *Ann Rheum Dis* 1976; 35: 206–212.
4. Moll JM, Wright V. Psoriatic arthritis. *Semin Arthritis Rheum* 1973; 3: 55–78.
5. Lawrence JS. *Rheumatism in populations*. London: William Heinemann Medical Books, 1977.
6. van Romunde LK, Cats A, Hermans J, Valkenburg HA. Psoriasis and arthritis. II. A cross-sectional comparative study of patients with 'psoriatic arthritis' and seronegative and seropositive polyarthritis: clinical aspects. *Rheumatol Int* 1984; 4: 61–65.
7. Symmons DP, Barrett EM, Bankhead CR, Scott DG, Silman AJ. The incidence of rheumatoid arthritis in the United Kingdom: results from the Norfolk Arthritis Register. *Br J Rheumatol* 1994; 33: 735–739.
8. Harrison BJ, Silman AJ, Barrett EM, Scott DGI, Symmons DPM. Presence of psoriasis does not influence the presentation of short term outcome of patients with early inflammatory polyarthritis. *J Rheumatol* 1997; 24: 1744–1749.
9. Scarpa R, Oriente P, Pucino A *et al.* The clinical spectrum of psoriatic spondylitis. *Br J Rheumatol* 1988; 27: 133–137.
10. Chamot AM, Benhamou CL, Kahn MF, Beraneck L, Kaplan G, Prost A. Acne-pustulosis-hyperostosis-osteitis syndrome. Results of a national survey. 85 cases. *Rev Rhum Mal Osteoartic* 1987; 54: 187–196.
11. Baker H. *The relationship between psoriasis, psoriatic arthritis and rheumatoid arthritis. An epidemiological, clinical and serological study*. Leeds University, 1965.
12. Arnett FC, Edworthy SM, Bloch DA *et al.* The American Rheumatism Association 1987 revised criteria for the classification of rheumatoid arthritis. *Arthritis Rheum* 1988; 31: 315–324.
13. Levin RW, Park J, Ostrov A, Reginato A, Baker DG. Clinical assessment of the 1987 American college of rheumatology criteria for rheumatoid arthritis. *Scand J Rheumatol* 1996; 25: 277–281.
14. Dougados M, van der Linden S, Juhlin R, Huitfeldt B, Amor B. The European spondylarthropathy study group preliminary criteria for the classification of spondylarthropathy. *Arthritis Rheum* 1991; 34: 1218–1227.
15. Amor B, Dougados M, Mijiyawa M. Criteria of the classification of spondyloarthropathies. *Rev Rhum Mal Osteoartic* 1990; 57: 85–89.
16. Salvarani C, Scocco GL, Macchioni P *et al.* Prevalence of psoriatic arthritis in Italian psoriatic patients. *J Rheumatol* 1995; 22: 1499–1503.
17. Kavli G, Forde OH, Arnesen E, Stenvold SE. Psoriasis: familial predisposition and environmental factors. *BMJ* 1985; 1384: 999–1000.
18. Lomholt G. *Psoriasis prevalence, spontaneous course and genetics. A census study on the prevalence of skin disease in the Faroe Islands*. Copenhagen: GEC Gad., 1963.
19. Hellgren L. *Psoriasis. The prevalence in sex, age and occupational groups in the total population in Sweden. Morphology, inheritance and association with other skin diseases*. Stockholm: Almquist and Wiksell, 1967.
20. Lawrence RC, Hochberg MC, Kelsey JL, McDuffie FC, Medsger TA. Estimates of the prevalence of selected arthritic and musculoskeletal diseases in the United States. *J Rheumatol* 1989; 16: 427–441.
21. Baker H. Epidemiological aspects of psoriasis and arthritis. *Br J Dermatol* 1966; 78: 249–261.
22. Falk ES, Vandbakk O. Prevalence of psoriasis in a Norwegian Lapp population. *Acta Derm Venereol (Stockh)* 1993; 182 (Suppl.): 6–9.
23. Farber EM, Carlsen RA. Psoriasis in childhood. *Calif Med* 1966; 105: 415–420.
24. Hellgren H. Association between rheumatoid arthritis and psoriasis in total populations. *Acta Rheumatol Scand* 1969; 15: 316–326.
25. Uramoto K, Shbeeb M, Sunku J *et al.* The epidemiology of psoriatic arthritis (PA) in Olmsted County 1980–91. *Arthritis Rheum* 1997; 40: 1100.
26. Erdes SH, Ibragimov S. Study of the prevalence of psoriatic arthritis in a population. *Vestn Dermatol Venerol* 1985; 5: 36–39.
27. Leczinsky CG. The incidence of arthropathy in a 10 year series of psoriasis cases. *Acta Derm* 1948; 28: 483–487.

28. Ingram JT. The approach to psoriasis. *BMJ* 1953; **2**: 591–594.

29. Molin L. Psoriasis. *Acta Derm Venereol* 1973; **53**: 36–69.

30. Maldonado Cocco JA, Porrini A, Garcia Morteo O. Prevalence of sacroiliitis and ankylosing spondylitis in psoriasis patients. *J Rheumatol* 1978; **5**: 311–313.

31. Green L, Meyers OL, Gordon W, Briggs B. Arthritis in psoriasis. *Ann Rheum Dis* 1981; **40**: 366–369.

32. Stern RS. The epidemiology of joint complaints in patients with psoriasis. *J Rheumatol* 1985; **12**: 315–321.

33. Kononen M, Torppa J, Lassus A. An epidemiological survey of psoriasis in the greater Helsinki area. *Acta Derm Venereol (Stockh)* 1986; **124** (Suppl): 1–10.

34. Zanolli MD, Wikle JS. Joint complaints in psoriasis patients. *Int J Dermatol* 1992; **31**: 488–491.

35. Barisic-Drusko I, Pasic A, Paljan D, Jukic Z, Basta-Juzbasic A, Marinovic B. Frequency of psoriatic arthritis in general population and among the psoriatics in department of dermatology. *Acta Derm Venereol (Stockh)* 1994; **186** (Suppl): 107–108.

36. Battistone MJ, Manaster BJ, Reda DJ, Clegg DO. The prevalence of sacroiliitis in psoriatic arthritis: new perspectives from a large, multicenter cohort. A department of veterans affairs cooperative study. *Skeletal Radiol* 1999; **28**: 196–201.

37. Kaipianen-Seppänen O. Incidence of psoriatic arthritis in Finland. *Br J Rheumatol* 1996; **35**: 1289–1291.

38. Lambert JR, Wright V. Psoriatic spondylitis: a clinical and radiological description of the spine in psoriatic arthritis. *QJM* 1974; **184**: 411–425.

39. Roberton D, Cabral D, Malleson P, Petty R. Juvenile psoriatic arthritis: follow-up and evaluation of diagnostic criteria. *J Rheumatol* 1996; **23**: 166–170.

40. Avila R, Pugh DG, Slocomb CH, Winklemann RK. Psoriatic arthritis: a roentgenological study. *Radiology* 1960; **75**: 691–701.

41. Thompson M, Holti G. Microcirculatory studies of the skin in the investigation of seronegative polyarthritis. In: *VI Congress Europa de Rheumatologia*. Lisboa, Portugal, 1967: 29.

42. Benevolenskaya LI, Boyer GS, Erdesz S *et al.* Spondylarthropathic disease in indigenous circumpolar populations of Russia and Alaska. *Rev Rhum Ed Eng* 1996; **63**: 815–822.

43. Thumboo J, Tham S, Tay Y *et al.* Patterns of psoriatic arthritis in Orientals. *J Rheumatol* 1997; **24**: 1949–1953.

44. Baker H, Golding DN, Thompson M. Psoriasis and arthritis. *Ann Int Med* 1963; **58**: 909–925.

45. Kammer GM, Soter NA, Gibson DJ, Schur PH. Psoriatic arthritis: a clinical, immunologic and HLA study of 100 patients. *Semin Arthritis Rheum* 1979; **9**: 75–97.

46. Moll JMH, Wright V. Familial occurrence of psoriatic arthritis. *Ann Rheum Dis* 1973; **32**: 181–201.

47. Alenius GM, Sojka BN, Nordmark L, Nordstrom S, Rantapaa Dahlqvist S. A multicase family with spondylarthropathies. *Scand J Rheumatol* 1997; **26**: 107–112.

48. Marcusson JA, Strom H, Lindvall N. Psoriasis peripheral arthritis, sacroiliitis and juvenile chronic arthritis: a family study in relation to segregation of HLA antigens. *J Rheumatol* 1983; **10**: 619–623.

49. Rahman P, Gladman D, Schentag C, Petronis A. Excessive paternal transmission in psoriatic arthritis. *Arthritis Rheum* 1999; **42**: 1228–1231.

50. Burden AD, Javed S, Bailey M, Hodgins M, Connor M, Tillman D. Genetics of psoriasis: paternal inheritance and a locus on chromosome 6p. *J Invest Dermatol* 1998; **110**: 958–960.

51. Gottlieb M, Calin A, Gale RP. Discordance for psoriatic arthropathy in monozygotic twins. *Clin J Am Rheum Assoc* 1979; **22**: 805–806.

52. Moll JMH, Johnson G, Wright V. Psoriatic arthritis: a unique family. *Rheumatol Rehabil* 1974; **13**: 154–157.

53. Jorgensen C, Bologna C, Sany J. Vasculitis and psoriatic arthritis associated with Down's syndrome. *Clin Exp Rheumatol* 1995; **13**: 749–751.

54. Brenner W, Gschnait F, Mayr WR. HLA B13, B17, B37 and Cw6 in psoriasis vulgaris: association with the age of onset. *Arch Dermatol Res* 1978; **262**: 337–339.

55. Tiilikainen A, Lassus A, Karvonen J, Vartiainen P, Julin M. Psoriasis and HLA-Cw6. *Br J Dermatol* 1980; **102**: 179–184.

56. Enerback C, Martinsson T, Inerot A *et al.* Evidence that HLA-Cw6 determines early onset of psoriasis, obtained using sequence-specific primers (PCR-SSP). *Acta Derm Venereol* 1997; **77**: 273–276.

57. Balendran N, Clough RL, Arguello JR *et al.* Characterization of the major susceptibility region for psoriasis at chromosome 6p21.3. *J Invest Dermatol* 1999; **113**: 322–328.

58. Trembath RC, Clough RL, Rosbotham JL *et al.* Identification of a major susceptibility locus on chromosome 6p and evidence for further disease loci revealed by a two stage genome-wide search in psoriasis. *Hum Mol Genet* 1997; **6**: 813–820.

59. Nair RP, Stuart P, Henseler T *et al.* Localization of psoriasis-susceptibility locus PSORS1 to a 60-kb interval telomeric to HLA-C. *Am J Hum Genet* 2000; **66**: 1833–1844.

60. Samuelsson L, Enlund F, Torinsson A *et al.* A genome-wide search for genes predisposing to familial psoriasis by using a stratification approach. *Hum Genet* 1999; **105**: 523–529.

61. Nair RP, Henseler T, Jenisch S *et al.* Evidence for two psoriasis susceptibility loci (HLA and 17q) and two novel candidate regions (16q and 20p) by genome-wide scan. *Hum Mol Genet* 1997; **6**: 1349–1356.

62. Capon F, Novelli G, Semprini S *et al.* Searching for psoriasis susceptibility genes in Italy: genome scan and evidence for a new locus on chromosome 1. *J Invest Dermatol* 1999; **112**: 32–35.

63. Russell TJ, Schultes LM, Kuban DJ. Histocompatibility (HLA) antigens associated with psoriasis. *N Engl J Med* 1972; **287**: 738–739.

64. White SH, Newcomer VD, Mickey MR, Terasaki PI. Disturbance of HLA antigen frequency in psoriasis. *N Engl J Med* 1972; **287**: 740–743.

65. Brewerton DA, Caffrey M, Nicholls A, Walters D, James DCO. HLA 27 and arthropathies associated with ulcerative colitis and psoriasis. *Lancet* 1974; **1**: 956–958.

66. Seignalet J, Sany J, Serre H. HLA antigens and arthropathies in psoriasis. *Lancet* 1974; **1**: 7870.

67. Metzger AL, Morris RI, Bluestone R, Terasaki PI. HLA W27 in psoriatic arthropathy. *Arthritis Rheum* 1975; **18**: 111–115.

68. Lambert JR, Wright V, Rajah SM, Moll JMH. Histocompatibility antigens in psoriatic arthritis. *Ann Rheum Dis* 1976; **35**: 526–530.

69. Espinoza LR, Vasey FB, Oh JH, Wilkinson R, Osterland CK. Association between HLA-BW38 and peripheral psoriatic arthritis. *Arthritis Rheum* 1978; **21**: 72–75.

70. Murray C, Mann DL, Gerber LN, Barth W, Perlmann S, Decker JL. Histocompatibility alloantigens in psoriasis and psoriatic arthritis. *J Clin Invest* 1980; **66**: 670–675.

71. Beaulieu AD, Roy R, Mathon G, Morissette J, Latulippe L, Lang JY. Psoriatic arthritis: risk factors for patients with psoriasis—a study based on histocompatibility antigen frequencies. *J Rheumatol* 1983; **10**: 633–636.

72. Armstrong RD, Panayi GS, Welsh KI. Histocompatibility antigens in psoriasis, psoriatic arthropathy, and ankylosing spondylitis. *Ann Rheum Dis* 1983; **42**: 142–146.

73. van Romunde LK, Cats A, Hermans J, Valkenburg HA, de Vries E. Psoriasis and arthritis. III. A cross-sectional comparative study of patients with 'psoriatic arthritis' and seronegative and seropositive polyarthritis: radiological and HLA aspects. *Rheumatol Int* 1984; **4**: 67–73.

74. Woodrow JC, Ilchysyn A. HLA antigens in psoriasis and psoriatic arthritis. *J Med Genet* 1985; **22**: 492–495.

75. Gladman DD, Anhorn KAB, Schachter RK, Mervart H. HLA antigens in psoriatic arthritis. *J Rheumatol* 1986; **13**: 586–592.

76. Salvarani C, Macchioni PL, Zizzi F *et al.* Clinical subgroups and HLA antigens in Italian patients with psoriatic arthritis. *Clin Exp Rheumatol* 1989; **7**: 391–396.

77. Hamilton ML, Gladman DD, Shore A, Laxer RM, Ed S. Juvenile psoriatic arthritis and HLA antigens. *Ann Rheum Dis* 1990; **49**: 694–697.

78. Lopez-Larrea C, Alonso JCT, Perez AR, Coto E. HLA antigens in psoriatic arthritis subtypes of a Spanish population. *Ann Rheum Dis* 1990; **49**: 318–319.

79. Fournié B, Granel J, Heraud A *et al.* HLA-B et rhumatisme psoriasique. Etude de 193 cas. *Rev Rhum Mal Osteoartic* 1991; **58**: 269–273.

80. Gladman D, Cheung C, Ng C, Wade J. HLA-C locus alleles in patients with psoriatic arthritis (PsA). *Hum Immunol* 1999; **60**: 259–261.

81. Gladman DD, Anhorn KAB. HLA and disease manifestations in rheumatoid arthritis—a Canadian experience. *J Rheumatol* 1986; **13**: 274–276.

82. Trabace S, Cappellacci S, Ciccarone P, Liaskos S, Polito R, Zorzin L. Psoriatic arthritis: a clinical, radiological and genetic study of 58 Italian patients. *Acta Derm Venereol (Stockh)* 1994; **186** (Suppl.): 69–70.

83. Hohler T, Schneider P, Ritter C, Hasenclever P, Mayer zum Buschenfelde K, Marker-Hermann E. LMP polymorphisms do not influence disease expression in psoriatic arthritis. *Clin Exp Rheumatol* 1996; **14**: 661–664.

84. Roux H, Mercier P, Maestracci D *et al.* Psoriatic arthritis and HLA antigens. *J Rheumatol* 1977; **3**: 64–65.

85. Eastmond CJ, Woodrow JC. The HLA system and the arthropathies associated with psoriasis. *Ann Rheum Dis* 1977; **36**: 112–120.

86. Gladman DD, Urowitz MB, Anhorn KAB, Chalmers A, Mervart H. Discordance between HLA-B27 and ankylosing spondylitis: a family investigation. *J Rheumatol* 1986; **13**: 129–136.

87. McHugh NJ, Laurent MR, Treadfwell BLJ, Tweed JM, Dagger.J. Psoriatic arthritis: clinical subgroups and histocompatibility antigens. *Ann Rheum Dis* 1987; **46**: 184–188.

88. Demaine AG, Panayi GS, Vaughan RW, Armstrong RD, Welsh KI. Immunoglobulin allotypes in psoriasis, psoriatic arthropathy and ankylosing spondylitis. *Exp Clin Immunogenet* 1984; **1**: 61–65.

89. Sakkas LI, Demaine AG, Panayi GS, Welsh KI. Arthritis in patients with psoriasis is associated with an immunoglobulin gene polymorphism. *Arthritis Rheum* 1988; **31**: 276–278.

90. Sakkas LI, Loqueman N, Bird H, Vaughan RW, Welsh KI, Panayi GS. HLA class II and T cell receptor gene polymorphisms in psoriatic arthritis and psoriasis. *J Rheumatol* 1990; **17**: 1487–1490.

91. Lombardini F, Taglione E, Riente L, Pasero G. Psoriatic arthritis with spinal involvement in a patient receiving alpha-interferon for chronic hepatitis C. *Scand J Rheumatol* 1997; **26**: 58–60.

92. O'Connell PG, Gerber LH, Digiovanna JJ, Peck GL. Arthritis in patients with psoriasis treated with gamma-interferon. *J Rheumatol* 1992; **19**: 80–82.

93. Taglione E, Vatteroni M, Martini P *et al.* Hepatitis C virus infection: prevalence in psoriasis and psoriatic arthritis. *J Rheumatol* 1999; **26**: 370–372.

94. Duvic M, Johnson TM, Rapini RP, Freese T, Brewton G, Rios A. Acquired immunodeficiency syndrome-associated psoriasis and Reiter's syndrome. *Arch Dermatol* 1987; **123**: 1622–1632.

95. Espinoza LR, Berman A, Vasey FB, Cahalin C, Nelson R, Germain BF. Psoriatic arthritis and acquired immunodeficiency syndrome. *Arthritis Rheum* 1988; **31**: 1034–1040.

96. Berman A, Espinoza LR, Diaz JD *et al.* Rheumatic manifestations of human immunodeficiency virus infection. *Am J Med* 1988; **85**: 59–64.

97. Solinger A, Hess E. Rheumatic disease and AIDS—is the association real? *J Rheumatol* 1993; **20**: 678–683.

98. Arnett FC, Reveille JD, Duvic M. Psoriasis and psoriatic arthritis associated with human immunodeficiency virus infection. *Rheum Dis Clin North Am* 1991; **17**: 59–78.

99. Cuellar ML, Silveira LH, Espinoza LR. Recent developments in psoriatic arthritis. *Curr Opin Rheumatol* 1994; **6**: 378–384.

100. Njobvu P, McGill P, Kerr H, Jellis J, Pobee J. Spondyloarthropathy and human immunodeficiency virus infection in Zambia. *J Rheumatol* 1998; **25**: 1553–1559.

101. Stein C, Davis P. Association with HIV infection in Zimbabwe. *J Rheumatol* 1996; **23**: 506–511.

102. Luxembourg A, Cailla H, Roux H, Roudier J. Do viruses play an etiologic role in ankylosing spondylitis or psoriatic arthritis? *Clin Immunol Immunopathol* 1987; **45**: 292–295.

103. Rodahl E, Asbakk K, Iversen OJ. Participation of antigens related to the Psoriasis associated antigen, pso p27, in immune complex formation in patients with ankylosing spondylitis. *Ann Rheum Dis* 1988; **47**: 628–633.

104. Vasey FB, Deitz C, Fenske NA, Germain BF, Espinoza LR. Possible involvement of group A streptococci in the pathogenesis of psoriatic arthritis. *J Rheumatol* 1982; **9**: 719–722.

105. Olivieri I, Gherardi S, Bini C, Trippi D, Ciompi ML, Pasero G. Trauma and seronegative spondyloarthropathy: rapid joint destruction in peripheral arthritis triggered by physical injury. *Ann Rheum Dis* 1988; **47**: 73–76.

106. Olivieri I, Gemignani G, Christou C, Pasero G. Trauma and seronegative spondyloarthropathy: report of two more cases of peripheral arthritis precipitated by physical injury. *Ann Rheum Dis* 1989; **48**: 520–521.

107. Vasey FB. Etiology and pathogenesis of psoriatic arthritis. In: Gerber LH, Espinoza LR, eds. *Psoriatic arthritis*. New York: Grune and Stratton, 1985: 45–47.

108. Williams KA, Scott JT. Influence of trauma on the development of chronic inflammatory polyarthritis. *Ann Rheum Dis* 1967; **26**: 532–537.

109. Goupille P, Soutie D, Valat JP. Psoriatic arthritis precipitated by physical trauma. *J Rheumatol* 1991; **18**: 633.

110. Langevitz P, Buskila D, Gladman DD. Psoriatic arthritis precipitated by physical trauma. *J Rheumatol* 1990; **17**: 695–697.

111. Sandorfi N, Freunlich B. Psoriatic and seronegative inflammatory arthropathy associated with traumatic onset: 4 cases and review of the literature. *J Rheumatol* 1997; **24**: 187–192.

112. Scarpa R, della Valle G, Del Puente A *et al*. Physical trauma triggers psoriasis in a patient with undifferentiated seronegative spondyloarthropathy. *Clin Exp Rheumatol* 1992; **10**: 100–102.

113. Thomachot B, Lafforgue P, Acquaviva PC. Posttraumatic psoriatic arthritis. 2 cases. *Presse Med* 1996; **25**: 21–24.

114. Scarpa R, Puente AD, Di GC, Valle GD, Lubrano EO. Interplay between environmental factors, articular involvement, and HLA-B27 in patients with psoriatic arthritis. *Ann Rheum Dis* 1992; **51**: 78–79.

115. Punzi L, Pianon M, Rizzi E, Rossini P, Todesco S. Prevalence of post-trauma psoriasic rheumatitis. *Presse Med* 1987; **26**: 420.

116. Punzi L, Pianon M, Bertazzolo N *et al*. Clinical, laboratory and immunogenetic aspects of post-traumatic psoriatic arthritis: a study of 25 patients. *Clin Exp Rheumatol* 1998; **16**: 277–281.

117. Punzi L, Rizzi E, Pianon M, Rossini P, Gambari PF. Tattooing-induced psoriasis and psoriatic arthritis. *Br J Rheumatol* 1997; **36**: 1133–1134.

118. Azzini M, Girelli D, Olivieri O *et al*. Fatty acids and antioxidant micronutrients in psoriatic arthritis. *J Rheumatol* 1995; **22**: 103–108.

5 | Ankylosing spondylitis and spondyloarthropathies

Alan J. Silman

Introduction

Ankylosing spondylitis and other related co-morbidities

It is now recognized that criteria for ankylosing spondylitis (AS) *per se* do not accurately reflect its co-occurrence with a number of other disorders, all of which can be characterized by an increased frequency of a spondyloarthritis which is pathologically and clinically identical to AS. This group of disorders, known collectively as spondyloarthropathies (SpAs) are perhaps best considered as a single entity for epidemiological purposes. The case for such a 'lumping' approach is strengthened by their common association with the HLA Class I allele B27—thus the disorders are frequently termed the **B-27 related spondyloarthropathies**.

The position is somewhat confusing as many of these co-morbid disorders, such as psoriasis, acute dysentery, inflammatory bowel disease, and acute anterior uveitis, are associated with a peripheral arthritis rather than axial involvement. Unlike rheumatoid arthritis, such peripheral arthritis is frequently asymmetrical, predominantly affects large lower limb joints, and is rheumatoid factor negative—these disorders are thus also termed **seronegative spondyloarthropathies**. This profusion of terms and concepts clearly adds to the confusion in attempting to describe the epidemiology of these disorders. In this volume, arthropathy associated with psoriasis (most of which is not B27/SpA related) is considered separately (Chapter 4). Similarly, post-dysenteric/urethritic reactive arthritis is also discussed separately (Chapter 6), though the overlap with AS is greater. The prevalence of AS in patients with psoriatic arthropathy is 20 per cent and those with Reiter's disease is 34 per cent; the prevalence of radiographic sacroiliitis in these two conditions is 22 per cent and 56 per cent respectively [1]. This chapter therefore provides a brief overview of the relationship between spondyloarthropathy and inflammatory bowel disease (IBD) and acute anterior uveitis.

Inflammatory bowel disease

Evidence for an association between arthritis and inflammatory bowel disease (IBD) has been recognized since White [2] described arthritis in association with ulcerative colitis. Since then, familial and other characteristics of patients with IBD and arthritis have been well documented. Approximately 17–20 per cent of patients with ulcerative colitis have radiographic evidence of sacroiliitis, and between 3 and 13 per cent have spondylitis [3,4]. In one series of 91 probands with ulcerative colitis, 20 per cent of males and 8 per cent of females had AS; in addition, 'definite' ankylosing spondylitis was diagnosed in 5 per cent of male and 3 per cent of female relatives compared to none in spouse controls [5]. In Crohn's disease, between 16 and 20 per cent of patients have radiographic sacroiliitis and 4–7 per cent have evidence of spondylitis [6–8]. In Crohn's disease, familial aggregation of sacroiliitis was found in 8 per cent of first degree relatives and 2 per cent of second degree relatives compared to none in spouse controls [7]. Since it has been postulated that neither IBD nor AS antedate each other, their co-occurrence is probably explained by a common aetiology [5], which could have a genetic basis.

Acute anterior uveitis

The association between acute anterior uveitis (or iritis) and AS has been confirmed by many studies too frequent to mention here, although less that 15 per cent of ankylosing spondylitics actually have uveitis [9]. However, in a recent survey of over 1300 people with AS, a much higher prevalence of uveitis (40 per cent) was reported [10], though this excess may be due to

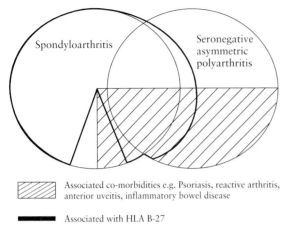

Associated co-morbidities e.g. Psoriasis, reactive arthritis, anterior uveitis, inflammatory bowel disease

Associated with HLA B-27

Fig. 5.1 Conceptual relationship between components of the seronegative spondyloarthropathy group of disorders.

confusion between uveitis and other minor and more common eye problems. Acute anterior uveitis (iritis) was clinical criterion for AS in the initial Rome proposals for diagnostic criteria (see below) [11]. However, since a reliable history of iritis is difficult to elicit because of possible confusion with more common eye disorders and because of a low specificity of iritis for AS, iritis was removed for the New York criteria set [12]. A diagrammatic representation aimed at helping the reader interpret the different studies is shown in Fig. 5.1.

Classification criteria

The first scheme for the classification of ankylosing spondylitis (AS) was proposed in 1963—the Rome Criteria (Table 5.1) which were useful for epidemiological studies as they did not require the use of poten-

Table 5.1 The Rome clinical criteria for the diagnosis of ankylosing spondylitis [11]

1. Low back pain and stiffness over 3 months duration which is not relieved by rest
2. Pain and stiffness in the thoracic region
3. Limited motion in the lumbar spine
4. Limited chest expansion
5. A history or evidence of iritis or its sequelae

The diagnosis is 'definite' if 4 out of 5 clinical criteria are fulfilled or if bilateral sacroiliitis and one other clinical criterion is satisfied

Table 5.2 The New York clinical criteria for ankylosing spondylitis [12]

1. Limitation of motion in the lumbar spine in all three planes—anterior flexion, lateral flexion, and extension
2. A history of or the presence of pain at the dorsolumbar junction or in the lumbar spine
3. Limited chest expansion to 2.5 cm or less, measured at the fourth intercostal space

'Definite' ankylosing spondylitis if (1) grade 3/ 4 bilateral sacroiliitis with at least one clinical criterion or (2) grade 3/ 4 unilateral sacroiliitis or grade 2 bilateral sacroiliitis associated with clinical criterion (1) or with both clinical criteria (2) and (3)

'Probable' ankylosing spondylitis for grade 3/ 4 bilateral sacroiliitis with no clinical criteria

tially harmful pelvic radiographics [11]. They were not, however, widely used as the lack of sacroiliac radiographic evidence of disease was considered too greater loss in specificity [13]. In 1968, a further set of criteria were proposed (the New York Criteria) (Table 5.2) [12], which required at least 'grade 2' bilateral radiographic sacroiliitis.

In population surveys, these criteria achieved widespread acceptability [14] though concerns about poor interobserver reliability in reading sacroiliac films were probably justified [15]. The criteria were modified by van der Linden (Table 5.3) [16,17] which provided greater specificity as well as introducing their extension to non-axial arthropathies. As discussed above, however, the lone concept of AS has been challenged and more recent criteria sets have attempted to be all-embracing, attempting to capture all the disorders

Table 5.3 Proposals for revision of diagnostic criteria for ankylosing spondylitis [17]

1. Insidious onset of low back pain, <45 years age, >3 months duration, associated with morning stiffness, relieved by rest
2. Occurrence in a relative of an AS proband or an HLA-B27 +ve individual
    (a) recurrent chest pain in the thoracic region
    (b) unilateral acute iritis with enthesopathy
    (c) seronegative oligoarthritis
3. Limitation of lumbar motion in 2 planes
4. Limited chest expansion, corrected for age and sex

'Definite' AS if grade 2+ bilateral sacroiliitis or grade 3/ 4 unilateral sacroiliitis with at least one clinical criteria present.

'Possible' AS if (1) any one clinical criteria satisfied, or (2) grade 2+ bilateral sacroiliitis or grade 3/ 4 unilateral sacroilliitis

Table 5.4 French criteria for spondyloarthropathy

Parameters	Scoring
A. Clinical symptoms or past history of:	
1. Lumbar or dorsal pain at night or morning stiffness of lumbar or dorsal pain	1
2. Asymmetrical oligoarthritis	2
3. Buttock pain	1
	or
If alternate buttock pain:	2
4. Sausage-like toe or digit	2
5. Heel pain or other well defined enthesiopathy	2
6. Iritis	1
7. Non-gonococcal uretritis or cervicitis within 1 month before the onset of arthritis	1
8. Acute diarrhoea within 1 month before the onset of arthritis	1
9. Psoriasis, balanitis, or inflammatory bowel disease (IBD) (ulcerative colitis or Crohn's disease	2
B. Radiological findings	
10. Sacroiliitis (bilateral grade 2 or unilateral grade 3)	3
C. Genetic background	
11. Presence of HLA B27 and /or family history of AS, reactive arthritis, uveitis, psoriasis, or IBD	2
D. Response to treatment	
12. Clear-cut improvement within 48 h after NSAID intake or rapid relaspe of the pain after their discontinuation	2

A patient is considered as suffering from a spondyloarthropathy if the sum is ≥ 6.
Source: [18,95].

Table 5.5 The European Spondyloarthropathy Study Group Criteria for the classification of spondylo-arthropathy

Inflammatory spinal pain
OR
Synovitis which is asymmetric AND/OR predominantly lower limb
AND ONE OF
1. Positive family history
2. Psoriasis
3. Inflammatory bowel disease (IBD)
4. Urethritis or acute diarrhoea
5. Alternating buttock pain
6. Enthesopathy
7. Radiographic sacroiliitis

Source: [19].

illustrated in Fig. 5.1. The Amor criteria [18] and more predominantly the European Spondyloarthropathy Study Group (ESSG) criteria sets [19] are now considered the most accepted way forward (Tables 5.4 and 5.5). A number of studies, from many different populations, show these criteria mirror clinical opinion (which is how they were derived) and distinguished the SpA group of disorders from other rheumatological disorders seen in clinical practice (Table 5.6). It is perhaps not surprising that the criteria perform well in this setting—their application to population surveys is, given their structure, likely to be more problematic. The AMOR and ESSG criteria have been validated in Japan and found to have a sensitivity of 84% and 84.6% respectively [121].

Table 5.6 Validation of spondyloarthropathy criteria sets in different populations

Reference	Country	Sensitivity		Specificity	
		Amor	ESSG	Amor	ESSG
[18]	France	90	N/A	87	N/A
[19]	Mixed European	N/A	87	N/A	87
[96]	US: Alaskan Eskimos	N/A	89	N/A	89
[97]	Spain	91	84	96	95
[98]	Brazil	N/A	99	N/A	89
[99]	Turkey	89	87	92	91
[100]	Lebanon	77	91	98	100

N/A = not assessed.

Occurrence

Incidence

Data on incidence of AS are sparse and are derived from data sources that capture diagnosed cases as they arise within a catchment population.

Data from Olmstead County (Minnesota, US), based on hospital attendance over a 50 year period (1935–1989), are shown in Table 5.7. Over the whole period, the incidence was approximately 1 per 10 000 males per year and a third of that in females [20]. One problem with interpreting such data is the strong likelihood that only a small population of cases come to clinical attention [21]. Interestingly, the Olmstead data shown no evidence of any secular increase (Fig. 5.2) which might have been expected in underascertainment, due to diagnostic uncertainty, might have been a problem in the earlier part of this period.

Another approach to estimating incidence came from studies of individuals in Finland eligible to receive free medication having been registered as having AS [22]. These data shown in Table 5.8 show increase in

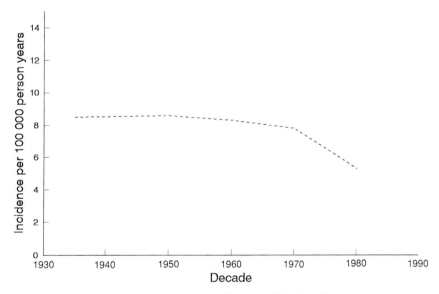

Fig. 5.2   Incidence of ankylosing spondylitis in Rochester, Minnesota, US, 1935–89.

Table 5.7   Incidence of AS[a] in Rochester, Minnesota, by age at onset and sex 1935–89

Age at onset	Males		Females		Combined rate
	No. cases	Rate[a]	No. cases	Rate[a]	
15–24	23	0.7	9	3.6	7.9
25–34	53	14.9	14	6.4	16.2
35–44	25	18.2	6	4.0	10.7
45–54	13	12.3	4	3.3	7.5
55–64	2	2.5	2	2.0	2.2
65+	3	3.8	2	1.4	2.2
Total	121	11.7[b]	37	2.9[b]	7.3[c]

Population based upon cases ascertained from hospital records.
[a] Per 100 000 person years.
[b] Age-adjusted to 1990 US Caucasians.
[c] Age and sex adjusted to 1990 US Caucasians.
Source: [20].

Table 5.8 Incidence of ankylosing spondylitis in Finland 1980–1990 based on disability registrations

Year	1980	1985	1990	Total
Total number of registrations	68	73	78	219
Incidence/100 000/year	6.6	6.9	7.3	6.9

Source: [23].

incidence between 1980 and 1990 but an average incidence of 7 per 100 000, virtually identical to the US data.

Age and gender

Both the Finnish [22] and the US [20] data confirm the male excess, which was greater in the latter. The US data, Table 5.7, also shows the peak onset in the third and fourth decades and increasing rarity after 55. Childhood cases are well described in a number of studies (for example [23,24]), but the incidence in childhood is harder to ascertain given the overlapping presentation with other childhood arthritides (see Chapter 3).

Time trends

As shown in Fig. 5.2 and Table 5.8, neither the Finnish or the US data suggest any recent change over time. Recent data suggest a decline in the delay to diagnosis with a halving of the time interval over the past 50 years from 15 to 7 years [25]. It has been suggested that the age at onset is increasing [26,27], but methodological difficulties make such observations difficult to interpret [28].

Prevalence

There have been several prevalence studies undertaken in a wide variety of populations. Many have been based on traditional cross-sectional surveys with combinations of questionnaire/interview physical examination, radiographic examination, and medical chart review being used. Thus some of the differences in occurrence might reflect methodological variation. One efficient strategy is to sample by HLA-B27 status, given that most cases occur in B27-positive individuals. Thus screening, for example of blood donors, for B27 is followed by follow-up of samples of positive and negative responders [29].

European populations

Earlier studies (Table 5.9) suggested a prevalence of 0.5–2/1000, including surveys based on large populations. The data used to derive the US incidence rates [20] have also been analysed to derive a prevalence estimate based on surviving current cases [30]. This yielded a prevalence of 1.9/1000 in males and 0.7/1000 in females in this population of Northern European extraction—figures remarkably similar to those from population surveys. The Berlin study of HLA-B27 positive and negative blood donors generated the highest recorded prevalence in a European population [29]. This might reflect selection bias in recruitment or, more probably, the use of MRI to screen for sacroiliitis—a technique much more sensitive than conventional survey methods.

Asian and middle-Eastern populations

Recent data from the Far East (Table 5.10) suggested prevalences higher than European data, based on very

Table 5.9 Prevalence in European populations

Reference	Country	Number studied	Criteria	Prevalence/1000
[101]	UK	N/S	N/S	0.5
[47]	Netherlands	2441	Clinical/X-ray	0.8
[102]	Finland	539	Clinical/X-ray	1.9
[103]	UK	2233	Clinical/X-ray	1.8
[104]	Netherlands	2957	New York	1.0
[105]	Finland	6176	X-ray	3.9
[106]	Norway	14539	New York	1.9
[107]	Norway (Lapps)	836	New York	1.8
[22]	Finland	7217	Clinical/X-ray	1.5
[29]	Germany	a	New York	9.0

a Based on screening B27+/B27– blood donors.

Table 5.10 Prevalence in Asian/Middle Eastern populations

Reference	Country	Number studied	Criteria	Prevalence/1000
[108]	Taiwan	2998	New York	5.4
		3000	New York	1.9
		3000	New York	4.0
[109]	China North	4192	New York	2.6
	China South	5047	New York	2.6

large sample surveys. By contrast, the disease is rare in Saudi Arabia [31] and the United Arab Emirates [32], populations in which the association with HLA-B27 is much weaker. The prevalence of AS in the Japanese population has recently been estimated to be <9.5/100,000 person-years [121].

Prevalence in Native American populations

Some native American populations have the highest recorded prevalences of AS in the world (Table 5.11). The Haida and Bella Indians have a prevalence of around 6 per cent [33], several times that of populations of European origin. The HLA-B27 frequency in these populations is also exceptionally high, at over 50 per cent [34]. Recent studies of the circum-polar Chukotkas in Siberia/Alaska have high frequency of both SpA in general and AS in particular [35,36], again explained by a high background frequency of HLA-B27. Other native populations such as Australian Aborigines do not appear to have AS [37].

Prevalence in African populations

Older studies suggested that populations of African origin only rarely had AS. Indeed Solomon [38] in a survey of 1300 African found only a single case. In a recent study of 900 male Gambians [39], again no cases were ascertained. It does seem generally accepted that AS is rare generally in Africa (Table 5.12), though when it does occur it is still associated with HLA-B27 [40].

Table 5.11 Prevalence in Native American populations

Reference	Population	Number studied	Criteria	Prevalence/1000
[13]	Pima	355	Rome	22.5 [a]
[33]	Bella Bella	158	New York	63.0 [a]
	Bella Coola	141	New York	27.0 [a]
	Itaida	209	New York	60.0 [a]
	Pima	1157	New York	54.0 [a]
[110]	Inupiat	2308	Rome	2.0 [a]
[111]	Yupile	13521	Rome	1.1
[35]	Chukotka [b]	355	New York	11.1
[112]	Papua New Guinea	109	Clinical	9.1

[a] Males only.
[b] Transpolar (Siberian Eskimos).

Table 5.12 Prevalence in African populations

Reference	Population	Number studied	Criteria	Prevalence/1000
[113]	Nigeria	1300	Clinical/X-ray	0.8
[38]	South African Black	1352	Clinical/X-ray	0
[114]	Jamaica	263	Clinical/X-ray	0
[39]	Gambia	900	Clinical/X-ray	0

Genetic factors

Familial aggregation

There is evidence of increased familial occurrence of disease. Across a large number of studies 4 per cent of relatives of probands have AS, though there is a wide variation between the published studies (Table 5.13). Such an increase was also observed recently in China [122]. Moller *et al.* [41,42] found that 10 per cent of relatives of diseased probands had AS, and when cases of 'probable AS' were included the figure rose to 20 per cent; all the relatives were HLA-B27 positive. Lochead *et al.* [43] reported a comparable figure. Emery and Lawrence [44] reported a 4 per cent increase in first degree relatives with clinical AS; when the extended (clinical) Rome criteria were applied the figure rose to 7 per cent [45]. Others have reported between 1 and 15 per cent of relatives of affected probands as having AS (Table 5.13). 'Familiarity', that is the proportion of probands with one or more relatives with AS, is approximately 14 per cent [46].

Relative risk estimates *per se* have been provided by only a few groups, which showed that the frequency of

AS among relatives of patients with disease was from 23 times higher [47] to 35 times higher [48] than in relatives of non-diseased patients. More recent data is lacking. Interestingly, early studies on familial aggregation in AS showed a lower degree of familial aggregation (less than 4 per cent on average) than more recent estimates (approximately 10 per cent) (see Table 5.13). The recent greater proportion of affected relatives observed today probably reflects different methods of case ascertainment as well as greater recognition of AS in females. In support of the latter argument, the early study by Hersh *et al.* [49] found twice as many male as female relatives of diseased probands had AS while later observation found similar percentages of male and female relatives of disease probands had AS [50].

In one study of sibling pairs [51], there was a greater similarity in calendar year of onset than in age at onset, suggested that shared environmental factors maybe more important that genetic ones in explaining familial aggregation.

Twin studies

A number of concordant monozygotic (MZ) twin pairs have been reported in the literature over several years [52–55]. There have been two recent studies [56,57] (Table 5.14), both small scale, comparing disease concordance between MZ and dizygotic (DZ) twins. Given the small sample sizes, the results were very similar with a five-fold increased concordance in the former. Genetic modelling of these data suggest that genetic, rather than environmental, factors explain most of the disease occurrence in these twins. Indeed in the UK study [57], genetic factors were thought to explain 97 per cent of the occurrence. An interesting study of discordant MZ twins [58] showed differences in responses to a number of microbial antigens between the affected and unaffected twin, though the exact identity of the putative agents remain to be elucidated (see below).

Table 5.13 Frequency of AS in relatives[a] of diseased probands

No. relatives	No. (%) with AS	Reference
247	7 (2.8)	[49]
428	16 (3.7)	[115]
2478	45 (1.8)	[47]
289	4 (1.4)	[116]
250	9 (3.6)	[44]
63	3 (4.8)	[117]
179	16 (8.9)	[43]
282	16 (5.7)	[118]
226	18 (7.9)	[119]
120	18 (15.0)	[120]
101	8 (7.8)	[104]
248	25 (10.1)	[41,42]
4991	185 (3.7)	All studies combined

[a] 1st, 2nd, and 3rd degree relatives combined.

Table 5.14 Twin concordance studies in ankylosing spondylitis

Reference	Monozygotic		Dizygotic	
	N	Concordant N (%)	N	Concordant N (%)
[56]	6	3 (50)	20	3 (15)
[57]	8	6 (75)	32	4 (13)
Pooled	14	9 (64)	52	7 (13.5)

Immunogenetics

The genetic basis to AS has been proven for 30 years with two landmark papers, published simultaneously in April 1973, reporting a spectacular association between the antigen HLA-B27 and AS [59–61]. The frequency of HLA-B27 in Caucasian AS patients ranged from 88–96 per cent as compared to 4–8 per cent of controls. This discovery of the HLA-B27 association revitalized the epidemiology of ankylosing spondylitis and helped broaden the clinical spectrum of the disease. Since this discovery there have been a wealth of papers discussing the HLA-B27 association to the extent that the epidemiology of AS may be described mainly by its immunogenetics.

There have been an enormous number of studies demonstrating a strong association in several diverse populations. Some 50 studies were published between 1973 and 1980 [62] with some key conclusions. Firstly, even in populations with a low, i.e. below 2 per cent, population frequency of HLA-B27, such as Japan [61], Indian [63], and Iraq [64], the associations were as strong. Secondly, in populations with a high frequency of HLA-B27, i.e. above 10 per cent, such as native Americans and Northern European, particularly Scandinavians [34,65,66], B27 was virtually ubiquitous amongst patients. Thirdly, the world-wide distribution of HLA-B27 mirrored the occurrence of the disease [67]. Thus as shown earlier, the disease is rare in South America, native Australian, and African populations—groups where HLA-B27 is also infrequent. Despite this, recent studies have confirmed an association with HLA-B27 even in these groups [68,69]. In African populations, there is a virtual absence of AS [39,70], though in the Gambia there is a B27 frequency of 6 per cent, but it is less than 1 per cent in Bantu. Formal linkage analysis in multicase families confirmed linkage to B27 with a maximal LOD score of 7.5 and consistent with an autosomal dominant inheritance with a penetrance of 20 per cent [71].

HLA-B27 subtypes

Recent advances in molecular genetics have identified at least nine B27 subtypes [72]. There is dispute as to whether some subtypes are more associated with AS than others. Thus in Danish patients only *2705 is found [73] and *2709 was not a susceptibility allele in Italians [72]. However, most studies have not found convincing differences [74]. Thus populations with a low prevalence of AS carry the same high proportion

with, for example, the *2705 allele that is thought to be the susceptibility allele in some populations [39]. The predominant subtype in affected individuals probably reflects the predominant subtype in the background population. In recent examples, *2704, a common Indian but rare European subtype, is the common subtype found in Indian AS patients [75]. By contrast, *2704 was positively associated and *2706 negatively associated with AS in Indonesians [76].

Influence of other MHC loci

Association with HLA-B27 might reflect linkage disequilibrium with other closely related loci. Studies of HLA-DRB1 alleles suggest positive, but weak, effects with susceptibility enhanced by DRB1 and DRB8 [57,77], effects which are independent of B27. In juvenile ankylosing spondylitis, DRB1*08 and DRB1*09 have been associated as well as the LMPZ b/b genotype [78].

Detailed investigation of other MHC loci including MICA and TNFα showed strong associations but these are entirely explained by linkage disequilibrium with B27 [79]. The presence of non-MHC genetic susceptibility factors in AS has recently been reported from a whole genome scan in 185 families containing 255 affected sib pairs. A number of loci of interest were revealed [123]. It seems unlikely however that any single gene will be found that has an effect anywhere near the magnitude of HLA-B27.

Non-genetic host factors

Pregnancy and sex hormones

Much attention has been devoted to investigating the role of male sex hormones in explaining the greater incidence in men. Cross-sectional studies are conflicting with some showing no alteration in testosterone levels in males with AS [80], whereas others have suggested low oestrogen levels in women [81]. It has also been suggested that the disease activity is influenced by exogenous sex hormones [82]. However, recent studies showed an alteration in androgens including testosterone, 17-β estradiol and androstenedione [83]. It was argued further that cross-sectional data are flawed either because of the effects of the disease, or its treatment (particularly phenylbutazone) on sex hormone levels.

Pregnancy has little effect on AS [84,85] suggestive of hormonal influences. However, one large study of

939 women with AS suggested that disease onset was related to pregnancy in 21 per cent [86]. Being a first born child and lower maternal age are also possible risk factors [124].

Other co-morbidities

These have been discussed earlier in relation to bowel, eye, and skin disease (see page 100). It certainly appears that the more intensive the bowel investigation, for example, the greater the likelihood that evidence of pathology will be found [87].

Environmental factors

Clearly HLA-B27 is not sufficient on its own to explain disease and the incomplete MZ twin concordance argues for an environmental trigger. Aside from other co-morbidities, most attention has focused on bowel infection, particularly with *Klebsiella pneumoniae*. This agent is present in faecal cultures to a greater extent when the disease is active. This was shown several years ago by Ebringer [88,89] and has been replicated recently by others finding an increase in IgA (but not IgG or IgM antibodies) in active versus inactive disease [90].

One model for the role of *K. pneumoniae* comes from Geczy and others [91,92] based on its cross-reactivity between HLA-B27. However, results are not consistent [93,94] and the evidence that Klebsiella infection is responsible for causing AS, rather than being associated with periods of disease activity, is not persuasive. Studies of disease-discordant twins do suggest, as mentioned above [58], that infection may be important, but the organism(s) involved remained to be identified.

References

1. Wright V. Relationship between ankylosing spondylitis and other spondarthritides. In: Moll JMH, ed. *Ankylosing spondylitis*. Edinburgh: Churchill Livingstone, 1980: 42–51.
2. White WH. Colitis. *Lancet* 1895; **1**: 537.
3. Rotstein J, Entel I, Zeviner B. Arthritis associated with ulcerative colitis. *Ann Rheum Dis* 1963; **22**: 194–197.
4. Woodrow JC. Genetics. In: Moll JMH, ed. *Ankylosing spondylitis*. Edinburgh: Churchill Livingstone, 1980: 26–41.
5. Macrae L, Wright V. A family study of ulcerative colitis. With particular reference to ankylosing spondylitis and sacroiliitis. *Ann Rheum Dis* 1973; **32**: 16–20.
6. Ansell BM, Wigley RAD. Arthritic manifestations in regional enteritis. *Ann Rheum Dis* 1964; **23**: 64–72.
7. Haslock I. Arthritis and Crohn's disease. A family study. *Ann Rheum Dis* 1973; **32**: 479–485.
8. Dekker-Saeys BJ, Meuwissen SGM, van den Berg-Loonen EM, de Haas WHD, Agenant D, Tytgat GNJ. Ankylosing spondylitis and inflammatory bowel disease. II. Prevalence of peripheral arthritis, sacroiliitis, and ankylosing spondylitis in patients suffering from inflammatory bowel disease. *Ann Rheum Dis* 1978; **37**: 33–35.
9. Rigby AS, Wood PHN. Observations on diagnostic criteria for ankylosing spondylitis. *Clin Exp Rheumatol* 1993; **11**: 5–12.
10. Edmunds L, Elswood J, Calin A. New light on uveitis in ankylosing spondylitis. *J Rheumatol* 1991; **18**: 50–52.
11. Kellgren JH, Jeffrey M, Ball J. *The epidemiology of chronic rheumatism*. Oxford: Blackwell Scientific, 1963.
12. Bennett PH, Wood PHN. *Population studies of the rheumatic diseases*. Amsterdam: Excerpta Medica, 1968.
13. Bennett PH, Burch TA. The epidemiological diagnosis of ankylosing spondylitis. In: Bennett PH, Wood PHN, eds. *Population studies of the rheumatic diseases*. Amsterdam: Excerpta Medica, 1968: 305–313.
14. Moll JMH. Diagnostic criteria and their evaluation. In: Moll JMH, ed. *Ankylosing spondylitis*. Edinburgh: Churchill Livingstone, 1980: 137–151.
15. Hollingsworth PN, Cheah PS, Dawkins RL, Owen ET, Calin A, Wood PHN. Observer variation in grading sacroiliac radiographs in HLA-B27 positive individuals. *J Rheumatol* 1983; **10**: 247–254.
16. van der Linden SM, Valkenberg HA, Cats A. Evaluation of diagnostic criteria for ankylosing spondylitis. A proposal for modification of the New York criteria. *Arthritis Rheum* 1984; **27**: 361–368.
17. van der Linden SM, Cats A, Goeithe HS, Khan MA. Proposals for the revision of diagnostic criteria for ankylosing spondylitis. *Arthritis Rheum* 1987; **30** (Suppl.): S75.
18. Amor B, Dougados M, Mijiyawa M. Criteria for the classification of spondyloarthropathies. *Rev Rhum Mal Osteoartic* 1990; **57**: 85–89.
19. Dougados M, van der Linden S, Juhlin R, *et al.* The European Spondyloarthropy Study Group preliminary criteria for the classification of spondyloarthropy. *Arthritis Rheum* 1991; **34**: 1218–1227.
20. Carbone LD, Cooper C, Michet CJEA. Ankylosing spondylitis in Rochester, Minnesota 1935–1989. Is the epidemiology changing? *Arthritis Rheum* 1992; **35**: 1476–1482.
21. Boyer GS, Templin DW, Bowler A, Lawrence RC, Heyse SP, Everett DF *et al.* Class I HLA antigens in spondyloarthropathy: Observations in Alaskan Eskimo patients and controls. *J Rheumatol* 1997; **24**: 500–506.
22. Kaipiainen SO, Aho K, Heliovaara M. Incidence and prevalence of ankylosing spondylitis in Finland. *J Rheumatol* 1997; **24**: 496–499.
23. Kaipiainen SO, Savolainen A. Incidence of chronic juvenile rheumatic diseases in Finland during 1980–1990. *Clin Exp Rheumatol* 1996; **14**: 441–444.

24. Gomez KS, Raza K, Jones SD, Kennedy LG, Calin A. Juvenile onset ankylosing spondylitis–more girls than we thought? *J Rheumatol* 1997; **24**: 735–737.

25. Feldtkeller E. [Age at disease onset and delayed diagnosis of spondyloarthropathies]Erkrankungsalter und Diagnoseverzogerung bei Spondylarthropathien. *Z Rheumatol* 1999; **58**: 21–30.

26. Calin A, Elswood J, Rigg S, Skevington SM. Ankylosing spondylitis—an analytical review of 1500 patients: the changing pattern of disease. *J Rheumatol* 1988; **15**: 1234–1238.

27. Will R, Calin A, Kirwan J. Increasing age at presentation for patients with ankylosing spondylitis [see comments]. *Ann Rheum Dis* 1992; **51**: 340–342.

28. Fries JF, Singh G, Bloch DA, Calin A. Editorial. The natural history of ankylosing spondylitis: is the disease really changing? *J Rheumatol* 1989; **16**: 860–863.

29. Braun J, Bollow M, Remlinger G, Eggens U, Rudwaleit M, Distler A et al. Prevalence of spondylarthropathies in HLA-B27 positive and negative blood donors. *Arthritis Rheum* 1998; **41**: 58–67.

30. Carter ET, McKenna CH, Brian DD, Kurland LT. Epidemiology of ankylosing spondylitis in Rochester, Minnesota, 1935–73. *Arthritis Rheum* 1979; **22**: 365–370.

31. al Arfaj A. Profile of ankylosing spondylitis in Saudi Arabia. *Clin Rheumatol* 1996; **15**: 287–289.

32. al Attia HM, Sherif AM, Hossain MM, Ahmed YH. The demographic and clinical spectrum of Arab versus Asian patients with ankylosing spondylitis in the UAE. *Rheumatol Int* 1998; **17**: 193–196.

33. Gofton JP, Bennett PH, Smythe H, Decker JL. Sacroiliitis and ankylosing spondylitis in North American Indians. *Ann Rheum Dis* 1972; **31**: 474–481.

34. Gofton JP, Chalmers A, Price GE, Reeve CE. HL-A 27 and ankylosing spondylitis in B. C. Indians. *J Rheumatol* 1975; **2**: 314–318.

35. Alexeeva L, Krylov M, Vturin V, Mylov N, Erdesz S, Benevolenskaya L. Prevalence of spondyloarthropathies and HLA-B27 in the native population of Chukotka, Russia. *J Rheumatol* 1994; **21**: 2298–2300.

36. Benevolenskaya LI, Boyer GS, Erdesz S, Templin DW, Alexeeva LI, Lawrence RC et al. Spondylarthropathic diseases in indigenous circumpolar populations of Russia and Alaska. *Rev Rhum Engl Ed* 1996; **63**: 815–822.

37. Cleland LG, Hay JAR, Milazzo S. Absence of HL-A27 and ankylosing spondylitis in Central Australian Aborigines. *Scand J Rheumatol* 1975; **4**(8 Suppl.): 30–35.

38. Solomon L, Beighton P, Valkenberg HA, Robin G, Soskolne CL. Rheumatic disorders in the South African Negro: part 1. Rheumatoid arthritis and ankylosing spondylitis. *S Afr Med J* 1975; **49**: 1292–1296.

39. Brown MA, Jepson A, Young A, Whittle HC, Greenwood BM, Wordsworth BP. Ankylosing spondylitis in West Africans—evidence for a non-HLA-B27 protective effect. *Ann Rheum Dis* 1997; **56**: 68–70.

40. Adebajo A, Davis P. Rheumatic diseases in African blacks. *Semin Arthritis Rheum* 1994; **24**: 139–153.

41. Moller P, Vinje O, Dale K, Berg K, Kass E. Family studies in Bechterew's syndrome (ankylosing spondylitis). I. Prevalence of symptoms and signs in relatives of HLA B27 positive probands. *Scand J Rheumatol* 1984; **13**: 1–10.

42. Moller P, Vinje O, Dale K, Berg K, Kass E. Family studies in Bechterew's syndrome (ankylosing spondylitis). II. Prevalence of symptoms and signs in relatives of HLA B27 negative probands. *Scand J Rheumatol* 1984; **13**: 11–14.

43. Lochead JA, Chalmers IM, Marshall WH, et al. HLA haplotypes in family studies of ankylosing spondylitis. *Arthritis Rheum* 1983; **26**: 1011–1016.

44. Emery AEH, Lawrence J. Genetics of ankylosing spondylitis. *J Med Genet* 1967; **4**: 239–244.

45. Bremner JM, Emery AEH, Kellgren JH, Lawrence J, Roth H. A family study of ankylosing spondylitis. In: Bennett PH, Wood PHN, eds. *Population studies of the rheumatic diseases*. Amsterdam: Excerpta Medica, 1968: 299–304.

46. Hochberg MC, Bias WB, Arnett FC. Family studies in HLA-B27 associated arthritis. *Medicine* 1978; **57**: 463–475.

47. de Blecourt JJ, Polman A, de Blecourt-Meindersma T. Hereditary factors on rheumatoid arthritis and ankylosing spondylitis. *Ann Rheum Dis* 1961; **20**: 215–223.

48. Stecher RM. Symposium on rheumatic diseases: hereditary factors in arthritis. *Med Clin NA* 1955; **39**: 499–508.

49. Hersh AH, Stecher RM, Solomon WM, Wolpaw R, Hauser H. Heredity in ankylosing spondylitis. A study of fifty families. *Am J Hum Genet* 1950; **2**: 391–408.

50. Khan MA, van der Linden SM, Kushner I, Valkenberg HA, Cats A. Spondylitic disease without radiologic sacroiliitis in relatives of HLA-B27 positive ankylosing spondylitis patients. *Arthritis Rheum* 1985; **28**: 40–43.

51. Calin A, Elswood J. Relative role of genetic and environmental factors in disease expression: sib pair analysis in ankylosing spondylitis. *Arthritis Rheum* 1989; **32**: 77–81.

52. Moesmann A. Hereditary and exogenous aetiological factors in ankylosing spondylitis. *Acta Rheumatol Scand* 1960; **50**: 140–145.

53. Kuthan F, Navratil J. Spondylarthrite ankylosante chez deux pairs de jumeaux homozygotes. *Rev Rhum* 1966; **33**: 211–214.

54. Truog P, Steiger V, Contu L, et al. Ankylosing spondylitis (AS): a population and family study usign HL-A serology and MLR. In: Kissemeyer-Nielson F, ed. *Histocompatibility testing*. Copenhagen: Munksgaard, 1975: 788.

55. Eastmond CJ, Woodrow JC. Discordance for ankylosing spondylitis in monozygotic twins. *Ann Rheum Dis* 1977; **36**: 360–364.

56. Jarvinen P. Occurrence of ankylosing spondylitis in a nationwide series of twins. *Arthritis Rheum* 1995; **38**: 381–383.

57. Brown MA, Kennedy LG, MacGregor AJ, Darke C, Duncan E, Shatford JL et al. Susceptibility to ankylosing spondylitis in twins: the role of genes, HLA, and the environment. *Arthritis Rheum* 1997; **40**: 1823–1828.

58. Hohler T, Hug R, Schneider PM, Krummenauer F, Gripenberg LC, Granfors K *et al*. Ankylosing spondylitis in monozygotic twins: studies on immunological parameters. *Ann Rheum Dis* 1999; **58**: 435–440.

59. Brewerton DA, Caffrey M, Hart FD, James DCO, Nicholls A, Sturrock RD. Ankylosing spondylitis and HL-A27. *Lancet* 1973; i: 904–907.

60. Schlosstein L, Terasaki PI, Bluestone R, Pearson CM. High association of an HLA antigen, W27, with ankylosing spondylitis. *New Engl J Med* 1973; **288**: 704–705.

61. Mitsui H, Juji T, Sonozaki H. Juvenile ankylosing spondylitis, its clinical features and HLA-B27. *Arch Orthop Unfall-Chir* 1977; **87**: 31–37.

62. Rigby AS. Ankylosing spondylitis. In: Silman AJ, Hochberg MC, eds. *Epidemiology of the rheumatic diseases*, 1st edn. Oxford: Oxford University Press, 1993: 105–147.

63. Bale UM, Methta NM, Contractor NM, Bhatia HM, Tilve GH. HLA antigens in ankylosing spondylitis: the association of HLA-B27. *Ind J Med Res* 1980; **71**: 96–103.

64. Al-Rawi ZS, Al-Shakarchi HA, Hasan F, Thewani AJ. Ankylosing spondylitis and its association with the histocompatibility antigen HL-A B27: an epidemiological and clinical study. *Rheumatol Rehab* 1978; **17**: 72–75.

65. Moller E, Olhagen B. Studies on the major histocompatibility system in patients with ankylosing spondylitis. *Tissue Antigens* 1975; **6**: 237–247.

66. Reiten T, Skavdal KO, Solheim BG. HLA B27 in ankylosing spondylitis. *J Rheumatol* 1977; **4**(Suppl. 3): 109.

67. Khan MA. Epidemiology of HLA-B27 and Arthritis. *Clin Rheumatol* 1996; **15**(Suppl 1): 10–12.

68. Nasution AR, Mardjuadi A, Suryadhana NG, Daud R, Muslichan S. Higher relative risk of spondyloarthropathies among B27 positive Indonesian Chinese than native Indonesians. *J Rheumatol* 1993; **20**: 988–990.

69. Rivera S, Hassanhi M, Marquez G, Fuenmayor A, Monzon J, Avila J. [Relation of spondylarthropathies and HLA-B27 antigen in patients from the state of Zulia, Venezuela]Estudio de la relacion existente entre las espondiloartropatias y el antigeno HLA-B27 en pacientes del estado Zulia de Venezuela. *Sangre Barc* 1996; **41**: 473–476.

70. Mbayo K, Mbuyi-Muamba JM, Lurhuma AZ, Halle L, Kaplan C, Dequeker J. Low frequency of HLA-B27 and scarcity of ankylosing spondylitis in a Zairean Bantu population. *Clin Rheumatol* 1998; **17**: 309–310.

71. Rubin LA, Amos CI, Wade JA, Martin JR, Bale SJ, Little AH *et al*. Investigating the genetic basis for ankylosing spondylitis. Linkage studies with the major histocompatibility complex region. *Arthritis Rheum* 1994; **37**: 1212–1220.

72. D'Amato M, Fiorillo MT, Carcassi C, Mathieu A, Zuccarelli A, Bitti PP *et al*. Relevance of residue 116 of HLA-B27 in determining susceptibility to ankylosing spondylitis. *Eur J Immunol* 1995; **25**: 3199– 3201.

73. Baech J, Schmidt OS, Steffensen R, Varming K, Grunnet N, Jersild C. Frequency of HLA-B27 subtypes in a Danish population and in Danish patients with ankylosing spondylitis. *Tissue Antigens* 1997; **49**: 499–502.

74. Feltkamp TEW. Non-HLA-B27 genetic factors in HLA-B27 associated diseases. *Clin Rheumatol* 1996; **15**: 40–43.

75. Kanga U, Mehra NK, Larrea CL, Lardy NM, Kumar A, Feltkamp TE. Seronegative spondyloarthropathies and HLA-B27 subtyes: a study in Asian Indians. *Clin Rheumatol* 1996; **15**(Suppl. 1): 13–18.

76. Nasution AR, Mardjuadi A, Kunmartini S, Suryadhana NG, Setyohadi B, Sudarsono D *et al*. HLA-B27 subtypes positively and negatively associated with spondyloarthropathy. *J Rheumatol* 1997; **24**: 1111–1114.

77. Brown MA, Kennedy LG, Darke C, Gibson K, Pile KD, Shatford JL *et al*. The effect of HLA-DR genes on susceptibility to and severity of ankylosing spondylitis. *Arthritis Rheum* 1998; **41**: 460–465.

78. Ploski R, Flato B, Vinje O, Maksymowych W, Forre O, Thorsby E. Association to HLA-DRB1*08, HLA-DPB1*0301 and homozygosity for an HLA-linked proteasome gene in juvenile ankylosing spondylitis. *Hum Immunol* 1995; **44**: 88–96.

79. Martinez-Borra J, Gonzalez S, Lopez-Vazquez A, Gelaz MA, Armas JB, Kanga U *et al*. HLA-B27 alone rather than B27-related class I haplotypes contributes to ankylosing spondylitis susceptibility. *Hum Immunol* 2000; **61**: 131–139.

80. Spector TM, Ollier W, Perry LA, Silman AJ, Thompson PW, Edwards A. Free and serum testosterone levels in 276 males: a comparative study of rheumatoid arthritis, ankylosing spondylitis, and healthy controls. *Clin Rheumatol* 1989; **8**: 37–41.

81. Jimenez-Balderas F, Tapia-Serrano R, Madero-Cervera J, Murrieta S, Mintz G. Ovarian function studies in active ankylosing spondylitis in women. Clinical response to Estrogen therapy. *J Rheumatol* 1990; **17**: 497–502.

82. Masi AT. Do sex hormones play a role in ankylosing spondylitis? *Rheum Dis Clin North Am* 1992; **18**: 153–176.

83. Giltay EJ, van Schaardenburg D, Gooren LJ, Popp SC, Dijkmans BA. Androgens and ankylosing spondylitis: a role in the pathogenesis? *Ann N Y Acad Sci* 1999; **876**: 340–364.

84. Husby G, Ostensen H, Gran JT. Ankylosing spondylitis and pregnancy. *Clin Exp Rheumatol* 1988; **6**: 165–167.

85. Ostensen M, Husby G. Ankylosing spondylitis and pregnancy. *Rheum Dis Clin North Am* 1989; **15**: 241–254.

86. Ostensen M, Ostensen H. Ankylosing spondylitis—the female aspect. *J Rheumatol* 1998; **25**: 120–124.

87. Leirisalo RM, Turunen U, Stenman S, Helenius P, Seppala K. High frequency of silent inflammatory bowel disease in spondylarthropathy. *Arthritis Rheum* 1994; **37**: 23–31.

88. Ebringer RW, Cawdell DR, Cowling P, Ebringer A. Sequential studies in ankylosing spondylitis. Association of *Klebsiella pneumoniae* with active disease. *Ann Rheum Dis* 1978; **37**: 146–151.

89. Ebringer R, Cawdell D, Ebringer A. *Klebsiella pneumoniae* and acute anterior uveitis in ankylosing spondylitis. *Br Med J* 1979; **1**: 383.

90. Tani Y, Tiwana H, Hukuda S, Nishioka J, Fielder M, Wilson C *et al*. Antibodies to Klebsiella, Proteus, and HLA-B27 peptides in Japanese patients with ankylosing spondylitis and rheumatoid arthritis. *J Rheumatol* 1997; **24**: 109–114.

91. Seager K, Bashir HV, Geczy AF, Edmonds J, de-Vere-Tyndall A. Evidence for a specific B27-associated cell surface marker on lymphocytes of patients with ankylosing spondylitis. *Nature* 1979; **277**: 68–70.

92. Geczy AF, Prendergast JK, Sullivan JS, *et al*. HLA-B27, molecular mimicry, and ankylosing spondylitis: popular misconceptions. *Ann Rheum Dis* 1987; **46**: 171–172.

93. Ferraz MB, Atra E, Trabulsi LR, Goldenberg J, Sato EI. A study of the gram-negative bacterial flora in patients with ankylosing spondylitis. *Braz J Med Biol Res* 1990; **23**: 29–36.

94. van Kregten E, Huber-Bruning O, Vandenbroucke JP, Willers JMN. No conclusive evidence of an epidemiological reaction between *Klebsiella* and ankylosing spondylitis. *J Rheumatol* 1991; **18**: 385–388.

95. Dougados M. Classification and diagnosis of seronegative spondylarthropathies—Comments. *Scand J Rheumatol* 1999; **28**: 336–339.

96. Boyer GS, Templin DW, Goring WP. Evaluation of the European Spondylarthropathy Study Group preliminary classification criteria in Alaskan Eskimo populations. *Arthritis Rheum* 1993; **36**: 534–538.

97. Collantes-Estevez E, Cisnaldel Mazo A, Gomariz E. Assessment of two systems of spondyloarthropy classification (Amor and ESSG) by a Spanish multicentre group. *J Rheumatol* 1995; **22**: 246–251.

98. Cury SE, Vilar MJ, Ciconelli RM, Ferraz MB, Atra E. Evaluation of the European Spondyloarthropathy Study Group (ESSG) preliminary classification criteria in Brazilian patients. *Clin Exp Rheumatol* 1997; **15**: 79–82.

99. Erturk M, Alaca R, Tosun E, Duruoz MT. Evaluation of the Amor and ESSG criteria in a Turkish population. *Rev Rhum* Engl Ed 1997; **64**: 293–300.

100. Baddoura R, Awada H, Okais J, Habis T, Attoui S, Abi SM. Validation of the European Spondylarthropathy Study Group and B. Amor criteria for spondylarthropathies in Lebanon. *Rev Rhum* Engl Ed 1997; **64**: 459–464.

101. West HF. The aetiology of ankylosing spondylitis. *Ann Rheum Dis* 1949; **8**: 143–148.

102. Julkunen H. Rheumatoid spondylitis: clinical and laboratory study of 149 cases compared with 182 cases of rheumatoid arthritis. *Acta Rheumatol Scand* 1962; **52**(Suppl.): 1–110.

103. Lawrence JS. The prevalence of arthritis. *Br J Clin Pract* 1963; **17**: 699–705.

104. van der Linden SM, Valkenberg HA, De Jong BM, Cats A. The risk of developing ankylosing spondylitis in HLA-B27 positive individuals. A comparison of relatives of spondylitis patients with the general population. *Arthritis Rheum* 1984; **27**: 241–249.

105. Julkunen H, Korpi J. Ankylosing spondylitis in three Finnish population samples. *Scand J Rheumatol* 1984; **52**(Suppl.): 16–18.

106. Gran JT, Hordvik M, Husby G. Roenterological features of ankylosing spondylitis. A comparison between patients attending hospital and cases selected through an epidemiological survey. *Clin Rheumatol* 1984; **3**: 467–472.

107. Johnsen K, Gran JT, Dale K, Husby G. The prevalence of ankylosing spondylitis among Norwegian Samis (Lapps). *J Rheumatol* 1992; **19**: 1591–1594.

108. Chou CT, Pei L, Chang DM, Lee CF, Schumacher HR, Liang MH. Prevalence of rheumatic diseases in Taiwan: a population study of urban, suburban, rural differences. *J Rheumatol* 1994; **21**: 302–306.

109. Wigley RD, Zhang NZ, Zeng QY, Shi CS, Hu DW, Couchman K *et al*. Rheumatic diseases in China: ILAR-China study comparing the prevalence of rheumatic symptoms in northern and southern rural populations. *J Rheumatol* 1994; **21**: 1484–1490.

110. Boyer GS, Lanier AP, Templin DW. Prevalence rates of spondyloarthropies, rheumatoid arthritis, and other rheumatic disorders in an Alaskan Inupiat Eskimo population. *J Rheumatol* 1988; **15**: 678–683.

111. Boyer GS, Lanier AP, Templin DW, Bulkow L. Spondyloarthropy and rheumatoid arthritis in Alaskan Yupik Eskimos. *J Rheumatol* 1990; **17**: 489–496.

112. Clunie GPR, Koki G, Prasad ML, Richens JE, Bhatia K, Keat A. HLA-B27, arthritis and sponylitis in an isolated community in Papua New Guinea. *Br J Rheumatol* 1990; **29**: 97–100.

113. Muller AS, Valkenberg HA, Greenwood BM. Rheumatoid arthritis in three West African populations. *East Afr Med J* 1972; **49**: 75–83.

114. Lawrence JS. *Rheumatism in populations*. London: Heinemann, 1977: 282–324.

115. O'Connell D. Heredity in ankylosing spondylitis. *Ann Int Med* 1959; **50**: 1115–1121.

116. Karten I, Di Tata D, McEwan C, Tanner M. A family study of rheumatoid (ankylosing) spondylitis. *Arthritis Rheum* 1962; **5**: 131–142.

117. Christiansen FT, Owen ET, Dawkins RL, Hanrahan P. Symptoms and signs among relatives of patients with HLA B27 positive ankylosign spondylitis: correlation between back pain, spinal movement, sacroiliitis and HLA antigens. *J Rheumatol* 1977; **4**(Suppl. 3): 11–17.

118. Calin A, Marder A, Becks E, Burns T. Genetic differences between B27 positive patients with ankylosing spondylitis and B27 positive healthy controls. *Arthritis Rheum* 1983; **26**: 1460–1464.

119. LeClerq SA, Chaput L, Russell AS. Ankylosing spondylitis: a family study. *J Rheumatol* 1983; **10**: 629–731.

120. Hammoudeh M, Khan MA. Genetics of HLA associated diseases: ankylosing spondylitis. *J Rheumatol* 1983; **10**: 301–304.

121. Hukuda S, Minami M, Saito T *et al*. Spondyloarthropathies in Japan: Nationwide questionnaire survey performed by the Japan Ankylosing Spondylitis Society. *J Rheumatol* 2001; **28**: 554–559.

122. Liu Y, Li J, Chen BT, Helenius H, Granfors K. Familial aggregation of ankylosing spondylitis in southern China. *J Rheumatol* 2001; **28**: 550–553.

123. Laval SH, Timms A, Edwards S *et al*. Whole-genome screening in ankylosing spondylitis: Evidence of non-MHC genetic-susceptibility loci. *Am J Hum Genet* 2001; **68**: 918–926.

124. Baudoin P, Horst-Bruinsma IE, Dekker-Saeys AJ, Weinreich S, Bezemer PD, Dijkmans BAC. Increased risk of developing ankylosing spondylitis among first-born children. *Arthritis Rheum* 2000; **43**: 2818–2822.

Reactive arthritis and Reiter's syndrome

Alan J. Silman

It is recognized that a chronic inflammatory arthritis can arise following infection at a distant site without evidence that the joint site itself is a site of actual infection. This phenomenon is referred to as reactive arthritis (ReA) [1]. Recent data suggest that there may be some evidence of infection within joint tissues [2]. However, unlike septic arthritis, the unifying concept behind ReA is that the original infection site is extra-articular, predominantly the urogenital and gastro-intestinal tracts.

The first descriptions of ReA were of a clinical syndrome, Reiter's syndrome. This syndrome is classically defined as the triad of non-gonococcal urethritis, conjunctivitis, and arthritis, the latter usually an asymmetric oligoarthritis predominantly involving lower extremity joints [3]. Brodie, in the early nineteenth century, described the relationship of urethritis with an episodic arthritis involving predominantly lower extremity joints and the co-occurrence of conjunctivitis [4,5]. The description by Reiter [6] of a young soldier with non-gonococcal urethritis, conjunctivitis, and severe arthritis following an episode of bloody diarrhoea focused attention on the syndrome in the European literature and highlighted the possible aetiological role of a dysenteric illness. Incomplete forms of Reiter's syndrome are now recognized [7]. Reiter's syndrome and ReA are now accepted as forming part of a spectrum of synovitis occurring as a consequence of infection. These conditions are also part of the spectrum of seronegative spondyloarthropathies [8–10].

Classification criteria

Separate classification criteria for Reiter's syndrome have been in use for over 20 years. Criteria for ReA are more recent and it is now accepted that the latter should be used to encompass cases of Reiter's [11]. It is relevant, however, to briefly describe the previous crite-ria for Reiter's syndrome as they have been used in earlier studies.

Criteria for Reiter's syndrome

In 1979, the Diagnostic and Therapeutic Criteria Committee of the American Rheumatism Association (ARA) proposed criteria for the classification of Reiter's syndrome: Reiter's syndrome consists of peripheral arthritis occurring in association with urethritis and/or cervicitis; the characteristic episode is of more than one month's duration [12]. This definition was later revised as follows: Reiter's syndrome consists of an episode of peripheral arthritis of more than one month's duration occurring in association with urethritis and/or cervicitis [13].

Of 83 patients with a clinical diagnosis of Reiter's syndrome seen at seven university-based rheumatology clinics, 70, or 84.3 per cent, fulfilled this criterion at their initial episode and 11 of the remaining 13 cases fulfilled this criterion during their subsequent attacks. Among the 166 controls with either ankylosing spondylitis ($N = 53$), psoriatic arthritis ($N = 53$), seronegative rheumatoid arthritis ($N = 33$), or gonococcal arthritis ($N = 27$), only three subjects, two with ankylosing spondylitis and one with gonococcal arthritis, fulfilled the criterion. Thus the specificity was 98.2 per cent overall. The addition of other common clinical features of Reiter's syndrome, such as conjunctivitis, balanitis, heel pain, fever, and weight loss, did not improve either the sensitivity or specificity of the criterion.

An alternative schema for the classification of Reiter's syndrome was proposed by Calin *et al.* [14] (Table 6.1). This schema is less specific than the ARA preliminary criteria in that subjects do not necessarily have clinical evidence of genitourinary infection. Indeed, persons with ReA following bacterial dysentery without urethritis would fulfil these criteria. These cri-

Table 6.1 Criteria for classification of Reiter's syndrome; adapted from [14]

Seronegative asymmetric arthropathy plus ≥ 1 of the following:
  Urethritis/cervicitis
  Inflammatory eye disease
  Dysentery
  Mucocutaneous disease
  Balanitis
  Oral ulceration
  Kerotodermia

Table 6.3 International consensus classification criteria for reactive arthritis; modified from Kingsley G, Sieper J. *Ann Rheum Dis* 1996; **55**: 564–584 [11] with permission from the BMJ Publishing group

Typical peripheral arthritis (predominantly lower limb, asymmetric oligoarthritis)
                        AND
Evidence of preceding infection
(a) Clear evidence of diarrhoea or urethritis in preceding
    4 weeks
                        OR
(b) Suggestive evidence of diarrhoea or urethritis in preceding
    4 weeks with laboratory confirmation

Exclusions: other known causes of mono/oligoarthritis
            other defined spondyloarthropathies
            septic arthritis
            crystal arthritis
            Lyme disease
            Streptococcal ReA

teria have been superseded by a number of criteria sets for ReA.

Criteria for reactive arthritis

The definition of ReA, as sterile joint inflammation due to infection elsewhere, has required modification in recent years due to the discovery of microbial antigens in joints of patients with ReA. Thus there is evidence of *Yersinia* [15–17], *Salmonella* [18], and *Chlamydia* infection [19–21]. The concept of ReA, in theory, should not only include arthritis following bacterial dysentery and genitourinary infection, but also arthritis in the setting of other micro-organisms such as *Borrelia burgdorferi* infection [22,23] and the human immunodeficiency virus [24]. Most criteria schemes for ReA restrict inclusion to the homogeneous entity of arthritis following urogenital or gastrointestinal infection. Perhaps reflecting the lack of agreed and practical

criteria for ReA, three-quarters of published studies do not use standard criteria [25] although a number of sets have been proposed.

The first criteria proposed by the French Society of Rheumatology [26] (Table 6.2) were not specific about verification of associated infection. These criteria had a sensitivity of 79 per cent and a specificity of 92 per cent when applied to a group of patients attending and early arthritis clinic [27]. An international consensus group [11] proposed criteria (Table 6.3) and subsequently published strict rules concerning evidence of previous infection (Table 6.4) [28]. An alternative criteria scheme (the Mexican) has also been recently published (Table 6.5) [25]. Neither of these recent sets has been validated in either a clinic or population setting.

Table 6.2 French Society of Rheumatology criteria for reactive arthritis; modified from [26] with permission of Springer-Verlag GmbH©

1. Asceptic arthritis with one of:
     Asymmetric oligoarthritis
     Lumbar, sacro-iliac, or heel pain
     Sausage fingers/toes
2. Diarrhoea in 4 weeks prior to arthritis
3. Conjunctivitis in 4 weeks prior to arthritis
4. Urethritis or cervicitis in 4 weeks prior to arthritis
5. Characteristic oral or genital lesions or psoriasis-like lesions or nail involvement
6. HLA-B27 or family history of ReA, ankylosing spondylitis, iritis, seronegative oligoarthritis
7. Triggering agent

4 criteria: definite ReA
Exclusions: rheumatic fever
            chronic bowel disease arthropathy
            Behçet's disease
            ankylosing spondylitis

Table 6.4 Evidence of preceding infection; modified from [28] with permission from the *Journal of Rheumatology*

Clinical diarrhoea or urethritis in preceding 4 weeks
                        OR
Positive stool culture
                        OR
Detection of *Chlamydia trachomatis* in early morning urine or urogenital swab
                        OR
Anti-*Yersinia* or anti-*Salmonella* antibodies to lipopolysaccharide or other specific antigens of IgG plus IgA or IgG plus IgM subtypes
                        OR
IgG, IgM and IgA antibodies to *Chlamydia trachomatis*
                        OR
Detection of *Chlamydial* DNA in joint by PCR

Table 6.5   Mexican classification criteria for reactive arthritis; reproduced with permission from the *Journal of Rheumatology* from [25]

Probable reactive arthritis
Musculoskeletal symptoms (one of)
   Arthritis
   Oligoarthritis
   Polyarthritis
   Arthropathy
                          AND EITHER
Extra-articular disease. One of:
   Mucositis (conjunctivitis, urethritis or cervicitis)
   Keratoderma blennorrhagica
   Balanitis circinata
   Uveitis
                          OR
Clinical features of infectious disease. One of:
   Urethritis
   Diarrhoea
No bacterial identification
Features in 4-6 weeks preceding symptoms

Definite reactive arthritis
Musculoskeletal symptoms (as above)
                          AND EITHER
Bacterial identification by culture at site of infection of an infectious disease (urethritis or diarrhoea) preceding symptoms
                          OR
Other evidence of bacterial infection in recent onset symptoms

The distinction in the Mexican criterion between 'probable' and 'definite' is unhelpful. Furthermore, unlike the International Consensus criteria, the Mexican criteria do not specify rules for previous infection.

Population occurrence

It is useful to distinguish between the occurrence of ReA in the general population and the incidence following 'outbreaks' of specific infections. The occurrence of ReA by definition reflects, in part, the underlying incidence of the predisposing infections.

Incidence

The incidence of Reiter's syndrome has been estimated in Olmsted County, MN, using data from the Rochester Epidemiology Program Project [29]. In that study, 16 cases of Reiter's syndrome occurred in residents of Rochester, MN, seen over a 30-year period,

Table 6.6   Age- and sex-specific incidence rates for Reiter's syndrome in UK general practice attenders

Age	Rate per 100 000		
	15–24	25–44	45–64
Males	13.2	31.0	13.0
Females	0	11.0	3.0
Both sexes	8.5	21.0	7.9

Source: [31].

from 1 January 1950 to December 1980; all cases were male and 10 (62.5 per cent) developed between the ages of 20 and 39. The incidence rate in men aged 49 and below, age-adjusted to the 1980 US white male population, was 3.5 per 100 000 per year (95 per cent confidence intervals: 1.8, 5.2). Incidence rates were greatest in the 20–29 year age group, 6.3 per 100 000. In a study of a Hispanic population the incidence rates between 1975 and 1989, at 2.66 and 0.65 per 100 00 in males and females respectively, are more similar to the Rochester data [30].

Data are also available from the UK based on attendances in general practice [31]. The rates in adults aged 15–64 were 21 and 6.8 per 100 000 in males and females respectively, substantially higher than the Rochester rates. The age- and sex-specific rates are shown in Table 6.6 and indicate the peak age of onset being between 25 and 44. The reason for the disparity in the UK study is not clear. The Rochester cases were all verified by review of hospital records whereas the UK data are based on the general practitioner recorded diagnosis provided after hospital referral. In a primary care-based study from Norway [32], the incidence of post-*Chlamydial* ReA was 4.6 per 100 000 adults aged 18 to 60, with an almost identical incidence of post-enteritic ReA: 5 per 100 000.

Prevalence

The prevalence of Reiter's syndrome was considered to be less than one per 10 000 individuals [110]. One group with a high prevalence of Reiter's syndrome is homosexual and/or bisexual young men. In a cohort of over 1000 homosexual and/or bisexual men with a median age of 33 years, Hochberg *et al.* [33] found a lifetime prevalence of Reiter's syndrome of 5 per 1000. Comparable estimates ranging from 1 to 4 per 1000 have been reported in other cohorts of similar sociodemographic distribution.

Time trends

There are no robust data of trends of ReA over time. Further trends are likely to reflect underlying trends in the incidence of precipitating infections. Hospitalization in the Netherlands for male patients with Reiter's syndrome fell 40 per cent between 1981 and 1987 [34]. Similarly, in a large military hospital in Greece, there were 27 cases admitted between 1980 and 1983 and this had fallen to four cases between 1989 and 1992. During this period there had been no decline in admissions with dysentery though a marked reduction in both gonococcal and non-gonococcal urethritis had been observed [35]. A trend towards a younger age of onset has been suggested [30,35] and children appear to be increasingly observed. Case series have implicated both *Salmonella enteritidis* [36] and *Yersinia enterocolitica* [37] in childhood disease onset.

Geographic and ethnic influences

ReA is well described in African American populations [38] in the context of sexually transmitted diseases. However, there are several non-Caucasian North American populations that have been recognized to have a higher prevalence and/or incidence of Reiter's syndrome than Caucasians; these include Navajo Indians with an estimated prevalence ratio of 6 per 1000 and an incidence rate of 133 per 100 000 in males [39], Greenland Inuit Eskimos with an estimated prevalence ratio of between 3.4 and 10 per 1000 and an incidence rate of between 100 and 380 per 100 000 in both sexes combined [40], Alaskan Inupiat Eskimos with an estimated prevalence ratio of 10 per 1000 in males [41], Alaskan Yupik Eskimos with an estimated prevalence ratio of 5 per 1000 in males [42], and Alaskan Indians of the south east coast with an estimated prevalence ratio of 3 per 1000 in males aged 20 and above [43]. This high prevalence and incidence of Reiter's syndrome is associated with a high frequency of HLA-B27 in all of these Native American populations, as well as high rates of epidemic shigellosis in the Navajos [39] and genitourinary infections in the Greenland Inuit Eskimos [40,44]. A high prevalence of Reiter's syndrome in males, exceeding 2 per cent, has also been reported among residents of Papua New Guinea, a population that also has a high prevalence of HLA-B27 [45].

Bardin and Lathrop [46] reviewed their studies of the clinical epidemiology of Reiter's syndrome in the Inuit population of Greenland. In three west coast villages studied in 1983, 60 persons were identified with Reiter's syndrome for an average prevalence of 6.6 per 1000. In three different south west coast villages studied in 1986, 65 cases were identified for an average prevalence of 8.4 per 1000. Ninety-six per cent of 79 cases were found to possess HLA-B27. Clusters of cases have been described amongst illegal Chinese immigrants to the US [47] but the interpretation of this is difficult.

A detailed prevalence study has been reported in the circumpolar region across Alaska and Siberia. In the Chukotka Eskimos the prevalence is similar in both the Alaskan and Siberian groups at 0.5 per cent [48,49] suggesting a strong genetic component in this group.

Risk factors: infection

Classical organisms

As discussed above ReA is traditionally considered to be a response to genitourinary infection with *Chlamydia* species. These include *Chlamydia trachomatis* [50–53]. Gastrointestinal infections with a number of different species include *Shigella flexneri* [54–62], *Salmonella* species [59,63–69], *Yersinia enterocolitica* [1,70–77], and *Campylobacter fetus jejuni* [78–84], which all produce bacterial dysentery. The hypothetical immune-mediated mechanisms by which these organisms cause Reiter's syndrome and ReA have recently been reviewed [21,85,86].

Occurrence following infection

The interest is in the frequency of arthritis following infection. Older studies of Reiter's syndrome suggest an attack rate of 0.5 to 2 per cent following non-gonococcal urethritis [87,88]. In a more recent study, 4 per cent of 271 African Americans attending a sexually transmitted disease clinic had objective evidence of ReA [38]. Given the nature of the exposure, obtaining robust estimates of ReA attack rates is difficult.

By contrast, there is substantially more data in relation to outbreaks of gastroenteritis. This rate varies by species and, presumably, by the underlying genetic predisposition. Data from some of the recent studies are shown in Table 6.7. There are some features of interest. The data from Bangladesh, of several thousand infected with *Shigella dysenteriae*, show that some *Shigella* species are associated with a very low or nonexistent risk [93]. The data suggesting high incidences

Table 6.7   Attack rates of reactive arthritis following infection

Reference	Organism	Number exposed	Cumulative incidence (%)
[89]	*S. enteritidis*	108	17
[90]	*S. enteritidis*	222	6
[91]	*S. bovismorbificans*	191	12
[92]	*Salmonella, Shigella, Campylobacter and Yersinia*	536	33[a]
[93]	*Shigella dysenteriae*	~12 000	nil
[94]	*S. typhimurium*	424	5
[95]	*Salmonella*	83	8
[96]	*Yersinia pseudotuberculosis*	16	56[a]

[a] Joint symptoms.

[92,96] have to be treated with caution given low follow-up participation rates and reliance on self-reported symptoms. It is, however, likely that some organisms, e.g. *Yersinia enterocolitica*, are more arthritogenic than others [97].

Human immunodeficiency virus

There has been considerable recent interest in the relationship between human immunodeficiency virus (HIV) infection and ReA. Any association could be explained, however, by (1) HIV being arthritogenic; (2) increased susceptibility to infection by arthritogenic bacteria in HIV positive subjects; or (3) the increased CD8 counts in HIV subjects contributing to the pathogenesis of ReA [98].

Data are not consistent. In three large cohorts of US males with HIV, numbering several thousands, ReA was rare affecting less than one per cent [99]. In that study, the authors ascribed any cases to infection with other known arthritogenic organisms. Arthritic symptoms are not uncommon in patients with AIDS and can be erroneously ascribed to ReA [100]. In a second study of 1100 HIV-positive subjects in the US, only one subject had ReA which antedated HIV infection [101].

In high HIV prevalence areas such as Congo-Brazzaville, HIV is the leading cause of arthritis and most rheumatology clinic attenders, who are HIV-positive, have an inflammatory arthritis [102]. There are a number of different clinical presentations of HIV-associated arthritis other than ReA [103]. In Zimbabwe, oligoarthritis suggestive of ReA is also the predominant arthritic disorder associated with HIV.

Other infectious triggers

Cases have been observed following immunisation for typhoid [104] and hepatitis B [105]. There have also been case reports of an association with *Helicobacter* infection [106]. A recent case report was linked to infection with *Giardia lamblia* [120]. In the absence of controlled epidemiological studies, these reports are difficult to interpret.

Genetic factors

The genetic predisposition to Reiter's syndrome and ReA is associated with the Class I major histocompatability antigen HLA-B27. This phenotype is present in at least three-quarters of patients with Reiter's syndrome [70,107,108] and ReA associated with *Shigella flexneri* [60], *Salmonella sp.* [64], *Yersinia enterocolitica* [70,74,75], and *Campylobacter fetus jejuni* [78].

The association with HLA-B27 varies between populations. Thus in Alaskan Eskimos, HLA-B27 is associated with a 13-fold increased risk of ReA [109], though this is much smaller rate than the 210-fold increased risk observed for ankylosing spondylitis in the same population. Within populations there is variation in strength of the association—thus over 75 per cent of 'clinic' cases were B27 positive in one Finnish study [70] compared to approximately 30–40% in others from that country [90,91]. There are some well-defined multicase families with ReA with no linkage to HLA-B27 [111]. HLA-B27 is also often unusual in some outbreaks of post-enteritic ReA (e.g. [94]), as well as other infectious causes [105]. Even in European HLA-B27 positive populations ReA is rare [112].

HLA-B27 is also in linkage disequilibrium with alleles at other loci with the MHC. Thus increases in C4A-Q0 and DRB1*04 have been observed—though no relationship has been found with DQA1*, DQB1*, or DPB1* alleles [113] or with a polymorphism in HSP-70 independent of B27 [114].

Laboratory studies suggest that the mechanism of this association is mediated through the process of molecular mimicry. Using monoclonal anti-HLA-B27 antibodies van Bohemen [115] identified antigens cross-reactive with HLA-B27M1 in *Yersinia enterocolitica* type 9 and *Klebsiella pnuemoniae* types K21 and K43 and with HLA-B27M2 in *Shigella flexneri*. These observations have been extended at the molecular level by the work of Schwimmbeck [116] and Steiglitz [117]. The former group identified a six-amino acid sequence homology between residues 72 and 77 of the α-1 domain of the most common B27 subtype, B27.1 or B*2705, and residues 188–193 of the nitrogenase reductase enzyme of *Klebsiella pnuemoniae*. The latter group sequenced a 2-mega-dalton plasmid from an arthritogenic strain of *Shigella flexneri* and identified a five-amino acid sequence homology with all B27 molecules which extends from residue 71 to 75 in the α-1 domain. Of great interest is the overlap in sequences between the *Klebsiella* protein and the *Shigella* plasmid with the same sequence in the hypervariable region of the α-1 domain of the B27 molecule.

An alternative explanation, as suggested by Benjamin and Parham [118], is that the HLA-B27 molecule presents bacterial antigen leading to the generation of Class 1 restricted cytotoxic T-cell response which is then amplified in the joints due to the presence of antigenic fragments of non-viable organisms in the synovial membrane. The observations that treatment with antibiotics, particularly tetracycline and/or its derivatives, both shortens the duration of and decreases the rate of recurrent attacks of arthritis in patients with *Chlamydia*-associated Reiter's syndrome [46,119] provides indirect support for the role of a persistent antigen and antigen-presentation in the development of arthritis in these patients.

References

1. Ahvonen P, Sievers K, Aho K. Arthritis associated with Yersinia enterocolitica infection. *Acta Rheum Scand* 1969; **15**: 232–253.

2. Inman RD. Classification criteria for reactive arthritis. *J Rheumatol* 1999; **26**: 1219–1221.

3. Bauer WF, Engleman EP. A syndrome of unknown etiology characterized by urethritis, conjunctivitis and arthritis (so-called Reiter's disease). *Trans Ass Am Phys* 1942; **57**: 307–313.

4. Brodie BC. Pathologic and surgical observations on diseases of the joints. London: Longman, 1818.

5. Brodie BC. Pathological and surgical observations on diseases of the joints with alterations and additions. London: Longman; 1836.

6. Reiter H. Ueber eine bisher unerkannte Spriochateninfektion (Spirochaetosis Arthritica). *Dtsch Med Wochenschr* 1916; **42**: 1535–1536.

7. Arnett FC, McClusky OE, Schacter BZ, Lordon RE. Incomplete Reiter's syndrome: discriminating features and HL-A W27 in diagnosis. *Ann Intern Med* 1976; **84**: 8–12.

8. Arnett FC. Seronegative spondylarthropathies. *Bull Rheum Dis* 1987; **37**: 1–12.

9. Khan MA, van der Linden SM. A wider spectrum of spondyloarthropathies. *Semin Arthritis Rheum* 1990; **20**: 107–113.

10. Moll JM, Haslock I, Macrae IF, Wright V. Associations between ankylosing spondylitis, psoriatic arthritis, Reiter's disease, the intestinal arthropathies, and Behcet's syndrome. *Medicine Baltimore* 1974; **53**: 343–364.

11. Kingsley G, Sieper J. Third international workshop on reactive arthritis. 23–26 September 1995, Berlin, Germany. Report and abstracts. *Ann Rheum Dis* 1996; **55**: 564–584.

12. Willkens RF, Arnett FC, Bitter T *et al.* Reiter's syndrome: evaluation of proposed criteria. *Ann Rheum Dis* 1979; **38** (Suppl.): 8–11.

13. Willkens RF, Arnett FC, Bitter T *et al.* Reiter's syndrome. Evaluation of preliminary criteria for definite disease. *Arthritis Rheum* 1981; **24**: 844–849.

14. Calin A, Fox R, Gerber RC, Gibson DJ. Prognosis and natural history of Reiter's syndrome. *Ann Rheum Dis* 1979; **38** (Suppl. 1): 29–31.

15. Granfors K, Jalkanen S, von Essen R *et al.* Yersinia antigens in synovial-fluid cells from patients with reactive arthritis. *N Engl J Med* 1989; **320**: 216–221.

16. Hammer M, Zeidler H, Klimsa S, Heesemann J. Yersinia enterocolitica in the synovial membrane of patients with Yersinia-induced arthritis. *Arthritis Rheum* 1990; **33**: 1795–1800.

17. Merilahti Palo R, Soderstrom KO, Lahesmaa Rantala R, Granfors K, Toivanen A. Bacterial antigens in synovial biopsy specimens in yersinia triggered reactive arthritis. *Ann Rheum Dis* 1991; **50**: 87–90.

18. Granfors K, Jalkanen S, Lindberg AA *et al.* Salmonella lipopolysaccharide in synovial cells from patients with reactive arthritis. *Lancet* 1990; **335**: 685–688.

19. Keat A, Thomas B, Dixey J, Osborn M, Sonnex C, Taylor Robinson D. Chlamydia trachomatis and reactive arthritis: the missing link. *Lancet* 1987; **1**: 72–74.

20. Schumacher HRJr, Magge S, Cherian PV *et al.* Light and electron microscopic studies on the synovial

membrane in Reiter's syndrome. Immunocytochemical identification of chlamydial antigen in patients with early disease. *Arthritis Rheum* 1988; **31**: 937–946.

21. Rahman MU, Hudson AP, Schumacher HR Jr. Chlamydia and Reiter's syndrome (reactive arthritis). *Rheum Dis Clin North Am* 1992; **18**: 67–79.

22. Arnett FC. The Lyme spirochete: another cause of Reiter's syndrome? *Arthritis Rheum* 1989; **32**: 1182–1184.

23. Weyand CM, Goronzy JJ. Immune responses to Borrelia burgdorferi in patients with reactive arthritis. *Arthritis Rheum* 1989; **32**: 1057–1064.

24. Winchester R, Bernstein DH, Fischer HD, Enlow R, Solomon G. The co-occurrence of Reiter's syndrome and acquired immunodeficiency. *Ann Intern Med* 1987; **106**: 19–26.

25. Pacheco Tena C, Burgos Vargas R, Vazquez Mellado J, Cazarin J, Perez Diaz JA. A proposal for the classification of patients for clinical and experimental studies on reactive arthritis. *J Rheumatol* 1999; **26**: 1338–1346.

26. Amor B. Reiter's syndrome and reactive arthritis. *Clin Rheumatol* 1983; **2**: 315–319.

27. Hulsemann JL, Zeidler H. Diagnostic evaluation of classification criteria for rheumatoid arthritis and reactive arthritis in an early synovitis outpatient clinic. *Ann Rheum Dis* 1999; **58**: 278–280.

28. Sieper J, Braun J. Problems and advances in the diagnosis of reactive arthritis. *J Rheumatol* 1999; **26**: 1222–1224.

29. Michet CJ, Machado EB, Ballard DJ, McKenna CH. Epidemiology of Reiter's syndrome in Rochester, Minnesota: 1950–1980. *Arthritis Rheum* 1988; **31**: 428–431.

30. Sanchez Burson JM, Gomez Rodriguez N, Rosales Rodriguez M, Aspe de la I, Grana Gil J, Atanes Sandoval A. Estudio epidemiologico del Sindrome de Reiter en un area sanitaria. *An Med Interna* 1992; **9**: 125–128.

31. Hay EM. Review of UK data on the rheumatic diseases-10: Reiter's syndrome and reactive arthritis. *Br J Rheumatol* 1991; **30**: 474–475.

32. Kvien TK, Glennas A, Melby K *et al*. Reactive arthritis: incidence, triggering agents and clinical presentation. *J Rheumatol* 1994; **21**: 115–122.

33. Hochberg MC, Fox R, Nelson KE, Saah A. HIV infection is not associated with Reiter's syndrome: data from the Johns Hopkins Multicenter AIDS Cohort Study. *AIDS* 1990; **4**: 1149–1151.

34. van Romunde LK, Stronks DL, Rijpma SE, Passchier J, Hunfeld JA, Stolz E. Het aantal opnamen voor de ziekte van Reiter (ICD-9-code 099.3) in Nederlandse ziekenhuizen over de periode 1981–1987. *Ned Tijdschr Geneeskd* 1993; **137**: 305–306.

35. Iliopoulos A, Karras D, Ioakimidis D *et al*. Change in the epidemiology of Reiter's syndrome (reactive arthritis) in the post-AIDS era? An analysis of cases appearing in the Greek Army. *J Rheumatol* 1995; **22**: 252–254.

36. Kanakoudi-Tsakalidou F, Pardalos G, Pratsidou Gertsi P, Kansouzidou-Kanakoudi A, Tsangaropoulou Stinga H. Persistent or severe course of reactive arthritis following Salmonella enteritidis infection—a prospective study of 9 cases. *Scand J Rheumatol* 1998; **27**: 431–434.

37. Taccetti G, Trapani S, Ermini M, Falcini F. Reactive arthritis triggered by Yersinia enterocolitica: a review of 18 pediatric cases. *Clin Exp Rheumatol* 1994; **12**: 681–684.

38. Rich E, Hook EW III, Alarcon GS, Moreland LW. Reactive arthritis in patients attending an urban sexually transmitted diseases clinic. *Arthritis Rheum* 1996; **39**: 1172–1177.

39. Morse HG, Rate RG, Bonnell MD, Kuberski T. High frequency of HLA-B27 and Reiter's syndrome in Navajo Indians. *J Rheumatol* 1980; **7**: 900–902.

40. Bardin T, Enel C, Lathrop M, Becker Christensen F. Reiter's syndrome in Greenland. A clinical and epidemiological study of two communities. *Scand J Rheumatol* 1985; **14**: 369–374.

41. Boyer GS, Lanier AP, Templin DW. Prevalence rates of spondyloarthropathies, rheumatoid arthritis, and other rheumatic disorders in an Alaskan Inupiat Eskimo population. *J Rheumatol* 1988; **15**: 678–683.

42. Boyer GS, Lanier AP, Templin DW, Bulkow L. Spondyloarthropathy and rheumatoid arthritis in Alaskan Yupik Eskimos. *J Rheumatol* 1990; **17**: 489–496.

43. Boyer GS, Templin DW, Lanier AP. Rheumatic diseases in Alaskan Indians of the southeast coast: high prevalence of rheumatoid arthritis and systemic lupus erythematosus. *J Rheumatol* 1991; **18**: 1477–1484.

44. Mardh PA, Lind I, From E, Andersen AL. Prevalence of Chlamydia trachomatis and Neisseria gonorrhoeae infections in Greenland. A seroepidemiological study. *Br J Vener Dis* 1980; **56**: 327–331.

45. Clunie GP, Koki G, Prasad ML, Richens JE, Bhatia K, Keat A. HLA-B27, arthritis and spondylitis in an isolated community in Papua New Guinea. *Br J Rheumatol* 1990; **29**: 97–100.

46. Bardin T, Lathrop GM. Postvenereal Reiter's syndrome in Greenland. *Rheum Dis Clin North Am* 1992; **18**: 81–93.

47. Solitar BM, Lozada CJ, Tseng CE *et al*. Reiter's syndrome among Asian shipboard immigrants: the case of The Golden Venture. *Semin Arthritis Rheum* 1998; **27**: 293–300.

48. Alexeeva L, Krylov M, Vturin V, Mylov N, Erdesz S, Benevolenskaya L. Prevalence of spondyloarthropathies and HLA-B27 in the native population of Chukotka, Russia. *J Rheumatol* 1994; **21**: 2298–2300.

49. Benevolenskaya LI, Boyer GS, Erdesz S *et al*. Spondylarthropathic diseases in indigenous circumpolar populations of Russia and Alaska. *Rev Rhum Engl Ed* 1996; **63**: 815–822.

50. Keat AC, Maini RN, Nkwazi GC, Pegrum GD, Ridgway GL, Scott JT. Role of Chlamydia trachomatis and HLA-B27 in sexually acquired reactive arthritis. *BMJ* 1978; **1**: 605–607.

51. Keat AC, Thomas BJ, Taylor Robinson D, Pegrum GD, Maini RN, Scott JT. Evidence of Chlamydia trachomatis infection in sexually acquired reactive arthritis. *Ann Rheum Dis* 1980; **39**: 431–437.

52. Kousa M, Saikku P, Richmond S, Lassus A. Frequent association of chlamydial infection with Reiter's syndrome. *Sex Transm Dis* 1978; **5**: 57–61.

53. Martin DH, Pollock S, Kuo CC, Wang SP, Brunham RC, Holmes KK. Chlamydia trachomatis infections in men with Reiter's syndrome. *Ann Intern Med* 1984; **100**: 207–213.

54. Young RH, McEwen EH. Bacillary dysentery as the cause of Reiter's syndrome (arthritis with nonspecific urethritis and conjunctivitis). *JAMA* 1947; **134**: 1456–1459.

55. Paronen I. Reiter's disease: a study of 344 cases observed in Finland. *Acta Med Scand* 1948; **131**: 1–114.

56. Berglot PE. Arthritis and intestinal infection. *Acta Rheum Scand* 1963; **9**: 141–149.

57. Noer HR. An 'experimental' epidemic of Reiter's syndrome. *JAMA* 1966; **198**: 693–698.

58. Davies NE, Haverty JR, Boatwright M. Reiter's disease associated with shigellosis. *South Med J* 1969; **62**: 1011–1014.

59. Aho K, Ahvonen P, Alkio P, *et al.* HLA 27 in reactive arthritis following infection. *Ann Rheum Dis* 1975; **34** (Suppl.): 29–30.

60. Calin A, Fries JF. An 'experimental' epidemic of Reiter's syndrome revisited. Follow-up evidence on genetic and environmental factors. *Ann Intern Med* 1976; **84**: 564–566.

61. Good AE, Schultz JS. Reiter's syndrome following Shigella flexneri 2a: a sequel to traveler's diarrhea. Report of a case with hepatitis. *Arthritis Rheum* 1977; **20**: 100–104.

62. Singsen BH, Bernstein BH, Koster-King KG, Glovsky MM, Hanson V. Reiter's syndrome in childhood. *Arthritis Rheum* 1977; **20**: 402–407.

63. Friis J, Svejgaard A. Salmonella arthritis and HLA 27. *Lancet* 1974; **1**: 1350.

64. Hâkansson U, Löw B, Eitrem R, Winblad S. HL-A27 and reactive arthritis in an outbreak of salmonellosis. *Tissue Antigens* 1975; **6**: 366–367.

65. Jones MB, Smith PW, Olnhausen RW. Reiter's syndrome after Salmonella infection: occurrence in HLA B27 positive brothers. *Arthritis Rheum* 1979; **22**: 1141–1142.

66. Jones RA. Reiter's disease after Salmonella typhimurium enteritis. *BMJ* 1977; **1**: 1391.

67. Stein HB, Abdullah A, Robinson HS, Ford DK. Salmonella reactive arthritis in British Columbia. *Arthritis Rheum* 1980; **23**: 206–210.

68. Vartiainen J, Hurri L. Arthritis due to Salmonella typhimurium: report of 12 cases of migratory arthritis in association with Salmonella typhimurium. *Acta Med Scand* 1964; **175**: 771–776.

69. Warren CP. Arthritis associated with Salmonella infections. *Ann Rheum Dis* 1970; **29**: 483–487.

70. Aho K, Ahvonen P, Lassus A, Sievers K, Tilikainen A. HLA 27 in reactive arthritis. A study of Yersinia arthritis and Reiter's disease. *Arthritis Rheum* 1974; **17**: 521–526.

71. Ahvonen P. Human yersiniosis in Finland. II. Clinical features. *Ann Clin Res* 1972; **4**: 39–48.

72. Jacobs JC. Yersinia enterocolitica arthritis. *Pediatrics* 1975; **55**: 236–238.

73. Laitenen O, Tuuhea J, Ahvonen P. Polyarthritis associated with Yersinia enterocolitica infection. Clinical features and laboratory findings in nine cases with severe joint symptoms. *Ann Rheum Dis* 1972; **31**: 34–39.

74. Laitinen O, Leirisalo M, Skylv G. Relation between HLA-B27 and clinical features in patients with yersinia arthritis. *Arthritis Rheum* 1977; **20**: 1121–1124.

75. Leirisalo M, Skylv G, Kousa M *et al.* Follow-up study on patients with Reiter's disease and reactive arthritis, with special reference to HLA-B27. *Arthritis Rheum* 1982; **25**: 249–259.

76. Marsal L, Winblad S, Wollheim FA. Yersinia enterocolitica arthritis in southern Sweden: a four-year follow-up study. *Br Med J Clin Res Ed* 1981; **283**: 101–103.

77. Winblad S. Arthritis associated with Yersinia enterocolitica infections. *Scand J Infect Dis* 1975; **7**: 191–195.

78. Kosunen TU. Reactive arthritis after Campylobacter jejuni enteritis in patients with HLA-B27. *Lancet* 1980; **1**: 1312–1313.

79. Békássy AN, Enell H, Schalén C. Severe polyarthritis following Campylobacter enteritis in a 12-year-old boy. *Acta Paediatr Scand* 1980; **69**: 269–271.

80. Gumpel JM, Martin C, Sanderson PJ. Reactive arthritis associated with campylobacter enteritis. *Ann Rheum Dis* 1981; **40**: 64–65.

81. Leung FY, Littlejohn GO, Bombardier C. Reiter's syndrome after Campylobacter jejuni enteritis. *Arthritis Rheum* 1980; **23**: 948–950.

82. Pönká A, Martio J, Kosunen TU. Reiter's syndrome in association with enteritis due to Campylobacter fetus ssp. jejuni. *Ann Rheum Dis* 1981; **40**: 414–415.

83. Teir W, Keat AC, Welsby PD, Brear G. Reactive arthritis associated with Campylobacter infection of the bowel. *J Infect* 1979; **1**: 281–284.

84. van de Putte LB, Berden JH, Boerbooms MT *et al.* Reactive arthritis after Campylobacter jejuni enteritis. *J Rheumatol* 1980; **7**: 531–535.

85. Granfors K. Do bacterial antigens cause reactive arthritis? *Rheum Dis Clin North Am* 1992; **18**: 37–48.

86. Kingsley G, Panayi G. Antigenic responses in reactive arthritis. *Rheum Dis Clin North Am* 1992; **18**: 49–66.

87. Csonka GW. The course of Reiter's syndrome. *BMJ* 1958; **1**: 1088–1092.

88. Laird SM. Figures and fancies. *Br J Vener Dis* 1958; **34**: 137–152.

89. Locht H, Kihlstrom E, Lindstrom FD. Reactive arthritis after Salmonella among medical doctors—study of an outbreak. *J Rheumatol* 1993; **20**: 845–848.

90. Mattila L, Leirisalo Repo M, Koskimies S, Granfors K, Siitonen A. Reactive arthritis following an outbreak of Salmonella infection in Finland. *Br J Rheumatol* 1994; **33**: 1136–1141.

91. Mattila L, Leirisalo Repo M, Pelkonen P, Koskimies S, Granfors K, Siitonen A. Reactive arthritis following an outbreak of Salmonella bovismorbificans infection. *J Infect* 1998; **36**: 289–295.

92. Thomson GTD, Blanchard J, Thomson BRJ, MacKay M, Cartageena R. Reactive arthritis (ReA) after sporadic cases of food poisoning: Incidence in a population. *Arthritis Rheum* 1997; **40**: 679–679.

93. Mazumder RN, Salam MA, Ali M, Bhattacharya MK. Reactive arthritis associated with Shigella dysenteriae type 1 infection. *J Diarrhoeal Dis Res* 1997; **15**: 21–24.

94. McColl GJ, Diviney MB, Holdsworth RF *et al.* HLA-B27 expression and reactive arthritis susceptibility in two patient cohorts infected with Salmonella typhimurium. *Aust N Z J Med* 2000; **30**: 28–32.

95. Thomson GT, Chiu B, De Rubeis D, Falk J, Inman RD. Immunoepidemiology of post-Salmonella reactive arthritis in a cohort of women. *Clin Immunol Immunopathol* 1992; **64**: 227–232.

96. Yli Kerttula T, Tertti R, Toivanen A. Ten-year follow up study of patients from a Yersinia pseudotuberculosis III outbreak. *Clin Exp Rheumatol* 1995; **13**: 333–337.

97. Keat A. Reiter's syndrome and reactive arthritis in perspective. *N Engl J Med* 1983; **309**: 1606–1615.

98. Altman EM, Centeno LV, Mahal M, Bielory L. AIDS-associated Reiter's syndrome. *Ann Allergy* 1994; **72**: 307–316.

99. Clark MR, Solinger AM, Hochberg MC. Human immunodeficiency virus infection is not associated with Reiter's syndrome. Data from three large cohort studies. *Rheum Dis Clin North Am* 1992; **18**: 267–276.

100. Hacbarth ET, Freire CA, Atra E. Manifestacoes reumaticas na sindrome de imunodeficiencia adquirida (AIDS). *Rev Assoc Med Bras* 1992; **38**: 90–94.

101. Solinger AM, Hess EV. Rheumatic diseases and AIDS—is the association real? *J Rheumatol* 1993; **20**: 678–683.

102. Bileckot R, Mouaya A, Makuwa M. Prevalence and clinical presentations of arthritis in HIV-positive patients seen at a rheumatology department in Congo-Brazzaville. *Rev Rhum Engl Ed* 1998; **65**: 549–554.

103. Olejarova M. Rheumatological manifestations of HIV infection. *Ceska Revmatol* 1998; **6**: 103–112.

104. Adachi JA, D'Alessio FR, Ericsson CD. Reactive arthritis associated with typhoid vaccination in travelers: report of two cases with negative HLA-B27. *J Travel Med* 2000; **7**: 35–36.

105. Gross K, Combe C, Kruger K, Schattenkirchner M. Arthritis after hepatitis B vaccination. *Scand J Rheumatol* 1995; **24**: 50–52.

106. Melby KK, Kvien TK, Glennas A. Helicobacter pylori—a trigger of reactive arthritis? *Infection* 1999; **27**: 252–255.

107. Brewerton DA, Caffrey M, Nicholls A, Walters D, Oates JK, James DC. Reiter's disease and HL-A 27. *Lancet* 1973; **2**: 996–998.

108. Woodrow JC, Treanor B, Usher N. The HLA system in Reiter's syndrome. *Tissue Antigens* 1964; **4**: 533–540.

109. Boyer GS, Templin DW, Bowler A *et al.* Class I HLA antigens in spondyloarthropathy: observations in Alaskan Eskimo patients and controls. *J Rheumatol* 1997; **24**: 500–506.

110. Lawrence JS. Rheumatism in populations. London: William Heinemann Medical Books Ltd; 1977.

111. Thomson GT, Minenko A, Schroeder ML. Host risk factors for the development of reactive arthritis: a family study. *J Rheumatol* 1993; **20**: 1350–1352.

112. Braun J, Bollow M, Remlinger G *et al.* Prevalence of spondylarthropathies in HLA-B27 positive and negative blood donors. *Arthritis Rheum* 1998; **41**: 58–67.

113. Wollenhaupt J, Zeidler H, Voegeler U *et al.* Frequency of HLA class II and non-HLA antigens in patients with chlamydia induced reactive arthritis. *Ann Rheum Dis* 1996; **55**: 584.

114. Westman P, Partanen J, Leirisalo Repo M, Koskimies S. HSP70-Hom Ncol polymorphism and HLA-associations in the finnish population and in patients with ankylosing-spondylitis or reactive arthritis. *Eur J Immunogenet* 1994; **21**: 81–90.

115. van Bohemen CG, Grumet FC, Zanen HC. Identification of HLA-B27M1 and -M2 cross-reactive antigens in Klebsiella, Shigella and Yersinia. *Immunology* 1984; **52**: 607–610.

116. Schwimmbeck PL, Yu DT, Oldstone MB. Autoantibodies to HLA B27 in the sera of HLA B27 patients with ankylosing spondylitis and Reiter's syndrome. Molecular mimicry with Klebsiella pneumoniae as potential mechanism of autoimmune disease. *J Exp Med* 1987; **166**: 173–181.

117. Stieglitz H, Fosmire S, Lipsky P. Identification of a 2-Md plasmid from Shigella flexneri associated with reactive arthritis. *Arthritis Rheum* 1989; **32**: 937–946.

118. Benjamin R, Parham P. HLA-B27 and disease: a consequence of inadvertent antigen presentation? *Rheum Dis Clin North Am* 1992; **18**: 11–21.

119. Lauhio A, Leirisalo Repo M, Lahdevirta J, Saikku P, Repo H. Double-blind, placebo-controlled study of three-month treatment with lymecycline in reactive arthritis, with special reference to Chlamydia arthritis. *Arthritis Rheum* 1991; **34**: 6–14.

120. Borman P, Seckin U, Ozoran K. Beaver fever – A rare cause of reactive arthritis. *J Rheumatol* 2001; **28**: 683.

PART II
Connective tissue diseases

7 | *Systemic lupus erythematosus*

Violeta Rus, Ali Hajeer, and Marc C. Hochberg

Classification criteria

In 1971, the American Rheumatism Association published preliminary criteria for the classification of systemic lupus erythematosus (SLE) [1]. At present, the American College of Rheumatology (ACR) 1982 revised criteria for the classification of SLE [2], as modified in 1997 [3], are used for case definition (Table 7.1). The original 1982 data set was reanalyzed by Edworthy *et al.*, using recursive partitioning, to generate two classification trees, in an attempt to identify simpler and more explicit rules to classify patients with SLE [4]. The resulting simple classification tree requires knowledge of only two variables: immunologic disorder and malar rash. A more complex tree requires knowledge of six variables, including serum complement levels, which is not included within the 1982 revised criteria. The sensitivity, specificity, and accuracy were 96 per cent for the 1982 revised criteria and 92 per cent for the simple classification tree

(Table 7.1). Perez-Gutthann *et al.* [5] compared the sensitivity of the 1982 revised criteria in the traditional format with both classification trees in 198 patients from the Johns Hopkins lupus cohort. The revised criteria were significantly more sensitive than the simple classification tree, correctly identifying 184 (93 per cent) compared with 168 cases (85 per cent), respectively (p = 0.016); the full classification tree correctly identified 186 cases (94 per cent). Thus, these data support the use of the 1982 revised criteria in the traditional format to classify patients with SLE.

Other groups have examined the relative value of individual criterion in selected patient populations using receiver operating characteristic curves [6] and Bayesian theory [7,8]; however, the use of weighted criterion scores has not proven to be more reliable in epidemiologic studies.

Recently, the Diagnostic and Therapeutic Criteria Committee of ACR has updated the 1982 criteria [3]. Within criterion 10, item (a) the positive LE cell test

Table 7.1 1982 Revised criteria for SLE

	Sensitivity	Specificity	Accuracy[a]
1. Malar rash	57	96	76
2. Discoid rash	18	99	57
3. Photosensitivity	43	96	68
4. Oral ulcers	27	96	60
5. Non-erosive arthritis	86	37	63
6. Pleuritis or pericarditis	56	86	70
7. Renal disorder	51	94	71
8. Seizures or psychosis	20	98	57
9. Hematologic disorder	59	89	73
10. Immunologic disorder	85	93	88
11. Positive antinuclear antibody	99	49	77
> 4 criteria	96	96	96
Simple classification tree	92	92	92
Full classification tree	97	95	96

[a] Accuracy is defined as the average of sensitivity and specificity. For definitions of individual criterion items, see [2]
Source: data from [2] and [4].

was deleted and item (d) was changed to positive test for antiphospholipid antibodies including: (1) an abnormal serum level of IgG or IgM anticardiolipin antibodies, (2) a positive test for lupus anticoagulant using a standard method, or (3) a false positive serologic test for syphilis known to be positive for at least 6 months and confirmed by *Treponema pallidum* immobilization or fluorescent treponemal antibody adsorption test. The updated version was more sensitive (78 per cent versus 72 per cent), but slightly less specific (88 per cent versus 91 per cent) than the 1982 criteria in a cohort of 346 patients with connective tissue disease [9].

None of the methods for classifying patients with SLE was designed for diagnostic purposes. These criteria should be used mainly for the purpose of classifying patients in clinical, epidemiologic, and pathogenetic studies of SLE. Assuring homogeneity of the case population is ideal for epidemiologic studies that address etiology or risk factors. However, classification criteria lack sensitivity for recognizing milder cases of SLE, which becomes a limitation for descriptive studies of morbidity and observational studies of prognosis, because subjects with a multisystem disease that is consistent with SLE will not be included if they fail to fulfill the criteria. Data from the Rochester study suggest that the prevalence of suspected SLE is comparable to that of definite SLE: 64 versus 54 per 100 000 in white females and 33 versus 40 per 100 000 overall, respectively [10]. For understanding the social burden of the disease and guiding health care and research policy, all patients should be included.

Criteria for classifying the subsets of neuropsychiatric SLE were developed by an ad hoc neuropsychiatric workshop group in 1990 [11]. An ad hoc multidisciplinary committee developed standard nomenclature as well as detailed diagnostic and exclusion criteria for 19 neuropsychiatric syndromes in 1997.

Occurrence

Prevalence

The overall prevalence of SLE in the continental United States and Hawaii has been reported to range between 14.6 and 122 cases per 100 000 persons (Table 7.2, [16]). Studies have varied over time and place and used different methods of case ascertainment [10,12–18]. The studies conducted in San Francisco, California, and Rochester, Minnesota used both inpatient and outpatient records for case identification and published criteria for case validation; the major differences were the sampling frame (members of Kaiser Foundation Health Plan and residents of Olmsted County, respectively) and racial composition of the populations (81 per cent and 99 per cent white, respectively). The sex- and race-specific prevalence estimates for white males and females, however, are comparable, because the 95 per cent confidence intervals for these ratios overlap. The most current estimate in blacks is that from the San Francisco study, but it is based on only 19 patients, 16 of whom were women. Thus, the confidence intervals are wide, limiting the reliability of this estimate.

Applying the rates obtained from the San Francisco study to the 1990 US population, the National Arthritis Data Workgroup estimated that 239 000 cases of suspected or definite SLE were present in the US: 4000 white males, 31 000 black males, 163 000 black females, and 41 000 white females [19]. Because of limited data on other racial and ethnic groups no estimates for Hispanics and Asians were attempted. Both of these groups have a higher reported prevalence of SLE than whites (see below). In a recent meta-analysis of 16 population-based prevalence studies from Europe and North America, Jacobson *et al.* estimated the weighted mean prevalence rate of SLE at 23.8/100 000. By applying these rates to the 1996 US census data the authors estimated that a total of 63 052 persons are afflicted with the disease [20].

Table 7.2 Prevalence of SLE by sex/race group in the United States[a]

Reference	Location	Year	WM	WF	BM	BF	Overall
[15]	New York	1965	3	17	3	56	14.6
[13]	San Francisco	1973	7	71	53	283	50.8
[10]	Rochester, MN	1980	19	54	ND	ND	40.0
[17]	Hawaii	1989	ND	ND	ND	ND	41.8

[a] Rates per 100 000 persons.
Abbreviations: BF = black females; BM = black males; ND = no data; WF = white females; WM = white males.

Two studies based on self-reported, physician-diagnosed SLE in the US using data from telephone screening [12,18] suggested that the prevalence of SLE might be much higher. In one study, the prevalence of SLE by unsubstantiated claim was 1 in 177 [18]. The prevalence reported by Hochberg *et al.* after validating the diagnosis of SLE by medical record review was 124 per 100 000 [12]. This increased prevalence was confirmed in the most recent study from Rochester, Minnesota, that reported age- and sex-adjusted prevalence rates as of January 1, 1993 to be 1.22 in 1000 [16].

Outside the United States, studies to estimate the prevalence of SLE have been conducted in Sweden [21,22], Finland [23], Iceland [24,25], New Zealand [26,27], Malaysia [28], England and Wales [29–32], China [33,34], Japan [35,36], the Caribbean island of Curacao [37], and Northern Ireland [38] (Table 7.3). Of the studies conducted in countries with predominantly white populations, prevalence estimates varied from a low of 12.5 per 100 000 females in England [32] to higher values as shown (Table 7.3). This variability may result from differences in methodology of case ascertainment, including use of general practice diagnostic registries [32], hospital discharge records [23,27,35], outpatient clinic records, surveys of physicians, or combinations thereof [22,25,29–31] as well as from differences in host and environmental factors among different populations. In comparing studies using similar methodologies for case identification and validation, the prevalence of SLE is almost identical. Studies from the United States and Sweden that used hospital records for case identification,

reported similar prevalence rates of about 40 per 100 000 [10,22] while studies from the United Kingdom using multiple case-finding methods found consistently lower prevalence rates of about 25 per 100 000 [29–31]. The lowest rate, at 12 per 100 000, was determined through use of general practice diagnostic registries [32]. True geographic differences in the prevalence of SLE among whites cannot however be excluded and may result from differences in genetic and other host or environmental factors [39].

Incidence

The average annual incidence of SLE in the continental United States has been estimated in several studies; incidence rates vary from 1.8 to 7.6 cases per 100 000 persons per year [10,13–16,40,41] (Table 7.4). International studies from Iceland [25], Sweden [21,31,42], the United Kingdom [30,31], Japan [36], and the Caribbean island of Curacao [37] reported incidence rates for SLE of similar magnitude (Table 7.5).

Age and gender

The variability in prevalence and incidence rates in different published studies may be explained in part by the effect of age, gender, and race. Overall, prevalence and incidence rates are higher in females compared to males, and higher in African-Americans, Afro-Carribeans, and Asians than in Caucasian populations.

Among white females, age-specific incidence rates have varied among studies and peak incidence rates per 100 000 per year occurred in the 15- to 44-year age

Table 7.3 Prevalence of SLE: selected international studies

Reference	Country	Year	Cases (n)	Rate[a]
[27]	New Zealand	1980	16	15
[21]	Sweden	1982	61	39
[23]	Finland	1978	1323	28
[32]	England	1982	20	12[b]
[35]	Japan	1984	NS	21
[25]	Iceland	1990	86	36
[29]	England	1992	50	26
[37]	Curacao	1992	69	48
[30]	England	1993	137	25
[51]	Australia	1993	22	52
[31]	England	1995	242	28
[38]	N Ireland	1993	467	254

[a] Rate per 100 000; both sexes combined.
[b] Females only, as no cases identified among males.
Abbreviation: NS = not stated.

Table 7.4   Incidence of SLE by sex/race group in the United States[a]

Reference	Location	Date	WM	WF	BM	BF	Overall
[15]	New York	1956–65	0.3	2.5	1.1	8.1	2.0
[13]	San Francisco	1965–73	ND	ND	ND	ND	7.6
[10]	Rochester, MN	1950–79	0.9	2.5	ND	ND	1.8
		1970–79	0.8	3.4	ND	ND	2.2
[40]	Baltimore, MD	1970–77	0.4	3.9	2.5	11.4	4.6
[41	Pittsburgh, PA	1985–90	0.4	3.5	0.7	9.2	2.4
[16]	Rochester, MN	1950–79	ND	ND	ND	ND	1.51
		1980–92	ND	ND	ND	ND	5.56

[a] Incidence rates per 100 000 persons per year.
Abbreviations: BF = black females; BM = black males; ND = no data; WF = white females; WM = white males.

Table 7.5   Incidence of SLE: selected international studies

Reference	Country	Date	Cases (n)	W	M	Overall[a]	95% CI
[21]	Sweden	1982	61	7.6	2.0	4.8	NS
[42]	Japan	1984	566	5.3	0.6	3.0	NS
[25]	Iceland	1990	76	5.8	0.8	3.3	NS
[37]	Curacao	1992	94	7.9	1.1	4.6	0.4–8.8
[30]	England	1993	23	6.1	1.3	3.7	NS
[31]	England	1995	33	6.8	0.5	3.8	2.5–5.1

[a] Rate per 100 000; both sexes combined.

group [15], the 20- to 39-year age group [41], the 25- to 44-year age group [10], the 35- to 54-year age group [40], the 45- to 64-year age group [22], the 50- to 74-year age group [25], the 50- to 59-year age group [30], and among those aged 18 and 19 years [31]. Median age at diagnosis for white females in these studies ranged from 37 to 50 years, emphasizing that SLE is not necessarily a disease of young women.

Age-specific incidence rates in white males are difficult to interpret because of the small numbers of cases. In those studies with adequate data, peak rates occurred in the 50- to 59-year age group [30] and in those aged 65 and older [10,15]. The later onset of SLE in white males compared with white females was also noted in the Baltimore study [40] and the Leicester, United Kingdom study [29].

Age-specific incidence rates in black females were greatest in the 15- to 44-year age group in New York City [15], the 20- to 39-year age group in Pittsburgh [41], and the 25- to 34-year age group in Baltimore [40] (Fig. 7.1) and Birmingham, United Kingdom [31], exceeding 20 per 100 000 per year. Age-specific rates in black males can be reliably estimated only from the Baltimore study and reached a peak in the 45- to 64-year age group of 5 per 100 000 per year [40]. Among Afro-Caribbeans on the island of Curacao,

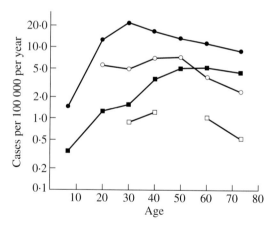

Fig. 7.1   Average annual age-specific incidence rates of systemic lupus erythematosus in Baltimore (city), 1970–1977, for white males (□), black males (■), white females (○), and black females (●). Note that the ordinate axis is a three-cycle logarithmic scale.

peak age-specific incidence rates occurred in the 45- to 64-year age group in women and among those aged 65 and older in men [37].

Age-specific prevalence rates for females in the United States are best estimated by the data of Fessel: approximately 1 and 4 per 1000 for white and black

Table 7.6 Female-to-male sex ratio at age of onset or diagnosis in SLE

Age of onset (y)	Female (n)	Male (n)	F:M ratio
0–9	39	19	2.0
10–19	220	39	5.6
20–29	369	49	7.5
30–39	298	37	8.0
40–49	183	35	5.2
50–59	98	25	3.9
60+	58	25	2.3
Total	1265	229	5.5

Source: adapted from [67].

women aged 15 to 64 years, respectively [13]. The prevalence of SLE among white women in southern Sweden, 99 per 100 000, is similar to that among white women in the United States [21]. Age-standardized prevalence among white women in Iceland was slightly lower, at 62 per 100 000 [25], while that among white women in the United Kingdom was markedly less, at 32 per 100 000 [29] and 36 per 100 000 [31].

Clinical studies have consistently demonstrated a female predominance approaching 90 per cent of SLE cases. This excess is especially noteworthy during the 10–49 year age groups wherein ratios of age- and sex-specific incidence rates show a five- to eight-fold female excess (Table 7.6). No such excess was noted in the 14 and younger or the 65 and older age groups in New York City [15], Rochester, Minnesota [10], Sweden [21], or Nottingham, UK [30]. A four-fold greater incidence rate in females age 65 and older than in males was found among whites but not blacks in Baltimore [40]. These age-related differences in the ratio of sex-specific incidence rates have been thought to relate to hormonal changes that occur during puberty and the childbearing years.

Time trends

Despite using different methods for case ascertainment, average annual incidence rates of SLE from 1985 to 1990 in Allegheny County, Pennsylvania [41], are quite similar to those reported in Baltimore during an earlier period [40]. Of particular interest are the differences in incidence reported by Kurland *et al.* [14], Michet *et al.* [10] and Uramoto *et al.* [16] for the same population using the identical medical record retrieval system. Michet *et al.* attributed these differences to changes in diagnostic classification. Nonetheless, a temporal trend in incidence among whites can be inferred from the

Rochester data. Rates nearly tripled from 1.5 in the 1950–1979 cohort to 5.56 per 100 000 in the 1980–1992 cohort [16]. Possible explanations for the increase in incidence is improved recognition of mild disease, increased exposure to hormones such as oral contraceptives and estrogen replacement therapy, and greater exposure to ultraviolet light because of depletion in the ozone layer.

Ethnicity

The relative increased frequency of SLE in people of African origin was examined by Symmons *et al.* [43] and more recently by Bae *et al.* [44]. A greater incidence and prevalence of SLE has consistently been found in blacks than in US whites [13,15,40,41]. Studies in both New York City [15] and San Francisco [13] found three- to four-fold greater prevalence in black females aged 15 to 64 than in white females (Table 7.2) and studies in Baltimore and Pittsburgh found a three-fold greater age-adjusted average annual incidence rate in black females compared with white females [40,41] (Table 7.4). A study in Birmingham, England, found higher age-adjusted incidence and prevalence rates in Afro-Caribbeans than in whites [31]. Age-adjusted incidence rates were 25.8 and 4.3 per 100 000 for Afro-Caribbeans and whites, respectively, and age-adjusted prevalence rates were 112 and 21 per 100 000 for Afro-Caribbeans and whites, respectively. Despite the apparent predilection for women of African origin in Northern Europe, North America, and the Caribbean, the frequency of SLE in West African countries, where most of their ancestors originated, as estimated from case reports and small series, is low [44]. This 'prevalence gradient' may be related to genetic and environmental factors as well as gene–environment interactions [44,45].

In a number of studies, the age distribution of incident cases differed significantly, with a younger median age and earlier peak incidence rates in women of African origin. Mean age in Afro-Caribbean females was of 34.5 years, compared with 41 years in white females, and, the peak incidence rate was in the 30- to 39-year age group compared with the 40- to 49-year age group, respectively [31]. These results are almost identical to those from a study in Baltimore, wherein the mean age of black females with SLE was 35.5 years, compared with 41.7 years for white females [40], and those from a study in Pittsburgh, wherein the mean age of black females was 35.2 years, compared with 39.8 years for white females [41]. The mean age at diagnosis was 31 years, with a peak age at diagnosis in the 21- to 30-year age group, in 93 Afro-Caribbean patients from Jamaica; no comparison with white patients was available [46]. On the island of Curacao, the mean age at diagnosis was 34 years, with a peak age at diagnosis in the 45- to 64-year age group, in 94 Afro-Caribbean patients; again, no comparison with whites was available [37].

Conflicting data exist regarding the excess prevalence of SLE among Asians compared with whites [26,29–31, 33–35,47–49]. In Hawaii, compared to Caucasians, the prevalence odds ratio was 1.3 for Japanese, 1.5 for Filipinos, 2.4 for Chinese, and 0.8 in Hawaiians [17]. An earlier study, performed by Serdula and Rhoads [47] from 1970 to 1975, reports an estimated age-adjusted prevalence of 5.8 per 100 000 in whites, compared with 17.0 per 100 000 among Asians (Chinese, Filipino, and Japanese). Age-adjusted prevalence rates of SLE in Auckland, New Zealand were 14.6 and 50.6 per 100 000 in whites and Polynesians, respectively [26]. Three studies from the United Kingdom [29–31], found higher age-adjusted incidence and prevalence rates of SLE in Asians (Indian, Pakistani, Bangladeshi) than in whites. In Leicester, England, the age-adjusted prevalence of SLE was 64.0 per 100 000 in Asians, compared with 26.1 per 100 000 in whites [29]. In Birmingham, England, the age-adjusted incidence and prevalence rates of SLE in Asians were 20.7 and 46.7 per 100 000 compared with 4.3 and 20.7 per 100 000 in whites, respectively [31]. Of interest, neither incidence nor prevalence rates differed by country of birth among Asians in this study.

Casting doubt on real differences between Asians, specifically Chinese, and whites are the findings of Fessel [13] and Nai-Zheng [33,34]. In the San Francisco study, the prevalence of SLE was not increased among Chinese compared with whites [13]. Data from China based on population surveys suggest a prevalence of SLE between 40 and 70 per 100 000 [34]. Finally, a survey in Taiwan identified only one case of

SLE among 1836 residents and no cases among 2000 female students [48]. Thus, population-based data in three countries fail to support an excess prevalence of SLE among Chinese compared with Caucasians. Prevalence data from Japan also fail to support the observations in Hawaii of an excess prevalence in Japanese compared with whites [35].

No published data exist about incidence rates in Hispanic-Americans, but an ongoing study is comparing genetic, clinical, and outcome features in Hispanics, African-Americans, and Caucasians [50].

The incidence and prevalence of SLE estimated in an Australian Aboriginal population in the Top End Northern Territory [51] were 11 per 100 000 per year and 52 per 100 000, respectively. The authors suggested these rates were higher than those for Australian whites; however, estimates for the European population in Australia are not available.

An excess incidence and prevalence of SLE among Native Americans compared with whites was suggested by three studies [52–54]. This excess was isolated to only three of 75 Native American tribes [52]; a single Pacific Northwest Native American population, the Nootka [53], and three different Native American groups, the Tlingit, Haida, and Tsimshian, living in coastal southeast Alaska [54]. Of interest, the prevalence of SLE among Alaskan Inuits is not increased over that which would be expected [55,56]. These isolated observations could represent chance findings; on the other hand, inbreeding and/or environmental factors may explain this clustering. Further studies of Native American populations could identify additional clusters with excess morbidity from SLE in an effort to test hypotheses regarding risk factors.

Population mortality

Population mortality rates can be used as a marker for the incidence of severe disease. Mortality attributed to SLE in the continental United States has been estimated

Table 7.7 Mortality rates from SLE by sex/race group in the United States[a]

Reference	Years	WM	WF	BM	BF
[15]	1956–65	1.6	6.6	4.4	20.0
[59]	1972–76	1.5	5.2	2.2	14.8
[58]	1972–76	1.2	4.5	1.9	13.1
[61][b]	1968–78	1.8	6.0	3.0	17.6

[a] Rates per 1 million persons per year.
[b] Includes deaths attributed to both discoid lupus erythematosus and SLE.
Abbreviations: BF = black females; BM = black males; WF = white females; WM = white males.

from community-based [15] as well as national data [57–60] (Table 7.7). Lopez-Acuna *et al.* [61] identified all deaths attributed to both discoid and systemic lupus erythematosus from National Center for Health Statistics (NCHS) data tapes for the period 1968 to 1978. A total of 11 156 deaths were identified, 2568 (23.0 per cent) of which were attributed to discoid lupus and 8588 (77.0 per cent) to SLE. There were no differences in the distribution of deaths from discoid lupus and SLE by sex/race, region, or year; therefore the authors combined results for their analysis. There were a total of 6452 deaths in white females, 2573 in black females, 1760 in white males, and 371 in black males, with average age-adjusted mortality rates of 6.0, 17.6, 1.8, and 3.0 per 1 million persons per year, respectively (Table 7.7). Age-specific average annual mortality rates showed a unimodal distribution for all sex/race groups, with maximum rates occurring in the 45- to 54-year age group for blacks and the 65- to 74-year age group for whites (Fig. 7.2).

Kaslow [62] analyzed a subset of these mortality records and examined deaths attributed to SLE alone from 1968 to 1976 in 12 states that contain 88 per cent of US residents of Asian descent. Mortality rates were three-fold greater among blacks and two-fold greater among Asians compared with whites: 8.4, 6.8, and 2.8 per 1 million person-years, respectively. Age- and sex-adjusted mortality rates for Chinese, Japanese, and Filipinos were 7.5, 6.8, and 5.1 per 1 million persons-years, respectively. Age- and sex-adjusted race-specific mortality rates in Hawaii were greatest among Filipinos and higher in the combined Asian group than

for the US mainland population, confirming previous observations [47]. A study from Hawaii reported that mortality rates were three times higher in non-Caucasian than Caucasians in 1985–1989 [17]. It is unclear whether the differences in mortality rates between Asians and whites mirror true differences in incidence rates as seen with blacks (see above).

Siegel and Lee [15] noted greater mortality and morbidity from SLE among Puerto Ricans compared with whites in New York City. Lopez-Acuna *et al.* [63] analyzed mortality from SLE in Puerto Rico from 1970 to 1977 as well as a subset of the NCHS data set for five southwestern states with the highest proportion of Hispanics: Arizona, California, Colorado, New Mexico, and Texas. A total of 92 deaths from SLE occurred in Puerto Rico; the average age-adjusted mortality rates of 7.5 and 2.0 deaths per 1 million person-years in females and males, respectively, were not significantly different from those noted among US whites over this period. A correlation between the proportion of Spanish-heritage population and county-specific mortality rates from SLE was noted for females but not males in these five states; the implications of this finding may reflect both ethnic/racial and socio-economic factors. Cause-specific mortality data from Latin American countries have not been reported.

Data on nationwide mortality from SLE have been reported from Finland [23], Iceland [25], England and Wales [64], and the island of Curacao [37]. Average mortality rates were 4.7, 2.5, and 17.0 per 1 million person-years in Finland, England and Wales, and Curacao, respectively. Patterns of age-specific mortality rates in Finland as well as England and Wales were similar to those in US whites. The four-fold greater age-adjusted mortality among English females compared with males is similar to that seen in the United States as well. Patterns of age-specific mortality rates in Curacao were similar to those in blacks, with a peak mortality rate in the 45- to 64-year age group and a four-fold greater mortality in women than in men [37].

Temporal trends in mortality rates have been examined in the United States [58,61] and in England and Wales [64]. In the United States, there was a significant decline in age-adjusted annual mortality rates between 1968 and 1978 for all sex/race groups [61] (Fig. 7.3). A significant temporal decline in age-adjusted annual mortality rates from SLE also was observed among females in England and Wales from 1974 to 1983 but not among males, probably because of the small numbers of deaths from SLE among males [64]. A similar decline in mortality was observed in the

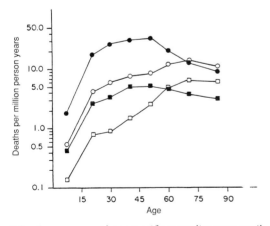

Fig. 7.2 Average annual age-specific mortality rates attributed to lupus erythematosus by sex/race groups in the US, 1968–78.   White males (□), white females (○), black males (■), black females (●).

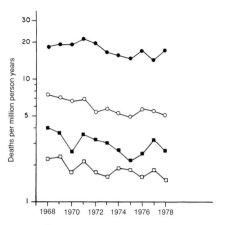

Fig. 7.3 Trends in age-adjusted annual mortality rates from lupus erythematosus by sex/race group in the US between 1968 and 1978. White males (□), white females (○), black males (■), black females (●).

Toronto Cohort, where estimated risk for death was compared for patients entered in the cohort between 1970–1977, 1978–1986, and 1987–1994 [65]. The standardized mortality ratios declined from 10.1 in the first group to 3.3 in the last group. The same decline was observed for the first two groups followed over the next time period. The decline in mortality rates observed in these developed countries is probably due to improved survival in patients with SLE, as reflected by: (1) a temporal increase in the mean age at death from SLE in the United States between 1968 and 1978 [61] (Fig. 7.4), and (2) 10-year cumulative survival rates approaching or exceeding 90 per cent in some studies [66] (see below).

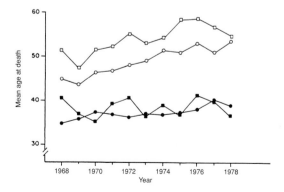

Fig. 7.4 Trends in mean age at death from lupus erythematosus by sex/race group in the US between 1968 and 1978. White males (□), white females (○), black males (■), black females (●).

Genetic factors

Familial clustering

The application of genetic epidemiology to SLE has generated strong evidence for a hereditary predisposition to this disorder [68,71]. Familial aggregation of SLE has been demonstrated in two studies [72,73]. Hochberg *et al.* [72] studied the occurrence of SLE among first-degree relatives of 77 patients with SLE and age-, sex-, and race-matched controls without a history of rheumatic disease. Eight (10.4 per cent) of the SLE probands had one or more first-degree relatives with SLE, compared with only one (1.3 per cent) of the controls (RR = 8, p = 0.03). SLE occurred in nine (1.67 per cent) of 541 first-degree relatives of SLE probands but in only one (0.18 per cent) of 540 first-degree relatives of controls (RR = 9, p = 0.01). Of the nine affected first-degree relatives of SLE probands, seven were female and two male, while the only affected control first-degree relative was female. The prevalence of SLE in female first-degree relatives was 2.64 per 100 for patients versus 0.40 per 100 for controls (RR = 6.8, p = 0.04).

Lawrence *et al.* [73] studied 41 consecutive patients with SLE, identified from hospital registers, who had 147 available first-degree relatives aged 15 and older, of whom 128 were fully evaluated with examinations and serologic studies. Control relatives were selected from family surveys of probands with osteoarthritis, psoriasis, and colitis. Definite SLE was found in five (3.9 per cent) of the first-degree relatives of SLE probands, compared with only one (0.8 per cent) of 128 matched first-degree relatives of controls: p = 0.001.

Twin studies

Twin studies have demonstrated a concordance rate among monozygotic twins ranging between 24 per cent and 69 per cent, compared to the 2 to 9 per cent concordance rate among dizygotic twins, providing further support for a genetic contribution to the mechanism of familial aggregation of SLE [74–77]. Block *et al.* [74] found a concordance for clinical SLE in four (57 per cent) of the seven monozygotic pairs and in none of the three dizygous pairs. Of the 12 monozygotic pairs in the literature, concordance for SLE was documented in seven (58 per cent). A more recent study, based on self-reported diagnoses of persons listed in a nationwide, chronic disease twin registry in the United States, found a lower rate of concordance in monozygous twin pairs [75]. Of 45 same-sex monozygous twin pairs, 11 (24 per cent) reported concordance for SLE, compared with only one (3 per cent) of 38 same-sex dizygous twin pairs. In a study from Finland, only one of nine monozygotic twin pairs was definitely concordant for SLE, while two additional monozygotic twin pairs probably were concordant for SLE (i.e. the co-twin fulfilled only three of the ACR classification criteria). None of 10 dizygotic twin pairs were concordant for SLE in yet another study [76]. Grennan *et al.* found that 25 per cent of monozygotic twins were concordant for SLE, while none of the 18 HLA identical, same-sex siblings of SLE probands had definite SLE, suggesting that most of the genetic predisposition to SLE may be attributed to genes outside the HLA region [77]. Arnett and Shulman [79] noted a striking concordance for clinical and laboratory features of SLE in monozygotic twin pairs compared with non-twin sib pairs. The concordance of autoantibody profiles in monozygotic twin pairs was recently confirmed by Reichlin *et al.* [80]. These observations also support a genetic influence on disease expression in SLE.

Genetic models

Two separate analyses support a polygenic mode for inheritance of SLE. Using Block's data on concordance for SLE in monozygotic twin pairs, Winchester and Nunez-Roldan [81] calculated that a multigenic hypothesis with either three or four dominant alleles best explained the familial inheritance of SLE. Lawrence *et al.* [73] determined that a pattern of polygenic inheritance with only moderate heritability best fit their family data. Advances in quantitative methods of segregation analysis, however, have allowed the study of single-gene effects in other conditions thought to have a polygenic mode of inheritance.

Segregation or pedigree analysis has been applied to SLE to determine the mode of Mendelian inheritance in multicase families. Arnett *et al.* [78] studied 19 multicase SLE families with 232 relatives, of whom 24 had SLE, 27 other autoimmune diseases, and 47 serologic abnormalities including high-titer antinuclear antibodies, antibody to single-stranded DNA, or a false-positive test for syphilis. They postulated a single, genetically determined autoimmune trait and applied segregation analysis to the family data. The results were consistent with Mendelian dominant inheritance pattern with a gene frequency of 0.06 and 91 per cent penetrance. The expression of autoimmunity was

modified by gender and age at the time of study, but not by HLA-DR phenotype. Further studies by this group estimated the population frequency of the autoimmune gene as 0.10, with penetrance of 92 per cent in females and 49 per cent in males [82]. Linkage of this autoimmune gene to other genetic markers was also studied by Bias *et al.*, but they failed to demonstrate linkage with any HLA phenotype, immunoglobulin allotype, or 21 other polymorphic genetic markers [82]. More recently, genome screens for human SLE by linkage analysis have indicated candidate genes on chromosome 1 and several other chromosomal regions [83,84,107].

Immunogenetics

The MHC region has been the target of several investigations. The highly polymorphic MHC cluster occurs on chromosome 6p21.3. It is characterized by the presence of multiple genes which play important role in the regulation of the immune response. It is divided into three major classes: class I, II, and III. Class I comprises of HLA A, B, and C. Class II comprises of HLA-DR, DP, and DQ. Class III comprises mainly of the complement system genes (C4A, C4B, C2, and Bf) and the tumor necrosis factor cluster (TNF-α and lymphotoxin α and β). Different alleles of different genes across the MHC region are tightly linked (allelic association or linkage disequilibrium). This presents as haplotypes, where alleles from different loci are in linkage disequilibrium and are passed from one generation to another with little recombination in between. This phenomenon makes it difficult to dissect out the primary associations with certain disease. Different MHC loci have been found to be associated with SLE [78]. Table 7.8 [111] presents the different MHC haplotypes found to be associated with SLE in different ethic groups. Whether any of the HLA loci or other genes within the MHC region such as C4A or C4B play a role in susceptibility to SLE is not clear.

Different association studies suggested a stronger association between genes within the MHC region and disease severity or markers of disease severity. For example in the UK Caucasoid population, TNF microsatellite polymorphisms were found to be associated with SLE, carrying odds ratios of 2 to 3 for TNF-α2, b1, and d3 alleles [95]. However, these alleles carried odds ratios of 2 to 7 in Ro+ and La+ subgroups [95]. No TNF microsatellite alleles were found to be associated with renal disease. In the Greek population, SLE was found to be associated with DRB1*1501,

Table 7.8 HLA extended haplotypes associated with SLE in different ethnic populations modified from [111]

Associated haplotype	Population
HLA-DQB1*-0201-DQA1*0501-DRB1*0301-C4A*Q0-TNF –308*A-HLA-B8	Northern European
HLA-DQB1*-0201-DQA1*0501-DRB1*0301-C4B*Q0-TNF –308*G-HLA-B18	Southern European and Mexicans
HLA-DQB1*-0602-DQA1*0102-DRB1*1501-TNF –308*G-HLA-B7	Western Europeans, Asians (Koreans, Chinese, Japanese), Blacks (DRB1*1503)
HLA-DQB1*-0402-DQA1*0401-DRB1*08	Native Americans (Mexican, Peruvians)

*1601, and *0701. TNF microsatellite a11 allele was in linkage disequilibrium with *1501; both *1501 and *1601 were associated with renal disease (OR = 4.6 and 3.3, respectively) [96]. In Spanish patients, only TNFc2 allele was associated with SLE; this was independent of DRB1 or C4B*Q0 alleles [97]. In this cohort, an increased DRB1*0301 was reported as well as an increased C4B*Q0 allele (OR = 6.0).

The TNF-308 (G/A) polymorphism was one of the first TNF markers to be reported in association with SLE [98]. The association between the –308*A allele and SLE was suggested to be due to linkage disequilibrium between this allele and the DRB1*0301-A1-B8 haplotype. Recent studies of different populations showed that the association between this TNF allele and SLE is independent of the DRB1 [99, 100].

Other markers

Mannose binding lectin (MBL), belongs to the acute phase proteins. The protein forms a trimer that represents C1q, which is capable of activating the complement pathways, classical and alternative. The MBL gene is located on chromosome 10q. Several polymorphisms have been described in the MBL gene; the most commonly studied are codon 54 and 57, which lead to MBL deficiency. The polymorphism at position 54 is rare or absent in Gambian (0.003) and Afro-Carribeans (0 per cent). However, codon 57 polymorphism was common in both populations [101]. In UK Caucasoids, the frequency of the codon 54 poly-

morphism was higher in SLE compared with controls (0.25 versus 0.19, respectively) [102]. In a group of 50 Spanish SLE patients and 49 controls, Davies *et al.* [103] found a significantly higher frequency of both codon 54 and 57 polymorphism. In Chinese, the frequency of codon 54 was higher in SLE patients (0.33) than in controls (0.23) [104]. In African-Americans, Sullivan *et al.* [105] found that the frequency of codon 54 was higher in SLE than controls (0.16 versus 0.09, respectively); similar results were seen for codon 57 (0.13 versus 0.05). In a group of 41 Greek SLE patients and 59 matched controls, MBL codon 54 mutation was found at higher frequency in SLE patients compared with controls (0.37 versus 0.24, respectively) [106].

Collectively these data suggest that MBL might be a risk factor involved in the susceptibility to SLE, though its penetrance could be low. Consistently, the mutant allele of the coding polymorphisms of MBL were shown to be marginally increased in SLE patients over controls in different populations.

Genetic linkage studies

Results from the mouse model of SLE presented the first evidence for genetic linkage to an area of chromosome 1 in the mouse. Tsao *et al.* [107] investigate the human syntenic region of the mouse chromosome 1 using 43 families with 52 affected sib pairs of mixed origins (approximately 50 per cent white, 30 per cent Asians, and 20 per cent black). They used seven microsatellite markers within the chromosome 1q41–42 and evidence for genetic linkage to the region was demonstrated for five out of the seven markers with D1S229 providing the strongest evidence of linkage.

Recently, several groups (Table 7.9) [84,83,112–114] attempted to investigate the genetics of SLE using the multicase families and genetic linkage analysis; whole genome screens (WGS) were carried out in different populations. The majority of these studies came from the US. Table 7.10 shows the results of positive linkage areas (in at least two studies) in the human genome from five different studies. However, one should exercise caution when analyzing these results. There are many variations between these studies including ethnic origins, sample size, differences in markers used, and type of analysis models employed.

It is interesting to note that many areas on chromosome 1 were positive in different studies; these are chromosome 1p36, 1q21–23, and 1q41–42. The area on 1q41–42 was studied extensively by Tsao *et al.* [107]; this is a syntenic region to the positive linkage

Table 7.9 Positive human SLE susceptibility loci identified in two or more mapping studies

Study parameters	[112]	[84]	[83]	[113]	[114)
Number of families	105	82	94	80	19
Type of study	Sib pair	Sib pair	Extended pedigrees	Extended pedigrees	Extended pedigrees
Number of affected individuals	220	179	220	188	44
Number of unaffected	155	101	313	246	52
Number of ethnic groups	5	4	2	2	2
Caucasian families	84	64	0	37	19
Mexican American families	0	0	0	43	0
African-American families	6	12	31	0	0
Hispanic families	8	5	0	0	0
European American families	0	0	55	0	0
Asian families	3	0	0	0	0
Mixed heritage	4	1	0	0	0
Number of loci analysed	341	366	312	350	336
Basis of linkage	LOD $\geq$ 1.0	LOD $\geq$ 1.0	LOD $\geq$ 1.5	Zlp> 1.5	LOD $\geq$1.0
Statistical methods	Non-parametric	Non-parametric	Model-based, then non-parametric	Non-parametric	Model-based

Table 7.10 Positive Human SLE susceptibility loci identified in two or more mapping studies

Locus	[112]	[84]	[83]	[113]	[114]
1p36	D1S234	D1S468	–	D1S468	–
1q23	–	–	FcgRIIA	D1S484	–
1q41-44	D1S235	–	D1S3462	D1S2785	–
2q32-37	–	D2S126	D2S1391	–	D2S125
3q11	D3S1271	–	D3S2406	–	–
4p15	–	D4S403	D4S403	–	–
4q28-31	D4S424	D4S413[a]	D4S2431	–	–
6p11-22	–	D6S426[a]	–	D6S276	–
14q11-23	D14S276	–	–	D14S258	–
16q12-13	D16S415	–	–	D16S3136	–
19q13	–	–	D19S246	–	–
20p12-13	D20S186	–	–	D20S115	–
20q11-13	D20S3119	–	D20S481	D20S195	–

[112]) 105 had affected sib pair families, 219 female and 1 male, 80 per cent white, 8 per cent Hispanics, 5 per cent black, 3 per cent Asian, 4 per cent mixed.
[84] 82 affected sib pair, 175 female and 4 males, 78 per cent white, 6 per cent Hispanic, 15 per cent Black, and 1 per cent mixed.
[83] 94 extended multiplex families, 55 white families, 31 black families.
[113] 80 multiplex families, 43 Mexican-American families, 37 white families.
[114] 19 multiplex families of Swedish (11 families) and Icelandic origin (8 families).
[a]Based on a combined analysis of 1 and 2.

area in the mouse spontaneous SLE model. Several genes of immunological importance are present within this region. Table 7.11 lists examples of these candidate genes. The majority of these genes have been implicated in the development of SLE in case–control studies. Recently, Tsao *et al*. [108] suggested that the PARP gene (poly ADP-ribose polymerase) was responsible for the positive linkage results on chromosome 1q41–42. They found that a microsatellite markers within the PARP gene promoter, allele (85 bp), was preferentially transmitted to affected offspring among 124 multiplex and simplex SLE families. Later, this study was not confirmed in a larger family collection of 746 (58 per cent European-American,

Table 7.11 Candidate genes within the SLE linkage areas on chromosome 1

Region	Candidate genes
1q21-23	FcgRIIA (CD32)
	FcgRIIIA (CD16)
	FcgRIA (CD64)
	IL-6R
	FasL
	CD3Z chain
	H3 and 4 histone family 2
	Amyloid serum protein
	C-reactive protein
	CD48
1q31-32	Complement component 4 binding protein alpha
	CR1
	CR2
	CD45
	Small ribonuclear protein
1q41-42	TGFB2
	ADPRT (ADP-ribosyl transerase factor-1)

17 per cent African-American, 12 per cent Hispanic-American, 10 per cent Asian-American, and 3 per cent others) [109]. Whether PARP is the gene responsible for the strong positive linkage results on chromosome 1 or other gene(s) still to be confirmed. It must be said that the original linkage area on chromosome 1q41–42 was narrowed down to 5 cM [91]. Risch [110], commenting on this PARP results controversy, argued that on the basis of the assumption that the human genome consists of 100 000 genes, a 5-cM region would be predicted to harbor 143 genes. He suggested that positional cloning and allelic variations within the region should be investigated to make any conclusions. Although the original data on PARP implicated the 85 bp allele in the linkage the disease, this can not exclude any linkage disequilibrium with other gene(s).

Non-genetic host factors

The strongest host factor for the development of SLE is female gender. In a review of five series of juvenile-onset and seven series of adult-onset SLE, totaling 317 and 1177 cases, respectively, Masi and Kaslow [67] showed that the sex ratio at age of onset or diagnosis rises with puberty from 2:1 to approximately 6:1, peaks in young adulthood at 8:1, and then declines with female menopause in the sixth decade of life (Table 7.6). The authors felt these data indicated that

study of sex-related factors offered a clue to the pathogenesis of SLE. Studies in the NZB/W F1 hybrid mouse, a murine model of SLE, support a role for female hormones in the modulation of autoantibody production, development of renal disease, and death [85]. Indeed, Lahita *et al.* as well as others have reported abnormalities in the metabolism of estrogens and androgens in both males and females with SLE [86, 87].

Two case–control studies have investigated the role of clinically recognizable endocrine factors in the etiology of SLE. Grimes *et al.* [88] found no association of age at menarche, parity, history of infertility, fetal wastage, or oral contraceptive usage with SLE. Hysterectomy appeared to be protective, with a crude OR = 0.55; however, after adjustment for age, the OR = 0.73 (95% CI 0.4–1.5) [88]. Simultaneous adjustment for age and race was not performed. A history of endometriosis was more common in women with SLE, but the odds ratio did not significantly differ from unity.

Hochberg and Kaslow [89] found no significant differences between cases and controls in age at menarche, age at first intercourse, and proportion with irregular menses, history of infertility, or usage of oral contraceptives. History of pregnancy ending in miscarriage was associated with SLE (OR = 2.7, 95% CI 1.4–5.2), as was being pregnant on one or more occasions without having a live birth (OR = 17.3, p = 0.006). Fetal–maternal microchimerism resulting from passage of the fetal cells in maternal circulation during pregnancy has not been found to be a risk factor for the development of SLE [90].

Sanchez-Guerrero *et al.* [91] used the Nurses' Health Study as a prospective cohort to study the role of the use of oral contraceptives in the development of SLE, and found that past use of oral contraceptives was associated with a slightly increased risk of developing SLE (RR = 1.4, 95% CI 1.1–3.3). The oral contraceptives used by this cohort in 1960–1970 contained higher estrogen doses than the oral contraceptives used currently. In two case-control studies, oral contraceptives use prior to diagnosis was not associated with an increased risk for lupus [88,92]. Overall, the current data do not definitely support an association between use of oral contraceptives and an increased risk for SLE. In a subset of nurses that were postmenopausal at entry into the cohort, Sanchez-Guerrero *et al.* analyzed the relation between postmenopausal hormone use and development of SLE [93]. An increase in the risk for SLE of 2.1 (95% CI 1.1–4.0) for ever-users, 2.5 (95 % CI 1.2–5.0) for current users, and 1.8 (95% CI 0.8–4.1) for past users was observed. The risk was proportionally related to the duration of use of postmenopausal hormones (test for trend, p= 0.011). The role of hormonal manipulation on disease activity is also an active area of investigation [94]. Large, prospective double-blind placebo controlled studies such as the Safety in Estrogens in Lupus Erythematosus-National Assessment (SELENA) trial should provide the basis for definitive recommendations.

Environmental factors

Infectious agents

Historically, SLE has been considered to probably have a viral etiology [115,116]. Despite several decades of investigation, however, no firm documentation of a definite viral etiology has been identified. Some studies have focused on human retroviruses, especially human T-lymphotropic virus type I (HTLV-I) and human immunodeficiency virus (HIV). Most studies have failed to demonstrate an association between antibodies to HTLV-I and SLE [117–120]. Talal *et al.* [121] found a higher incidence of antibodies to the human immunodeficiency virus but this finding was not confirmed in other populations [122].

Antibodies to specific viruses have been shown to cross-react with autoantigens such as vesicular stomatitis virus with Ro [123] and Epstein–Barr virus with Sm antigen [124]. Hardgrave *et al.* [123] found that a greater proportion of patients with SLE than controls had antibodies against the viral proteins of vesicular stomatitis virus. Also, in SLE patients the antibodies displayed a different binding pattern that included the internal viral matrix and nucleocapsid proteins.

Blomberg *et al.* [125] examined the frequency of antibodies cross-reactive with purified C-type retrovirus particles and with synthetic retroviral peptides in patients with SLE and population controls; they found that a greater proportion of patients with SLE reacted with viral proteins, including whole baboon endogenous virus and murine leukemia virus, and that reactivity with whole baboon endogenous virus correlated with the presence of antibodies to U1 ribonucleoproteins.

James *et al.* [124] have reported a higher rate of seroconversion to Epstein–Barr virus in young patients with SLE compared with controls (OR = 49.9, 95% CI 9.3–102.5) and Rider *et al.* [126] reported an increased prevalence for CMV in SLE patients compared with normal controls (OR = 14.53, 95% CI 6.39–33.04). In both studies, no difference was found in the seroconversion rates against other herpes viruses. However, in a case–control study by Strom *et al.* [92] the occurrence of herpes zoster before the diagnosis of SLE was associated with a risk of developing SLE (age-, sex-, and race-adjusted OR = 6.4, 95% CI 1.4–28.0). The implications for a viral etiology of SLE are, however, unclear.

The presence of a transmissible agent, presumably viral, was hypothesized to explain the co-occurrence of human and canine SLE in the same household [127]. One study found no association of dog ownership with SLE [89] and another study found no excess cases of SLE or asymptomatic subjects with anti-DNA antibodies among household contacts of index dogs [128]. In one study, less than half of the dogs owned by patients with SLE had abnormal serum protein electrophoresis and elevated titers of anti-DNA antibodies compared with none of the control dogs [129]. However, the control dogs, owned by pharmaceutical companies, were housed in special environments and were not comparable to the pets owned by the patients.

Chemical exposures

The most likely non-infectious environmental factors with an etiologic role in SLE are chemicals. The syndrome of drug-induced lupus, most commonly reported with hydralazine, procainamide, and isoniazid [130], and environmental lupus syndromes [131] provide models to study the possible effects of chemicals, especially aromatic amines [132]. In one initial case–control study, Freni-Titulaer *et al.* [133] found an association between use of hair dyes and connective tissue diseases, including SLE (OR = 7.2, 95% CI 1.9–26.9), but two subsequent case–control studies [134,135] and one cohort study [136] failed to demonstrate an association between use of hair products and the development of SLE.

Reidenberg [132] hypothesized that slow acetylation was a risk factor for the development of SLE as an explanation for drug-induced lupus and the possible association of exposure to aromatic amines with SLE. Several studies, however, failed to confirm an independent association of slow acetylation with SLE [57,60,134]. Thus, data from controlled epidemiologic studies fail to support a role for environmental in the etiology of idiopathic SLE.

Several epidemiologic studies have examined the association between SLE and silica dust exposure. A high SLE prevalence of 93 per 100 000 found in male uranium workers [137], a higher than expected number of SLE and SLE overlap syndrome cases among workers at a silica-containing scouring powder plant [138], and a significantly increased number of hospitalizations for treatment of SLE among silicotic men (RR = 23.8, 95% CI 11.9–86.3) [139], suggest that workers occupationally exposed to silica have a higher probability of developing clinical manifestations of SLE. Other putative environmental or occupational triggers and the mechanisms underlying their possible association with SLE have been recently reviewed [140].

Four case–control and four cohort studies have examined the association between breast implants and connective tissue diseases including SLE [141–148]. In a recent meta-analysis of these studies, Janowsky *et al.* found a summary, unadjusted OR of 0.63 (95% CI 0.44–0.86) [68]. When the data were reanalyzed after limiting the analysis to five studies that provided an adjusted estimate, the adjusted relative risk for SLE was 1.01, hence silicon breast implants do not appear to be associated with a risk for SLE [69].

Dietary factors including antioxidants were explored by Comstock *et al.* in a nested case–control study of six SLE patients and 24 controls. Although the number of cases was too small to allow definite conclusions, the levels of α-tocopherol, β-carotene, and retinol measured in serum that was collected more than 2 years prior to the onset of disease were 13–20 per cent lower in SLE patients compared to controls [70]. As dietary factors are potentially modifiable risk factors, future epidemiologic studies should investigate their possible association with SLE.

References

1. Cohen AS, Reynolds WE, Franklin EC et al. Preliminary criteria for the classification of systemic lupus erythematosus. *Bull Rheum Dis* 1971; **21**: 643–648.
2. Tan EM, Cohen AS, Fries JF et al. The 1982 revised criteria for the classification of systemic lupus erythematosus. *Arthritis Rheum* 1982; **25**: 1271–1277.
3. Hochberg MC. Updating the American College of Rheumatology revised criteria for the classification of systemic lupus erythematosus. *Arthritis Rheum* 1997; **40**: 1725.
4. Edworthy SM, Zatarain E, McShane DJ, Bloch DA. Analysis of the 1982 ARA lupus criteria data set by recursive partitioning methodology: new insights into the relative merit of individual criteria. *J Rheumatol* 1988; **15**: 1493–1498.
5. Perez-Gutthann S, Petri M, Hochberg MC. Comparison of different methods of classifying patients with systemic lupus erythematosus. *J Rheumatol* 1991; **18**: 1176–1179.
6. Manu P. Receiver operating characteristic curves of the revised criteria for the classification of systemic lupus erythematosus. *Arthritis Rheum* 1983; **26**: 1054–1055.
7. Clough JD, Elrazak M, Calabrese LH, Valenzuela R, Braun WB, Williams GW. Weighted criteria for the diagnosis of systemic lupus erythematosus. *Arch Intern Med* 1984; **144**: 281–285.
8. Somogyi L, Cikes N, Marusic M. Evaluation of criteria contributions for the classification of systemic lupus erythematosus. *Scand J Rheumatol* 1993; **22**: 58–62.
9. Gilboe IM, Husby G. Application of the 1982 revised criteria for the classification of systemic lupus erythematosus on a cohort of 346 Norwegian patients with connective tissue disease. *Scand J Rheumatol* 1999; **28**: 81–87.
10. Michet CJ Jr, McKenna CH, Elveback LR, Kaslow RA, Kurland LT. Epidemiology of systemic lupus erythematosus and other connective tissue diseases in Rochester, Minnesota, 1950 through 1979. *Mayo Clin Proc* 1985; **60**: 105–113.
11. Singer J, Denburg JA. Diagnostic criteria for neuropsychiatric systemic lupus erythematosus: the results of a consensus meeting. The Ad Hoc Neuropsychiatric Lupus Workshop Group. *J Rheumatol* 1990; **17**: 1397–1402.
12. Hochberg MC, Perlmutter DL, Medsger TA et al. Prevalence of self-reported physician-diagnosed systemic lupus erythematosus in the USA. *Lupus* 1995; **4**: 454–456.
13. Fessel WJ. Systemic lupus erythematosus in the community. Incidence, prevalence, outcome, and first symptoms; the high prevalence in black women. *Arch Intern Med* 1974; **134**: 1027–1035.
14. Kurland LT, Hauser WA, Ferguson RH, Holley KE. Epidemiologic features of diffuse connective tissue disorders in Rochester, Minn., 1951 through 1967, with special reference to systemic lupus erythematosus. *Mayo Clin Proc* 1969; **44**: 649–663.
15. Siegel M, Lee SL. The epidemiology of systemic lupus erythematosus. *Semin Arthritis Rheum* 1973; **3**: 1–54.
16. Uramoto KM, Michet CJ Jr, Thumboo J, Sunku J, O'Fallon WM, Gabriel SE. Trends in the incidence and mortality of systemic lupus erythematosus, 1950–1992. *Arthritis Rheum* 1999; **42**: 46–50.
17. Maskarinec G, Katz AR. Prevalence of systemic lupus erythematosus in Hawaii: is there a difference between ethnic groups? *Hawaii Med J* 1995; **54**: 406–409.
18. Lahita RG. Special report: adjusted lupus prevalence. Results of a marketing study by the Lupus Foundation of America. *Lupus* 1995; **4**: 450–453.
19. Lawrence RC, Helmick CG, Arnett FC et al. Estimates of the prevalence of arthritis and selected musculoskeletal disorders in the United States. *Arthritis Rheum* 1998; **41**: 778–799.
20. Jacobson DL, Gange SJ, Rose NR, Graham NM. Epidemiology and estimated population burden of selected autoimmune diseases in the United States. *Clin Immunol Immunopathol* 1997; **84**: 223–243.
21. Nived O, Sturfelt G, Wollheim F. Systemic lupus erythematosus in an adult population in southern Sweden: incidence, prevalence and validity of ARA revised classification criteria. *Br J Rheumatol* 1985; **24**: 147–154.

22. Jonsson H, Nived O, Sturfelt G. Outcome in systemic lupus erythematosus: a prospective study of patients from a defined population. *Medicine* (Baltimore) 1989; **68**: 141–150.

23. Helve T. Prevalence and mortality rates of systemic lupus erythematosus and causes of death in SLE patients in Finland. *Scand J Rheumatol* 1985; **14**: 43–46.

24. Teitsson I, Thorsteinsson J. Systemic lupus erythematosusu in Iceland. *Iceland Med J* 1978; **64**(Suppl): 116.

25. Gudmundsson S, Steinsson K. Systemic lupus erythematosus in Iceland 1975 through 1984. A nationwide epidemiological study in an unselected population. *J Rheumatol* 1990; **17**: 1162–1167.

26. Hart HH, Grigor RR, Caughey DE. Ethnic difference in the prevalence of systemic lupus erythematosus. *Ann Rheum Dis* 1983; **42**: 529–532.

27. Meddings J, Grennan DM. The prevalence of systemic lupus erythematosus (SLE) in Dunedin. *N Z Med J* 1980; **91**: 205–206.

28. Frank AO. Apparent predisposition to systemic lupus erythematosus in Chinese patients in West Malaysia. *Ann Rheum Dis* 1980; **39**: 266–269.

29. Samanta A, Roy S, Feehally J, Symmons DP. The prevalence of diagnosed systemic lupus erythematosus in whites and Indian Asian immigrants in Leicester city, UK. *Br J Rheumatol* 1992; **31**: 679–682.

30. Hopkinson ND, Doherty M, Powell RJ. The prevalence and incidence of systemic lupus erythematosus in Nottingham, UK, 1989–1990. *Br J Rheumatol* 1993; **32**: 110–115.

31. Johnson AE, Gordon C, Palmer RG, Bacon PA. The prevalence and incidence of systemic lupus erythematosus in Birmingham, England. Relationship to ethnicity and country of birth. *Arthritis Rheum* 1995; **38**: 551–558.

32. Hochberg MC. Prevalence of systemic lupus erythematosus in England and Wales, 1981–2. *Ann Rheum Dis* 1987; **46**: 664–666.

33. Nai-Zheng C. Rheumatic diseases in China. *J Rheumatol* 1983; **10**(Suppl 10): 41–44.

34. Nai-Zheng Z. Epidemiology of systemic lupus erythematosus (SLE) in China. In: *Proceedings of the Second International Conference on Systemic Lupus Erythematosus*. Tokyo, 1989: 29–31.

35. Nakae K, Furusawa F, Kasukawa R. A nationwide epidemiological survey on diffuse collagen diseases: estimation of prevalence rates in Japan. In: Kakusawa R, Missouri GC, eds. *Mixed connective tissue disease and antinuclear antibodies*. Amsterdam: Elsevier, 1987: 9–20.

36. Iseki K, Miyasato F, Oura T, Uehara H, Nishime K, Fukiyama K. An epidemiologic analysis of end-stage lupus nephritis. *Am J Kidney Dis* 1994; **23**: 547–554.

37. Nossent JC. Systemic lupus erythematosus on the Caribbean island of Curacao: an epidemiological investigation. *Ann Rheum Dis* 1992; **51**: 1197–1201.

38. Gourley IS, Patterson CC, Bell AL. The prevalence of systemic lupus erythematosus in Northern Ireland. *Lupus* 1997; **6**: 399–403.

39. Hopkinson N. Epidemiology of systemic lupus erythematosus. *Ann Rheum Dis* 1992; **51**: 1292–1294.

40. Hochberg MC. The incidence of systemic lupus erythematosus in Baltimore, Maryland, 1970–1977. *Arthritis Rheum* 1985; **28**: 80–86.

41. McCarty DJ, Manzi S, Medsger TA, Jr. *et al.* Incidence of systemic lupus erythematosus. Race and gender differences. *Arthritis Rheum* 1995; **38**: 1260–1270.

42. Jonsson H, Nived O, Sturfelt G, Silman A. Estimating the incidence of systemic lupus erythematosus in a defined population using multiple sources of retrieval. *Br J Rheumatol* 1990; **29**: 185–188.

43. Symmons DP. Frequency of lupus in people of African origin. *Lupus* 1995; **4**: 176–178.

44. Bae SC, Fraser P, Liang MH. The epidemiology of systemic lupus erythematosus in populations of African ancestry: a critical review of the 'prevalence gradient hypothesis'. *Arthritis Rheum* 1998; **41**: 2091–2099.

45. Polednak AP. Connective tissue responses in blacks in relation to disease: further observations. *Am J Phys Anthropol* 1987; **74**: 357–371.

46. Wilson WA, Hughes GR. Rheumatic disease in Jamaica. *Ann Rheum Dis* 1979; **38**: 320–325.

47. Serdula MK, Rhoads GG. Frequency of systemic lupus erythematosus in different ethnic groups in Hawaii. *Arthritis Rheum* 1979; **22**: 328–333.

48. Chou CT, Lee FT, Schumacher HR. Modification of a screening technique to evaluate systemic lupus erythematosus in a Chinese population in Taiwan. *J Rheumatol* 1986; **13**: 806–809.

49. Catalano MA, Hoffmeier M. Frequency of systemic lupus erythematosus in different ethnic groups of Hawaii. *Arthritis Rheum* 1989; **22**: 328–333.

50. Reveille JD, Moulds JM, Ahn C *et al.* Systemic lupus erythematosus in three ethnic groups: I. The effects of HLA class II, C4, and CR1 alleles, socioeconomic factors, and ethnicity at disease onset. LUMINA Study Group. Lupus in minority populations, nature versus nurture. *Arthritis Rheum* 1998; **41**: 1161–1172.

51. Anstey NM, Bastian I, Dunckley H, Currie BJ. Systemic lupus erythematosus in Australian aborigines: high prevalence, morbidity and mortality. *Aust N Z J Med* 1993; **23**: 646–651.

52. Morton RO, Gershwin ME, Brady C, Steinberg AD. The incidence of systemic lupus erythematosus in North American Indians. *J Rheumatol* 1976; **3**: 186–190.

53. Atkins C, Reuffel L, Roddy J, Platts M, Robinson H, Ward R. Rheumatic disease in the Nuu-Chah-Nulth native Indians of the Pacific Northwest. *J Rheumatol* 1988; **15**: 684–690.

54. Boyer GS, Templin DW, Lanier AP. Rheumatic diseases in Alaskan Indians of the southeast coast: high prevalence of rheumatoid arthritis and systemic lupus erythematosus. *J Rheumatol* 1991; **18**: 1477–1484.

55. Boyer GS, Lanier AP. Spondyloarthropathy and Rheumatoid Arthritis in Alaskan Yupik Eskimos. *J Rheumatol* 1990; **17**: 489–496.

56. Boyer GS, Lanier AP, Templin DW. Prevalence rates of spondyloarthropathies, rheumatoid arthritis, and other rheumatic disorders in an Alaskan Inupiat Eskimo population. *J Rheumatol* 1988; **15**: 678–684.

57. Baer AN, Woosley RL, Pincus T. Further evidence for the lack of association between acetylator phenotype

and systemic lupus erythematosus. *Arthritis Rheum* 1986; **29**: 508–514.

58. Gordon MF, Stolley PD, Schinnar R. Trends in recent systemic lupus erythematosus mortality rates. *Arthritis Rheum* 1981; **24**: 762–769.

59. Kaslow RA, Masi AT. Age, sex, and race effects on mortality from systemic lupus erythematosus in the United States. *Arthritis Rheum* 1978; **21**: 473–479.

60. Ong ML, Mant TG, Veerapen K *et al*. The lack of relationship between acetylator phenotype and idiopathic systemic lupus erythematosus in a South-east Asian population: a study of Indians, Malays and Malaysian Chinese. *Br J Rheumatol* 1990; **29**: 462–464.

61. Lopez-Acuna D, Hochberg MC, Gittelsson AM. Mortality from discoid and systemic lupus erythematosus in the United States,1968–1978. *Arthritis Rheum* 1982; **25**(Suppl): S80.

62. Kaslow RA. High rate of death caused by systemic lupus erythematosus among U. S. residents of Asian descent. *Arthritis Rheum* 1982; **25**: 414–418.

63. Lopez-Acuna D, Hochberg MC, Gittelson AM. Do persons of Spanish-heritage have an increased mortality from systemic lupus eryhtematosus compared to other Caucasians?. *Arthritis Rheum* 1982; **25**(Suppl): S67.

64. Hochberg MC. Mortality from systemic lupus erythematosus in England and Wales, 1974–1983. *Br J Rheumatol* 1987; **26**: 437–441.

65. Urowitz MB, Gladman DD, Abu-Shakra M, Farewell VT. Mortality studies in systemic lupus erythematosus. Results from a single center. III. Improved survival over 24 years. *J Rheumatol* 1997; **24**: 1061–1065.

66. Roubenoff K, Hochberg MC. Systemic lupus erythematosus. In: Bellamy N, ed. *Prognosis in the rheumatic diseases*. Lancaster: Kluwer Academic, 1991: 193–212.

67. Masi AT, Kaslow RA. Sex effects in systemic lupus erythematosus: a clue to pathogenesis. *Arthritis Rheum* 1978; **21**: 480–484.

68. Hochberg MC. Genetic epidemiology of systemic lupus erythematosus. In: *Proceedings of the second international conference on systemic lupus erythematosus*. Tokyo, 1989: 9–19.

69. Janowsky EC, Kupper LL, Hulka BS. Meta-analyses of the relation between silicone breast implants and the risk of connective-tissue diseases. *N Engl J Med* 2000; **342**: 781–790.

70. Harbige LS. Nutrition and immunity with emphasis on infection and autoimmune disease. *Nutr Health* 1996; **10**: 285–312.

71. Hochberg MC. The application of genetic epidemiology to systemic lupus erythematosus. *J Rheumatol* 1987; **14**: 867–869.

72. Hochberg MC, Florsheim F, Scott J, Arnett F. Familial aggregation of systemic lupus erythematosus. *Am J Epidemiol* 1985; **122**: 526–527.

73. Lawrence JS, Martins CL, Drake GL. A family survey of lupus erythematosus. 1. Heritability. *J Rheumatol* 1987; **14**: 913–921.

74. Block SR, Winfield JB, Lockshin MD, D'Angelo WA, Christian CL. Studies of twins with systemic lupus erythematosus. A review of the literature and presentation of 12 additional sets. *Am J Med* 1975; **59**: 533–552.

75. Deapen D, Escalante A, Weinrib L *et al*. A revised estimate of twin concordance in systemic lupus erythematosus. *Arthritis Rheum* 1992; **35**: 311–318.

76. Jarvinen P, Kaprio J, Makitalo R, Koskenvuo M, Aho K. Systemic lupus erythematosus and related systemic diseases in a nationwide twin cohort: an increased prevalence of disease in MZ twins and concordance of disease features. *J Intern Med* 1992; **231**: 67–72.

77. Grennan DM, Parfitt A, Manolios N *et al*. Family and twin studies in systemic lupus erythematosus. *Dis Markers* 1997; **13**: 93–98.

78. Arnett FC, Reveille JD, Wilson RW, Provost TT, Bias WB. Systemic lupus erythematosus: current state of the genetic hypothesis. *Semin Arthritis Rheum* 1984; **14**: 24–35.

79. Arnett FC, Shulman LE. Studies in familial systemic lupus erythematosus. *Medicine* (Baltimore) 1976; **55**: 313–322.

80. Reichlin M, Harley JB, Lockshin MD. Serologic studies of monozygotic twins with systemic lupus erythematosus. *Arthritis Rheum* 1992; **35**: 457–464.

81. Winchester RJ, Nunez-Roldan A. Some genetic aspects of systemic lupus erythematosus. *Arthritis Rheum* 1982; **25**: 833–837.

82. Bias WB, Reveille JD, Beaty TH, Meyers DA, Arnett FC. Evidence that autoimmunity in man is a Mendelian dominant trait. *Am J Hum Genet* 1986; **39**: 584–602.

83. Moser KL, Neas BR, Salmon JE *et al*. Genome scan of human systemic lupus erythematosus: evidence for linkage on chromosome 1q in African-American pedigrees. *Proc Natl Acad Sci USA* 1998; **95**: 14869–14874.

84. Gaffney PM, Ortmann WA, Selby SA *et al*. Genome screening in human systemic lupus erythematosus: results from a second Minnesota cohort and combined analyses of 187 sib-pair families. *Am J Hum Genet* 2000; **66**: 547–556.

85. Roubinian JR, Talal N, Greenspan JS, Goodman JR, Siiteri PK. Effect of castration and sex hormone treatment on survival, anti-nucleic acid antibodies, and glomerulonephritis in NZB/NZW F1 mice. *J Exp Med* 1978; **147**: 1568–1583.

86. Jungers P, Nahoul K, Pelissier C, Dougados M, Tron F, Bach JF. Low plasma androgens in women with active or quiescent systemic lupus erythematosus. *Arthritis Rheum* 1982; **25**: 454–457.

87. Lahita RG. The connective tissue diseases and the overall influence of gender. *Int J Fertil Menopausal Stud* 1996; **41**: 156–165.

88. Grimes DA, LeBolt SA, Grimes KR, Wingo PA. Systemic lupus erythematosus and reproductive function: a case-control study. *Am J Obstet Gynecol* 1985; **153**: 179–186.

89. Hochberg MC, Kaslow RA. Risk factors for the development of systemic lupus erythematosus: A case control study. *Clin Res* 1983; **153**: 179–186.

90. Rus V, Luzina IG, Atamas SP, Flores R, Handwerger BS, Via CS. Is micro-engraftment of fetal cells a risk factor for the development of systemic lupus erythematosus? *Arthritis Rheum* 1999; **42** 9S: A1438.

91. Sanchez-Guerrero J, Karlson EW, Liang MH, Hunter DJ, Speizer FE, Colditz GA. Past use of oral contra-

ceptives and the risk of developing systemic lupus erythematosus. *Arthritis Rheum* 1997; **40**: 804–808.

92. Strom BL, Reidenberg MM, West S, Snyder ES, Freundlich B, Stolley PD. Shingles, allergies, family medical history, oral contraceptives, and other potential risk factors for systemic lupus erythematosus. *Am J Epidemiol* 1994; **140**: 632–642.

93. Sanchez-Guerrero J, Liang MH, Karlson EW, Hunter DJ, Colditz GA. Postmenopausal estrogen therapy and the risk for developing systemic lupus erythematosus. *Ann Intern Med* 1995; **122**: 430–433.

94. Petri M, Robinson C. Oral contraceptives and systemic lupus erythematosus. *Arthritis Rheum* 1997; **40**: 797–803.

95. Hajeer AH, Worthington J, Davies EJ, Hillarby MC, Poulton K, Ollier WE. TNF microsatellite a2, b3 and d2 alleles are associated with systemic lupus erythematosus. *Tissue Antigens*. 1997; **49**: 222–227.

96. Tarassi K, Carthy D, Papasteriades C *et al*. HLA-TNF haplotype heterogeneity in Greek SLE patients. *Clin Exp Rheumatol*. 1998; **16**: 66–68.

97. Naves M, Hajeer AH, Teh LS *et al*. Complement C4B null allele status confers risk for systemic lupus erythematosus in a Spanish population. *Eur J Immunogenet* 1998; **25**: 317–320.

98. Wilson AG, Gordon C, di Giovine FS *et al*. A genetic association between systemic lupus erythematosus and tumor necrosis factor alpha. *Eur J Immunol* 1994; **24**: 191–195.

99. Rood MJ, van Krugten MV, Zanelli E *et al*. TNF-308A and HLA-DR3 alleles contribute independently to susceptibility to systemic lupus erythematosus. *Arthritis Rheum* 2000; **43**: 129–134.

100. Sullivan KE, Wooten C, Schmeckpeper BJ, Goldman D, Petri MA. A promoter polymorphism of tumor necrosis factor alpha associated with systemic lupus erythematosus in African-Americans. *Arthritis Rheum* 1997; **40**: 2207–2211.

101. Lipscombe RJ, Beatty DW, Ganczakowski M *et al*. Mutations in the human mannose-binding protein gene: frequencies in several population groups. *Eur J Hum Genet* 1996; **4**: 13–19.

102. Davies EJ, Snowden N, Hillarby MC *et al*. Mannose-binding protein gene polymorphism in systemic lupus erythematosus. *Arthritis Rheum* 1995; **38**: 110–114.

103. Davies EJ, Teh LS, Ordi-Ros J *et al*. A dysfunctional allele of the mannose binding protein gene associates with systemic lupus erythematosus in a Spanish population. *J Rheumatol* 1997; **24**: 485–488.

104. Lau YL, Lau CS, Chan SY, Karlberg J, Turner MW. Mannose-binding protein in Chinese patients with systemic lupus erythematosus. *Arthritis Rheum* 1996; **39**: 706–708.

105. Sullivan KE, Wooten C, Goldman D, Petri M. Mannose-binding protein genetic polymorphisms in Black patients with systemic lupus erythematosus. *Arthritis Rheum* 1996; **39**: 2046–2051.

106. Carthy D, Hajeer A, Ollier B *et al*. Mannose-binding lectin gene polymorphism in Greek systemic lupus erythematosus patients. *Br J Rheumatol* 1997; **36**: 1238–1239.

107. Tsao BP, Cantor RM, Kalunian KC *et al*. Evidence for linkage of a candidate chromosome 1 region to human systemic lupus erythematosus. *J Clin Invest* 1997; **99**: 725–731.

108. Tsao BP, Cantor RM, Grossman JM *et al*. PARP alleles within the linked chromosomal region are associated with systemic lupus erythematosus. *J Clin Invest* 1999; **103**: 1135–1140.

109. Criswell LA, Moser KL, Gaffney PM *et al*. PARP alleles and SLE: failure to confirm association with disease susceptibility. *J Clin Invest* 2000; **105**: 1501–1502.

110. Risch N. Searching for genes in complex diseases: lessons from systemic lupus erythematosus. *J Clin Invest* 2000; **105**: 1503–1506.

111. Tan FK, Arnett FC. The genetics of lupus. *Curr Opin Rheumatol* 1998; **10**: 399–408.

112. Gaffney PM, Kearns GM, Shark KB *et al*. A genome-wide search for susceptibility genes in human systemic lupus erythematosus sib-pair families. *Proc Natl Acad Sci U S A* 1998 ; **95**: 14875–14879.

113. Shai R, Quismorio FP Jr, Li L *et al*. Genome-wide screen for systemic lupus erythematosus susceptibility genes in multiplex families. *Hum Mol Genet* 1999; **8**: 639–644.

114. Lindqvist AK, Steinsson K, Johanneson B *et al*. A susceptibility locus for human systemic lupus erythematosus (hSLE1) on chromosome 2q. *J Autoimmun* 2000; **14**: 169–178.

115. Pincus T. Studies regarding a possible function for viruses in the pathogenesis of systemic lupus erythematosus. *Arthritis Rheum* 1982; **25**: 847–856.

116. Phillips PE. The potential role of microbial agents in the pathogenesis of systemic lupus erythematosus. *J Rheumatol* 1981; **8**: 344–347.

117. Boumpas DT, Popovic M, Mann DL, Balow JE, Tsokos GC. Type C retroviruses of the human T cell leukemia family are not evident in patients with systemic lupus erythematosus. *Arthritis Rheum* 1986; **29**: 185–188.

118. Koike T, Kagami M, Takabayashi K, Maruyama N, Tomioka H, Yoshida S. Antibodies to human T cell leukemia virus are absent in patients with systemic lupus erythematosus. *Arthritis Rheum* 1985; **28**: 481–484.

119. McDougal JS, Kennedy MS, Kalyanaraman VS, McDuffie FC. Failure to demonstrate (cross-reacting) antibodies to human T lymphotropic viruses in patients with rheumatic diseases. *Arthritis Rheum* 1985; **28**: 1170–1174.

120. Murphy EL Jr, De Ceulaer K, Williams W *et al*. Lack of relation between human T-lymphotropic virus type I infection and systemic lupus erythematosus in Jamaica, West Indies. *J Acquir Immune Defic Syndr* 1988; **1**: 18–22.

121. Talal N, Flescher E, Dang H. Are endogenous retroviruses involved in human autoimmune disease? *J Autoimmun* 1992; 5 (Suppl A): 61–66.

122. Kalden JR, Gay S. Retroviruses and autoimmune rheumatic diseases. *Clin Exp Immunol* 1994; **98**: 1–5.

123. Hardgrave KL, Neas BR, Scofield RH, Harley JB. Antibodies to vesicular stomatitis virus proteins in patients with systemic lupus erythematosus and in normal subjects. *Arthritis Rheum* 1993; **36**: 962–970.

124. James JA, Kaufman KM, Farris AD, Taylor-Albert E, Lehman TJ, Harley JB. An increased prevalence of Epstein-Barr virus infection in young patients suggests a possible etiology for systemic lupus erythematosus. *J Clin Invest* 1997; **100**: 3019–3026.

125. Blomberg J, Nived O, Pipkorn R, Bengtsson A, Erlinge D, Sturfelt G. Increased antiretroviral antibody reactivity in sera from a defined population of patients with systemic lupus erythematosus. Correlation with autoantibodies and clinical manifestations. *Arthritis Rheum* 1994; **37**: 57–66.

126. Rider JR, Ollier WE, Lock RJ, Brookes ST, Pamphilon DH. Human cytomegalovirus infection and systemic lupus erythematosus. *Clin Exp Rheumatol* 1997; **15**: 405–409.

127. Beaucher WN, Garman RH, Condemi JJ. Familial lupus erythematosus. Antibodies to DNA in household dogs. *N Engl J Med* 1977; **296**: 982–984.

128. Reinertsen JL, Kaslow RA, Klippel JH *et al.* An epidemiologic study of households exposed to canine systemic lupus erythematosus. *Arthritis Rheum* 1980; **23**: 564–568.

129. Jones DR, Hopkinson ND, Powell RJ. Autoantibodies in pet dogs owned by patients with systemic lupus erythematosus. *Lancet* 1992; **339**: 1378–1380.

130. Yung RL, Richardson BC. Drug-induced lupus. *Rheum Dis Clin North Am* 1994; **20**: 61–86.

131. Hess EV. Environmental lupus syndromes. *Br J Rheumatol* 1995; **34**: 597–599.

132. Reidenberg MM. Aromatic amines and the pathogenesis of lupus erythematosus. *Am J Med* 1983; **75**: 1037–1042.

133. Freni-Titulaer LW, Kelley DB, Grow AG, McKinley TW, Arnett FC, Hochberg MC. Connective tissue disease in southeastern Georgia: a case-control study of etiologic factors. *Am J Epidemiol* 1989; **130**: 404–409.

134. Reidenberg MM, Drayer DE, Lorenzo B *et al.* Acetylation phenotypes and environmental chemical exposure of people with idiopathic systemic lupus erythematosus. *Arthritis Rheum* 1993; **36**: 971–973.

135. Petri M, Allbritton J. Hair product use in systemic lupus erythematosus. A case-control study. *Arthritis Rheum* 1992; **35**: 625–629.

136. Sanchez-Guerrero J, Karlson EW, Colditz GA, Hunter DJ, Speizer FE, Liang MH. Hair dye use and the risk of developing systemic lupus erythematosus. *Arthritis Rheum* 1996; **39**: 657–662.

137. Conrad K, Mehlhorn J, Luthke K, Dorner T, Frank KH. Systemic lupus erythematosus after heavy exposure to quartz dust in uranium mines: clinical and serological characteristics. *Lupus* 1996; **5**: 62–69.

138. Sanchez-Roman J, Wichmann I, Salaberri J, Varela JM, Nunez-Roldan A. Multiple clinical and biological autoimmune manifestations in 50 workers after occupational exposure to silica. *Ann Rheum Dis* 1993; **52**: 534–538.

139. Brown LM, Gridley G, Olsen JH, Mellemkjaer L, Linet MS, Fraumeni JF Jr. Cancer risk and mortality patterns among silicotic men in Sweden and Denmark. *J Occup Environ Med* 1997; **39**: 633–638.

140. Cooper GS, Dooley MA, Treadwell EL, St.Clair EW, Parks CG, Gilkeson GS. Hormonal, environmental, and infectious risk factors for developing systemic lupus erythematosus. *Arthritis Rheum* 1998; **41**: 1714–1724.

141. Goldman JA, Greenblatt J, Joines R, White L, Aylward B, Lamm SH. Breast implants, rheumatoid arthritis, and connective tissue diseases in a clinical practice. *J Clin Epidemiol* 1995; **48**: 571–582.

142. Hennekens CH, Lee IM, Cook NR *et al.* Self-reported breast implants and connective-tissue diseases in female health professionals. A retrospective cohort study. *JAMA* 1996; **275**: 616–621.

143. Strom BL, Reidenberg MM, Freundlich B, Schinnar R. Breast silicone implants and risk of systemic lupus erythematosus. *J Clin Epidemiol* 1994; **47**: 1211–1214.

144. Edworthy SM, Martin L, Barr SG, Birdsell DC, Brant RF, Fritzler MJ. A clinical study of the relationship between silicone breast implants and connective tissue disease. *J Rheumatol* 1998; **25**: 254–260.

145. Friis S, Mellemkjaer L, McLaughlin JK *et al.* Connective tissue disease and other rheumatic conditions following breast implants in Denmark. *Ann Plast Surg* 1997; **39**: 1–8.

146. Nyren O, Yin L, Josefsson S *et al.* Risk of connective tissue disease and related disorders among women with breast implants: a nation-wide retrospective cohort study in Sweden. *BMJ* 1998; **316**: 417–422.

147. Sanchez-Guerrero J, Colditz GA, Karlson EW, Hunter DJ, Speizer FE, Liang MH. Silicone breast implants and the risk of connective-tissue diseases and symptoms. *N Engl J Med* 1995; **332**: 1666–1670.

148. Teel WB. *A population-based case-control study of risk factors for connective tissue diseases.* Ph.D. dissertation. Seattle: University of Washington, 1997.

8 | *Scleroderma*

Alan J. Silman

Disease definition and criteria

Scleroderma in the strictest sense refers to a pathological thickening and tethering of skin. In the broader sense, the disease is characterized by abnormal fibrosis, autoimmunity, and vascular damage. Scleroderma, localized to the skin, as in morphoea and linear scleroderma, does not form part of a multisystem disease and will not be considered further in this chapter. The epidemiology of these disease entities has been described recently for the first time. Interestingly, there is no evidence that patients with these disorders have decreased survival rates [1]. Systemic sclerosis, sometimes prefixed with the term 'progressive' is an alternative term used in the literature to relate to the combination of sclerodermatous skin change and internal organ involvement. However, the current preferred term is scleroderma and for classification purposes it is usefully subdivided into *limited* and *diffuse cutaneous* forms [2]. The diffuse form requires skin involvement proximal to the hands and feet, an increased risk of internal organ involvement, and a high frequency of the antitopoisomerase-1 antibody. By contrast the limited form, by definition, has skin involvement limited to the extremities, has low risk of internal

Table 8.1 Classification criteria for scleroderma

I	Proximal skin scleroderma
	OR 2 of
II	Sclerodactyly
	Digital pitting scars/pulp loss
	Bibasilar pulmonary fibrosis
Definitions	
Skin scleroderma	Tightness, thickening, and non-pitting induration excluding local forms of scleroderma
Sclerodactyly	Scleroderma skin change involving the fingers or toes
Pulp loss	Loss of substance of digital finger pad

Source: [3].

organ involvement, and a high frequency of the anticentromere antibody. One typical syndrome of limited cutaneous scleroderma is the CREST syndrome. This comprised of calcinosis, Raynaud's, oesophageal hypomotility, sclerodactyly (see Table 8.1) [3], and telangiectasia. The clinical and serological differences between these two forms are not absolute and, for epidemiological purposes, it is more usual and perhaps appropriate to consider scleroderma as a single disease entity.

Classification criteria

There is not a single diagnostic test for scleroderma and studies prior to 1980 relied on clinician's opinion. Indeed it is argued that the disease is sufficiently obvious and distinct clinically to obviate the need for specific criteria. A subcommittee of the American Rheumatism Association (now American College of Rheumatology) undertook a study of 264 patients with 'definite' scleroderma from 29 centres and compared the clinical findings with some 400 patients with SLE, dermato- or polymyositis, or Raynaud's phenomenon [3]. All patients studied were within 2 years of onset. The resulting criteria were not surprising (Table 8.1) and these criteria were 97 per cent sensitive and had a specificity of 98 per cent (99 per cent compared to the SLE and 94 per cent compared to the Raynaud's patients). The single criterion of proximal scleroderma was 100 per cent specific and 91 per cent sensitive. There is a problem here in that such a feature is, by definition, absent from patients with the limited cutaneous form of the disease and thus the criteria are likely to be insensitive for that group, who account for approximately 50 per cent of patients in published clinical series. Thus in 57 consecutive new patients from New Zealand, the ARA criteria were only 79 per cent sensitive [4,5]. By contrast, in a heavily selected population of 47 Belgian patients the criterion of proximal scleroderma was present in all [6]. There is also the problem that there is considerable subjectivity in assessing whether skin is involved even with experienced observers [7]. There have, however, been no recent attempts to develop alternative criteria. The sensitivity of the ACR criteria is however markedly increased when severe nailfold capillaroscopy abnormalities are added. The suspicion remains that clinical opinion is still widely used for case definition in epidemiological studies.

Occurrence

Scleroderma is too rare a disease for population surveys to be undertaken easily to ascertain either the prevalence of the disorder from a population sample or the incidence of new cases as they arise within the community. Virtually all of the estimates of occurrence are derived from either prospective or retrospective review of patients diagnosed and attending health service institutions serving a defined denominator population.

Incidence

There have been a large number of published reports of scleroderma incidence from Western populations (Table 8.2). The published rates vary between 2 and

30 per million, with higher rates from North America compared to Europe. Most studies have relied on ascertaining cases from a number of incompletely overlapping sources such as inpatient registers and laboratory records. Data derived from patients attending the Mayo Clinic, Rochester, Minnesota [9,19] have the advantage that the nature of the health care system is such that all patients within their denominator population are likely to be ascertained. However, that population is small and thus the confidence intervals for their estimates were wide: e.g. males 0–6 per million, females 7–25 per million [9].

Age and sex

There is consistent female excess in all populations with ratios (Table 8.2) although the extent of this varies from 3:1 to 14:1. In studies with available data, this female excess is most apparent in early adult life [8,15] although the absolute excess increases with increasing age (Fig. 8.1). There are few studies with sufficient data to quantify the effect of age. However, the data from Pittsburgh (Fig. 8.1), show the rarity of the disease under the age of 25 and the increasing incidence in age to the seventh decade. Scleroderma can occur, albeit

Table 8.2 Population incidence studies of scleroderma

Country/region	Place	Period	Source of cases	Incidence/million adults			Female : Male ratio	Reference	Comments
				Males	Females	Both			
US	Tennessee	1947–52	Hospital record review	0.0	0.0		–	[8]	Data presented on whites only
		1953–57		1.5	1.1		0.7		
		1958–62		2.1	6.5		3.1		
		1963–68		1.5	6.9		4.6		
	Minnesota	1950–79	Hospital record review	0.2	1.6		8.0	[9]	
	Nationwide	1963–68	Veteran hospitals' record review	2.3			N/A	[10]	
	Pittsburgh	1963–67	Hospital record review	5.3	14.4		2.7	[11]	Data presented on whites only
		1968–72		4.6	11.7		2.5		
		1973–77		9.4	27.7		2.9		
		1978–82		8.3	27.2		3.3		
	Detroit	1989–91	Multiple sources	7.5	28.6		3.8	[12]	Nurses cohort
	Nationwide	1976–90	Screening		12.0			[13]	
Europe	Slovakia Piestany	1961–69	Hospital record review			7.0		[14]	
	UK, West Midlands	1980–85	Multiple sources	1.1	6.2		5.6	[15]	
	Finland	1990	Sickness benefit registration			3.7		[16]	
	Iceland	1975–90	Multiple sources	0.5	7.0		14.0	[17]	
Oceania	New Zealand	1950–73	Hospital record review			2.0		[4]	Estimate
	New Zealand	1970–79	Hospital record review			6.3		[18]	

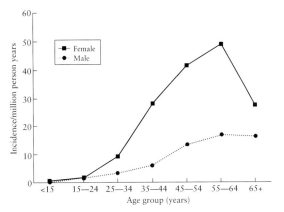

Fig. 8.1 Influence of age and gender on incidence of scleroderma: data from Allegheny County, Philadelphia 1963–1982. Data are from whites only. Reproduced with permission of Lippincott Williams and Wilkins from Steen VD, Oddis C, Conte CG, Janoski J, Casterline GZ, Medsger TA, Jr. *Arthritis Rheum* 1997; 40: 441–445 [11].

rarely, in childhood and the features in this group are well described [20–22]. The CREST form is particularly rare [23] and many children have localized scleroderma [21]. By contrast, scleroderma is not infrequent in the very elderly (age 80+) [24]. In this group though the CREST form is the typical pattern [25]. This observation might reflect the relatively late or missed presentation of those forms of the disease associated with slow progression and high survival. It does therefore seem likely that age modifies the clinical expression.

Time trends

There are few populations with repeat estimates of incidence over time. The data gathered in Allegheny County, Pittsburgh, between 1963 and 1987 [11] are

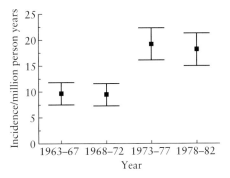

Fig. 8.2 Trends in incidence (age-adjusted) of scleroderma in Allegheny County, Philadelphia 1963–1982. Data from [11].

shown in Fig. 8.2. There was a doubling in incidence during 1973 to 1982. However, whether the increase in this period represents better case ascertainment is unknown. Data from Sydney [26], gathered between 1974 and 1988, suggested a rise in incidence based on changes in prevalence and mortality. Against these trends, older data from New Zealand showed a decline in incidence between 1963 and 1972 [4].

Mortality

In a disease like scleroderma, with a subsequent and relatively stable case fatality rate, mortality rates may be used as a surrogate for incidence, particularly in relation to measuring trends. The advantages of using mortality data are that they are readily available for national and other large population groups. There are inaccuracies in data derived from death certificates both in standardization of the diagnosis and in the variable inclusion of the diagnosis on the certificate. There have been six population mortality studies [10,26–30] and these are shown in Table 8.3 and Fig. 8.3. All studies have produced very similar results, with male rates at around one per million and female rates at two to three per million. The age-specific population mortality curves for both the US and the UK are shown in Fig. 8.4 and demonstrate the rarity of the disease under the age of 25 and the relatively slow increase in mortality with increasing age until the seventh decade. There are, however, no population mortality data from the past decade. Annual data analysed from Sydney [26], collected between 1974 and 1988, showed a trend of increasing mortality in both males and females during this period (Fig. 8.3). The clinical assumption is that the improved treatment of hypertensive renal crisis will, however, reduce mortality dramatically and thus, in the future, trends in mortality may not be an appropriate surrogate for underlying trends in incidence.

Table 8.3 Population mortality rates from scleroderma

Reference	Country	Period	Mortality rate/million	
			Males	Females
[27]	US	1959–61	1.0	2.1
[28]	US	1949–63	1.3	2.2
[10]	US[a]	1963–68	1.4	
[29]	US	1969–77	1.5	3.5
[30]	UK	1974–85	0.9	3.8

[a] Rates from veterans.

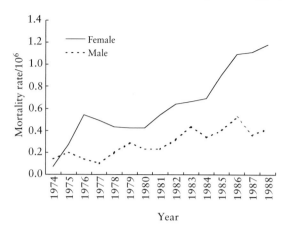

Fig. 8.3 Mortality rates from scleroderma, Sydney 1974–1988. Data from [26].

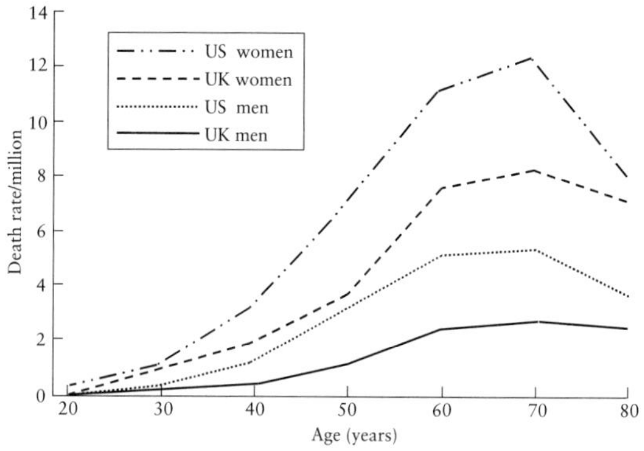

Fig. 8.4 Age specific population mortality curves for the US and the UK.

Table 8.4 Population prevalence studies of scleroderma

Country/ region	Place	Case ascertainment	Prevalence/ million adults					Reference	Comments
			Prevalence date (period)	Males	Females	Both	Female : male ratio		
US	Detroit	Multiple sources for diagnosed cases	1989–91	80	386	242	4.8	[31]	
	Rochester	Hospital record review	1968			105		[19]	
	Tennessee	Hospital record review	1947–52 1953–57 1958–62 1963–68			4 7 21 28		[8]	Based on new cases only subject to error
	South Carolina	Multistage population survey				290ᵃ– 1130		[32]	Only 2 definite cases ascertained
	Rochester	Hospital record review	1980	0	253ᵇ	138	N/A	[9]	Only 8 cases ascertained
Europe Iceland	Nationwide	Multiple source diagnosed cases	1990	15	119	71	8.0	[17]	
Denmark	Nationwide	Hospital record review	1977–79			126		[33]	All ages, figure is estimate
UK	West Midlands	Multiple sources	1986	13	48	31	3.7	[15]	
Germany (former DDR)	Leipzig	Hospital record review	1980–81			100		[34]	
Estonia	Two towns	Multistage population survey	Not stated			350		[35]	Only 2 definite cases ascertained
Oceania Australia	South Australia	Hospital record review	1993			208		[36]	Figure allowed for under ascertainment
Australia	Sydney	Multiple sources	1974–1988			45– 86			
Japan	Nationwide	Not stated	1974–76			7	6:1	[37]	Methods not clear

ᵃ Minimum estimate.
ᵇ No male cases detected.

Prevalence

Estimates of prevalence are a more difficult measure to derive from the available sources. This reflects the lack of population surveys and the requirement to estimate prevalence from retrospective ascertainment of patients attending clinic facilities who are alive at a particular date. The difficulties inherent in such an approach are illustrated by the wide variation in rates shown in Table 8.4. As an example, no male case was alive at 'prevalence day' in the Mayo Clinic data [9]. The data from Tennessee are derived from incidence rates [8]. The UK data were derived using multiple methods of ascertainment including primary care and the patient self-help organizations in addition to hospital clinics [15]. The most robust data came from two recent studies, one from Detroit [31], the other from Sydney [26]. The prevalence in the former was high, at 1 in 4000 adults, whereas the latter had a prevalence a third of that figure. Under-ascertainment is a major concern in deriving prevalence estimates from diagnosed cases from registers. Interestingly, in another study from Australia [36], after allowing for under-ascertainment, the prevalence approached the US figure (Table 8.4).

There have been true population surveys using a multistage screening strategy with an initial questionnaire for the symptoms of Raynaud's phenomenon and follow-up of subsamples of both the positive and negative respondents [32,35]. With this strategy, the authors could only derive estimates of prevalence under a series of assumptions about the occurrence of scleroderma in those not sampled. In the South Carolina study of 7000 residents [32], only two cases were observed, a minimum prevalence (subject to a wide confidence interval) of 290 per million. In addition, a further five patients with 'scleroderma spectrum disorders' were detected, that is patients unable to satisfy the ARA criteria but who had some clinical features of scleroderma. In a similar study of 14 500 subjects from Estonia, again only two subjects had scleroderma with a further six with the more broadly defined disorder [35]. The not surprising conclusion from this work is that, as with most other disorders, scleroderma varies in severity and hospital-based epidemiological studies, or indeed any study based on only diagnosed cases, will underestimate the true occurrence of pathology in the community. However, robust estimates of occurrence, particularly by age and gender, have to rely on ascertained cases from a much larger population than could practically be screened.

Ethnic influences on incidence

Populations of African origin

The disease is not rare in black African populations in the US, with recent data suggesting that the incidence is higher than in white Americans. Thus, data from Pittsburgh [11] (Table 8.5) showed that the excess in black Americans was restricted to males and, in that group, the difference has narrowed recently. These data are consistent with rates amongst male army veterans published some 20 years ago [10] which showed an incidence that was substantially higher in black Americans compared to white Americans (7.1 vs. 1.9 per million respectively). These data contrast with the results of limited information from African populations from Africa. There are, however, differences in the age influences on incidence between African and white American women [38] with a younger peak age at onset in the former group as well as a greater predominance of diffuse disease (Fig. 8.5). In Lomé, scleroderma was seen four times as frequently as systemic lupus [39]. The disease is also seen in black

Table 8.5 Ethnic factors and scleroderma

Years	Incidence/ million Males		Females	
	Whites	Blacks	Whites	Blacks
1963–72	5.0	12.2	16.3	13.0
1973–82	8.8	8.8	27.5	28.5

Source: [11].

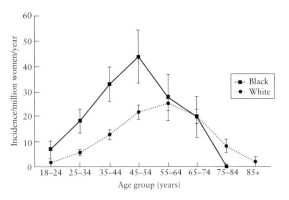

Fig. 8.5 Ethnic factors and scleroderma: age specific incidence of scleroderma in women, Michigan 1985–1991. Vertical bars are one standard error above and below point estimate. Reproduced with permission of Lippincott Williams and Wilkins from Laing TJ, Gillespie BW, Toth MB *et al. Arthritis Rheum* 1997; **40**: 734–742 [38].

South Africans with a predominance of diffuse disease [40]. Others have suggested that limited disease is the more frequent [41] perhaps because of selection bias. The Nigerian experience, by contrast, would suggest that scleroderma in black African groups is rare as judged by its absence at the main connective tissue disease centre [42]. A case series from Togo, however, suggested that the diffuse disease was the more frequent [43].

South East Asia populations

Scleroderma has been described in a number of South East Asian populations, with some of the highest rates coming from Japan. Early studies suggested that the prevalence of scleroderma in Japan was around seven per million, that is at a level much lower than seen in Western countries [37]. However, more recent studies based on population survey techniques, admittedly with small samples, suggest that the prevalence was much higher. Thus, in one study, based on examination of over 1000 individuals, scleroderma was ascertained in approximately 3 per cent of the population who were found to have Raynaud's phenomenon, this is equivalent to an overall prevalence of some 900 per million [44]. Another small study of some 731 individuals in Gifu Prefecture in Japan suggested that the prevalence was almost 4000, far higher than suggested in any other population studied [45]. The disease is also well described in India. In that population there is also a marked female excess but the peak age of onset is in the third and fourth decades [46]. This, however, possibly reflects the demographic structure of that country. There are interesting regional differences in disease type, with diffuse disease being relatively more common in Northern India. The disease is well described in Polynesians living in New Zealand [18] and in that population the rate of disease is similar to that seen in those of European extraction living in New Zealand. By contrast, no cases were diagnosed in Aborigines amongst a personal series of 179 Australian patients [47].

Other population groups

Scleroderma has been well described in Latin America, including Mexico [48], and was said to occur at a frequency equivalent to approximately 0.1 per cent of all new rheumatological attendees in Brazil and 0.6 per cent of such attendees in Peru [49]. Potentially the most interesting population studied is the Choctaw native Americans in Oklahoma [50]. The results from that population (Table 8.6) show that full blooded Choctaws from Oklahoma have the highest recorded prevalence whereas other Choctaw in the same population have a higher occurrence than other native Americans but substantially lower than their full blooded counterparts. Choctaws from outside Oklahoma do not have an excess risk. These data suggest a potential genetic effect in this localized group.

Geographic influences on incidence

Studies within countries have shown some variation in rates, although there does not appear to be any urban/rural difference in occurrence [10]. In a study of US male veterans there was an increase, after adjustment for race, in those living in the South Atlantic and East South Central (sic) regions of the US. The same phenomenon was also found in the national mortality analysis [29]. This area was subject to a more detailed analysis of mortality from 995 counties in 12 South Eastern states [51]. This suggested three localized clusters for white males and for black males but no evidence of clustering in females. In the UK, rates in South and West London were higher than those described in the West Midlands. Further analysis at electoral ward level of those areas showed a non-random distribution with a clustering of cases in some small areas. One hypothesis from that study was the apparent

Table 8.6 Prevalence of scleroderma in Native American populations

Population studied	N	No. cases	Prevalence (95% CI) per 100 000
Oklahoma Choctaw			
Full blooded	1704	8	469 (203–930)
Other	19 551	6	
Non-Oklahoma Choctaw			
Full blooded	4500	0	–
Other Oklahoma Native Americans	210 811	20	9.5 (5.8–14.6)

Source: [50].

concentration in those areas adjacent to major international airports [30]. A geographical cluster of patients with a variety of connective tissue diseases was also described from Georgia but formal analysis could not confirm a significant increase in prevalence [52]. Another cluster has been described near Rome in Italy [53], with five cases identified in a population of some 572 adults with others displaying non-specific features of connective tissue disease. The existence of such geographical clustering in scleroderma is interesting, though may be artifactual. If true, it highlights the need for local investigation of possible environmental triggers.

Non-genetic host factors

There are two 'host' areas of interest that have been investigated in scleroderma. The first is in relation to a possible link with cancer, the second is the relationship to reproductive and gynaecological factors in women.

Association with cancer

There have been some interesting suggestions of specific cancer risks with scleroderma with over 300 cases cited in the literature between 1886 and 1996 [54]. One report of an unexpected cluster of breast cancer cases in women with scleroderma [55] was followed by a formal epidemiological study that could not confirm an excess of breast cancer but did

suggest a temporal relationship between the onset of the two diseases in some women [56]. Case reports of the simultaneous co-occurrence of scleroderma with ovarian cancer [57] are of interest but the possibility that this is a random event cannot be ruled out. There is also an increased rate of lung cancer in scleroderma patients [56]. This seems to be independent of cigarette smoking but related to the presence of pulmonary fibrosis [58]. This is perhaps not a surprising result given the association of lung cancer with pulmonary fibrosis from occupational causes.

A record review of 248 patients [59] suggested twice the frequency of cancer compared to the background population. Data from other recent epidemiological studies are summarized in Table 8.7. Swedish data, as with the other data, are consistent with either of the alternative hypothesis: scleroderma increases the risk of cancer and vice versa. The data from the case–control study of relatives [62], although subject to both subject and interviewer bias, would support common genetic or environmental links between these disorders. In one large, uncontrolled study of 599 patients, 52 developed a non-skin malignancy, including four with primaries at more than one site [63].

Reproductive and gynaecological factors

The female excess described above has been the starting point for a number of studies looking for possible reproductive and gynaecological factors in disease susceptibility. Clinical case series of women with estab-

Table 8.7 Epidemiological studies of scleroderma and malignancy

Reference	Country	Approach	Results
[60]	Sweden 1965–1983	Record linkage between hospital discharge data of scleroderma and cancer registry	Standardized incidence ratios (SIR) Site SIR (95% CI) All 1.5 (1.2–1.9) Lung 4.9 (2.8–8.1) Liver 3.3 (1.1–7.6) Non-melanoma skin 4.2 (1.4–9.8)
[61]	Sweden, Uppsala Health Region 1955–1984	Record linkage between hospital discharge data of scleroderma and cancer registry	Standardized incidence ratios (SIR) Site SIR (95% CI) All 2.4 (1.5–3.6) Lung 7.8 (2.5–18.2) Non-Hodgkin lymphoma 9.6 (1.1–34.5)
[62]	US	Comparison of incidence in first degree relatives of 166 scleroderma cases and matched controls	Odds ratio (95% CI) for all reported cases of cancer relatives of cases vs. controls 3.75 (2.2–6.7)

lished scleroderma have suggested an increased reproductive loss because of the disease, although this might not be as large as originally thought [64]. The work discussed below refers to the converse hypothesis: that is reproductive problems might be a marker or indeed casually related to the *subsequent* development of scleroderma. The problem, even in prospective epidemiological studies, is that dating disease onset is very difficult and thus it is not possible to exclude a long latent or subclinical period during which adverse reproductive events may occur.

Fertility and conception

Scleroderma patients appear to have a reduced fertility prior to disease presentation [65–67]. The latter study was of interest in that two control groups were used although reduced fertility was only observed in comparison to a community control group. There were no differences in comparison to a group of Raynaud's women. This is consistent with the recent observations of reduced fertility in women with apparently primary Raynaud's [68,69]. The authors of the latter study suggested that the vasospasm induced by Raynaud's could impair fertility. Thus the fertility problem in women pre-onset of scleroderma can be explained by their often having Raynaud's for some years prior to disease onset. Women with scleroderma who are able to conceive also have an increased rate of delayed (more than 1 year) conception compared to normal controls [67]. A more recent report [70] found only a marginal suggestion of increased infertility in women with scleroderma prior to disease onset although that study did not specifically bring on pre-morbid reproductive experience. Interestingly, and unexplained, is the higher occurrence of male partner infertility in scleroderma women [70].

Reproductive loss

A second avenue of enquiry has been the possibility that there is an increased rate of early reproductive loss (spontaneous abortion) in women prior to the onset of their scleroderma. Those studies with available data are reviewed in Table 8.8. The results are not consistent with the most recent studies finding no increase in this loss. Thus the frequency of miscarriage prior to disease onset was identical in 214 women with scleroderma compared to 167 women with rheumatoid arthritis [70]. The study by Englert *et al.* [67] also suggested an increased rate of low birth weight babies but this might be a reflection of the vasospasm mentioned above. The frequency of premature and low birth weight babies was also similar in the scleroderma/RA comparison study discussed above.

Microchimerism and graft-versus-host disease

The data on reproductive histories in women with scleroderma have recently become of greater interest given the fascinating hypothesis that scleroderma is the consequence of a type of chronic graft-versus-host disease

Table 8.8 Results of case–control studies of spontaneous abortion rates prior to clinical onset of scleroderma

Reference	Cases			Controls			
	Women N	Pregnancies N	Abortions (%) spontaneous	Women N	Pregnancies N	Abortions (%) spontaneous	Odds ratio (95% CI)
[71]	22	47	28	(no control group)			N/A
[72]	86	299	16.7	86	332	9.6	1.9 (1.2–3.0)
[66]	115		28.7	115		17.4[b]	1.9 (1.0–3.6)
[64][a]	48	47	15	48[d]	77	15	0.9 (0.3–2.6)
[73]	28	63	33[f]	117[d]	264	15[c]	2.8 (1.5–5.7)
[67]	204	331	14.8	233[e]	310	18.1	0.8 (0.5–1.2)
				189[f]	221	12.7	1.2 (0.7–2.0)
[74]	13	26	15.0	20	61	8.0	2.0 (0.5–7.7)

[a] Includes only women who had pregnancy both before and after disease onset.
[b] Percentage of women.
[c] All pregnancy losses.
[d] Controls were rheumatoid arthritis women.
[e] Raynaud's controls.
[f] Community controls.

resulting from persistence in the maternal circulation of fetal stem cells from pregnancies occurring many years earlier. Two recent studies tend support to this hypothesis. In the first, Y chromosome sequences (presumed to be the consequence of a pregnancy with a male fetus) were found in 46 per cent of 69 women with scleroderma and only 4 per cent of 25 controls. Data from biopsies provided a similar conclusion and the Y chromosome material was virtually restricted to those with a male offspring [75]. In a similar study, the mean number of male cell DNA equivalents was 11.1 in scleroderma women who had a male offspring, compared to 0.4 in 16 controls [76]. This persistence of fetal cells, or microchimerism, was supported by the observation that HLA class II compatibility of offspring was greater in scleroderma patients than in controls [77].

Hormonal factors

There is no association between oral contraceptive use and scleroderma though hormonal replacement therapy, particularly when taken without progesterone, is a significant risk factor [78].

Genetics

Familial and twin aggregation

Familial aggregation scleroderma is a rare disease and the occurrence of multiple cases within a family would be of interest, though unless a sufficiently large pedigree was available such families are consistent with both shared genetic and/or environmental factors. A number of multicase families have been reported but it is impossible to determine from such sporadic reports whether there is an excess compared to random expectations. Nonetheless a considerable number of such reports have emerged over the past 40 years [79–89] together with many reports in the non-English literature. These data have limited epidemiological value and attempts within these families to demonstrate linkage with HLA or other genetic markers were either unsuccessful [89] or inappropriate. There have been a few surveys of large series of scleroderma probands (Table 8.9). The most obvious conclusion is that the number of such probands with an affected relative is extremely few. In the most recent study of three large patient cohorts [93], the familial incidence was very similar and the authors estimated that the increased

Table 8.9 Frequency of multicase families in scleroderma probands

Reference	No. of probands	No. (%) with affected relative
[90]	727	0
[87]	154	1 (0.6)
[91]	164	0
[92]	30	1 (3.3)
[93]	190	3 (1.6)
	119[a]	2 (1.7)
	338	11 (3.3)

[a] Disease duration < 5 years.

risk in first-degree relatives (λ) ranges from 11 to 27. Thus, linkage-based approaches to identifying possible susceptibility genes are almost impossible. There is an increased occurrence of disease markers in the relatives, such as ANA positivity [94] and evidence of chromosome breakage (a characteristic feature of sclero-derma) [95]. The presence of these phenomena could also represent shared environmental exposure particularly given the increased ANA positive rate (24 per cent) in one report of 38 spouses of scleroderma probands [96].

Twin aggregation

Reports of concordance for scleroderma in adult pairs of monozygotic twins are fairly recent [97,98]. The largest twin series has only been presented in an abstract [99]. This series of 34 twin parts yielded only two (6 per cent) who were concordant. Disease discordant monozygotic twins have been investigated for abnormalities in the immune response. The non-affected twins did not show the immunological abnormalities displayed by the scleroderma co-twins [100,101]. These data suggest that the immunological abnormality may not be genetic in origin.

Immunogenetics

As with the other autoimmune disorders, there has been considerable interest in the role of HLA genes in leading to susceptibility to scleroderma. An overall summary would be that the results have only showed relatively weak relationships with the disease overall. Stronger associations have been found in relation to the production of specific autoantibodies, specifically antitopoisomerase or anticentromere antibodies and their clinical correlates of diffuse and limited scleroderma respectively.

Table 8.10   Recent results of association studies with alleles in the MHC region

Locus	Reference	Disease type	Number cases	Number controls	Results Allele : odds ratio (95% CI)	Comments
HLA-DRB1	[102]	Diffuse 134 Limited 103	237	200	Association with DR1 (both disease types) DR3 (limited) DR5 (diffuse)	
	[103]	Not stated	35[a]	1094[b]	DR1:2.1 DR3: 1.9 DR5: 2.1	Caucasian
	[104]	Not stated	18	36	DRw15 (DRB1*1501 *1502) : 4.0	Japanese
	[105]	Limited (62) Diffuse (53)	115	142	DR3 : 1.9 DR11: 2.5	Possibly primary association with DQA2
	[106]	All	16	104	DRB1*1502:5.5 DRB1*0802	
	[107]	Diffuse (19) Limited (51) 'Overlap' (21)	94	50	No consistent association in relation to anticentromere antibody production	Japanese Patients
	[108]	All	41	85	DR5: 3.3 (1.3–8.3) DRB1*1104: 4.3 (CI not stated)	Mexican patients
	[109]	Diffuse Limited	20 35	95	See below in relation to TAP	
	[50]	Mostly diffuse	12	48	Haplotype B35-Cw4-DRB1*1601–DQA1*0501–DQB1*0301 : 21	Choctaw Native Americans (similar data presented by [112])
	[110]	Limited Diffuse			Association with DR3 Association with DR11	
	[111]	Limited Diffuse	61 69	602	No relationship with anticentromere antibody DRB1*11 associated with antitopoisomerise antibody	Analysis mainly by serological/ clinical status
	[112]	Not stated	18	76	DRB1*1602:6.8 (1.4–64.3)	Choctaw Native Americans
DPB	[113]	Not stated	52	70	No association with DPB1*01	
DQ	[107]	See above	94	50	Association between anticentromere antibody production and DQB1*0501	Japanese patients
	[50]	See above	12	48	Association with DQB1*0301	Choctaw Native Americans
	[105]	Limited (62) Diffuse (53)	115	142	DQAZ Odds ratio 2.5	Possibly explained by linkage disequilibrium with DR11
	[111]	See above	130	602	Association with DQB1*0201 and anti-RNA polymerase antibodies	

Table 8.10 (*continued*)

Locus	Reference	Disease type	Number cases	Number controls	Results Allele:odds ratio (95% CI)	Comments
C4	[114]	Not stated	25	42	C4AQO:8.9	
	[115]	Not stated	17	144	C4BQO seen in 12 patients significantly higher than controls	
	[105]	Limited (39) Diffuse (41)	80	307	C4AQO Odds ratio : 2.8	
	[110]	Diffuse Limited	21 26	45	No increase with C4AQO Non-significant increase with C4AQO	Data does not permit calculation of odds ratios
TAP	[109]	Diffuse Limited	20 35	95	TAP1A and TAP2A significantly increased in diffuse disease	In linkage disequilibrium with DRB1*15Q in Japanese patients
Microsatellites on 15q	[116]	Not stated	18	77	2 cM haplotype containing fibrillarin gene strongly associated	Choctaw Native Americans

[a] Blood donor panels.
[b] White cases only.

The major studies, with a particular emphasis on the more recent ones where DNA typing methods have been used, are shown in Table 8.10. Most interest has centred around alleles at DRB1, DPB, DQA and DQB, and C4A and C4B. As the results show, there is a substantial linkage disequilibrium between alleles at these various loci and it is often difficult to ascertain the source of primary linkage. There have been an insufficient number of multicase families to undertake formal linkage analysis. In one study of two large pedigrees [117], no relationship was found between disease and HLA. Conversely, in a study of five families with affected sib pairs, in four families there was evidence of increased HLA type sharing [118]. In one other review of four multicase families, again there was no consistent evidence of HLA explaining the occurrence [119]. However, such small numbers mean no robust conclusions can be drawn. Interestingly, as regards familial risk, in one study comparing the siblings and offspring of probands, there was an increased occurrence of unstable variable number tandem repeats occurring at a frequency of approximately 20 per cent compared to less than 1 per cent in the control population [120]. The most consistent finding within HLA has been with HLA-DRB1*1104. In studies with less precise HLA-DR typing, similar results have been found with HLA-DR11 and, in older studies, with DR5. This consistent finding does seem specifically centred around diffuse scleroderma. Data from other loci within the MHC region are less convincing, although HLA-DQA1*0501 is associated with scleroderma, particularly in males [121]. The most interesting data comes from the small study of the Chocktaw Indians [112]. In this population, with the highest published occurrence of scleroderma, there is a very strong relationship between HLA-DRB1*1602 and also with a region on chromosome 15 corresponding to a similar region in the tight skin mouse (which has been linked to scleroderma) containing the gene for fibrillarin. There is a strong association with the development of scleroderma in this group. Other loci of interest include TNF-β: a polymorphism within the first intron of that gene has been associated with scleroderma in the Japanese [122].

One of the more intriguing aspects of the epidemiology of scleroderma has been the interaction between genetics and environment. As discussed elsewhere in this chapter, there are fairly strong environmental links with the development of this disease and similar diseases. Detailed investigations have suggested that the putative environmental agents were effecting those with genetic susceptibility, the latter being particularly related to the HLA status. Thus, in the study of vinyl chloride disease, those who are likely to develop severe disease were more likely to carry HLA-DR5 [123]. Similarly, HLA and TNF gene status was important in determining the autoantibody response in individuals with scleroderma who had been exposed to silica dust [124]. Similarly there is an association with the development of antitopoisomerise antibodies in relation to DPB1*1301 in uranium miners with scleroderma [125].

Environmental factors

Unlike many of the rheumatic and connective tissue disorders, there is a considerable literature investigating the possibility that environmental agents are linked to the development of scleroderma. The major groups of exposures investigated are (i) silica; (ii) silicone, particularly from medical implants; (iii) organic solvents; and (iv) drugs. In addition, there are two specific symptoms related to, but not identical with, scleroderma that are of interest: (i) eosinophilia—myalgia symptoms related to tryptophan ingestion and (ii) disonic phase of the (Spanish) toxic oil syndrome, thought to be related to the consumption of adulterated rapeseed oil.

Silica

Crystalline silica is probably capable of inducing disease when inhaled at particles smaller then 5 μm [126]. At this size it is taken up by macrophages to which it is toxic. This leads to macrophagacitosis. On macrophage death, the macrophages release cytokines such as TNF, IL1, and IL6, which are likely to induce fibrosis. In addition, in mitosis experiments, silica dust can induce lymphocyte proliferation [127].

The first description linking exposure to silica with diffuse scleroderma came from case reports of Scottish stone masons [128]. Subsequent case series from South African gold miners [129] and other silica-exposed workers [130,131] have been very suggestive of links. There have been a number of epidemiological studies comparing exposure to silica in both male and female patients with scleroderma to that in controls and the results are consistently persuasive in favour of a link (Table 8.11).

The first study by Rodnan *et al.* [135], of 60 male patients, showed that 16 were miners and, in a controlled study, found that the rates of chronic exposure to silica in male cases was twice as high compared to both hospital and relative controls. Very large relative risks have been observed from studies of miners in East Germany. In one study, 77 per cent of 86 patients had been exposed to silica dust of whom 45 per cent actually had silicosis. The occupations of these men included miners, quarrymen, sandblasters, and sandstone sculptors and grinders. It was estimated from this study that there was a 25-fold increased risk of developing scleroderma with this degree of exposure [136]. A further study from East Germany suggested a relative risk of 74. Other European studies have also shown a very high prevalence of silica exposure amongst male cases with scleroderma. Thus, in a recent French study, 44 per cent of males were exposed to silica although there was a mean interval between first exposure and disease onset of some 25 years.

Studies of other mining populations in Europe have been less impressive. Thus, reports from West Germany showed only one in six of male cases with scleroderma having definite silica exposure although a further 22 per cent had possible exposure. In a study of scleroderma from males in the UK, none of 56 patients had definite exposure to silica and there was no increase in that group compared to population-based controls. There is a suggestion, however, that silica exposure may be responsible for some diseases in females. In the largest case–control study, five per cent of 274 female cases had exposure, which was non-

Table 8.11 Epidemiological studies of silica exposure and scleroderma

Reference	Study design	Results
[132]	Comparison of silica exposure in 79 gold miners with scleroderma to 79 'control' gold miners	Cases had a higher accumulated dust exposure
[133]	Case control study of 274 women compared to 1184 population controls	Adjusted odds ratio for all silica exposure 1.50 (0.76–2.93)
[134]	Case control study of 16 female and 5 male cases compared to 2 age/sex matched hospital controls	Suggestion of increased exposure, study too small
[135]	Case control study comparing 47 male cases with 2 groups of hospital controls and male relatives of female cases	Higher frequency of chronic exposure (47%) in the cases than in either hospital control group (19%, 16%) or relative group (27%)

significantly greater than a 3 per cent occurrence in almost 1200 population controls [133].

It has been suggested that there may be a genetic predisposition to the development of scleroderma in patients exposed to silica dust and part of this genetic predisposition may lie within the HLA class II region [124,125]. Further suggestions have been that those who are exposed to silica might develop anticentromere antibodies as an early marker of disease [137]. Some of the data on miners may have to be treated with caution. It has been suggested [138] that some miners who have developed hand arm vibration syndrome and pulmonary fibrosis as a consequence of the work have been misclassified as having scleroderma.

Silicone implants

In contrast to silica, silicones are a class of synthetic polymers consisting of alternating atoms of silicone and oxygen with various organic groups attached to silicone atoms via carbon–silicone bonds. The most common silicone polymer in medical use is poly(dimethylsiloxane). This is produced in both a gel and an elastomer form, which has been widely used in medicine, particularly in relation to silicone breast implants. There have been a large number of case reports and other series suggesting that silicone breast implants are linked to the development of a wide variety of morbidities with specific emphasis on features of connective tissue disease, including cases of scleroderma. The initial reports mainly came from Japan [139] and a series of 18 patients with presumed connective tissue disease resulting from silicone breast implants were reviewed in 1984 [140]. As a consequence of the major public health interest, fuelled in large part by medicolegal considerations, there have been a large number of epidemiological studies, both case–control and cohort studies aiming to investigate

Table 8.12 Cohort studies of scleroderma in women with breast implants

Reference	Implants		Non-implants			Relative risk	
	No.	No. (%) with scleroderma	Source	No.	No. (%) with scleroderma	95% CI	
[141][a]	749	5 (0.7)	Medical evaluation within 2 years of case breast implantation	1 498	10 (0.7)	1.06 (0.34–2.97)	
[142]	1 576	0 (0)	Other cosmetic surgery	727	3 (0.4)	–	
[13]	1 183	0 (0)	Non-implanted nurses	86 318	14 (0.016)	–	
[143]	2 570	1 (0.04)	National hospital discharges	11 023	1 (0.009)	–	
[144]	7 442	0 (0)	Breast reduction surgery	3 353	3 (0.09)	–	
[145]	10 830	10 (0.09)	Female health professionals	384 713	314 (0.08)	1.84 (0.98–3.46)	

[a] Any connective tissue disease

Table 8.13 Case–control studies of silcone implant exposure in scleroderma

Reference	Cases		Controls		
	No.	No. (%) with implants	Source	No. (%)	Odds ratio (95% CI)
[133]	274	2 (0.7)	Random digit dialing telephone sampling Frequency matched by race and age (5-year intervals)	12 (1.01)	1.30 (0.27–6.23)
[146]	286	3 (1.05)	General practice	2 (0.8)	1.00 (0.16–6.16)
[147]	837	11 (1.3)	Race matched Random digit dialing Frequency matched on age	31 (1.2)	1.07 (0.53–2.13)
[148]	189	1 (0.5)	Random selection from medical record review	10 (0.96)	1.01 (0.13–8.15)
Quoted in [149]	55	0 (0)	–	–	–

whether there is an increased risk of scleroderma, specifically in connective tissue disease in general following silicone gel breast implantation.

A summary of the main results from these studies is presented in Table 8.12 and Table 8.13. There are certain key observations. Firstly, silicone gel implants were very common in some populations and the overall majority of women receiving such an implant do not develop scleroderma. Similarly, the overall majority of women with scleroderma have not had an implant. Given the rarity of the disease and of the exposure, it is very difficult to conduct an epidemiological study which can produce a definitive result in either direction. A number of meta-analyses have, however, been conducted attempting to pool the results from different studies. These overviews [149–152] have shown no evidence of an increased risk of scleroderma following silicone breast implantation.

The most detailed study investigating silicone exposure and risk of scleroderma was a case–control study comparing 274 confirmed cases of scleroderma with 1184 controls who were given an intensive interview about all possible exposures to silicone [133]. This study showed no evidence overall of an increased risk from silicone breast implants but there were some suggestions that some occupations, for example, individuals who were involved in window manufacture and those that used silicone based glues, sealants, and caulks, might

have an increased risk of scleroderma. However, many other occupations and exposures, both medically and non-medically, did not show an increased risk and the possibility of type 1 error needs to be considered.

Organic solvents

Data linking the development of scleroderma to organic solvent exposure comes from a number of types of reports. Predominantly, these are single case reports in which a patient presenting with scleroderma had prior exposure to solvents although massive exposure, for example due to accidental immersion, and a strong temporal relationship has suggested a causal link. Such individual case reports have to be treated with caution. There have, indeed, been a number of case reports linking organic solvent exposure to scleroderma and these are listed in Table 8.14.

There have, however, been some epidemiological studies, predominantly of the case–control design. One of the problems with many of these studies is the difficulty in verifying exposure based on self report, differential recall between those with and without scleroderma, and small sample sizes, which result in estimates that are subject to random error. There have been four such studies and these are shown in Table 8.15. Broadly, they have all been consistent in showing a substantial increased risk in the development

Table 8.14   Case reports linking organic solvent exposure to scleroderma

Reference	Exposure	Type of disorder	Comments
[153]	Trichloroethylene	Scleroderma Raynaud's phenomenon Symptoms of faintness related to exposure Some improvement on stopping exposure	2 years of exposure
[154]	Trichloroethylene Carbon tetrachloride	Scleroderma Raynaud's phenomenon Neuropathy Steroid responsive	Long exposure (25 years); onset over 1 year
[155]	Trichloroethylene	Fatigue, muscle pain, and weakness Joint pains and scleroderma leading to rapid death	Massive exposure with symptom onset after few days
[156]	Multiple solvents	Raynaud's phenomenon Neuropathy	32 years of exposure
[157]	Trichloroethylene	Scleroderma Raynaud's phenomenon	2 years of exposure
[158]	Multiple solvents	Probable scleroderma with heart and chest problems Initially steroid responsive	Lone exposure (23 years); slow onset
[159]	Multiple solvents including trichloroethylene	Raynaud's phenomenon Pain Scleroderma	Mild exposure for 10 years

Table 8.15 Case–control studies of organic solvent exposure and development of connective tissue disease

Reference	Type	Cases No	Source	Controls No	Exposure investigated	Risk – expressed as odds ratio (95% CI)	Comments
[160]	Scleroderma (males)	56	GP panel	56	Organic solvents	1.7 (0.7–4.1)	Self-report
			Friends	41	Organic solvents	2.3 (0.9–6.2)	Self-report
[134]	Scleroderma	21	Other non-rheumatic disorders	62	Trichloroethylene Trichloroethane	9.3 (1.1–244)	Self-report
[161]	Scleroderma	33	Other rheumatic disorders	246	Perchloroethylene Trichloroethane	11.8[a] 15.3[a]	Small numbers exposed
[162]	Scleroderma (males)	37	Other rheumatic disorders	62	Trichloroethylene Trichloroethane	3.3 (1.0–10.3) 2.7[a]	Exposure based on maximum intensity

[a] Confidence intervals not provided.

of scleroderma compared to population or other rheumatic disease controls. Although organic solvents can be investigated as a group, the two most common solvents involved in disease are trichloroethylene and trichloroethene.

Drugs

There have been a number of case reports linking the development of scleroderma to the use of specific drugs and these are listed in Table 8.16. The most widely studied group of drugs has been appetite suppressants. A number of such agents have been implicated, as shown in the table. However, there are a number of problems in interpreting the data from these appetite suppressants. In these case reports, the duration and the use of these drugs is considerable [182,183]. Secondly, a large number of different appetite suppressants have been implicated and, although many of them do share common properties, the drugs themselves are distinct. Thirdly, as with all case reports, if these drugs were in widespread use in the population, a number of cases are likely to have occurred by chance. However, an interesting proposal [183] is that appetite suppressants might link with the development of scleroderma in so far as they are sympathomimetic and the drugs also have serotonergic properties.

Tryptophan

In one case report [186], scleroderma developed following treatment with carbidopa and L-5-hydroxytryptophan (L-5HTP). Interestingly, carbidopa inhibits the conversion of 5-hydroxytryptophan to 5-hydroxytryptamine. The alternative pathway for the metabolism of tryptophan results in an increased synthesis of kynurenine. In further studies, it was shown that scleroderma itself is associated with increased kynurenine levels and it has been proposed that the pathogenesis of scleroderma might, in part, be related to an enzyme defect that leads to elevated kynurenine levels.

Bleomycin

A number of reports [184,185] have linked the development of scleroderma to bleomycin intake. Bleomycin is known to stimulate collagen production in normal skin fibroblasts.

Analgesic abuse

Reports have occurred of scleroderma developing following pentazocine [187] and cocaine [188,189] although the explanation of these links is unclear.

Toxic oil syndrome

In May 1981, in Spain, there was an epidemic of a previously unrecognized multisystem disease with fever, malaise, myalgia, headaches, eosinophilia, pulmonary oedema, and rashes. An association with cooking oil was established [190] which was subse-

Table 8.16 Environmental agents implicated in scleroderma: case reports and series

Agent	Exposure group	Reference
Silica dust	Stone masons	[128]
	Gold miners	[129]
		[130]
		[131]
	Coal miners	[135]
		[136]
		[34]
	Uranium miners	[164]
		[165]
		[166]
	Scouring powder	[167]
		[168]
		[169]
	Various workers	[126]
		[170]
Organic solvents:		
Trichloroethylene		[153]
		[154]
		[155]
Perchloroethylene		[171]
Mixed solvents		[172]
		[173]
		[157]
		[134]
Meta-phenylenediamine		[174]
Benzene		[175]
Vinyl chloride		[176]
	Air conditioning workers	[177]
Urea-Formaldehyde	Foam in solution	[178]
Bis (4-amino-3-methyl-cycloheryl methane)	Epoxy resins	[179]
	Welders	[180]
		[181]
Drugs		
Appetite suppressants		
Phenmetrazine		[182]
Amphetamine		[183]
Dexamphetamine		
Diethylpropion hydrochloride		
Fenproporex		
Bleomycin		[184]
L-5 hydroxytryptophan		[185]
Pentazocine	Abuser	[186]
Cocaine	Abusers	[187]
		[188]
		[189]

quently found to be explained by aniline adulterated rapeseed oil and further cases in other parts of Spain have supported this [191]. A chronic phase of the disease occurs several months after exposure, which, in 30 per cent, includes a scleroderma-like illness [192]. The relationship between toxic oil syndrome and scleroderma is still a matter of debate. There are some epidemiological similarities including the marked excess in premenopausal females and the link with HLA-DR3 [193].

L-Tryptophan

L-tryptophan is a naturally occurring amino acid, though it has been manufactured and marketed for the treatment of depression and premenstrual symptoms.

In October 1989, three patients in New Mexico were diagnosed with eosinophilia–myalgia syndrome, thought to be due to the ingestion of this drug [194]. Subsequently, another nine US patients with the same syndrome were described [195].

The association does not appear to be due to chance. A case–control study was undertaken in New Mexico [196] comparing all 11 cases of eosinophilia–myalgia found by a review of haematology records between May and October 1989. Their rates of L-tryptophan ingestion were compared to that recalled by 22 age and sex matched community controls. The extremely clear result was that all 11 cases had consumed the drug compared to only two of the 22 controls, there being no difference in any of the other exposures sought. The nature of the toxic factor is not completely clear, though suggestions include the quinolinic metabolites of the drug or toxic products produced by the manufacturing process which are unrelated to the amino acid. The latter seems the most likely given that all cases seem to be associated with a single manufacturer whose process involves fermentation with *Bacillus amyloliquefaciens* [197]. There are similarities between this syndrome and toxic oil syndrome which are both distinct clinically from scleroderma. The skin lesions are similar to those of morphoea or localized scleroderma and the other findings 'do not resemble the cutaneous and visceral abnormalities of systemic sclerosis' [198].

Other environmental factors

There are few data on other lifestyle factors. There was an excess rate of smoking prior to disease onset in one study of US males and there was an increased rate of moderate alcohol consumption when compared to a similarly drawn control group [10]. Other findings of note include the, as yet, uncorroborated suggestion that there is a higher rate of pet ownership (cats and dogs), particularly those owning more than one pet [199] and the possibility that trauma including road traffic accidents and assaults might precipitate disease onset.

References

1. Peterson LS, Nelson AM, Daniel Su WP, Mason T, O'Fallon WM, Gabriel SE. The epidemiology of morphea (localized scleroderma) in Olmsted County 1960–1993. *J Rheumatol* 1997; **24**: 73–80.

2. LeRoy EC, Black C, Fleischmajer R *et al.* Scleroderma (systemic sclerosis): classification, subsets and pathogenesis. *J Rheumatol* 1988; **15**: 202–205.

3. Subcommittee for scleroderma criteria of the American Rheumatism Association Diagnostic and Therapeutic Criteria Committee. Preliminary criteria for the classification of systemic sclerosis (scleroderma). *Arthritis Rheum* 1980; **23**: 581–590.

4. Wigley R, Borman B. Medical geography and the aetiology of the rare connective tissue diseases in New Zealand. *Soc Sci Med* 1980; **14D**: 175–183.

5. Tan PLJ, Wigley RD, Borman GB. Clinical criteria for systemic sclerosis. *Arthritis Rheum* 1981; **24**: 1589–1590.

6. Janssens X, Herman L, Mielants H, Verbruggen G, Veys EM. Disease manifestations of progressive systemic sclerosis: sensitivity and specificity. *Clin Rheumatol* 1987; **6**: 532–538.

7. Brennan P, Silman A, Black C *et al.* Reliability of skin involvement measures in scleroderma. *Br J Rheumatol* 1992; **31**: 457–460.

8. Medsger TA, Masi AT. Epidemiology of systemic sclerosis (scleroderma). *Ann Intern Med* 1971; **74**: 714–721.

9. Michet CJ, McKenna CH, Elveback LR, Kaslow RA, Kurland LT. Epidemiology of systemic lupus erythematosus and other connective tissue diseases in Rochester, Minnesota, 1950 through 1979. *Mayo Clin Proc* 1985; **60**: 105–113.

10. Medsger TA, Masi AT. The epidemiology of systemic sclerosis (scleroderma) among male U.S. veterans. *J Chronic Dis* 1978; **31**: 73–85.

11. Steen VD, Oddis C, Conte CG, Janoski J, Casterline GZ, Medsger TA, Jr. Incidence of systemic sclerosis in Allegheny County, Pennsylvania. *Arthritis Rheum* 1997; **40**: 441–445.

12. Mayes MD. Epidemiology of systemic sclerosis and related diseases. *Curr Opin Rheumatol* 1997; **9**: 557–561.

13. Sánchez-Guerrero J, Colditz MA, Karlson EW, Hunter DJ, Speizer FE, Liang MH. Silicone breast implants and the risk of connective-tissue diseases and symptoms. *N Engl J Med* 1995; **332**: 1666–1670.

14. Bosmansky K, Zitnan D, Urbanek T, Svec U. Incidence of diffuse disorders of the connective tissue with special reference to SLE in a selected district in the years 1961–69. *Fysiatr Rheumatol Vestn* 1971; **49**: 267–272.

15. Silman AJ, Jannini S, Symmons D, Bacon P. An epidemiological study of scleroderma in the West Midlands. *Br J Rheumatol* 1988; **27**: 286–290.

16. Kaipianen-Seppänen O, Aho K. Incidence of rare systemic rheumatic and connective tissue diseases in Finland. *J Intern Med* 1996; **240**: 81–84.

17. Geirsson AJ, Steinsson K, Gudmundsson S, Sigurdsson V. Systemic sclerosis in Iceland. A nationwide epidemiological study. *Ann Rheum Dis* 1994; **53**: 502–505.

18. Eason RJ, Tan PL, Gow PJ. Progressive systemic sclerosis in Auckland: a ten year review with emphasis on prognostic features. *Aust N Z J Med* 1981; **11**: 657–662.

19. Kurland LT, Hauser WA, Ferguson RH, Holley KE. Epidemiologic features of diffuse connective tissue disorders in Rochester, Minn., 1951 through 1967, with special reference to systemic lupus erythematosus. *Mayo Clin Proc* 1969; **44**: 649–663.

20. Black CM. Scleroderma in children. *Adv Exp Med Biol* 1999; **455**: 35–48.

21. Bodemer C, Belon M, Hamel-Teillac D *et al.* Scleroderma in childhood: a retrospective study of 70 cases. *Ann Dermatol Venereol* 1999; **126**: 691–694.

22. Ansell BM. *Clinics in rheumatic diseases. rheumatic disorders in childhood.* London: WB Saunders Company Limited, 1976.

23. Burge SM, Ryan TJ, Dawber RPR. Case report: juvenile onset systemic sclerosis. *J R Soc Med* 1984; **77**: 793–794.

24. Dalziel JA, Wilcox GK. Progressive systemic sclerosis in the elderly. *Postgrad Med J* 1979; **55**: 192–193.

25. Kyndt X, Launay D, Hebbar M *et al.* Influence of age on the clinical and biological features of systemic sclerosis. *Rev Med Interne* 1999; **20**: 1088–1092.

26. Englert H, Small-McMahon J, Davis K, O'Connor H, Chambers P, Brooks P. Systemic sclerosis prevalence and mortality in Sydney 1974–1988. *Aust N Z J Med* 1999; **29**: 42–50.

27. Cobb S. *The frequency of rheumatic diseases.* Cambridge, MA: Harvard University Press, 1971.

28. Masi AT, D'Angleo WA. Epidemiology of fatal systemic sclerosis (diffuse scleroderma). *Ann Intern Med* 1967; **66**: 870–875.

29. Hochberg MC, Lopez-Acuna D, Gittlesohn AM. Mortality from systemic sclerosis (scleroderma) in the United States, 1969–85. In: Black CM, Myers AR, eds. *Systemic sclerosis.* New York: Gower, 1985.

30. Silman AJ, Howard Y, Hicklin AJ, Black C. Geographical clustering of scleroderma in South and West London. *Br J Rheumatol* 1990; **29**: 92–96.

31. Mayes MD. Scleroderma epidemiology. *Rheum Dis Clin North Am* 1996; **22**: 751–764.

32. Maricq HR, Weinrich MC, Keil JE *et al.* Prevalence of scleroderma spectrum disorders in the general population of South Carolina. *Arthritis Rheum* 1989; **32**: 998–1006.

33. Asboe-Hansen G. Epidemiology of progressive systemic sclerosis in Denmark. In: Black CM, ed. *Current Topics in Rheumatology,* 1985.

34. Haustein UF, Ziegler V. Environmentally induced systemic sclerosis-like disorders. *Internat J Dermatol* 1985; **24**: 147–151.

35. Valter I, Saretok S, Maricq HR. Prevalence of scleroderma spectrum disorders in the general population of Estonia. *Scand J Rheumatol* 1997; **26**: 419–425.

36. Chandran G, Smith M, Ahern MJ, Roberts-Thomson PJ. A study of scleroderma in South Australia: prevalence, subset characteristics and nailfold capillaroscopy. *Aust N Z J Med* 1995; **25**: 688–694.

37. Shinkai H. Epidemiology of progressive systemic sclerosis in Japan. In: Black CM, Myers AR, eds. *Systemic sclerosis (scleroderma).* New York: Gower, 1985.

38. Laing TJ, Gillespie BW, Toth MB *et al.* Racial differences in scleroderma among women in Michigan. *Arthritis Rheum* 1997; **40**: 734–742.

39. Mijiyawa M, Amanga K, Oniankitan OI, Pitche P, Tchangai-Walla K. Les connectivites en consultation hospitaliere a Lome (Togo). *Rev Med Interne* 1999; **20**: 13–17.

40. Tager RE, Tikly M. Clinical and laboratory manifestations of systemic sclerosis (scleroderma) in Black South Africans. *Rheumatology* 1999; **38**: 397–400.

41. Mody GM. Rheumatoid arthritis and connective tissue disorders: Sub-Saharan Africa. *Baillieres Clin Rheumatol* 1995; **9**: 31–44.

42. Somorin AO, Mordi VIN. Connective tissue disease in Nigeria with emphasis on scleroderma. *Cent Afr J Med* 1980; **26**: 59–63.

43. Pitche P, Amanga Y, Koumouvi K, Oniankitan O, Mijiyawa M, Tchangai-Walla K. Scleroderma in a hospital setting in Togo. *Med Trop* 1998; **58**: 65–68.

44. Inaba R, Maeda M, Fujita S *et al.* Prevalence of Raynaud's phenomenon and specific clinical signs related to systemic sclerosis in the general population of Japan. *Int J Dermatol* 1993; **32**: 652–655.

45. Maeda M, Ichiki Y, Shikano Y, Mori S, Kitajima Y. Detection of scleroderma with capillaroscopic abnormalities of nailfolds. *Int J Dermatol* 1996; **35**: 857–861.

46. Chanderasekaran A, Radhakrishna B. Rheumatoid arthritis and connective tissue disorders: India and South-East Asia. *Baillieres Clin Rheumatol* 1995; **9**: 45–57.

47. Barnett AJ. Epidemiology of systemic sclerosis (scleroderma) in Australia. In: Black CM, Myers AR, eds. *Systemic sclerosis.* New York: Gower, 1985.

48. de Kasep GI, Alarcón-Segovia D. Preliminary epidemiologic data on progressive systemic sclerosis. In: Black CM, Myers AR, eds. *Systemic sclerosis.* New York: Gower, 1985.

49. Ferraz MB. Tropical rheumatology. epidemiology and community studies: Latin America. *Baillieres Clin Rheumatol* 1995; **9**: 1–9.

50. Arnett FC, Howard RF, Tan F *et al.* Increased prevalence of systemic sclerosis in a Native American tribe in Oklahoma. *Arthritis Rheum* 1996; **39**: 1362–1370.

51. Walsh SJ, Fenster JR. Geographical clustering of mortality from systemic sclerosis in the Southeastern United States, 1981–90. *J Rheumatol* 1997; **24**: 2348–2352.

52. Freni-Titulaer LWJ, Kelley DB, Grow AG, McKinley TW, Arnett F, Hochberg MC. Connective tissue disease in South Eastern Georgia: a case-control study of etiologic factors. *Am J Epidemiol* 1989; **130**: 404–409.

53. Valesini G, Litta A, Bonavita MS *et al.* Geographical clustering of scleroderma in a rural area of the province of Rome. *Clin Exp Rheumatol* 1993; **11**: 41–47.

54. Bielefeld P, Meyer P, Caillot D *et al.* Systemic sclerosis and cancer: 21 new cases and review of literature. *Rev Med Interne* 1996; **17**: 810–813.

55. Lee P, Alderdice C, Wilkinson S, Keystone EC, Urowitz MB, Gladman DD. Malignancy in progressive systemic sclerosis—association with breast carcinoma. *J Rheumatol* 1983; **10**: 665–666.

56. Roumm AD, Medsger TA, Jr. Cancer and systemic sclerosis: an epidemiologic study. *J Rheumatol* 1985; **12**: 1336–1340.

57. Young R, Towbin B, Isern R. Scleroderma and ovarian carcinoma. *Br J Rheumatol* 1990; **29**: 314.

58. Peters-Golden M, Wise RA, Hochberg M, Stevens MB, Wigley FM. Incidence of lung cancer in systemic sclerosis. *J Rheumatol* 1985; **12**: 1136–1139.

59. Abu-Shakra M, Guillemin F, Lee P. Cancer in systemic sclerosis. *Arthritis Rheum* 1993; **36**: 460–464.

60. Rosenthal AK, McLaughlin JK, Gridley G, Nyren O. Incidence of cancer among patients with systemic sclerosis. *Cancer* 1995; **76**: 910–914.

61. Rosenthal AK, McLaughlin JK, Linet MS, Persson I. Scleroderma and malignancy: an epidemiological study. *Ann Rheum Dis* 1993; **52**: 531–533.

62. Sakkas LI, Moore DF, Akritidis NC. Cancer in families with systemic sclerosis. *Am J Med Sci* 1995; **310**: 223–225.

63. Jimenez SA, Sakkas I, Rasheed M, Artlett C, Cox L. A prospective study of the association of malignancy with systemic sclerosis. *Arthritis Rheum* 1999; **42**: 712.

64. Steen VD, Conte C, Day N, Ramsey-Goldman R, Medsger TA, Jr. Pregnancy in women with systemic sclerosis. *Arthritis Rheum* 1989; **32**: 151–157.

65. Ballou SP, Morley JJ, Kushner I. Pregnancy and systemic sclerosis. *Arthritis Rheum* 1984; **27**: 295–298.

66. Silman AJ, Black C. Increased incidence of spontaneous abortion and infertility in women with scleroderma before disease onset: a controlled study. *Ann Rheum Dis* 1988; **47**: 441–444.

67. Englert H, Brennan P, McNeil D, Black C, Silman AJ. Reproductive function prior to disease onset in women with scleroderma. *J Rheumatol* 1992; **19**: 1575–1579.

68. de Trafford JC, Lafferty K, Potter CE, Roberts VC, Cotton LT. An epidemiological survey of Raynaud's phenomenon. *Eur J Vasc Surg* 1988; **2**: 167–170.

69. Kahl LE, Blair C, Ramsey-Goldman R, Steen VD. Pregnancy outcomes in women with primary Raynaud's phenomenon. *Arthritis Rheum* 1990; **33**: 1249–1255.

70. Steen VD, Medsger TA, Jr. Fertility and pregnancy outcome in women with systemic sclerosis. *Arthritis Rheum* 1999; **42**: 763–768.

71. Serup J, Hagdrup HK. Age at menopause of females with systemic sclerosis. *Acta Derm Venereol* 1983; **63**: 71–73.

72. Giordano M, Valentini G, Lupoli S, Giordano A. Pregnancy and systemic sclerosis. *Arthritis Rheum* 1985; **28**: 237–238.

73. McHugh NJ, Reilly PA, McHugh LA. Pregnancy outcome and autoantibodies in connective tissue disease. *J Rheumatol* 1989; **16**: 42–46.

74. Jimenez FX, Simeon CP, Fonollosa V et al. Systemic sclerosis and pregnancy: obstetric complications and effect of pregnancy on the evolution of the disease. *Med Clin* 1999; **113**: 761–764.

75. Artlett C, Smith B, Jimenez A. Identification of fetal DNA and cells in skin lesions from women with systemic sclerosis. *N Engl J Med* 1998; **338**: 1186–1191.

76. Nelson J, Furst DE, Maloney S et al. Microchimerism and HLA-compatible relationships of pregnancy in scleroderma. *Lancet* 1998; **351**: 559–562.

77. Artlett CM, Welsh KI, Black CM, Jimenez SA. Fetal-maternal HLA compatibility confers susceptibility to systemic sclerosis. *Immunogenetics* 1997; **47**: 17–22.

78. Beebe JL, Lacey JV, Mayes MD et al. Reproductive history, oral contraceptive use, estrogen replacement therapy and the risk of developing scleroderma. *Arthritis Rheum* 1997; **40**: 419.

79. Rees RB, Bennett J. Localized scleroderma in father and daughter. *Arch Dermatol* 1953; **68**: 360.

80. Orabona ML, Albano O. Systemic progressive sclerosis. *Acta Med Scand* 1958; **160**: 128–161.

81. Blanchard RE, Speed EM. Scleroderma: periodontal membrane manifestations in two brothers. *Peridontics* 1965; **3**: 77–80.

82. McAndrew GM, Barnes EG. Familial scleroderma. *Ann Phys Med* 1965; **8**: 128–131.

83. Burge KM, Perry HO, Stickler GB. 'Familial' scleroderma. *Arch Dermatol* 1969; **99**: 681–687.

84. Rendall JR, McKenzie AW. Familial scleroderma. *Br J Dermatol* 1974; **91**: 517–522.

85. Greger RE. Familial progressive systemic scleroderma. *Arch Dermatol* 1975; **11**: 81–85.

86. Mund DJ, Greenwald RA. The CREST syndrome variant of scleroderma in a mother-daughter pair. *J Rheumatol* 1978; **5**: 307–310.

87. Sheldon WB, Lurie DP, Maricq HR et al. Three siblings with scleroderma (systemic sclerosis) and two with Raynaud's phenomenon from a single kindred. *Arthritis Rheum* 1981; **24**: 668–676.

88. Soppi E, Lehtonen A, Toivanen A. Familial progressive systemic sclerosis (scleroderma): immunological analysis of two patients and six siblings from a single kindred. *Clin Exp Immunol* 1982; **50**: 275–282.

89. McGregor AR, Watson A, Yunis E et al. Familial clustering of scleroderma spectrum disease. *Am J Med* 1988; **84**: 1023–1032.

90. Tuffanelli DL, Winklemann RK. Systemic scleroderma: clinical study of 727 cases. *Arch Dermatol* 1961; **84**: 359–371.

91. Giordano M, Valentini G, Vatti M, Tirri G, Gualdieri L, Lupoli S. Epidemiology of systemic sclerosis in Italy. *Conn Tiss Dis* 1984; **3**: 3–16.

92. Pereira S, Black C, Welsh K et al. Autoantibodies and immunogenetics in 30 patients with systemic sclerosis and their families. *J Rheumatol* 1987; **14**: 760–765.

93. Aguilar MB, Cho M, Reveille JD, Mayes M, Arnett FC. Prevalences of familial systemic sclerosis and other autoimmune diseases in three US cohorts. *Arthritis Rheum* 1999; **42**: 696.

94. Tuffanelli DL. Scleroderma, immunological and genetic disease in three families. *Dermatologica* 1969; **138**: 93–104.

95. Emerit I, Housset E, Feingold J. Chromosomal breakage and scleroderma: studies in family members. *J Lab Clin Med* 1976; **88**: 81–86.

96. Maddison PJ, Skinner RP, Pereira RS et al. Antinuclear antibodies in the relatives and spouses of patients with systemic sclerosis. *Ann Rheum Dis* 1986; **45**: 793–799.

97. Guseva NG, Folomeeva OM, Oskilko TG. Familial systemic sclerosis: a follow up study of concordant monozygotic twins. *Ter Arkh* 1981; **53**: 43–47.

98. Cook NJ, Silman AJ, Propert J, Cawley MID. Features of systemic sclerosis (scleroderma) in an identical twin pair. *Br J Rheumatol* 1993; **32**: 926–928.

99. Feghali CA, Wright TM. Epidemiologic and clinical study of twins with scleroderma. *Arthritis Rheum* 1995; **38**: S308.

100. Dustoor MM, McInerney MM, Mazanec DJ, Cathcart MK. Abnormal lymphocyte function in scleroderma: a study on identical twins. *Clin Immunol Immunopathol* 1987; **44**: 20–30.

101. McHugh NJ, Harvey GR, Whyte J, Dorsey JK. Segregation of autoantibodies with disease in monozygotic twin pairs discordant for systemic sclerosis. *Arthritis Rheum* 1995; **38**: 1845–1850.

102. Lynch CJ, Singh G, Whiteside TL, Rodnan GP, Medsger TA, Jr., Rabin BS. Histocompatibility antigens in progressive systemic sclerosis (PSS;scleroderma). *J Clin Immunol* 1982; **2**: 314–318.

103. Livingston JZ, Scott TE, Wigley FM *et al*. Systemic sclerosis (scleroderma): clinical, genetic, and serologic subsets. *J Rheumatol* 1987; **14**: 512–518.

104. Jazwinska EC, Olive C, Dunckley H, Naito§ S, Kuseba T, Serjeantson SW. HLA-DRw15 is increased in frequency in Japanese scleroderma patients. *Dis Markers* 1990; **8**: 323–326.

105. Briggs D, Stephens C, Vaughan R, Welsh K, Black C. A molecular and serological analysis of the major histocompatibility complex and complement component C4 in systemic sclerosis. *Arthritis Rheum* 1993; **36**: 943–954.

106. Takeuchi F, Nakano K, Yamada H *et al*. Association of HLA-DR with progressive systemic sclerosis in Japanese. *J Rheumatol* 1994; **21**: 857–863.

107. Kuwana M, Okano Y, Kaburaki J, Inoko H. HLA class II genes associated with anticentromere antibody in Japanese patients with systemic sclerosis (scleroderma). *Ann Rheum Dis* 1995; **54**: 983–987.

108. Vargas-Alarcón G, Granados J, Ibañez de Kasep G, Alcocer-Varela J, Alarcón-Segovia D. Association of HLA-DR5 (DR11) with systemic sclerosis (scleroderma) in Mexican patients. *Clin Exp Rheumatol* 1995; **13**: 11–16.

109. Takeuchi F, Kuwata S, Nakano K *et al*. Association of TAP1 and TAP2 with systemic sclerosis in Japanese. *Clin Exp Rheumatol* 1996; **14**: 513–521.

110. Venneker GT, van der Hoogen FHJ, van Meegen M *et al*. Molecular heterogeneity of second and fourth components of complement and their genes in systemic sclerosis and association of HLA alleles A1, B8 and DR3 with limited and DR5 with diffuse systemic sclerosis. *Exp Clin Immunogenet* 1998; **15**: 90–99.

111. Fanning GC, Welsh KI, Bunn C, Du Bois R, Black CM. HLA associations in three mutually exclusive autoantibody subgroups in UK systemic sclerosis patients. *Br J Rheumatol* 1998; **37**: 201–207.

112. Tan FK, Stivers DN, Arnett FC, Chakraborty R, Howard R, Reveille JD. HLA haplotypes and microsatellite polymorphisms in and around the major histocompatibility complex region in a native American population with a high prevalence of scleroderma (systemic sclerosis). *Tissue Antigens* 1999; **53**: 74–80.

113. Stephens CO, Briggs DC, Vaughan RW, Hall MA, Welsh KI, Black CM. The HLA-DP locus in systemic sclerosis—no primary association. *Tissue Antigens* 1993; **42**: 144–145.

114. Briggs DC, Welsh K, Pereira RS, Black CM. A strong association between null alleles at the C4A locus in the major histocompatibility complex and systemic sclerosis. *Arthritis Rheum* 1986; **29**: 1274–1277.

115. Mollenhauer E, Schmidt R, Heinrichs M, Rittner C. Scleroderma: possible significance of silent alleles at the C4B locus. *Arthritis Rheum* 1984; **27**: 711–712.

116. Tan FK, Stivers DN, Foster MW *et al*. Association of microsatellite markers near the fibrillin 1 gene on human chromosome 15q with scleroderma in a native American population. *Arthritis Rheum* 1998; **41**: 1729–1737.

117. de Juan MD, Belzunegui J, Belmonte I *et al*. An immunogenetic study of familial scleroderma. *Ann Rheum Dis* 1994; **53**: 614–617.

118. Manolios N, Dunckley H, Chivers T, Brooks P, Englert H. Immunogenetic analysis of 5 families with multicase occurrence of scleroderma and/or related variants. *J Rheumatol* 1995; **22**: 85–92.

119. Stephens CO, Briggs DC, Whyte J *et al*. Familial scleroderma—evidence for environmental versus genetic trigger. *Br J Rheumatol* 1994; **33**: 1131–1135.

120. Artlett CM, Black CM, Briggs DC, Stephens C, Welsh KI. DNA Allelic alterations within VNTR loci of scleroderma families. *Br J Rheumatol* 1996; **35**: 1216–1222.

121. Lambert NC, Furst DE, Distler O *et al*. HLA-DQA1*0501 is associated with risk of systemic sclerosis in men. *Arthritis Rheum* 1999; **42**: 805.

122. Pandey JP, Takeuchi F. TNF-alpha and TNF-beta gene polymorphisms in systemic sclerosis. *Hum Immunol* 1999; **60**: 1128–1130.

123. Black CM, Welsh KI, Walker AE *et al*. Genetic susceptibility to scleroderma-like syndrome induced by vinyl chloride. *Lancet* 1983; **1**: 53–55.

124. Frank KH, Füssel M, Conrad K *et al*. Different distribution of HLA Class II and tumour necrosis factor alleles (TNF-308.2, TNFa2 microsatellite) in antitopoisomerase 1 responders among scleroderma patients with and without exposure to quartz/metal dust. *Arthritis Rheum* 1998; **41**: 1306–1311.

125. Rihs HP, Conrad K, Mehlhorn J *et al*. Molecular analysis of HLA-DPB1 alleles in idiopathic systemic sclerosis patients and uranium miners with systemic sclerosis. *Int Arch Allergy Immunol* 1996; **109**: 216–222.

126. Ziegler V, Pampel W, Zshunke E. Kristalliner quarz (eine) ursache der progressiven sklerodermie? Epidemiologische untersuchungen zum gemeinsamen auftreten der progressiven sklerodermie und der silikose. *Dermato Monatsschr* 1982; **168**: 398–401.

127. Haustein UF, Herrmann K. Environmental scleroderma. *Clin Dermatol* 1994; **12**: 467–473.

128. Bramwell B. Diffuse scleroderma: its frequency, its occurrence in stone masons; its treatment by fibrolysin-elevations of temperature due to fibrolysin injections. *Edinburgh Med J* 1914; **12**: 387–401.

129. Erasmus LD. Scleroderma in gold miners on the Witzwaterzrand with particular reference to pulmonary manifestations. *J Lab Clin Med* 1957; **3**: 209–231.

130. Bernstein R, Prinsloo I, Zwi S, Andrew MJA, Dawson B, Jenkins T. Chromosomal aberrations in occupation-associated progressive systemic sclerosis. *S Afr Med J* 1980; **58**: 235–237.

131. Cowie RL. Silica-dust-exposed mine workers with scleroderma (systemic sclerosis). *Chest* 1987; **92**: 260.

132. Sluis-Cremer GK, Hessel PA, Nizdo EH, Churchill AR, Zeiss EA. Silica, silicosis, and progressive systemic sclerosis. *Br J Ind Med* 1985; **42**: 838–843.

133. Burns CJ, Laing TJ, Gillespie BW *et al.* The epidemiology of scleroderma among women: assessment of risk from exposure to silicone and silica. *J Rheumatol* 1996; **23**: 1904–1911.

134. Bovenzi M, Barbone F, Betta A, Tommasini M, Versini W. Scleroderma and occupational exposure. *Scand J Work Environ Health* 1995; **21**: 289–292.

135. Rodnan GP, Benedek TG, Medsger TA, Jr., Cammaratta RJ. The association of progressive systemic sclerosis (scleroderma) with coal miners' pneumoconiosis and other forms of silicosis. *Ann Intern Med* 1967; **66**: 323–334.

136. Ziegler V, Haustein UF, Mehlhorn J, Münzberger H, Rennau H. Quarzinduzierte sklerodermie. Sklerodermie-ahnliches syndrom oder echte progressive sklerodermie? *Dermato Monatsschr* 1986; **172**: 86–90.

137. Conrad K, Stahnke G, Liedvogel B. Anti-CENP-B response in uranium miners exposed to quartz dust and patients with possible development of scleroderma (systemic sclerosis). *J Rheumatol* 1995; **22**: 1286–1294.

138. Degens P, Baur X. Zur epidemiologie und statistik der sklerodermie als mögliche berufskrankheit. *Arbeitsmed Sozialmed Umweltmed Sonderheft* 1994; **22**: 27–33.

139. Miyoshi K, Miyaoka T, Kobayashi Y *et al.* Hypergammaglobulinemia by prolonged adjuvanticity in man: disorders developed after augmentation mammoplasty. *Ijishimpo* 1964; **2122**: 9–14.

140. Kumagai Y, Shiokawa Y, Medsger TA, Jr., Rodnan GP. Clinical spectrum of connective tissue disease after cosmetic surgery. *Arthritis Rheum* 1984; **27**: 1–12.

141. Gabriel SE, O'Fallon WM, Kurland LT, Beard CM, Woods JE, Melton LJ, III. Risk of connective-tissue diseases and other disorders after breast implantation. *N Engl J Med* 1994; **330**: 1697–1702.

142. Edworthy SM, Martin L, Barr SG, Birdsell DC, Brant RF, Fritzler MJ. A clinical study of the relationship between silicone breast implants and connective tissue disease. *J Rheumatol* 1998; **25**: 254–260.

143. Friis S, Mellemkjaer L, McLaughlin JK *et al.* Connective tissue disease and other rheumatic conditions following breast implants in Denmark. *Ann Plast Surg* 1997; **39**: 1–8.

144. Nyren O, Yin L, Josefsson S *et al.* Risk of connective tissue disease and related disorders among women with breast implants: a nationwide retrospective cohort study in Sweden. *BMJ* 1998; **316**: 417–422.

145. Hennekens CH, Lee IM, Cook NR *et al.* Self-reported breast implants and connective-tissue diseases in female health professionals. A retrospective cohort study. *JAMA* 1996; **275**: 616–621.

146. Englert H, Morris D, March L. Scleroderma and silicone gel breast prostheses–the Sydney study revisited. *Aust N Z J Med* 1996; **26**: 349–355.

147. Hochberg MC, Perlmutter DL, Medsger TA, Jr. *et al.* Lack of association between augmentation mammoplasty and systemic sclerosis (scleroderma). *Arthritis Rheum* 1996; **39**: 1125–1131.

148. Lacey JV, Laing TJ, Gillespie BW, Schottenfeld D. Epidemiology of scleroderma among women: assessment of risk from exposure to silicone and silica—reply. *J Rheumatol* 1997; **24**: 1854–1855.

149. Janowskyy EC, Kupper LL, Hulka BS. Meta-analyses of the relation between silicone breast implants and the risk of connective-tissue diseases. *N Engl J Med* 2000; **342**: 781–790.

150. Hochberg MC, Perlmutter DL. The association of augmentation mammoplasty with connective tissue disease, including systematic sclerosis (scleroderma): a meta-analysis. *Curr Top Microbiol Immunol* 1996; **210**: 411–417.

151. Perkins LL, Clark BD, Klein PJ, Cook RR. A meta-analysis of breast implants and connective tissue disease. *Ann Plast Surg* 1995; **35**: 561–570.

152. Wong O. A critical assessment of the relationship between silicone breast implants and connective tissue diseases. *Regul Toxicol Pharmacol* 1996; **23**: 74–85.

153. Reinl W. Sclerodermia caused by trichlorethylene. *Zent f Arbeitsmed u Arbeitsschutz* 1957; **7**: 58–60.

154. Saihan EM, Burton JL, Heaton KW. A new syndrome with pigmentation, scleroderma, gynaecomastia, Raynaud's phenomenon and peripheral neuropathy. *Br J Dermatol* 1978; **99**: 437–440.

155. Lockey JE, Kelly CR, Cannon GW, Colby TV, Aldrich V, Livingston GK. Progressive systemic sclerosis associated with exposure to trichloroethylene. *J Occup Med* 1987; **29**: 493–496.

156. Bottomley WW, Sheehan-Dare RA, Hughes P, Cunliffe WJ. A sclerodermatous syndrome with unusual features following prolonged occupational exposure to organic solvents. *Br J Dermatol* 1993; **128**: 203–206.

157. Czirják L, Pócs E, Szegedi G. Localized scleroderma after exposure to organic solvents. *Dermatology* 1994; **89**: 399–401.

158. Garcia-Zamalloa AM, Ojeda E, Gonzalez-Beneitez C, Goni J, Garrido A. Systemic sclerosis and organic solvents: early diagnosis in industry. *Ann Rheum Dis* 1994; **53**: 618.

159. Altomonte A, Mirone L, Zoli A, Magnavita N. Scleroderma-like disease following occupational exposure to organic solvents. *Clin Rheumatol* 1996; **15**: 416–417.

160. Silman AJ, Jones S. What is the contribution of occupational environmental factors to the occurrence of scleroderma in men? *Ann Rheum Dis* 1992; **51**: 1322–1324.

161. Goldman JA. Connective tissue disease in people exposed to organic chemical solvents: Systemic sclerosis (scleroderma) in dry cleaning plant and aircraft industry workers. *Arthritis Rheum* 1996; **39**: 739–739.

162. Nietert PJ, Sutherland SE, Silver RM *et al.* Is occupational organic solvent exposure a risk factor for scleroderma? *Arthritis Rheum* 1998; **41**: 1111–1118.

163. Lonzetti LS, Joyal F, Raynauld JP *et al.* Updating the American College of Rheumatology preliminary classifi-

cation criteria for systemic sclerosis: addition of severe nailfold capillaroscopy abnormalities markedly increases the sensitivity for limited scleroderma. *Arthritis Rheum* 2001; **44**: 735–736.

164. Mehlhorn J. Quarzinduzierte progressive systemische scklerodermie—exposition, klinische beobachtungen, lungenfunktion. *Arbeitsmed Sozialmed Umweltmed Sonderheft* 1994; **22**: 8–11.

165. Dirschka T, Jansen A, Hoffmann K, Altmeyer P. Klinisch-dermatologische befunde. *Arbeitsmed Sozialmed Umweltmed Sonderheft* 1994; **22**: 12–13.

166. Seeman U, Hillenbach C. Auswertung von autopsiefällen aus dem Uranerzbergbau. *Arbeitsmed Sozialmed Umweltmed Sonderheft* 1994; **22**: 14.

167. Mehlhorn VJ, Gerlach CH, Ziegler V. Occupational progressive systemic sclerosis through scouring powder. *Dermatosen* 1990; **38**: 180–185.

168. Koeger AC, Marre JP, Rozenberg S, Gutmann L, Bourgeois P. Maladies auto-immunes après expositions inhabituelles à la silice ou aux silicones. *Ann Med Interne* 1992; **143**: 165–170.

169. Sanchez-Roman J, Wichmann I, Salaberri J, Varela JM, Nuñez-Rolden A. Multiple clinical and biological autoimmune manifestations in 50 workers after occupational exposure to silica. *Ann Rheum Dis* 1993; **52**: 534–538.

170. Schiele R, Hanslik A, Weltle D. Progressive systemische Sklerodermie und berufliche Quarzstaubexposition. *Arbeitsmed Sozialmed Praventivmed* 1990; **25**: 252–255.

171. Sparrow GP. A connective tissue disorder similar to vinyl chloride disease in a patient exposed to perchlorethylene. *Clin Exp Dermatol* 1977; **2**: 17–22.

172. Walder BK. Do solvents cause scleroderma? *Int J Dermatol* 1983; **22**: 157–158.

173. Czirják L, Dankó K, Schlammadinger J, Surányi P, Tamási L, Szegedi GY. Progressive systemic sclerosis occurring in patients exposed to chemicals. *Int J Dermatol* 1987; **26**: 374–378.

174. Owens GR, Medsger TA. Systemic sclerosis secondary to occupational exposure. *Am J Med* 1988; **85**: 114–116.

175. Czirják L, Szegedi G. Benzene exposure and systemic sclerosis. *Ann Intern Med* 1987; **107**: 118.

176. Lilis R, Anderson H, Nicholson WJ, Daum S, Fischbein AS, Selikoff IJ. Prevalence of disease among vinyl chloride and polyvinyl chloride workers. *Ann N Y Acad Sci* 1975; **246**: 22–41.

177. Mark ME, Kaplan BL, Mayes MD. Scleroderma in heating and air conditioning workers—possible occupational link. *Arthritis Rheum* 1992; **35**: R32.

178. Rush PJ, Chaiton A. Scleroderma, renal failure and death associated with exposure to urea formaldehyde foam insulation. *J Rheumatol* 1986; **13**: 475.

179. Yamakage A, Ishikawa H, Saito Y, Hattori A. Occupational scleroderma-like disorder occurring in men engaged in the polymerization of epoxy resins. *Dermatologica* 1980; **161**: 33–44.

180. Fessel WJ. Scleroderma and welding. *N Engl J Med* 1977; **296**: 1537.

181. Pelmear PL, Roos JO, Maehle WM. Occupationally-induced scleroderma. *J Occup Med* 1992; **34**: 20–25.

182. Aeschlimann A, de Truchis P, Kahn MF. Scleroderma after therapy with appetite suppressants. *Scand J Rheumatol* 1990; **19**: 87–90.

183. Tomlinson IW, Jayson MI. Systemic sclerosis after therapy with appetite suppressants. *J Rheumatol* 1984; **11**: 254.

184. Finch WR, Rodnan GP, Buckingham RB, Prince RK, Winkelstein A. Bleomycin-induced scleroderma. *J Rheumatol* 1980; **7**: 651–659.

185. Kerr LD, Spiera H. Scleroderma in association with the use of bleomycin: a report of 3 cases. *J Rheumatol* 1992; **19**: 294–296.

186. Sternberg EM, Van Woert MH, Young SN *et al.* Development of a scleroderma-like illness during therapy with L-5-hydroxytryptophan and carbidopa. *N Engl J Med* 1980; **303**: 782–787.

187. Palestine RF, Millns JL, Spigel GT, Schroeter AL. Skin manifestations of pentazocine abuse. *J Am Acad Dermatol* 1980; **2**: 47–55.

188. Trozak DJ, Gould WM. Cocaine abuse and connective tissue disease. *J Am Acad Dermatol* 1984; **10**: 525.

189. Kilaru P, Kim W, Sequeira W. Cocaine and scleroderma: is there an assocation? *J Rheumatol* 1991; **18**: 1753–1755.

190. Tabuenca JM. Toxic-allergic syndrome caused by ingestion of rapeseed oil denatured with aniline. *Lancet* 1981; **2**: 567–568.

191. Posada M, Castro M, Kilbourne EM *et al.* Toxic-oil syndrome: case reports associated with the ITH oil refinery in Sevilla. *Food Chem Toxicol* 1987; **25**: 87–90.

192. Kilbourne EM, Rigau-Perez JG, Heath CW *et al.* Clinical epidemiology of toxic-oil syndrome: manifestations of a new illness. *N Engl J Med* 1983; **309**: 1408–1414.

193. Alonso-Ruiz A, Zea-Mendoza AC, Salazar-Vallinas JM, Rocamora-Ripoll A, Beltran-Gutierrez J. Toxic oil syndrome: a syndrome with features overlapping those of various forms of scleroderma. *Semin Arthritis Rheum* 1986; **15**: 200–212.

194. Hertzman PA, Blevins W, Mayer J, Greenfield B, Ting M, Gleich GJ. Association of the eosinophilia-myalgia syndrome with the ingestion of tryptophan. *N Engl J Med* 1990; **322**: 869–873.

195. Silver RM, Heyes EP, Maize JC, Quearry B, Vionnet-Fuasset M, Sternberg EM. Scleroderma, fasciitis and eosinophilia associated with the ingestion of tryptophan. *N Engl J Med* 1990; **322**: 874–881.

196. Eidson M, Philen RM, Sewell CM, Voorhees R, Kilbourne EM. L-tryptophan and eosinophilia-myalgia syndrome in New Mexico. *Lancet* 1990; **335**: 645–648.

197. Belongia EA, Hedberg CW, Gleich GJ *et al.* An investigation of the cause of the eosinophilia-myalgia syndrome associated with tryptophan use. *N Engl J Med* 1990; **323**: 357–365.

198. Medsger TA. Tryptophan induced eosinophilia-myalgia syndrome. *N Engl J Med* 1990; **322**: 926–928.

199. Silman AJ, Jones S. Pet ownership: a possible risk factor for scleroderma. *Br J Rheumatol* 1990; **29**: 494.

9 | Polymyositis/dermatomyositis

Alan J. Silman

Polymyositis is an acquired, inflammatory myopathy of unknown aetiology involving striated skeletal and, less commonly, cardiac muscle. Associated clinical features include skin rash (dermatomyositis), dysphagia, arthritis, Raynaud's phenomenon, interstitial lung disease, and other visceral manifestations; however, proximal limb girdle muscle weakness is the dominant feature of this disorder [1,2]. Although epidemiologically polymyositis and dermatomyositis are frequently considered as part of the same disease entity this might be inappropriate. Pathologically polymyositis is a T-cell driven disorder whereas dermatomyositis is predominantly a microangiopathic vascular disease [3]. The epidemiology of polymyositis was reviewed by Cronin and Plotz [4]. This chapter will summarize current knowledge of classification criteria, descriptive and analytic epidemiology, and the relationship of malignancy with polymyositis/dermatomyositis.

Classification criteria

The problems inherent in the diagnosis of polymyositis/dermatomyositis were reviewed by Bohan and Peter [5,6]. They proposed five major criteria to define polymyositis and dermatomyositis, primarily for purposes of clinical research (Table 9.1). These authors qualified the criteria by stating 'the diagnosis of polymyositis or dermatomyositis is not necessarily excluded by failure to meet them'. Furthermore, they enumerated several exclusion criteria including congenital muscular dystrophies, central or peripheral neurologic disease, infectious myositis, metabolic/endocrine myopathies, and myasthenia gravis.

Several authors have estimated the sensitivity of these criteria in cohorts of patients with polymyositis/dermatomyositis [7–14]. Based on almost 900 cases, two-thirds and slightly over one-fifth of subjects fulfilled criteria for definite and probable disease respect-

Table 9.1 Diagnostic criteria for polymyositis and dermatomyositis; source: [4]

Item No.	Description
1	Symmetrical weakness of the limb-girdle muscles and anterior neck flexors
2	Muscle biopsy evidence of myositis
3	Elevation in serum of skeletal muscle enzymes, particularly creatine kinase
4	Typical electromyographic features of myositis
5	Typical rash of dermatomyositis including heliotrope lids and Gottron's papules

Polymyositis:	Definite	All of items 1 through 4
	Probable	3 of items 1 through 4
	Possible	2 of items 1 through 4
Dermatomyositis:	Definite	Item 5 plus 3 of items 1–4
	Probable	Item 5 plus 2 of items 1–4
	Possible	Item 5 plus 1 of items 1–4

Table 9.2 Sensitivity[a] of diagnostic criteria for polymyositis and dermatomyositis

Reference	No. of patients	Polymyositis/dermatomyositis Definite (%)	Probable (%)
[11]	76	56 (74)	20 (26)
[8]	153	140 (92)	11 (7)
[7]	92	46 (50)	26 (28)
[9]	107	87 (81)	15 (14)
[15]	27	17 (63)	6 (22)
[14]	105	47 (45)	30 (29)
[10]	120	88 (73)	23 (19)
[13]	25	16 (64)	9 (36)
[12]	177	86 (49)	56 (32)
Total	882	583 (66)	196 (22)

[a] Sensitivity = number of patients who fulfil criteria/total number of patients with disease in study

ively (Table 9.2). The specificity of the criteria, when validated against a combined control group of 172 patients with systemic lupus erythematosus and 264 patients with systemic sclerosis, was 93 per cent [10].

Table 9.3 Classification schema for polymyositis and dermatomyositis; source: [4]

Type	Category
I	Typical polymyositis
II	Typical dermatomyositis
III	Typical dermatomyositis or polymyositis associated with malignancy
IV	Childhood dermatomyositis
V	Polymyositis associated with another connective tissue disease (most often Sjogren's syndrome, systemic sclerosis, or systemic lupus erythematosus)

The generally accepted classification scheme for polymyositis is that proposed by Pearson [16] (Table 9.3); adult-onset disease is separated from childhood-onset disease, and, among adults, polymyositis is separated from dermatomyositis. In addition, the occurrence of myositis in the setting of malignancy (see page 168) or with an associated connective tissue disease, most often systemic sclerosis, Sjögren's syndrome, or systemic lupus erythematosus are recognized as clinical subtypes. The major flaw in these criteria is they do not distinguish between polymyositis and dermatomyositis [3]. A suggested scheme for distinguishing these disorders is shown in Table 9.4 and seems highly discriminating [17].

Investigators from the National Institutes of Health have suggested an alternative approach to classification based on the presence of myositis-specific anti-

Table 9.4 Japanese criteria for distinguishing polymyositis from dermatomyositis; reproduced with the permission of the *Journal of Rheumatology* from [17]

Skin features	Other features
1. Heliotrope rash	1. Proximal muscle weakness
2. Gottron's papules	2. Elevated creatine kinase or aldolase
3. Erythema/purpura on extensor surfaces	3. Myopathy on EMG
	4. Anti-Jo1 antibody
	5. Non-erosive arthritis/arthralgia
	6. Abnormal muscle biopsy

Dermatomyositis:	1 skin and 4 other features	
Polymyositis:	4 other features	
	Sensitivity %	Specificity %
Dermatomyositis	94	90
Polymyositis	99	95

bodies [18]. They studied 212 patients with probable or definite polymyositis or dermatomyositis or inclusion body myositis (IBM); one-third had a myositis-specific autoantibody. Their classification scheme subdivides the group having autoantibodies into four subsets, those with antisynthetase antibodies (most commonly antiJo1), antibodies to signal recognition particles, antiMi2, and antiMAS antibodies; the remaining two-thirds had no myositis-specific auto-antibodies. Half of patients with primary polymyositis or dermatomyositis belonged to the former group while over 90 per cent of patients associated with either connective tissue disease or malignancy and all patients with IBM belonged in the latter group. Finally, the patients with antibodies to either signal recognition particles or antisynthetase antibodies had cumulative survival rates significantly lower than those of patients with myositis specific antibodies. The validity of this classification scheme will need to be determined in an alternative cohort of patients with sufficient longitudinal data to assess clinical outcomes in addition to survival.

Descriptive epidemiology

Incidence

There have been a number of studies of incidence based predominantly on ascertaining diagnosed cases attending specialist centres and relating these to the presumed catchment population of these centres. Numerator/denominator errors and the difficulty in retrospective studies in validating diagnosis from contemporary medical records all lead to considerable scope for error and may explain differences between populations. Studies have been reported on both childhood and adult populations and these are considered separately.

Childhood

A number of studies have been undertaken in the past 10 years and the results are shown in Table 9.5; predominantly in this age group dermatomyositis rather than polymyositis is the major form. The data from North America, Europe, and Japan are remarkably consistent although there are some interesting and difficult to explain differences. Thus in Finland the boy:girl ratio was 1:1 [21], whereas in the UK it was 1:6 [22]. The latter study also suggested a cluster of onsets in the spring [22].

Table 9.5   Incidence of polymyositis/ dermatomyositis in children

Reference	Period	Diagnosis	Country	Survey method	Incidence/100 000
[19]	1948–72	PM/DM	US	Hospital discharge	0.3
[12]	1963–82	PM/DM	US	Hospital discharge	0.25
[20]	1984–92	PM/DM	US	Hospital register	0.4
[21]	1983–86	PM/DM	Finland	Hospital discharge register	0.3
[22]	1992–93	DM	UK	Prospective notification	0.2 (0.14–0.26)
[23]	1991–92	DM	Canada	Hospital registers	0.15 (0.09–0.29)
[24]	1994	PM/DM	Japan	Questionnaire to hospitals	0.16

Table 9.6   Incidence of polymyositis/ dermatomyositis in adults

Reference	Period	Diagnosis	Country	Study method	Incidence/100 000
[25]	1951–67	PM	US	Hospital admission	0.6[a]
[26]	1947–48	PM	US	Hospital admission	0.5
	1963–68				0.8
[27]	1960–76	PM/DM	Israel	Hospital discharge	0.2
[28]	1988–92	PM/DM	Japan	Hospital registers	1.0
[29]	1990	PM/DM	Finland	National disability register	0.4
[30]	1984–93	PM/DM	Sweden	Special register	0.8

[a] Based on only 6 cases.

Adulthood

The results of the major studies are summarized in Table 9.6. The data from Medsger *et al.* [26] provide the first robust estimates based on cases admitted to hospitals in Memphis and Shelby county in Tennessee between 1947 and 1968. As shown in Table 9.6, the incidence was higher in the last 5 years of that period. Other studies from Israel, Japan, and Scandinavia have shown remarkably similar incidence rates. It should be noted that none of these data are age standardized.

Age and gender

The data from adults and children have already been described. As shown above, the incidence of dermato-myositis in childhood, at around 0.2–0.3 per 100 000, is around half that seen in adult studies. The data from Allegheny County, US [12] did show strong evidence of increasing incidence with age (Table 9.7). Older data from Tennessee [26] had suggested a childhood peak at 0.4 per 100 000 between 5 and 14 years and an adult peak of 1 per 100 000 between 45 and 64 again confirming this adult/child ratio of 2.5:1.

The gender ratio varies between studies. The unexplained difference in the paediatric series between Finland and the UK has already been discussed. In both the Tennessee and Allegheny County studies, there was

Table 9.7   Number of cases and average annual age-specific incidence rates per million population of polymyositis in Allegheny County, PA, 1963–82; modified from [12]

Age group	Number of cases	Rate
<15	16	2.5
15–24	12	2.5
25–34	16	3.3
35–44	19	5.5
45–54	32	8.9
55–64	37	9.8
≥65	45	10.5
Total	177	5.5

a female: male excess of approximately 2:1 in adults (Table 9.8).

Ethnicity and geography

Interestingly, in both the US studies [12,26], there were substantially higher incidence rates in African American populations compared to whites. There are no other data comparing ethnic groups within a population. In one report based on small numbers and anecdotal reports of case numbers, there was a suggestion of increasing prevalence with increasing latitude [31] (Fig. 9.1).

Table 9.8   Influence of gender and ethnic background on incidence

| Reference | Population | Incidence/100 000 | | | |
| | | Whites | | African Americans | |
		Males	Females	Males	Females
[26]	Tennessee, US	0.4	0.6	1.0	1.8
[12]	Allegheny County, PA, US[a]	0.3	0.6	1.1	1.7

[a] Data are age adjusted

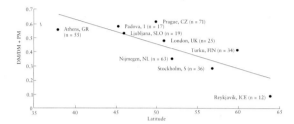

Fig. 9.1   Relative prevalence of DM (DM/DM + PM) as a function of geographical latitude. DM = dermatomyositis, PM = polymyositis, GR = Greece, I = Italy, SLO = Slovenia, CZ = Czech Republic, UK = United Kingdom, NL = Netherlands, S = Sweden, FIN = Finland, and ICE = Iceland. Reproduced from Hengstman GJD, van Venrooij WJ, Vencovsky J, Moutsopoulos HM, van Engelen BGM. *Ann Rheum Dis* 2000; 59: 141–142 [31] with permission of BMJ Publishing Group.

Time trends

Data on trends over time come from the studies from Tennessee [26] and Pennsylvania [12]. In the latter study, overall age-adjusted average annual incidence rates increased from 2.3 to 10.2 cases per million from the 5-year interval 1963–7 to 1978–82. This increased incidence was present in all sex–race groups. Possible explanations suggested by the authors and others [4] include: (1) increased availability of automated testing for serum levels of skeletal muscle enzymes; (2) increased physician awareness of polymyositis due to promulgation of classification criteria and other educational activities; and (3) a true increase in incidence. There may also be a seasonal influence on incidence as discussed previously [22].

Mortality

In a disease such as polymyositis with a relatively high mortality, population mortality rates can be used to infer trends regarding occurrence, for example between genders or ethnic groups. Hochberg *et al.* [32] reported the age-, sex-, and race-specific mortality rates for polymyositis/dermatomyositis in the US between 1968 and 1978 using nation-wide data from the National Centre for Health Statistics. A total of 1986 deaths were attributed to polymyositis and/or dermatomyositis over that 11-year period: 1004 in white females, 563 in white males, 291 in non-white females, and 168 in non-white males. Age-adjusted average annual mortality per million person-years were 0.6, 0.9, 1.2, and 2.2 for white males, white females, non-white males, and non-white females respectively, reflecting the differences in incidence discussed above. Furthermore, as with the incidence rates, there was evidence of synergistic interaction between sex and race in producing the highest mortality rates in non-white females as assessed by Rothman's synergy index.

In contrast to the pattern observed with age-specific incidence rates, age-specific average annual mortality rates showed a unimodal distribution with maximum

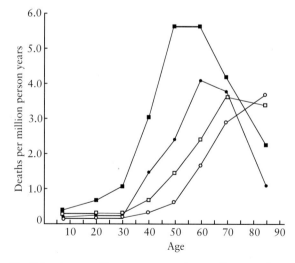

Fig. 9.2   Age-specific average annual mortality rates from polymyositis/ dermatomyositis by sex–race group in the US, 1968–78. ○ = white males, □ = white females, ● = non-white males, ■ = non-white females. Reprinted with permission of Lippincott Williams and Wilkins from [32].

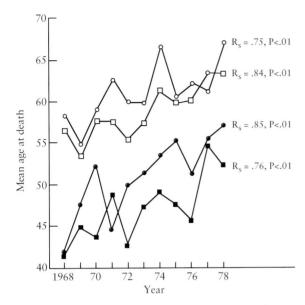

Fig. 9.3 Mean age at death by sex–race group and year, from 1968 to 1978. ○ = white males, □ = white females, ● = non-white males, ■ = non-white females. Reprinted with permission of Lippincott Williams and Wilkins from [32].

rates in the 45–64 year age-group for non-white females, 55–64 year age-group for non-white males, 65–74 year age group for white females, and 75 and above age group for white males (Fig. 9.2).

Analysis of secular trends in annual age-adjusted mortality rates from 1968 to 1978 revealed significant increases in both white males and white females which was attributed, by the authors, to increased physician awareness and diagnosis of these conditions and/or a 'true' increase in incidence of polymyositis. Finally, analysis of secular trends in mean age at death from 1968 to 1978 revealed significant increase in mean age at death among all sex–race groups which was felt to be most consistent with improvement in prognosis over time and a concomitant decrease in mortality rates in childhood onset and young adult cases rather than an increase in age at diagnosis of polymyositis (Fig. 9.3).

Prevalence

Prevalence is a much less useful measure of occurrence than incidence but, where appropriate, can give an indication of the number of subjects with evidence of disease at a single point in time—a proportion of use in planning health care delivery. Based only on three living cases, Kurland [25] estimated the prevalence of polymyositis to be 6 per 100 000 in January 1968.

Data from Japan suggested a similar figure of 5 per 100 000 [33]. More recent Japanese data suggested a higher prevalence of 10 per 100 000 [28] but whether this represents increased incidence or longer disease duration, because of lower case fatality, is unclear.

Genetics

Polymyositis/dermatomyositis does not appear to demonstrate familial aggregation as has been reported in systemic lupus erythematosus [34] and rheumatoid arthritis [35]. Familial occurrence has only rarely been reported [36,37].

There have been a number of immunogenetic studies. Early studies were broadly consistent in demonstrating an association between the A1 B8 DR3 'autoimmune' haplotype and disease. Thus Hirsch *et al.* [38] studied 53 patients with myositis; all were typed for HLA-A, B, C, and DR antigens and results were compared to local controls. HLA-B8 was found in seven (54 per cent) of 13 whites with polymyositis compared to 19 per cent of over 1400 controls (*P* = 0.005) while HLA-DR3 was found in eight (75 per cent) of 12 whites with polymyositis compared to 23 per cent of over 100 controls (*P* = 0.003). HLA-B7 was found in six (67 per cent) and HLA-DRw6 in seven (78 per cent) of nine black patients with polymyositis compared to 26 per cent of 89 (*P* = 0.02) and 46 (*P* = 0.005) controls respectively. No HLA specificities were increased in frequency in the seven white and nine black patients with dermatomyositis.

Friedman *et al.* [39] reported results of HLA-A and B locus typing in 67 white patients with juvenile dermatomyositis, of whom 36 were also typed for HLA-DR antigens [40]. HLA-B8 was found in 37 per cent of patients compared to 17.5 per cent of controls (*P* < 0.01) while DR3 was found in 53 per cent of patients compared to 22.7 per cent of controls (*P* < 0.01). The association of DR3 but not B8 with juvenile dermatomyositis was also found in Latin American and black patients studied by the authors. Plotz *et al.* [2] noted that DR3 was present in 48 per cent of 52 white patients with polymyositis or dermatomyositis, but was only 'slightly increased' in 23 black patients.

Recent immunogenetic studies using PCR based molecular methods have attempted to focus down on the most likely susceptibility allele after allowing for linkage disequilibrium. HLA-DQA1*0501 is in strong linkage with HLA-DRB1*03 (DR3) and in juvenile dermatomyositis it appears that this allele is the site of the strongest association. Indeed, an association was observed in non-DR3, DQA1*0501 bearing haplotypes [41]. This association has been replicated in juvenile dermatomyositis patients from three ethnic groups in the US: Europeans, Hispanics, and Africans with the weakest effects in those of European origin [42]. No association was seen in Japanese patients in whom the predominant DRB1 associated allele was DRB1*08 [43]. In that study there were differences in HLA class I associations between dermatomyositis and polymyositis—a reduction in HLA-A24/B52 and an increase in Cw3 in the latter compared to the former.

Arnett *et al.* [44] noted an association between the presence of HLA-DR3 and anti-Jo1 antibody; seven of 11 patients with antoJo1 antibody were positive for DR3 compared to eight of 36 patients without antiJo1 antibody. This association was confirmed by Plotz *et al.* [2] who found DR3 in 12 of 15 white and four of eight black patients with antiJo1 antibody. More recent studies by Goldstein *et al.* [45] and the group from the National Institutes of Health [18] demonstrate that the vast majority of patients with antiJo1 and other antisynthetase antibodies as well as antibodies to signal recognition particles have HLA-DRw52 while patients with antiMi2 antibodies uniformly had the HLA-DRw53 specificity. Thus, genetic factors appear to identify distinct serologic subsets of polymyositis/ dermatomyositis with different clinical features and, possibly, different responses to treatment and prognoses [18]. The agents, if any, which trigger the autoantibody responses in these genetically susceptible individuals remain to be identified.

Non-genetic host factors

The most important non-genetic host factor of interest is the co-occurrence of poly/dermatomyositis with

Table 9.9 Frequency of malignancy in patients with adult-onset polymyositis and/or dermatomyositis; modified from [56]

Reference	Number of cases	No. (%) with malignancy
[8]	142	13 (9)
[48]	25	5 (20)
[49]	58	8 (14)
[50]	27	3 (11)
[9]	86	7 (8)
[51]	50	11 (22)
[52]	27	5 (19)
[15]	27	2 (7)
[53]	36	4 (11)
[14]	105	16 (15)
[54]	71	17 (24)
[11]	76	6 (8)
[55]	115	29 (25)
[13]	25	1 (4)
[12]	117	20 (17)
[18]	212	13 (6)
Total	1259	160 (13)

malignancy, particularly adenocarcinomas and other solid tumours. This topic has been extensively reviewed, see for example [46,47].

There are a large number of case series suggesting a high prevalence of malignancy in patients with these disorders (Table 9.9). In 10 of the 16 studies shown, data are provided separately for polymyositis and dermatomyositis. A 'meta-analysis' of these studies yielded a cancer prevalence of 20 per cent for dermatomyositis and one of 13 per cent for polymyositis [56].

The only true test of an association is one of a comparison between the onset of cancer in subjects with poly/dermatomyositis and a control population, which ideally should be the expected age and sex adjusted incidence in the population base from which the

Table 9.10 Analytical studies of the association between cancer and poly/dermatomyositis

Reference	Country	Control group	Relative risk (Odds Ratio) (95% CI) of cancer		
			Polymyositis	Dermatomyositis	Pooled
[54]	Canada	Mixed rheumatic diseases	5.8 (1.8–18.5)	11.3 (3.6–35.0)	8.0 (2.9–22.0)
[55]	US	Population	1.8 (0.9–3.7)	1.3 (0.6–3.0)	1.6 (0.8–3.0)
[58]	US	Closest living same-sexed siblings	N/A	N/A	1.6 (0.27–13.0)
[57]	Sweden	Males[a]	1.8 (1.1–2.7)	2.4 (1.6–3.6)	
		Females[a]	1.7 (1.0–2.5)	3.4 (2.4–4.7)	
[60]	Finland	National data	1.0 (0.5–1.8)	6.5 (3.9–10.0)[b]	2.1 (1.4–2.9)
[61]	Denmark	National data	1.7 (1.1–2.4)	3.8 (2.6–5.4)[c]	

[a] Comparison with expected national rates.
[b] Risk in first year after diagnosis 26 (12–48).
[c] Risk in first/second year after diagnosis were 5.9 (3.8–8.7) and 2.5 (1.1–4.8) respectively.

cases arose. A meta-analysis of four published studies up to 1992 [54,55,57,58] combined data from 565 polymyositis and 513 dermatomyositis patients [59]. The individual data from those four studies and two other recent studies is shown in Table 9.10.

The studies clearly show: (1) a substantial increased risk of cancer, (2) a much greater risk in dermatomyositis than polymyositis, and (3) a higher risk in the period close to diagnosis with dermatomyositis. These data suggest a common aetiology rather than the malignancy being a consequence of the disease. Indeed, as shown, the cancer incidence was also raised prior to diagnosis of dermatomyositis. A range of solid tumours are increased including ovarian [62,63], rectal [64], and nasopharynx [65]. The latter report was interesting given the high population incidence of nasopharyngeal carcinoma in that country (Singapore).

Environmental factors

Two groups of environmental factors have been linked to the development of polymyositis/dermatomyositis. These are infection and exposure to chemicals and other agents.

Infection

Three groups of organisms have been studied: Toxoplasma, bacteria including mycobacteria, and viruses.

Toxoplasma

Kagen *et al.* [66] first presented evidence of an association between toxoplasmosis and adult-onset polymyositis. They found titres of 1:1024 or above in the Sabin–Feldman dye test in six of 10 adult patients with polymyositis compared to two of seven adults with dermatomyositis and only one of 35 adult hospital controls. Positive complement fixation antibody tests were found, in five, one, and one patient in each of these three groups, respectively. Among the polymyositis patients, positive serologic findings correlated with disease duration of 1 year or less and no prior or concurrent steroid therapy. The authors interpreted their results as consistent with either recently acquired or activated Toxoplasma infection in patients with recent onset polymyositis. Subsequently, Phillips *et al.* [67] studied 20 patients with polymyositis, 25 with dermatomyositis, and 25 with myositis associated with

another connective tissue disease and 69 controls matched on age, sex, race, and hospital. Complement fixing antibodies to *T. gondii* were found in seven (35 per cent) of polymyositis patients compared to none of the 20 matched controls and only two of the total 69 controls. No differences were noted in the frequency of positive Sabin–Feldman dye tests; however, myositis patients had higher antibody titres against Epstein–Barr virus than controls. These authors interpreted their results as supporting the findings of Kagen *et al.* [66] and consistent with a role for Toxoplasma infection, either primary or reactivated, in the pathogenesis of polymyositis.

More recently, Magid and Kagen [68] found positive Sabin–Feldman dye tests in 19 (76 per cent) of 25 patients with polymyositis compared to 10 (30 per cent) of 33 patients with dermatomyositis ($P = 0.001$). IgM antiToxoplasma antibodies, indicative of recent infection, were detected in seven patients in each of the two myositis groups for a total of 24 per cent of those studied. The authors felt their data supported the hypothesis that *Toxoplasma gondii* may be aetiologically related to polymyositis. This is supported by a recent case report of co-existent toxoplasmic myocarditis and polymyositis which responded to antitoxoplasmic treatment [69].

Bacteria

There is a recent case report of polymyositis developing after *Mycoplasma pneumonia* infection [70]. Five cases of polymyositis/dermatomyositis developing tuberculosis, mycobacterium TB being isolated in most cases, are also of interest but this probably represents the increased occurrence of an opportunistic infection in an immunocompromised host [70,71].

Viruses

Indirect support for the role of viral infection comes from the observations of seasonal clustering during the winter months in some series [26,72] and spring months in another series [22] of onset of symptoms in cases of childhood-onset dermatomyositis and seasonal patterns in onset of adult patients with myositis-specific autoantibodies [73]. However, a case–control study of 42 cases of childhood-onset myositis failed to confirm seasonal clustering of onset [74].

A large number of different viruses have been implicated including Coxsackie, Hepatitis B, and C and retroviruses. Coxsackie virus B1 Tucson strain produced a polymyositis-like illness in infected CD1 Swiss mice [75]. Christensen *et al.* [72] performed a case-control study measuring complement-fixing and neutralizing antibodies to Coxsackie types B1-B6 in 12 children with juvenile dermatomyositis, 24 children with juvenile rheumatoid arthritis matched on age, sex, and date of rheumatology clinic visit, and 2192 hospitalized controls with suspected viral infections. Ten (83 per cent) of the children with juvenile dermatomyositis had significant levels of IgG complement-fixing antibody to at least one Coxsackie B antigen compared to four (17 per cent) of the arthritic controls and less than 25 per cent of the hospital controls. Neutralizing antibodies were also more common in dermatomyositis than arthritis clinic patients. No differences were found in results of tests for antibodies to 13 other viral antigens between these two groups. In a more recent study, elevated antibody titres to Coxsackie virus types A7, B3 and B4 were observed in adult patients with polymyositis, dermatomyositis, and mixed poly/dermatomyositis with malignancy subgroups respectively, suggesting that different viral subtypes are associated with different clinical phenotypes [76]. However, even in recent-onset disease with strong serological evidence of Coxsackie infection (IgM positive), it has proved difficult to reveal Coxsackie virus in muscle either using PCR or *in situ* hybridization techniques [77,78].

Cases have been rarely described following infection with Hepatitis B and C [79–81]. In a recent case series of 90 Hepatitis C virus infected patients from Israel, only one subject with polymyositis was revealed, confirming the weakness of the association [82].

The role of retroviruses has also been investigated with reports of patients with the co-occurrence of polymyositis and acquired immunodeficiency syndrome [1,83–86]. Other cases have been described following HTLV-1 infection [87]. In one uncontrolled series from Jamaica, 11 of 13 adult patients were IgG positive [88]. It is difficult, however, to demonstrate a direct myopathic role for HTLV-1 though it might act by triggering autoaggressive T cells [89].

There is a single case report of polymyositis developing after cytomegalovirus infection [90]. Finally, one case report of disease following bone marrow transplantation might be due to infection or through graft-versus-host disease is another explanation [91], as suggested by others [92].

The observations of Walker and Jeffrey [93] also have profound implications concerning the molecular basis of the viral aetiology of polymyositis. They demonstrated sequence homologies between histidyl-tRNA synthetase, the autoantigen against which the Jo1 antibody is directed, the light chain of myosin, and a hypothetical EC-RF4 protein of Epstein–Barr virus, as well as between alanyl-tRNA synthetase, tropomyosin, and four different viral proteins including two from influenza species and one each from Epstein–Barr virus and adenovirus. These sequence homologies support the hypothesis of molecular mimicry, that antibodies initially directed against foreign viral antigens may cross-react with muscle protein and produce myositis [94,95].

Exposure to chemicals and other agents

Cases have been described following drug use such as d-penicillamine and more recently tiopronine [96]. Other drugs linked to polymyositis in case reports include pentazocine, after prolonged use [97].

Recent interest has focused on both collagen and silicone implants. Bovine collagen implants, although raised as a potential risk factor, are not associated with any increased susceptibility. Indeed the number of cases observed after implants are 25–50 per cent of the number expected [98,99]. In one large series no case of polymyositis was observed in women with silicone breast implants [100]. In a very large retrospective study of over 10 000 women with an implant, a small but statistically insignificant increased risk was observed [101]. In a recent study comparing risk between 7442 silicone implanted women and 3353 women having breast reduction surgery, again there was no evidence of any significant risk [102].

References

1. Dalakas MC. Polymyositis, dermatomyositis and inclusion-body myositis. *N Engl J Med* 1991; **325**: 1487–1498.
2. Plotz PH, Dalakas M, Leff RL, Love LA, Miller FW, Cronin ME. Current concepts in the idiopathic inflammatory myopathies: polymyositis, dermatomyositis, and related disorders. *Ann Intern Med* 1989; **111**: 143–157.
3. Leteurtre E, Hachulla E, Janin A, Hatron PY, Brouillard M, Devulder B. Dermatomyositis and polymyositis are thought to have a distinct pathogenetic mechanism. *Rev Med Interne* 1994; **15**: 800–807.
4. Cronin ME, Plotz PH. Idiopathic inflammatory myopathies. *Rheum Dis Clin North Am* 1990; **16**: 655–665.
5. Bohan A, Peter JB. Polymyositis and dermatomyositis (second of two parts). *N Engl J Med* 1975; **292**: 403–407.

6. Bohan A, Peter JB. Polymyositis and dermatomyositis (first of two parts). *N Engl J Med* 1975; **292**: 344–347.

7. Benbassat J, Gefel D, Larholt K, Sukenik S, Morgenstern V, Zlotnick A. Prognostic factors in polymyositis/dermatomyositis. A computer-assisted analysis of ninety-two cases. *Arthritis Rheum* 1985; **28**: 249–255.

8. Bohan A, Peter JB, Bowman RL, Pearson CM. Computer-assisted analysis of 153 patients with polymyositis and dermatomyositis. *Medicine Baltimore* 1977; **56**: 255–286.

9. Henriksson KG, Sandstedt P. Polymyositis—treatment and prognosis. A study of 107 patients. *Acta Neurol Scand* 1982; **65**: 280–300.

10. Medsger TAJr. Polymyositis and dermatomyositis. In: Lawrence RC, Shulman LE, editors. *Epidemiology of the rheumatic diseases*. New York: Gower; 1984: 176–180.

11. Hochberg MC, Feldman D, Stevens MB. Adult onset polymyositis/dermatomyositis: an analysis of clinical and laboratory features and survival in 76 patients with a review of the literature. *Semin Arthritis Rheum* 1986; **15**: 168–178.

12. Oddis CV, Conte CG, Steen VD, Medsger TA. Incidence of polymyositis-dermatomyositis: a 20 year study of hospital diagnosed cases in Allegheny county, PA 1963–1982. *J Rheumatol* 1990; **17**: 1329–1334.

13. Ramirez G, Asherson RA, Khamashta MA, Cervera R, D'Cruz D, Hughes GR. Adult-onset polymyositis-dermatomyositis: description of 25 patients with emphasis on treatment. *Semin Arthritis Rheum* 1990; **20**: 114–120.

14. Tymms KE, Webb J. Dermatopolymyositis and other connective tissue diseases: a review of 105 cases. *J Rheumatol* 1985; **12**: 1140–1148.

15. Hoffman GS, Franck WA, Raddatz DA, Stallones L. Presentation, treatment, and prognosis of idiopathic inflammatory muscle disease in a rural hospital. *Am J Med* 1983; **75**: 433–438.

16. Pearson CM. Patterns of polymyositis and their responses to treatment. *Ann Intern Med* 1963; **59**: 827–838.

17. Tanimoto K, Nakano K, Kano S *et al.* Classification criteria for polymyositis and dermatomyositis. *J Rheumatol* 1995; **22**: 668–674.

18. Love LA, Leff RL, Fraser DD *et al.* A new approach to the classification of idiopathic inflammatory myopathy: myositis-specific autoantibodies define useful homogeneous patient groups. *Medicine Baltimore* 1991; **70**: 360–374.

19. Hanissian AS, Masi AT, Pitner SE, Cape CC, Medsger TA Jr. Polymyositis and dermatomyositis in children: an epidemiologic and clinical comparative analysis. *J Rheumatol* 1982; **9**: 390–394.

20. Denardo BA, Tucker LB, Miller LC, Szer IS, Schaller JG. Demography of a regional pediatric rheumatology patient population. Affiliated Children's Arthritis Centers of New England. *J Rheumatol* 1994; **21**: 1553–1561.

21. Pelkonen PM, Jalanko HJ, Lantto RK *et al.* Incidence of systemic connective tissue diseases in children: a nation-wide prospective study in Finland. *J Rheumatol* 1994; **21**: 2143–2146.

22. Symmons DP, Sills JA, Davis SM. The incidence of juvenile dermatomyositis: results from a nation-wide study. *Br J Rheumatol* 1995; **34**: 732–736.

23. Malleson PN, Fung MY, Rosenberg AM. The incidence of pediatric rheumatic diseases: results from the Canadian Pediatric Rheumatology Association Disease Registry. *J Rheumatol* 1996; **23**: 1981–1987.

24. Fujikawa S, Okuni M. A nationwide surveillance study of rheumatic diseases among Japanese children. *Acta Paediatr Jpn* 1997; **39**: 242–244.

25. Kurland LT, Hauser WA, Ferguson RH, Holley KE. Epidemiologic features of diffuse connective tissue disorders in Rochester, Minn., 1951 through 1967, with special reference to systemic lupus erythematosus. *Mayo Clin Proc* 1969; **44**: 649–663.

26. Medsger TAJr, Dawson WMJr, Masi AT. The epidemiology of polymyositis. *Am J Med* 1970; **48**: 715–723.

27. Benbassat J, Geffel D, Zlotnick A. Epidemiology of polymyositis-dermatomyositis in Israel, 1960–76. *Isr J Med Sci* 1980; **16**: 197–200.

28. Kusumi M, Nakashima K, Nakayama H, Takahashi K. Epidemiology of inflammatory neurological and inflammatory neuromuscular diseases in Tottori Prefecture, Japan. *Psychiatry Clin Neurosci* 1995; **49**: 169–174.

29. Kaipiainen Seppanen O, Aho K. Incidence of rare systemic rheumatic and connective tissue diseases in Finland. *J Intern Med* 1996; **240**: 81–84.

30. Weitoft T. Occurrence of polymyositis in the county of Gavleborg, Sweden. *Scand J Rheumatol* 1997; **26**: 104–106.

31. Hengstman GJD, van Venrooij WJ, Vencovsky J, Moutsopoulos HM, van Engelen BGM. The relative prevalence of dermatomyositis and polymyositis in Europe exhibits a latitudinal gradient. *Ann Rheum Dis* 2000; **59**: 141–142.

32. Hochberg MC, Lopez Acuna D, Gittelsohn AM. Mortality from polymyositis and dermatomyositis in the United States, 1968–1978. *Arthritis Rheum* 1983; **26**: 1465–1471.

33. Araki S, Uchino M, Yoshida O. Epidemiologic study of multiple sclerosis, myasthenia gravis and polymyositis in the city of Kumamoto, Japan. *Rinsho Shinkeigaku* 1983; **23**: 838–841.

34. Hochberg MC. The application of genetic epidemiology to systemic lupus erythematosus. *J Rheumatol* 1987; **14**: 867–869.

35. Grennan DM, Sanders PA. Rheumatoid arthritis. *Baillieres Clin Rheumatol* 1988; **2**: 585–601.

36. Lambie IA, Duff IF. Familial occurence of dermatomyositis: case reports and a family survey. *Ann Intern Med* 1963; **59**: 839–847.

37. Lewkonia RM, Buxton PH. Myositis in father and daughter. *J Neurol Neurosurg Psychiatry* 1973; **36**: 820–825.

38. Hirsch TJ, Enlow RW, Bias WB, Arnett FC. HLA-D related (DR) antigens in various kinds of myositis. *Hum Immunol* 1981; **3**: 181–186.

39. Friedman JM, Pachman LM, Maryjowski ML *et al.* Immunogenetic studies of juvenile dermatomyositis.

HLA antigens in patients and their families. *Tissue Antigens* 1983; **21**: 45–49.

40. Friedman JM, Pachman LM, Maryjowski ML *et al.* Immunogenetic studies of juvenile dermatomyositis: HLA-DR antigen frequencies. *Arthritis Rheum* 1983; **26**: 214–216.

41. Reed AM, Pachman L, Ober C. Molecular genetics studies of major histocompatability complex genes in children with juvenile dermatomyositis—increased risk associated with HLA-DQA1–0501. *Hum Immunol* 1991; **32**: 235–240.

42. Reed AM, Stirling JD. Association of the HLA-DQA1*0501 allele in multiple racial groups with juvenile dermatomyositis. *Hum Immunol* 1995; **44**: 131–135.

43. Furuya T, Hakoda M, Higami K *et al.* Association of HLA class I and class II alleles with myositis in Japanese patients. *J Rheumatol* 1998; **25**: 1109–1114.

44. Arnett FC, Hirsch TJ, Bias WB, Nishikai M, Reichlin M. The Jo-1 antibody system in myositis: relationships to clinical features and HLA. *J Rheumatol* 1981; **8**: 925–930.

45. Goldstein R, Duvic M, Targoff IN *et al.* HLA-D region genes associated with autoantibody responses to histidyl-transfer RNA synthetase (Jo-1) and other translation-related factors in myositis. *Arthritis Rheum* 1990; **33**: 1240–1248.

46. Callen JP. Dermatomyositis and malignancy. *Clin Dermatol* 1993; **11**: 61–65.

47. Callen JP. Relationship of cancer to inflammatory muscle diseases—dermatomyositis, polymyositis and inclusion body myositis. *Rheum Dis Clin North Am* 1994; **20**: 943–953.

48. Scaling ST, Kaufman RH, Patten BM. Dermatomyositis and female malignancy. *Obstet Gynecol* 1979; **54**: 474–477.

49. Callen JP, Hyla JF, Bole GGJr, Kay DR. The relationship of dermatomyositis and polymyositis to internal malignancy. *Arch Dermatol* 1980; **116**: 295–298.

50. Ogle S. Retrospective study of polymyositis in Auckland over 10 years. *N Z Med J* 1980; **92**: 433–435.

51. Herson S, Degoulet P, Piette JC, Herreman G, Godeau P. Factors affecting prognosis in adult polymyositis/dermatomyositis (PM/DM): a 287 patient years survey. *Arthritis Rheum* 1982; **25**: S49.

52. Black KA, Zilko PJ, Dawkins RL, Armstrong BK, Mastaglia GL. Cancer in connective tissue disease. *Arthritis Rheum* 1982; **25**: 1130–1133.

53. Holden DJ, Brownell AK, Fritzler MJ. Clinical and serologic features of patients with polymyositis or dermatomyositis. *Can Med Assoc J* 1985; **132**: 649–653.

54. Manchul LA, Jin A, Pritchard KI *et al.* The frequency of malignant neoplasms in patients with polymyositis-dermatomyositis. A controlled study. *Arch Intern Med* 1985; **145**: 1835–1839.

55. Lakhanpal S, Bunch TW, Ilstrup DM, Melton LJ. Polymyositis-dermatomyositis and malignant lesions: does an association exist? *Mayo Clin Proc* 1986; **61**: 645–653.

56. Masi AT, Hochberg MC. Temporal association of polymyositis-dermatomyositis with malignancy: methodo-

logic and clinical considerations. *Mt Sinai J Med* 1988; **55**: 471–478.

57. Sigurgeirsson B, Lindelof B, Edhag O, Allander E. Risk of cancer in patients with dermatomyositis or polymyositis. A population-based study. *N Engl J Med* 1992; **326**: 363–367.

58. Lyon MG, Bloch DA, Hollak B, Fries JF. Predisposing factors in polymyositis-dermatomyositis—results of a nationwide survey. *J Rheumatol* 1989; **16**: 1218–1224.

59. Zantos D, Zhang Y, Felson D. The overall and temporal association of cancer with polymyositis and dermatomyositis. *J Rheumatol* 1994; **21**: 1855–1859.

60. Airio A, Pukkala E, Isomaki H. Elevated cancer incidence in patients with dermatomyositis: a population based study. *J Rheumatol* 1995; **22**: 1300–1303.

61. Chow WH, Gridley G, Mellemkjaer L, McLaughlin JK, Olsen JH, Fraumeni JFJr. Cancer risk following polymyositis and dermatomyositis: a nationwide cohort study in Denmark. *Cancer Causes Control* 1995; **6**: 9–13.

62. Cherin P, Piette JC, Herson S *et al.* Dermatomyositis and ovarian cancer: a report of 7 cases and literature review. *J Rheumatol* 1993; **20**: 1897–1899.

63. Davis MDP, Ahmed I. Ovarian malignancy in patients with dermatomyositis and polymyositis: A retrospective analysis of fourteen cases. *J Am Acad Dermatol* 1997; **37**: 730–733.

64. Pautas E, Cherin P, Piette JC *et al.* Features of polymyositis and dermatomyositis in the elderly: a case-control study. *Clin Exp Rheumatol* 2000; **18**: 241–244.

65. Leow YH, Goh CL. Malignancy in adult dermatomyositis. *Int J Dermatol* 1997; **36**: 904–907.

66. Kagen LJ, Kimball AC, Christian CL. Serologic evidence of toxoplasmosis among patients with polymyositis. *Am J Med* 1974; **56**: 186–191.

67. Phillips PE, Kassan SS, Kagen LJ. Increased toxoplasma antibodies in idiopathic inflammatory muscle disease. A case-controlled study. *Arthritis Rheum* 1979; **22**: 209–214.

68. Magid SK, Kagen LJ. Serologic evidence for acute toxoplasmosis in polymyositis-dermatomyositis. Increased frequency of specific anti-toxoplasma IgM antibodies. *Am J Med* 1983; **75**: 313–320.

69. Montoya JG, Jordan R, Lingamneni S, Berry GJ, Remington JS. Toxoplasmic myocarditis and polymyositis in patients with acute acquired toxoplasmosis diagnosed during life. *Clin Infect Dis* 1997; **24**: 676–683.

70. Aihara Y, Mori M, Kobayashi T, Yokota S. A pediatric case of polymyositis associated with Mycoplasma pneumoniae infection. *Scand J Rheumatol* 1997; **26**: 480–481.

71. Hernandez Cruz B, Sifuentes Osornio J, Ponce de Leon Rosales S, Ponce de Leon Garduno A, Diaz Jouanen E. Mycobacterium tuberculosis infection in patients with systemic rheumatic diseases. A case-series. *Clin Exp Rheumatol* 1999; **17**: 289–296.

72. Christensen ML, Pachman LM, Schneiderman R, Patel DC, Friedman JM. Prevalence of Coxsackie B virus antibodies in patients with juvenile dermatomyositis. *Arthritis Rheum* 1986; **29**: 1365–1370.

73. Leff RL, Burgess SH, Miller FW *et al*. Distinct seasonal patterns in the onset of adult idiopathic inflammatory myopathy in patients with anti-Jo-1 and anti-signal recognition particle autoantibodies. *Arthritis Rheum* 1991; **34**: 1391–1396.

74. Koch MJ, Brody JA, Gillespie MM. Childhood polymyositis: a case-control study. *Am J Epidemiol* 1976; **104**: 627–631.

75. Strongwater SL, Dorovini Zis K, Ball RD, Schnitzer TJ. A murine model of polymyositis induced by coxsackievirus B1 (Tucson strain). *Arthritis Rheum* 1984; **27**: 433–442.

76. Nishikai M. Coxsackievirus infection and the development of polymyositis/dermatomyositis. *Rheumatol Int* 1994; **14**: 43–46.

77. Fox SA, Finklestone E, Robbins PD, Mastaglia FL, Swanson NR. Search for persistent enterovirus infection of muscle in inflammatory myopathies. *J Neurol Sci* 1994; **125**: 70–76.

78. Kummerle Deschner J, Kandolf R, Enders G, Labay F, Niethammer D, Dannecker G. Coxsackie-B-virus-infection. A possible cause of dermatomyositis? *Monatsschr Kinderh* 1997; **145**: 23–25.

79. Nishikai M, Miyairi M, Kosaka S. Dermatomyositis following infection with hepatitis C virus. *J Rheumatol* 1994; **21**: 1584–1585.

80. Nojima T, Hirakata M, Sato S *et al*. A case of polymyositis associated with hepatitis B infection. *Clin Exp Rheumatol* 2000; **18**: 86–88.

81. Weidensaul D, Imam T, Holyst MM, King PD, McMurray RW. Polymyositis, pulmonary fibrosis and hepatitis-C. *Arthritis Rheum* 1995; **38**: 437–439.

82. Buskila D, Shnaider A, Neumann L *et al*. Musculoskeletal manifestations and autoantibody profile in 90 hepatitis C virus infected Israeli patients. *Semin Arthritis Rheum* 1998; **28**: 107–113.

83. Dalakas MC, Pezeshkpour GH, Gravell M, Sever JL. Polymyositis associated with AIDS retrovirus. *JAMA* 1986; **256**: 2381–2383.

84. Wiley CA, Nerenberg M, Cros D, Soto Aguilar MC. HTLV-1 polymyositis in a patient also affected with the human immunodeficiency virus. *N Engl J Med* 1989; **320**: 992–995.

85. Dalakas MC, Pezeshkpour GH, Flaherty M. Progressive nemaline (rod) myopathy associated with HIV infection. *N Engl J Med* 1987; **317**: 1602–1603.

86. Simpson DM, Bender AN. Human immunodeficiency virus-associated myopathy: analysis of 11 patients. *Ann Neurol* 1988; **24**: 79–84.

87. Cartier L, Prina L. Polymyositis associated to HTLV-1 infection. *Rev Med Chil* 1996; **124**: 461–464.

88. Morgan OS, Mora C, Rodgers Johnson P, Char G. HTLV-1 and polymyositis in Jamaica. *Lancet* 1989; **2**: 1184–1186.

89. Leonmonzon M, Illa I, Dalakas MC. Polymyositis in patients infected with human T-cell leukemia virus type 1—the role of the virus in the cause of the disease. *Ann Neurol* 1994; **36**: 643–649.

90. Maeda M, Maeda A, Wakiguchi H *et al*. Polymyositis associated with primary cytomegalovirus infection. *Scand J Infect Dis* 2000; **32**: 212–214.

91. Ascensao JL, Mascarenhas RB, Mittelman A, Ahmed T. Case-report—acute polymyositis in a patient with chronic graft vs host disease. *Med Oncol Tumor Pharmacother* 1992; **9**: 149–150.

92. Tse S, Saunders EF, Silverman E, Vajsar J, Becker L, Meaney B. Myasthenia gravis and polymyositis as manifestations of chronic graft-versus-host-disease. *Bone Marrow Transplant* 1999; **23**: 397–399.

93. Walker EJ, Jeffrey PD. Polymyositis and molecular mimicry, a mechanism of autoimmunity. *Lancet* 1986; **2**: 605–607.

94. Mathews MB, Bernstein RM. Myositis autoantibody inhibits histidyl-tRNA synthetase: a model for autoimmunity. *Nature* 1983; **304**: 177–179.

95. Plotz PH. Autoantibodies are anti-idiotype antibodies to antiviral antibodies. *Lancet* 1983; **2**: 824–826.

96. Cacoub P, Sbai A, Azizi P, Gatfosse M, Godeau P, Piette JC. Tiopronine-induced polymyositis. *Presse Med* 1999; **28**: 911–912.

97. Kim HA, Song YW. Polymyositis developing after prolonged injections of pentazocine. *J Rheumatol* 1996; **23**: 1644–1646.

98. Hanke CW, Thomas JA, Lee WT, Jolivette DM, Rosenberg MJ. Risk assessment of polymyositis/dermatomyositis after treatment with injectable bovine collagen implants. *J Am Acad Dermatol* 1996; **34**: 450–454.

99. Rosenberg MJ, Reichlin M. Is there an association between injectable collagen and polymyositis/dermatomyositis? *Arthritis Rheum* 1994; **37**: 747–753.

100. Goldman JA, Greenblatt J, Joines R, White L, Aylward B, Lamm SH. Breast implants, rheumatoid arthritis, and connective tissue disease in a clinical practice. *J Clin Epidemiol* 1995; **48**: 571–582.

101. Hennekens CH, Lee IM, Cook NR *et al*. Self-reported breast implants and connective-tissue diseases in female health professionals. A retrospective cohort study. *JAMA* 1996; **275**: 616–621.

102. Nyren O, Yin L, Josefsson S *et al*. Risk of connective tissue disease and related disorders among women with breast implants: a nation-wide retrospective cohort study in Sweden. *BMJ* 1998; **316**: 417–422.

10 | Systemic vasculitis

Alan J. Silman

Introduction

The systemic vasculitic disorders are a heterogeneous group of conditions characterized by inflammation of blood vessel walls leading to necrosis and subsequent tissue damage. Vasculitis can occur as a secondary phenomenon to infections such as HIV or syphilis or in the context of other connective tissue disorders such as rheumatoid arthritis, SLE, or Sjögren's syndrome [1]. In this chapter, however, only those disorders where the vasculitis is considered to be the primary event will be reviewed, though this distinction is somewhat arbitrary reflecting ignorance concerning the aetiology of these disorders. Giant cell arteritis (syns, temporal arteritis, cranial arteritis) is discussed in Chapter 11 but should be considered as one of the primary group of vasculitic disorders affecting large arteries (see below). The other group of disorders not considered in this chapter are those vasculitides predominantly restricted to the skin and without significant risk of serious systemic involvement. These cutaneous vascular disorders include Henoch–Schönlein purpura and hypersensitivity vasculitis, classification criteria for both of which have been proposed by the American College of Rheumatology [2,3]. Others have suggested that the latter be referred to as cutaneous leukocytoclastic angiitis [4]. The classification and epidemiology of these disorders have been recently reviewed elsewhere [5].

Classification and criteria

As stated, the systemic vasculitis group of disorders are heterogeneous and attempts have been made to classify them into mutually exclusive subgroups and provide criteria of high discriminate ability that can be used to allocate patients to these individual subtypes. However, in clinical series, possibly up to one-third of cases can not be so classified and are considered as undifferentiated systemic vasculitis [6].

The historical approaches used in the classification of these disorders will not be considered in detail and modern classification schemes have developed as a consequence of evolving clinical experience and discovery of specific autoantibodies, predominantly

Table 10.1 Classification schemes for primary systemic vasculitis

	Chapel Hill		Scott and Watts
Vessels involved	Disorders	Vessels involved	Disorders
Large arteries	Giant cell arteritis	Large arteries	Giant cell arteritis
	Takayasu arteritis		Takayasu arteritis
Medium arteries	PAN	Medium arteries	PAN
	Kawasaki Disease		Kawasaki disease
Small vessels	WG	Small vessels and	WG
	Churg–Strauss Syndrome	medium arteries (ANCA	Churg Strauss syndrome
	MPA	associated)	MPA
	Henoch–Schönlein purpura		
	Cutaneous Leukocytoclastic angiitis	Small vessels	Leukocytoclastic

those designated as antineutrophil cytoplasmic anti-bodies (ANCAs). There are two broad staining patterns detected: cytoplasmic directed against proteinase 3 and perinuclear directed against myeloperoxidase, possibly with differing specialities for the different disorders. ANCA presence is considered as a key feature dis-criminating large and medium sized vessel from small vessel disease [1,7].

Two very similar classification schemes have been proposed: those from an international consensus con-ference—the Chapel Hill [4]—and those from Scott and Watts [8] (Table 10.1). The major difference is that the latter consider the ANCA related small vessel diseases as a separate group. The key aspect of both these schemes is the classification by the predominant sized vessel involved. Watts and Scott [1] emphasize the practical or therapeutic advantages of their scheme is that large vessel vasculitic disorders are controlled by high-dose corticosteroids and leukocytoclastic disorders by low-dose corticosteroids, whereas those disorders involving medium and small sized vessels require more extensive immunosuppression.

Criteria for individual disorders

Classification criteria have been proposed for the indi-vidual vasculitic disorders using two approaches. In the first, analytical, approach over 1000 cases with various forms of vasculitis were identified (Table 10.2). Criteria were developed from data acquired from a standard-ized set of clinical and laboratory variables: the American College of Rheumatology (ACR) criteria [9]. The criteria sets derived in both a conventional x/y and a decision tree approach were tested for their specificity and sensitivity against the other identified disorders (Table 10.3 to 10.6) [10–13]. As discussed by Watts and Scott, the disadvantage of this approach is that the results can not be extrapolated to the classification of unselected cases including those with undifferentiated

Table 10.2 Patients used in derivation of ACR criteria; modified from [9]

Disease	Number	%
Giant cell arteritis	214	20.9
Secondary vasculitis	141	13.8
Non-specific vasculitis	129	12.6
PAN	118	11.6
Hypersensitivity vasculitis	93	9.1
WG	85	8.3
Henoch–Schönlein purpura	85	8.3
Takayasu's disease	63	6.2
Kawasaki disease	52	5.1
Churg–Strauss syndrome	20	2.0
Other	20	2.0

forms that would be ascertained in a population survey [1]. As an example of the problem, polyarteritis nodosa (PAN) in theory would be classified as being present in a subject with weight loss together with mild elevation of blood pressure and urea (Table 10.4). In the 'open population' such an individual is very unlikely to have that disorder.

The second approach—the Chapel Hill Consensus Criteria (CHCC)—was based on the consensus of experts which ensured the face and content validity [4] but, as shown (Table 10.7), are not easy to use in prac-tice. The definitions are not mutually exclusive and may not include all patients. Nonetheless, these criteria have achieved widespread acceptance. One key disad-vantage of the ACR criteria is the lack of separation of PAN from microscopic polyangiitis (MPA) [14]. Not surprisingly, therefore, these criteria sets detect differ-ing individuals. PAN is virtually non-existent using the strict CHCC criteria [14]. In one report of 15 patients satisfying ACR criteria for Wegener's granulomatosis (WG), only five satisfied the CHCC definition [15].

Criteria for Takayasu's arteritis have also been defined separately, predominantly from the Japanese

Table 10.3 American College of Rheumatology criteria for Takayasu arteritis; modified from [10]

Individual criteria	Classification rule	Sensitivity %	Specificity %
1. Age <40 2. Claudication of extremities 3. Decreased brachial artery pulse 4. Distolic blood pressure difference between arms >10 mmHg 5. Subclavian or aortic bruit 6. Abnormal arteriogram	3/6	90.5	97.8

Table 10.4 American College of Rheumatology criteria for PAN; modified from [12]

Individual criteria	Classification rule	Sensitivity %	Specificity %
1. Weight loss >4 kg 2. Livido reticularis 3. Testicular pain/tenderness 4. Myalgia/muscle weakness 5. Mono/polyneuropathy 6. Diastolic blood pressure >90 mmHg 7. Elevated blood urea >40 mg/dl or creatinine >1.5 mg/dl 8. Evidence of hepatitis B infection 9. Abnormal arteriogram 10. Positive arterial biopsy	3/10	82.2	86.6

Table 10.5 American College of Rheumatology criteria for WG; modified from [11]

Individual criteria	Classification rule	Sensitivity %	Specificity %
1. Nasal/oral inflammation 2. Chest X-ray nodules/infiltrates 3. Microhaematuria or red cell casts 4. Granuloma on biopsy	3/4	88.2	92.0

Table 10.6 American College of Rheumatology criteria for Churg–Strauss syndrome; modified from [13]

Individual criteria	Classification rule	Sensitivity %	Specificity %
1. Asthma 2. Eosinophilia 3. Mono/polyneuropathy 4. Transitory lung infiltrates 5. Paranasal sinus problems 6. Eosinophils on tissue or arterial biopsy	4/6	85.0	99.7

Table 10.7 Chapel Hill consensus definitions for various forms of systemic vasculitis; modified from [4]

Disorder	Definition
Takayasu's Disease	Granulomatous infiltration of aorta and branches usually in patients under 50
Classic PAN	Necrotizing inflammation of medium sized or small arteries without glomerulonephritis or vasculities in small sized vessels
WG	Granulomatous inflammation involving respiratory tract and necrotizing vasculitis affecting small to medium sized vessels with frequent occurrence of glomerulonephritis
Churg–Strauss syndrome	Eosinophil rich and granulomatous inflammation involving the respiratory tract, necrotizing vasculitis affecting small to medium sized vessels and associated with asthma and eosinophilia
MPA	Necrotizing vasculitis with few or no immune deposits affecting small vessels though may involve medium sized arteries. Necrotizing glomerulonephritis is common as is pulmonary capillaritis

experience with this disorder. The first criteria set proposed by Ishikawa [16] included obligatory age of onset of below 40 years and consisted of major criterion of subclavian stenosis and nine minor criteria. Sharma *et al.* [17] proposed a variation of those criteria with three major and ten minor criteria, predominantly to allow for perhaps 30 per cent of patients in South-East Asia having disease confined to the aorta and renal arteries [18,19]. In one study of 106 patients with Takayasu's arteritis from India, the sensitivity of the Ishikawa criteria was only 60 per cent and the ACR criteria was 77 per cent. By contrast, the Sharma criteria had a sensitivity of 93 per cent [17]. However, these latter criteria may lack specificity.

In summary, it is reasonable to consider the epidemiology of these disorders individually. Giant cell arteritis is reviewed, together with polymyalgia rheumatica in Chapter 11. In the remaining part of this chapter epidemiology data are reviewed on the following disorders: large vessel—Takayasu's arteritis; medium vessel—PAN; small (and medium) vessel—MPA, WG, and Churg–Strauss syndrome. However, given the confusion in the literature regarding the separate identity of MPA and PAN, these two diagnostic groups are considered together.

Large vessel disease: Takayasu's arteritis

Incidence

There have been very few systematic studies of the incidence of Takayasu's arteritis. Most estimates have been derived from ascertaining a relatively small number of cases and extrapolating back to a presumed catchment population. Pooled data from a number of studies are summarized in Table 10.8.

In two European reports, no new cases were ascertained in relatively large tertiary referral centres in the United Kingdom and north-west Spain—suggesting the rarity of this disorder in Europe [24,25]. A study from Sweden identified 15 cases occurring between 1969 and 1976, approximately equivalent to one per million population [20]. Data from Japan, based on a large number of cases (150) suggested a similar incidence [22] but such an approach is methodologically fraught and suggests considerable underascertainment. Underascertainment is also possible in Western populations due to the lack of sensitivity of classification criteria, particularly the obligatory onset under the age of 40 [26]. It is also questionable as to whether published incidence rates derived from only 32 cases, as in the US [21], have any value.

Age and gender

The relative occurrence by age and gender is based on clinical series and no robust estimates exist on the actual age and gender rates. In addition, the age criterion (discussed above) arbitrarily sets the ceiling at age 40. Possibly up to one in six have an older age onset [27]. It is widely reported that the onset is mainly in the second and third decades [28] with a median age of onset of 25 in one series. Onset in childhood is well described [29].

Although the disease is described as having a strong female preponderance [28], this varies between countries and a female excess of approximately 2:1 is typical in countries such as India [30] and Kuwait [23].

Time trends

There are no robust data on time trends. An anecdotal report from Japan suggests a possible decrease in incidence [31], which is of interest given the recent rarity of cases in Europe.

Table 10.8   Incidence studies of Takayasu arteritis

Reference	Country	Population studied	Period	No. cases	Incidence/10⁶/year
[20]	Sweden		1969–1975		0.8
[21]	US	Olmsted County	1971–1983	3	2.6
[22]	Japan	Country estimate		150	1.2
[23]	Kuwait	All	1989–1994	13	2.2
		Age <40			3.3
[24]	UK	Norwich	1988–1990	0	–
[25]	Spain	North-west Spain	1988–1997	0	–

Prevalence

No systemic prevalence survey has been undertaken and is unlikely to be considered given the rarity of the disease. A post-mortem series of 300 000 from Japan revealed 90 cases, equivalent to a prevalence of 300/million [32]. Selection factors and diagnostic error may be important. Such data do, however, suggest either an important underascertainment and/or the existence of mild subclinical forms of the disease.

Race and geography

As already intimated, there are major geographical differences in the reported incidence of this disorder [28]. The disease is thus well described in South-East and South Asian populations such as Japan, China, Korea, Thailand, India, and Singapore [19]. Interestingly, it also appears to be (relatively) common in central and South America [19]. A recent report, for example, describes a reasonable sized case series from Columbia [33]. Although these data might suggest a Hispanic influence, as described above, the disease is very rare in Spain (Table 10.8).

Within a country there may be important differences. In Israel, for example, the disease appears confined to Sephardi, and is not seen in Ashkenazi, Jews [34], thereby suggesting a genetic influence. The disease is apparently different between countries, for reasons which are not clear. Thus, in Indian subjects abdominal vessels are more frequently involved than in Japanese subjects [30].

Genetics—family aggregation

Reports of familial aggregation are restricted to anecdotal reports of multicase families. The rarity of the disease would suggest that any clustering within families is unlikely to be random. There are reports of 21 familial cases from Japan including three pairs of disease concordant monozygotic twins [35].

Immunogenetics

Overall, only weak associations have been reported with HLA class II genes [27]. There have been a number of associations with HLA class I genes, particularly HLA-B5 in Indian populations and HLA-B52 in Japanese Korean groups [19,36]. There is a linkage disequilibrium between class I and class II alleles. Thus,

the haplotype A24-B52-DR2 is the most frequent and the primacy of the B locus can clearly not be established from the above data [37]. Similarly, other associations with HLA-DRB1* 1502 and 0901 revealed from DNA typing methods can be explained by linkage disequilibrium with HLA-B52 [37]. An independent association with HLA-B39.2 has also been established [37] and, interestingly, both B52 and B39.2 have a similar molecular structure at their antigen binding site [38]. These relationships are not the complete genetic story as only 60 per cent of cases carry either of these B alleles [37].

Host factors: co-morbidity

Few host factors for Takayasu's arteritis have been described. A number of case reports have suggested the co-occurrence of the disease with disorders such as ankylosing spondylitis [39], sarcoidosis [40], and inflammatory bowel disease [41].

Environmental factors

The geographical data described do suggest environmental influences and the most studied hypothesis is the role of mycobacterium TB, consistent with the granulomatosus nature of this disorder [42,43]. In one study, an IgG antibody was found in patients' sera which recognized a 38-kD glycoprotein which is a specific antigen in the human immune response to mycobacterium TB. It has also been postulated that BCG immunization, in a susceptible host, is the cause.

Case reports suggest other infectious antecedents. As an example, one case was described following immunization with Hepatitis B vaccine [44].

Medium and small vessel disease: PAN and MPA

Introduction

As discussed above, the data on the epidemiology of these disorders from older literature is confusing given the relatively recent identification of MPA as a separate entity based on the identification of ANCA [45]. As Watts *et al.* [46] pointed out, the epidemiology of these disorders can only be sensibly considered against the disease entities included in the study. A useful definition and distinction proposed by Lhote *et al.* [47] is that MPA is a systemic necrotizing vasculitis that clinically and histologically affects small-sized vessels, without granulomata, and is associated with necrotizing glomerulonephritis. It is not always distinguishable from PAN but, unlike the latter disorder, previous Hepatitis B infection is rare and most cases are ANCA positive.

Incidence

Data on the incidence of PAN/MPA from a number of studies are summarized in Table 10.9. One important source of cases is regional renal biopsy registers [54–58] where all cases of biopsy proven necrotizing vasculitis on glomerular biopsy were used as a source for case ascertainment. Studies using this source

Table 10.9   Incidence studies of PAN and MPA

Reference	Case ascertainment	Period	Place	Disease	Criteria	No. cases	Incidence/ million/year	95% CI
[48]			Olmsted County, US	PAN			9	
[49]		1972–80	Bath/Bristol, UK	PAN		80	4.6	
[50]		1980–86	Leicester, UK	MPA	Fauci [a]	5	0.5	
		1987–89				13	3	
[24]	Multiple sources	1988–94	Norfolk, UK	PAN	ACR	8	2.4	0.9–5.3
				PAN	CHCC	0	0	0–1.5
				MPA	CHCC	13	3.6	1.7–6.9
[25]		1988–97	Lugo, Spain	PAN	ACR		6.6	
				CHCC			1.1	
				CHCC			5.8	
[51]		1993–96	Kuwait	PAN	CHCC		16	
				MPA	CHCC		24	
	All renal vasculitis						45	27–64
[52]		1992–96	Kristainsand, Norway	PAN	ACR		6.6	
[53]		1957–71	Michigan, US	PAN			2	
[54]	Survey of necrotizing vasculitis from renal biopsy	1984–89	Heidelberg, Germany	MPA		7	1.5	
[55]	Survey of necrotizing vasculitis from renal biopsy		Sweden				2.5	
[56]	Survey of necrotizing vasculitis from renal biopsy	1986–92	Sweden				8	
[b]			Japan	MPA			10	
				PAN			1	
[57]	Survey of necrotizing vasculitis from renal biopsy		Italy				1.6	
[58]	Survey of necrotizing vasculitis from renal biopsy	1992–96		MPA			7.9	
				PAN			4.4	
[59]	Survey of paediatricians	1986–94	New England, US	PAN			2	

[a] See: [117].
[b] Quoted in [24].

suggest an annual incidence of between one and 10/million person years, depending on criteria used (Table 10.9). The scope for underascertainment is large. Thus it is interesting to note that studies of ascertainment based on clinically diagnosed cases generate similar estimates (Table 10.9).

As shown in Table 10.9, most studies are based on very small numbers of cases and it is therefore very difficult to derive robust estimates of the incidence by age and gender. PAN clearly occurs in children [59–61] though in general terms, combining all forms of ANCA-associated vasculitis, the incidence probably increases with increasing age [24,60]. In the latter report, the incidence of all forms of ANCA-associated vasculitis based on an inpatient register was 63/million in men aged 55 to 64. There are also few quantitative estimates of the effects of gender. These disorders are reported to be more frequent in males [47]. In some series with specific causes such as HTLV-1 infection (see below), females may be the predominant gender group affected [62]. In one large series of 29 patients, 60 per cent were males with a mean age (SD) of onset of 46 (17) years [63]. Extrapolating from such clinical series to population estimates is impossible in the absence of denominator data.

Prevalence

Prevalence is a far less useful concept than incidence in a disorder with a relapsing and remitting clinical course and few data are available. One survey in Norway [52] suggested a prevalence of 33/million, approximately five times the annual incidence.

Time trends

Small numbers of cases and changing case definition limit the usefulness of data on time trends. The introduction of tests such as ANCA can have a profound affect on the assessment of the incidence of MPA, for example. Thus, Andrews *et al.* [50] showed a six-fold rise in incidence after 1986. Watts and Scott [24], who have undertaken the most methodologically sound studies in this area, suggest that overall ANCA associated vasculitic disorders are increasing though there maybe a cyclical pattern [61]. The complete absence of PAN in recent series [24] might be due, in part, to changes in classification but is also likely to be due to a decline in hepatitis B infection rates [64]. There are some suggestions from more tightly undertaken, recent studies that there may be a modest increase [61].

Geographical trends

The data in Table 10.9 cover a broad range of European, Asian, and North American populations with few obvious differences in occurrence. The incidence in Kuwait is particularly high [51] but in that population many of the affected individuals were non-Kuwaiti nationals. The highest recorded incidence was in a study from Alaskan Indians. In a small population of 14 000 individuals, the incidence rate of PAN was estimated to be 77/million person years, substantially higher than any other group [65]. All cases had recent hepatitis B infection, which might be the explanation.

Genetics—family aggregation

Given the rarity of the disorder, it is not surprising that there are few definitive reports of familial aggregation. A father–son pair has been described occurring in the context of hepatitis B infection [66]. A second pair of siblings of Asian origin has also been described developing the disease 8 years apart [67].

Immunogenetics

There are also very few studies of immunogenetics and most have been negative. In the family mentioned above [66], the father and son both shared HLA haplotypes which was not the case with a second son, who was also infected with hepatitis B but who did not develop vasculitis. No association in case–control studies has been found with either HLA-DR or DQ [68]. In one study of 17 subjects with PAN, no patient had HLA-DR3 compared to 16 per cent in controls [63]; the authors suggesting that this allele may be protective, unlike its susceptibility influence on other autoimmune disorders.

Host factors—co-morbidity

There are a large number of case reports which, by definition, the authors argue, suggest an association between PAN and other co-morbidities (Table 10.10). These disorders can be divided into autoimmune conditions such as SLE/sarcoidosis [69,70] and malignant disorders of various organs and types (Table 10.10). In truth, however, these case reports add little to the aetiology hypothesis. The only exception might be the association with hairy-cell leukaemia where a large case series has been reported [76], which presumably must be beyond chance given the rarity of these disorders.

Table 10.10　Co-morbid conditions associated with PAN/MPA

Co-morbidity	Reference	Comments
SLE	[69]	Case report
Sarcoidosis	[70]	Case report
Familial mediterranean fever	[71]	Case report
Gastric cancer	[72]	Case report
Multiple myeloma	[73]	Case report
	[74]	Case report
Chronic myelomonocytic leukaemia	[75]	Case report
Hairy cell leukaemia	[76]	Case series of 17 cases

Environmental factors

Infection

There appears to be a well accepted association between hepatitis B virus (HBV) infection and PAN. Some recent studies are summarized in Table 10.11. Reference has already been made to the high occurrence of PAN in Alaska, thought to be associated with the high prevalence of HBV [65]. The disease may respond to antiviral therapy [77]. The majority of current cases are HBV –ve [25,63] but it has been claimed that PAN has declined because of declining HBV infection rates in many populations [65,87]. Other virus linked to PAN include hepatitis C, HIV, HTLV1, and herpes zoster, but these have been predominantly proposed based on isolated case reports (Table 10.11).

Table 10.11　Infectious agents in recent reports associated with PAN/MPA

Agent	Reference	Comments
Hepatitis B	[77]	Responds well to antiviral treatment
	[78]	Case series
	[63]	5/22 (23%) positive
	[25]	2/13 (15%) positive
Hepatitis C	[79]	11/56 (20%) positive
	[80]	Presented after IFN treatment
	[81]	Case report
HIV	[82]	Prostitute case report
	[84]	Case report
HTLV1	[62]	Case series of 6 patients
Parvovirus	[83]	2 cases in children
Streptococcus	[85]	Coincidence of disease episodes with *Streptococcus* infection
Herpes-zoster	[86]	Developed after zoster infection in case

Other agents

In one small study (16 cases matched to two controls) there was a 14-fold increased reporting of exposure to silica. The cases in this series all had rapidly progressive glomerulonephritis and there have been no subsequent studies on this hypothesis [88].

Small vessel disease: WG

The epidemiology of Wegener's granulomatosis (WG) needs to be considered in relation to the discovery of ANCA in 1985, despite its first description in the 1930s [89]. The wide availability of ANCA as a diagnostic tool has undoubtedly increased the number of cases diagnosed, as illustrated in the observations by Andrews *et al.* [50]. It is for this reason that epidemiological studies prior to 1986 could be unreliable.

Incidence

The data on the incidence of WG are derived predominantly from the same studies reporting on the incidence of the other vasculitis (see for example Table 10.9). Unlike PAN/MPA, necrotizing glomerulonephritis is not a predominant feature, thus case ascertainment has to rely on clinically diagnosed cases. The available data (Table 10.12) show a great and reassuring similarity in the recent (post-ANCA) rates from Europe and North America at around five per one million person years based on the ACR criteria.

The gender and age pattern has also been described. In the Norwich data set of only 21 cases, the incidence was 50 per cent higher in males [50,91]. By contrast, in the nation-wide study of 10 000 hospitalizations in the US, the number of episodes in each of the genders was similar.

There are, as with the other rare vasculitides, no robust data on the incidence rates by age but the available data suggest a very rare onset in children and a peak age at onset in the sixth or seventh decades [91,92].

Time trends

As discussed above, the advent of ANCA testing has influenced diagnosis and an increase in incidence after 1986 was only to be expected (Table 10.12). Similarly,

Table 10.12 Incidence of WG

Reference	Case ascertainment	Period	Place	Criteria	No. cases	Incidence/million/year
[49]		1972–80	Bath, Bristol, UK		4	0.5
[50]		1980–86	Leicester, UK	Fauci[a]	6	0.7
		1987–87	Leicester, UK		11	2.8
[55]		1971–93		ACR		2.1
[52]		1992–96	Kristainsand, Norway	ACR		6.6
[24]	Multiple clinics and histology records	1988–97	Norwich, UK	ACR		9.7
[25]		1988–97		ACR		4.8
[90]				ACR		4.0
[91]	Multiple clinics and histology records	1988–94		ACR		10.8 (5.8–18.2)[b]
				ACR		6.2 (2.7–12.3)[c]

[a] See: [117].
[b] Male adults.
[c] Female adults.

the number of deaths ascribed to WG between 1979 and 1988 in the US doubled [92]. It remains to be determined whether there is a true increase in incidence.

By contrast, there has been considerable interest in the possibility that there is a seasonal influence on the occurrence of WG with a number of reports suggesting a winter peak and a summer trough [91,93,94]. Data from Norfolk, UK, admittedly from a small number of total cases, revealed none arising in the autumn (Table 10.13). Other reports have not confirmed any seasonality. In one study, there was no greater seasonality in WG patients onset than in other rheumatic diseases and in that study of 101 cases, 29 had a summer onset [95]. There was also no influence of season on hospitalization for WG [92] but such data can not be used to make inferences about incidence. In northern Norway the annual incidence/million people has increased from 5.2 (95% CI 2.7–9.0) during 1984–88 to 12.0 (95% CI 8.0–17.3) during 1994–98 [118]. However, no seasonal variation in the onset of WG was found in this study.

Race and geography

There are little data on WG from non-European Caucasoid groups. The disease does occur in African blacks in South Africa [96]. The hospitalization occurrence is lower in US blacks compared to whites, relative to their population distribution [92]. Whether this reflects bias in diagnosis/hospitalization or a true difference in occurrence is unknown. A single case report from Bahrain [97] is likely to be followed by descriptions of the occurrence of the disorder in other non-European populations.

On a micro level, the distribution of cases within different countries in New York State was examined to determine 'pockets' of increased occurrence [92]. Five-year period prevalences varied between zero and 17/100 000. Clearly, some of this variation would be expected by chance and, in that report, no formal cluster analysis was undertaken to determine whether the distribution was non-random. WG was slightly higher in northern than in southern Germany with 58 and 42 cases/million inhabitants respectively [119].

Table 10.13 Onset of symptoms of WG by season; reproduced with permission of Oxford University Press from [91]

Period	Winter (Dec–Feb)	Spring (March–May)	Summer (June–August)	Autumn (Sep–Nov)
No. patients (n = 21)	9	5	7	0
%	42.9	23.8	33.3	0

Genetics

There are few data on genetic aspects of this disorder, reflecting its rarity and the difficulty in collecting a sufficiently large series of patients. Two cases occurring within one family have been reported, but they occurred within 2 months and are perhaps more suggestive of shared environment [97]. In support of this, a second multicase family reported consisted of father and stepson, again with a relatively close time of onset [98].

There have been a few immunogenetic studies. An older (pre-ANCA) serological study suggested an association with HLA-B8 [99] (part of the autoimmune A1-B8-DR3 haplotype). This common allele was also shared by the father/stepson pair discussed above [98]. WG has been associated with HLA-DR1 (and not DR3) in a case control study of Greek patients [63]. Hereditary C4 deficiency has also been linked to the development of WG in one family [100].

Host factors: co-morbidity

Associations with various malignancies have been described including, for example, Hodgkin's disease [101]. The most impressive study comes from a comparison of 477 WG patients with 479 rheumatoid arthritis (RA) controls [102]. Although there was no statistically significant overall increased association with malignancy in general, there was a nine-fold increased risk of renal cell carcinoma. Further simultaneous onset of both malignancy and disease was observed in 14 of the WG cases (including 5/7 with renal cancer) and only one of the RA cases (OR 18.0, 95% CI 2.3–140).

Other case reports of co-morbidities include Hashimoto's thyroiditis [103] and giant cell arteritis [104].

Environmental factors

There have been some cases linked to various infectious agents including one case following pneumonia with *Staphylococcus aureus* and *Candida* [105], parvovirus B19 [106], and following nematode infection with *Angiostrongylus* species [107]. The seasonal and familial clustering data would point to an infectious cause but apart from the case reports above, there are few data.

The other environmental agents investigated are inhaled toxins; silica dust was implicated, for example, in one case [108]. There has been one formal epidemiological study comparing the self-reported inhalation histories, at work and outside, between 101 WG cases, 54 normal controls, and 69 with other diseases [95]. Many exposures in the year preceding onset were investigated and were high in all populations. There were some significant differences, with WG patients having more exposure to fumes at work and at home and were more likely to have been exposed to pesticides and carpet cleaning chemicals.

Small vessel disease: Churg–Strauss syndrome

Churg–Strauss syndrome is the rarest of the vasculitic group of disorders discussed in this chapter and thus data on its occurrence are based on very imprecise estimates.

Incidence

The major data on incidence are summarized in Table 10.14 and the low incidence of this disorder is approximately one per million person years. As Watts and Scott have pointed out [1], the Chapel Hill criteria

Table 10.14 Incidence of Churg–Strauss syndrome

Reference	Period	Place	Criteria	No. cases	Incidence/ million/ year	95% CI
[48]	1976–79	Olmsted County, US		1	4.0	0.1–22.3
[1]	1988–95	Norwich, UK	CHCC	1	0.3	0.0–1.7
			ACR	6	1.8	0.7–.3.9
[24]	1988–97	Norwich, UK	ACR		2.8	
[25]	1988–97	Lugo, Spain	ACR		1.1	
[61]	1975–95	Orebro, Sweden	CHCC	2	0.4	

are less sensitive and incidence estimates based on their use are therefore much lower. Two cases were ascertained in a Norwegian county of population size 150 000 equivalent to a prevalence of 13/million [52].

Data from Norwich, UK [1] suggest an incidence in males and females of 4.3 and 2.3/million respectively. These incidence rates are based on clinical criteria and are thus not consistent with the incidence data calculated using either the ACR or CHCC definitions. There are no data on the influence of age.

Similarly there are no useful data on trends or geographical distribution. Cases have been described from Spain [25], UK [24], Sweden [61], Greece [63], and Japan [109] amongst other countries.

Risk factors

There are no good genetic data though the disease appears to be unrelated to HLA-DR3. A case has been described in association with non-Hodgkin's lymphoma [110]. Most interest has been centred on the role of allergens. The disease frequently presents as asthma with an associated eosinophilia and thus the rate of inhaled allergens may be important. In one study of eight patients, all had a history of allergy based on self-report [6] including five with skin allergy, five with rhinitis, and four with food allergy. The numbers were small but were significantly different from controls. Case reports have suggested other allergens may be important in some people, such as pigeon droppings [111]. A recent report raised the possibility that the drug zafirlukast may have been responsible for eight cases [112] but the cause–effect relationship is uncertain [113–115]. Immunization may act as an initiating event with cases reported after tetanus [111] and hepatitis B [116] immunization.

There are few data on other environmental factors though some drugs, including sulphonamides, penicillin, anticonvulsants, and thiazide diuretics, have been reported to be linked to the disease [24].

References

1. Watts RA, Scott DGI. Classification and epidemiology of the vasculitides. *Baillieres Clin Rheumatol* 1997; **11**: 191–217.
2. Calabrese LH, Michel AM, Bloch DA *et al*. The American College of Rheumatology 1990 criteria for the classification of hypersensitivity vasculitis. *Arthritis Rheum* 1990; **33**: 1108–1113.
3. Mills JA, Michel BA, Bloch DA *et al*. The American College of Rheumatology 1990 criteria for the classification of Henoch-Schonlein purpura. *Arthritis Rheum* 1990; **33**: 1114–1121.
4. Jennette JC, Falk RJ, Andrassy K *et al*. Nomenclature of systemic vasculitides. Proposal of an international consensus conference. *Arthritis Rheum* 1994; **37**: 189–192.
5. Watts RA, Jolliffe VA, Grattan CEH, Elliott J, Lockwood M, Scott DGI. Cutaneous vasculitis in a defined population—clinical and epidemiological associations. *J Rheumatol* 1998; **25**: 920–924.
6. Cuadrado MJ, D'Cruz D, Lloyd M, Mujic F, Khamashta MA, Hughes GRV. Allergic disorders in systemic vasculitis: a case-controlled study. *Br J Rheumatol* 1994; **33**: 749–753.
7. Guillevin L, Lhote F, Amouroux J, Gherardi R, Callard P, Casassus P. Antineutrophil cytoplasmic antibodies, abnormal angiograms and pathological findings in polyarteritis nodosa and Churg-Strauss syndrome: indications for the classification of vasculitides of the polyarteritis nodosa group. *Br J Rheumatol* 1996; **35**: 958–964.
8. Scott DGI, Watts RA. Classification and epidemiology of systemic vasculitis. *Br J Rheumatol* 1994; **33**: 897–900.
9. Bloch DA, Michel BA, Hunder GG *et al*. The American College of Rheumatology 1990 criteria for the classification of vasculitis. Patients and methods. *Arthritis Rheum* 1990; **33**: 1068–1073.
10. Arend WP, Michel BA, Bloch DA *et al*. The American College of Rheumatology 1990 criteria for the classification of Takayasu arteritis. *Arthritis Rheum* 1990; **33**: 1129–1134.
11. Leavitt RY, Fauci AS, Bloch DA *et al*. The American College of Rheumatology 1990 criteria for the classification of Wegener's granulomatosis. *Arthritis Rheum* 1990; **33**: 1101–1107.
12. Lightfoot RWJ, Michel BA, Bloch DA *et al*. The American College of Rheumatology 1990 criteria for the classification of polyarteritis nodosa. *Arthritis Rheum* 1990; **33**: 1088–1093.
13. Masi AT, Hunder GG, Lie JT *et al*. The American College of Rheumatology 1990 criteria for the classification of Churg-Strauss syndrome (allergic granulomatosis and angiitis). *Arthritis Rheum* 1990; **33**: 1094–1100.
14. Watts RA, Jolliffe VA, Carruthers DM, Lockwood M, Scott DGI. Effect of classification on the incidence of polyarteritis nodosum and microscopic polyangiitis. *Arthritis Rheum* 1996; **39**: 1208–1212.
15. Bruce IN, Bell AL. Effect of classification on the incidence of polyarteritis nodosum and microscopic polyangiitis. *Arthritis Rheum* 1997; **40**: 1183.
16. Ishikawa K. Diagnostic approach and proposed criteria for the clinical diagnosis of Takayasu's arteriopathy. *J Am Coll Cardiol* 1988; **12**: 964–972.
17. Sharma BK, Jain S, Suri S, Numano F. Diagnostic criteria for Takayasu arteritis. *Int J Cardiol* 1996; **54**: 141–147.
18. Hata A, Noda M, Moriwaki R, Numano F. Angiographic findings of Takayasu arteritis: new classification. *Int J Cardiol* 1996; **54**: 155–163.

19. Numano F. Differences in clinical presentation and outcome in different countries for Takayasu's arteritis. *Curr Opin Rheumatol* 1997; **9**: 12–15.

20. Waern AU, Andersson P, Hemmingsson A. Takayasu Arteritis: a hospital-region based study on occurrence, treatment and prognosis. *Angiology* 1983; **34**: 311–320.

21. Hall S, Barr W, Lie JT, Stanson AW, Kazmier FJ, Hunder GG. Takayasu Arteritis: a study of 32 North American patients. *Medicine* 1985; **64**: 89–99.

22. Koide K. Takayasu arteritis in Japan. *Heart Vessels* 1992; **7**: 48–54.

23. El Reshaid K, Varro J, Al Duwairi Q, Anim JT. Takayasu's arteritis in Kuwait. *J Trop Med Hyg* 1995; **98**: 299–305.

24. Watts RA, Scott DG. Epidemiology of vasculitis. In: Ball GV, Bridges SL, editors. *Vasculitis*. Oxford University Press, 2000.

25. González-Gay M, García-Porrúa C. Systemic vasculitis in adults in northwestern Spain, 1988–1997. Clinical and epidemiologic aspects. *Medicine* 1999; **78**: 292–308.

26. Sharma BK, Siveski Iliskovic N, Singal PK. Takayasu arteritis may be underdiagnosed in North America. *Can J Cardiol* 1995; **11**: 311–316.

27. Kerr G. Takayasu's arteritis. *Curr Opin Rheumatol* 1994; **6**: 32–38.

28. Cid MC, Font C, Coll-Vinent B, Grau JM. Large vessel vasculitides. *Curr Opin Rheumatol* 1998; **10**: 18–28.

29. Fujikawa S. Epidemiological studies of rheumatic diseases among Japanese children. *Ryumachi* 1998; **38**: 555–561.

30. Moriwaki R, Noda M, Yajima M, Sharma BK, Numano F. Clinical manifestations of Takayasu arteritis in India and Japan. New classification of angiographic findings. *Angiology* 1997; **48**: 369–379.

31. Tanabe T. Intractable vasculitis syndromes—incidence and epidemiology. *Nippon Rinsho* 1994; **52**: 1987–1991.

32. Emmerich J, Fiessinger JN. Epidemiologie et facteurs etiologiques des arterites a cellules geantes (maladie de Horton et maladie de Takayasu). *Ann Med Interne* 1998; **149**: 425–432.

33. Canas CA, Jimenez CA, Ramirez LA *et al*. Takayasu arteritis in Columbia. *Int J Cardiol* 1998; **66**: S73-S79.

34. Deutsch V, Wexler L, Deutsch H. Takayasu's arteritis. An angiographic study with remarks on ethnic distribution in Israel. *Am J Roentgenol Radium Ther Nucl Med* 1974; **122**: 13–28.

35. Numano F, Kobayashi Y, Maruyama Y, Kakuta T, Miyata T, Kishi Y. Takayasu arteritis: clinical characteristics and the role of genetic factors in its pathogenesis. *Vasc Med* 1996; **1**: 227–233.

36. Mehra NK, Rajalingam R, Sagar S, Jain S, Sharma BK. Direct role of HLA-B5 in influencing susceptibility to Takayasu aortoarteritis. *Int J Cardiol* 1996; **54**: 71–79.

37. Kimura A, Kitamura H, Date Y, Numano F. Comprehensive analysis of HLA genes in Takayasu arteritis in Japan. *Int J Cardiol* 1996; **54**: 61–69.

38. Yoahida M, Kimura A, Katsuragi K, Numano F, Sasazuki T. DNA typing of HLA-B gene in Takayasu's arteritis. *Tissue Antigens* 1993; **42**: 87–90.

39. Soubrier M, Dubost JJ, Demarquilly F, Therre T, Boyer L, Ristori JM. Maladie de Takayasu et spondylarthrite ankylosante: une association probablement non fortuite. *Presse Med* 1997; **26**: 610.

40. Kerr GS, Hallahan CW, Giordano J *et al*. Takayasu arteritis. *Ann Intern Med* 1994; **120**: 919–929.

41. Oyanagi H, Ishihata R, Ishikawa H *et al*. Ulcerative colitis associated with Takayasu's disease. *Intern Med* 1994; **33**: 127–129.

42. Kothari SS. Aetiopathogenisis of Takayasu's arteritis and BCG vaccination: the missing link? *Med Hypotheses* 1995; **45**: 227–230.

43. Hernandez Pando R, Espitia C, Mancilla R, Reyes PA. Arteritis de Takayasu. Prueba seroinmunologica de su relacion con infeccion por micobacterias. *Arch Inst Cardiol Mex* 1994; **64**: 331–337.

44. Castresana Isla CJ, Herrera Martinez G, Vega Molina J. Erythema nodosum and Takayasu's arteritis after immunization with plasma derived hepatitis B vaccine. *J Rheumatol* 1993; **20**: 1417–1418.

45. Murakami M, Ozaki S, Nakao K. Polyarteritis nodosa. *Nippon Rinsho* 1999; **57**: 349–354.

46. Watts RA, Carruthers DM, Scott DGI. Epidemiology of systemic vasculitis: changing incidence or definition? *Semin Arthritis Rheum* 1995; **25**: 28–34.

47. Lhote F, Cohen P, Genereau T, Gayraud M, Guillevin L. Microscopic polyangiitis: clinical aspects and treatment. *Ann Med Interne* 1996; **147**: 165–177.

48. Kurland LT, Chuang TY, Hunder GG. The epidemiology of systemic arteritis. In: Lawrence RC, editor. *The epidemiology of the rheumatic diseases*. New York: Gower Publishing, 1984: 196–205.

49. Scott DG, Bacon PA, Elliott PJ, Tribe CR, Wallington TB. Systemic vasculitis in a district general hospital 1972–1980: clinical and laboratory features, classification and prognosis of 80 cases. *QJM* 1982; **51**: 292–311.

50. Andrews M, Edmunds M, Campbell A, Walls J, Feehally J. Systemic vasculitis in 1980s—is there an increasing incidence of Wegener's granulomatosis and microscopic polyarteritis? *J R Coll Physicians Lond* 1990; **24**: 284–288.

51. El Reshaid K, Kapoor MM, El Reshaid W, Madda JP, Varro J. The spectrum of renal disease associated with microscopic polyangiitis and classic polyarteritis nodosa in Kuwait. *Nephrol Dial Transplant* 1997; **12**: 1874–1882.

52. Haugeberg G, Bie R, Bendvold A, Storm Larsen A, Johnsen V. Primary vasculitis in a Norwegian community hospital: a retrospective study. *Clin Rheumatol* 1998; **17**: 364–368.

53. Sack M, Cassidy JT, Bole GG. Prognostic factors in polyarteritis. *J Rheumatol* 1975; **2**: 411–420.

54. Andrassy K, Küster S, Waldherr R, Ritz E. Rapidly progressive glomerulonephritis: analysis of prevalence and clinical course. *Nephron* 1991; **59**: 206–212.

55. Westman KW, Bygren PG, Olsson H, Ranstam J, Wieslander J. Relapse rate, renal survival, and cancer morbidity in patients with Wegener's granulomatosis or microscopic polyangiitis with renal involvement. *J Am Soc Nephrol* 1998; **9**: 842–852.

56. Pettersson EE, Sundelin B, Heigl Z. Incidence and outcome of pauci-immune necrotizing and crescentic glomerulonephritis in adults. *Clin Nephrol* 1995; **43**: 141–149.

57. Schena FP. Survey of the Italian Registry of Renal Biopsies. Frequency of the renal diseases for 7 consecutive years. The Italian Group of Renal Immunopathology. *Nephrol Dial Transplant* 1997; **12**: 418–426.

58. Lane SE, Scott DGI, Heaton A, Watts RA. Primary renal vasculitis in Norfolk—increasing incidence or increasing recognition? *Nephrol Dial Transplant* 2000; **15**: 23–27.

59. Denardo BA, Tucker LB, Miller LC, Szer IS, Schaller JG. Demography of a regional pediatric rheumatology patient population. Affiliated children's arthritis centers of New England. *J Rheumatol* 1994; **21**: 1553–1561.

60. Maeda M, Kobayashi M, Okamoto S *et al.* Clinical observation of 14 cases of childhood polyarteritis nodosa in Japan. *Acta Paediatr Jpn* 1997; **39**: 277–279.

61. Tidman M, Olander R, Svalander C, Danielsson D. Patients hospitalized because of small vessel vasculitides with renal involvement in the period 1975–95: organ involvement, anti-neutrophil cytoplasmic antibodies patterns, seasonal attack rates and fluctuation of annual frequencies. *J Intern Med* 1998; **244**: 133–141.

62. Vernant JC, Smadja D, Deforge Lasseur C *et al.* Vascularites et manifestations neurologiques liees au HTLV-1. *Presse Med* 1994; **23**: 1421–1425.

63. Boki KA, Dafni U, Karpouzas GA, Papasteriandes C, Drosos AA, Mountsopoulos HM. Necrotizing vasculitis in Greece: clinical, immunological and immunogenetic aspects. A study of 66 patients. *Br J Rheumatol* 1997; **36**: 1059–1066.

64. Mouthon L. Periarterite noueuse liee au virus de l'hepatite B. *Pathol Biol* 1999; **47**: 237–244.

65. McMahon BJ, Heyward WL, Templin DW, Clement D, Lanier AP. Hepatitis B-associated polyarteritis nodosa in Alaskan Eskimo's: clinical and epidemiological features and long-term follow-up. *Hepatology* 1989; **9**: 97–101.

66. Reveille JD, Goodman RE, Barger BO, Acton R. Familial polyarteritis nodosa. *J Rheumatol* 1989; **16**: 181–185.

67. Mason JC, Cowie MR, Davies KA *et al.* Familial polyarteritis nodosa. *Arthritis Rheum* 1994; **37**: 1249–1253.

68. Zhang L, Jayne DR, Zhao MH, Lockwood CM, Oliveira DB. Distribution of MHC class II alleles in primary systemic vasculitis. *Kidney Int* 1995; **47**: 294–298.

69. Vivancos J, Soler Carrillo J, Ara del Rey J, Font J. Development of polyarteritis nodosa in the course of inactive systemic lupus erythematosus. *Lupus* 1995; **4**: 494–495.

70. Kwong T, Valderrama E, Paley C, Ilowite N. Systemic necrotizing vasculitis associated with childhood sarcoidosis. *Semin Arthritis Rheum* 1994; **23**: 388–395.

71. Kocak H, Cakar N, Hekimoglu B, Atakan C, Akkok N, Unal S. The coexistence of familial Mediterranean fever and polyarteritis nodosa; report of a case. *Pediatr Nephrol* 1996; **10**: 3–17.

72. Poveda F, Gonzalez Garcia J, Picazo ML *et al.* Systemic polyarteritis nodosa as the initial manifestation of a gastric adenocarcinoma. *J Intern Med* 1994; **236**: 679–683.

73. Birchmore D, Sweeney C, Choudhury D, Konwinski MF, Carnevale K, D'Agati V. IgA multiple myeloma presenting as Henoch-Schonlein purpura/polyarteritis nodosa overlap syndrome. *Arthritis Rheum* 1996; **39**: 698–703.

74. Seelen MA, de Meijer PH, Arnoldus EP, van Duinen SG, Meinders AE. A patient with multiple myeloma presenting with severe polyneuropathy caused by necrotizing vasculitis. *Am J Med* 1997; **102**: 485–486.

75. Rosen AM, Haines K, Tallman MS, Hakimian D, Ramsey Goldman R. Rapid Progressive cutaneous vasculitis in a patient with chronic myelomonocytic leukemia. *Am J Hematol* 1995; **50**: 310–312.

76. Hasler P, Kistler H, Gerber H. Vasculitides in hairy cell leukemia. *Semin Arthritis Rheum* 1995; **25**: 134–142.

77. Guillevin L, Lhote F, Leon A, Fauvelle F, Vivitski L, Trepo C. Treatment of polyarteritis nodosa related to hepatitis B virus with short term steroid therapy associated with antiviral agents and plasma exchanges. A prospective trial in 33 patients. *J Rheumatol* 1993; **20**: 289–298.

78. Guillevin L, Lhote F, Cohen P *et al.* Polyarteritis nodosa related to hepatitis B virus. A prospective study with long-term observation of 41 patients. *Medicine* 1995; **74**: 238–253.

79. Carson CW, Conn DL, Czaja AJ, Wright TL, Brecher ME. Frequency and significance of antibodies to hepatitis C virus in polyarteritis nodosa. *J Rheumatol* 1993; **20**: 304–309.

80. Pateron D, Fain O, Sehonnou J, Trinchet JC, Beaugrand M. Severe necrotizing vasculitis in a patient with hepatitis C virus infection treated by interferon. *Clin Exp Rheumatol* 1996; **14**: 79–81.

81. Tohme A, Haddad F, Malek N, Ghayad E. Manifestations extra-hepatiques du virus de l'hepatite C. *J Med Liban* 1998; **46**: 84–88.

82. Angulo JC, Lopez JI, Garcia ME, Peiro J, Flores N. HIV infection presenting as renal polyarteritis nodosa. *Int Urol Nephrol* 1994; **26**: 637–641.

83. Finkel TH, Torok TJ, Ferguson J *et al.* Chronic parvovirus B19 infection and systemic necrotising vasculitis: opportunistic infection or aetiological agent? *Lancet* 1994; **343**: 1255–1258.

84. Gisselbrecht M. Les vascularites au cours de l'infection par le virus de l'immunodeficience acquise. *Pathol Biol* 1999; **47**: 245–247.

85. Albornoz MA, Benedetto AV, Korman M, McFall S, Tourtellotte CD, Myers AR. Relapsing cutaneous polyarteritis nodosa associated with streptococcal infections. *Int J Dermatol* 1998; **37**: 664–666.

86. Rodreguez Pereira C, Suarez Penaranda JM, del Rio E, Forteza Villa J. Cutaneous granulomatous vasculitis after zoster infection showing polyarteritis nodosa-like features. *Clin Exp Dermatol* 1997; **22**: 274–276.

87. Guillevin L. Virus-associated vasculitides. *Rheumatology* 1999; **38**: 588–590.

88. Gregorini G, Ferioli A, Donato F *et al.* Association between silica exposure and necrotizing crescentic

glomerulonephritis with p-ANCA and anti-MPO antibodies: a hospital-based case-control study. *Adv Exp Med Biol* 1993; **336**: 435–440.

89. Kerkow J, Gross WL. Conference report: Wegener's granulomatosis and ANCA -associated diseases in 1992. *Br J Rheumatol* 1993; **32**: 150–153.

90. Michet CJ. Epidemiology of vasculitis. *Rheum Dis Clin North Am* 1990; **16**: 261–268.

91. Carruthers DM, Watts RA, Symmons DPM, Scott DGI. Wegener's granulomatosis increased incidence or increased recognition. *Br J Rheumatol* 1996; **35**: 142–145.

92. Cotch MF, Hoffman GS, Yerg DE, Kaufman G, Targonski P, Karslow RA. The epidemiology of Wergener's granulomatosis: estimates of the five year period prevalence, annual mortality, and geographic disease distribution from population-based data sources. *Arthritis Rheum* 1996; **39**: 87–92.

93. Falk RJ, Hogan S, Carey TS, Jennette JC. Clinical course of anti-neutrophil cytoplasmic autoantibody-associated glomerulonephritis and systemic vasculitis. The Glomerular Disease Collaborative Network. *Ann Intern Med* 1990; **113**: 656–663.

94. Raynauld JP, Bloch DA, Fries JF. Seasonal variation in the onset of Wegener's Granulomatosis, Polyarteritis Nodosa and Giant Cell Arteritis. *J Rheumatol* 1993; **20**: 1524–1526.

95. Duna GF, Cotch MF, Galperin C, Hoffman DB, Hoffman GS. Wegener's granulomatosis: role of environmental exposures. *Clin Exp Rheumatol* 1998; **16**: 669–674.

96. Mody GM. Rheumatoid arthritis and connective tissue disorders: sub-Saharan Africa. *Baillieres Clin Rheumatol* 1995; **9**: 31–44.

97. Sewell RF, Hamilton DV. Time-associated Wegener's granulomatosis in two members of a family. *Nephrol Dial Transplant* 1992; 7: 882.

98. Barrett TG, Thomason P. Environmental trigger for anti-neutrophil cytoplasmic antibodies? *Lancet* 1993; **342**: 369–370.

99. Katz P, Alling DW, Haynes BF, Fauci AS. Association of Wegener's granulomatosis with HLA-B8. *Clin Immunol Immunopathol* 1979; **14**: 268–270.

100. Lhotta K, Kronenberg F, Joannidis M, Feichtinger H, Koing P. Wegener's granulomatosis and Henoch-Schonlein purpura in a family with hereditary C4 deficiency. *Adv Exp Med Biol* 1993; **336**: 415–418.

101. Gratadour P, Fouque D, Laville M *et al.* Wegener's granulomatosis with antiproteinase-3 antibodies occurring after Hodgkin's disease. *Nephron* 1993; **64**: 456–461.

102. Tatsis E, Reinhold Keller E, Steindorf K, Feller AC, Gross W. Wegener's granulomatosis associated with renal cell carcinoma. *Arthritis Rheum* 1999; **42**: 751–756.

103. Masor JJ, Gal AA, Li Volsi VA. Case report: Hashimoto's thyroiditis associated with Wegener's granulomatosis. *Am J Med Sci* 1994; **308**: 112–114.

104. Nishino H, De Remee RA, Rubino FA, Parisi JE. Wegener's granulomatosis associated with vasculitis of the temporal artery: report of five cases. *Mayo Clin Proc* 1993; **68**: 115–121.

105. Valenti S, Vignolo C, Benevolo E, Braido F. Mixed infection by staphylococcus and candida, and Wegener's granulomatosis. *Monaldi Arch Chest Dis* 1996; **51**: 387–390.

106. Nikkari S, Mertsola J, Korvenranta H, Vainionpaa R, Toivanen P. Wegener's granulomatosis and parvovirus B19 infection. *Arthritis Rheum* 1994; **37**: 1707–1708.

107. Pirisi M, Gutierrez Y, Minini C *et al.* Fatal human pulmonary infection caused by an Angiostrongylus-like nematode. *Clin Infect Dis* 1995; **20**: 59–65.

108. Neyer U, Woss E, Neuweiler J. Wegener's granulomatosis associated with silicosis. *Nephrol Dial Transplant* 1994; **9**: 559–561.

109. Kobayashi A, Maeda K, Fu A *et al.* Allergic granulomatosis angiitis in a patient with positive reactions on serological tests for parasite antigens. *Nippon Kyobu Shikkan Gakkai Zasshi* 1996; **34**: 1130–1135.

110. Calonje JE, Greaves MW. Cutaneous extravascular necrotizing granuloma (Churg-Strauss) as a paraneoplastic manifestation of non-Hodgkin's B-cell lymphoma. *J R Soc Med* 1993; **86**: 549–550.

111. Guillevin L, Amouroux J, Arbeille B, Boura R. Churg-Strauss angiitis. Arguments favoring the responsibility of inhaled antigens. *Chest* 1991; **100**: 1472–1473.

112. Wechsler ME, Garpestad E, Flier SR *et al.* Pulmonary infiltrates, eosinophilia, and cardiomyopathy following corticosteroid withdrawal in patients with asthma receiving zafirlukast. *JAMA* 1998; **279**: 455–457.

113. Churg J, Churg A. Zafirlukast and Churg-Strauss syndrome. *JAMA* 1998; **279**: 1949–1950.

114. Honsinger RW. Zafirlukast and Churg-Strauss syndrome. *JAMA* 1998; **279**: 1949.

115. Katz RS, Papernik M. Zafirlukast and Churg-Strauss syndrome. *JAMA* 1998; **279**: 1949.

116. Vanoli M, Gambini D, Scorza R. A case of Churg-Strauss vasculitis after hepatitis B vaccination. *Ann Rheum Dis* 1998; **57**: 256–257.

117. Fauci AS, Haynes BF, Katz P, Wolff SM. Wegener's granulomatosis: prospective clinical and therapeutic experience with 85 patients for 21 years. *Ann Intern Med* 1983; **98**: 76–85.

118. Koldingsnes W, Nossent H. Epidemiology of Wegener's granulomatosis in northern Norway. *Arthritis Rheum* 2000; **43**: 2481–2487.

119. Reinhold Keller E, Zeidler A, Gutfleisch J, Peter HH, Raspe HH, Gross WL. Giant cell arteritis is more prevalent in urban than in rural populations: results of an epidemiological study of primary systemic vasculitides in Germany. *Rheumatology* 2000; **39**: 1396–1402.

11 | Polymyalgia rheumatica and giant cell arteritis

Alan J. Silman

Disease definition and criteria

Relationship between the disorders

Polymyalgia rheumatica (PMR) and giant cell (syn. temporal) arteritis (GCA) are two related disorders which, for epidemiological purposes, are best considered together. The nomenclature in epidemiological literature is, however, confusing with some recent authors using the terms (i) temporal arteritis for those with a biopsy-proven arteritis and (ii) GCA for those with either PMR or GCA [1]. PMR is a relatively ill defined clinical syndrome of limb girdle pain and stiffness in association with systemic features such as pyrexia and a raised erythrocyte sedimentation rate (ESR), though these may be absent in a small proportion [2]. Diagnosis depends on the presence of combinations of the relevant features in the absence of another pathology such as rheumatoid arthritis, malignancy, or infection. By contrast, GCA is a vasculitic disorder, which can be widely disseminated, affecting the medium and large arteries and whose diagnosis is pathological, classically based on the microscopic appearance of granulomatous change with Langerhans giant cells. There is, however, considerable overlap between the two disorders with a variable proportion of patients with PMR, depending on the study, with a positive biopsy of the temporal artery. Similarly series of patients have shown that a variable proportion of

patients with GCA satisfy the clinical grounds for the diagnosis of PMR. The degree of overlap between the two depends on the referral practice of the reporting centre, the frequency with which temporal artery biopsy is undertaken, and the length of follow-up. The latter is important as cross-sectional studies will underestimate the true co-occurrence rate. Thus in one series, 42 per cent of 66 patients presenting with PMR developed GCA 1 month to 9 years after presentation, whereas 27 per cent of PMR patients who did not progress to GCA also had a positive temporal artery biopsy [3]. There are also clinical differences in PMR patients with and without GCA [4]. There have been some large population-based studies where attempts have been made to ascertain all cases with either disorder [5–8]. The overlap between the two disorders and the relationship to the temporal artery biopsy result from these cross sectional studies are shown in Table 11.1. The results suggest that between 20 and 30 per cent of cases have features of both diseases and that isolated PMR accounts for over 50 per cent. These proportions are lower in series from North America where biopsy positive proportions are as low as 1 per cent [8]. Further complicating the position is that up to 50 per cent of clinically-presumed GCA cases are temporal artery biopsy negative [9]. Variability in biopsy technique and histological examination would influence these data. However, these population data underscore the belief of others

Table 11.1 Overlap between PMR and GCA in population based surveys

Reference	Total No of cases	GCA N (%)	Biopsy +ve (%)	PMR N (%)	Biopsy +ve (%)	Both GCA and PMR N (%)	Biopsy +ve (%)
[5]	116	26 (22)	96	67 (58)	31	23 (20)	87
[6]	45	3 (7)	67	31 (69)	16	10 (22)	60
[7]	56	14 (25)	57	24 (46)	0[a]	16 (29)	44

[a] A positive biopsy was considered as GCA.

that the two disorders can be considered as a single entity.

Diagnostic criteria

GCA

The diagnosis of GCA, as stated above, is pathologically based on the presence of inflammation in the arterial wall which may be granulomatous with giant cells or, more frequently, non-specific or even fibrotic from resolved inflammatory change [10]. The diagnosis of GCA in the biopsy-negative patients is based on the presence of clinical abnormality in the temporal arteries with other features of the disease such as jaw claudication. Criteria are available which distinguish GCA from other forms of vasculitis and did not necessitate a positive biopsy [11] (Table 11.2A,B). These criteria were derived from a statistical analysis and two formats were derived: a traditional format (Table 11.2A) and one based on a classification tree approach (Table 11.2B). Interestingly, the latter excluded ESR and indeed age of onset over 50 and temporal artery tenderness was sufficient. It should be born in mind

that these criteria were designed to distinguish GCA from other forms of vasculitis and will presumably be too non-specific and possibly insensitive for epidemiological purposes. The criteria have been shown to be very sensitive (>91 per cent) [12], though others have found poor discriminate ability in the clinic [13]. Criteria for biopsy-negative GCA were derived from a series of French patients and had a sensitivity of 85 per cent, though the nature of the gold standard in such studies is unclear [14]. A novel approach to criteria derivation using neural networks did not show any obvious superiority over the classification tree approach [15].

PMR

There are two sets of criteria for PMR that have been formulated: from the UK [16] the other from Japan [17]. The UK (Table 11.3A) and Japanese criteria sets (Table 11.3B) are based on the discrimination between PMR and similar conditions, which in the Japanese criteria was restricted to rheumatoid arthritis. The UK criteria were derived from 146 patients and then validated in a further 140. The sensitivity was 92 per cent for the derivation sample and 82 per cent for the validation

---

Table 11.2 American College of Rheumatology criteria for GCA

A Traditional format
1 Age onset ≥50 years
2 New onset headache of localized headache (different from previous headache)
3 Tenderness or decreased pulsation in at least one of the temporal arteries
4 ESR ≥50 mm/hour (Westergren)
5 Abnormal artery biopsy with either mononuclear cell infiltrate or granulomatous inflammation (with giant cells)
  To classify a patient as having GCA the patient has to meet at least 3 of the 5 criteria

B Classification tree
1 Age onset ≥50 years
2 New onset headache
3 Claudication of jaw or tongue on mastication and swallowing
4 Tenderness or decreased pulsation in temporal artery
5 Abnormal artery biopsy with either mononuclear cell infiltrate or granulanatous inflammation (with giant cells)
  Positive sets =
    (1) 1 and 4
    (2) 1 and 5 (4 absent)
    (3) 1 and 3 (4 and 5 absent)

Source: [11].

Table 11.3A UK criteria for PMR

1. Bilateral shoulder pain and, or stiffness
2. Delay from onset to maximal symptoms <2 weeks
3. Initial ESR ≥40 mm/hour
4. Morning stiffness >1 hour
5. Age >65
6. Depression and, or loss of weight
7. Upper arm tenderness bilaterally

Positive = >3 criteria
Source: [16].

Table 11.3B Japanese criteria for PMR

1. Bilateral muscular pain for at least 2 weeks in at least 2 of the following:
      neck
      shoulders/shoulder girdle
      upper arms
      hips
      pelvic
2. Normal muscle enzymes
3. ESR >40 mm/hour
4. No hand joint swelling

All 4 criteria to be present.
Source: [17].

Table 11.3C United States criteria for PMR

1. Age ≥50 years
2. Severe and bilateral pain associated with morning stiffness (lasting ≥30min) for more than 1 month in at least 2 of 3 areas:
   neck or torso
   shoulders or proximal regions of arms
   hips or proximal aspects of the thighs
3. ESR at the time of diagnosis ≥ 40 mm/hour
4. Exclusion of other diseases that may present with polymyalgia manifestations or mimic polymyalgia rheumatica, except GCA

Source: [18].

sample. Specificity rates were 80 per cent and 75 per cent respectively. The Japanese criteria were 93 per cent sensitive and 98 per cent specific against the rheumatoid arthritis control panel. These criteria have not been validated in a subsequent sample but were surprisingly discriminatory. The high sensitivity might reflect their current diagnostic process and lower rates may be found when applied to other series of patients considered to have PMR. A further set of criteria were used in a US study of PMR (Table 11.3C) but their performance has not been subject to the same evaluation [18]. Other tests, such as a low CD8 positive lymphocyte count, would appear to show good discrimination between PMR/CGA and other disorders [19] but are probably not sufficiently widely available to be useful for classification.

Occurrence

The variable nature of the disorders and their tendency to remit and relapse, particularly in relation to steroid therapy, makes assessments of point prevalence difficult to interpret and incidence rates for both conditions are a more robust guide. The latter are, however, almost always derived retrospectively from ascertained cases. Prospective notification by general practitioners [1] and population surveys both suggest a considerable proportion of undiagnosed patients with PMR in the elderly community [20,21]. The data for GCA are more robust [1].

Mortality

PMR/GCA are an uncommon cause of mortality and, indeed, are not associated with decreased sur-

vival [22,23]. Therefore published mortality statistics have little to offer in considering the occurrence of this disorder. By contrast, post-mortem examination of the temporal arteries can reveal at least the extent of pathological change independent of clinical presentation during life. In the one series reported [24], the prevalence of GCA at post-mortem was 1.7 per cent in 889 consecutive autopsies. Interestingly, of the 15 cases discovered only two had been diagnosed during life.

Incidence

There have been some 'quasi'-epidemiological studies where observers have attempted to relate their caseload to their local population. Thus observations from a UK general practitioner of nine cases of GCA over a 4.5-year period suggested an incidence of 54/100 000 total population [25]. Similarly, Alestig [26] estimated the incidence of PMR to be 2.7/100 000 derived from 10 cases over a 1.5-year period; Hamrin [27] estimated rates of 1.5 and 13/100 000 for PMR and GCA respectively, based on 52 and six cases respectively seen over a 4-year period. There have been a number of more formal incidence studies and the results from the major ones from Europe and North America are described in Table 11.4. These studies are broadly comparable insofar as the results presented are restricted to those over the age of 50. However, there is a marked age and sex gradient in this disorder and some of the differences observed may be accounted for by differences in the demographic structure of the populations studied over the age of 50.

Six of the studies have been from the Olmsted County population served by the Mayo Clinic [18,28–32] with successive reports updating previous estimates and providing information on trends. More recent reports have usefully age adjusted the rates to the US white population [31,32] and provided confidence limits for the estimates. Broadly, incidence rates for GCA alone range from below one to 30/100 000 population 50+ and for PMR from 10–110/100 000. Those surveys that attempt to identify cases prospectively recorded higher incidence rates [1,33] suggesting more complete ascertainment using this approach. A recent study from Northern Spain [34] was useful in demonstrating that approximately one-quarter of incident cases also satisfied criteria for GCA and that the incidence of pure PMR can be derived accordingly.

Table 11.4 Incidence rates per 100 000 of PMR/GCA in populations aged 50+

Reference	Country	Period	Disease group	Incidence in		
				Males	Females	All
North America						
[28]	US[a]	1951–67	GCA	–	–	13.0
[29]	US	1950–74	GCA	–	–	11.7
[18]	US[a]	1970–79	PMR	37.9	65.5	53.7
[41][b,c]	US	1971–80	GCA	0.65	3.38	2.24
[30]	US[a]	1950–85	GCA	7.4	23.4	17.0
[32]	US	1970–91	PMR	40 (30–49)	62 (52–71)	53 (50–59)
[31]	US	1950–91	GCA	8 (5–12)	24 (20–29)	18 (15–21)
Europe						
[104]	Denmark	1973–83	PMR/GCA	7.7	15.9	11.8
[6]	Denmark	1982–83	PMR/GCA	28.0	120.8	76.6
[109]	Denmark	1982–94	PMR	–	–	41 (30–67)
			GCA	–	–	20 (19–23)
[125]	England	1976–83	PMR/GCA	–	–	40.0
[33]	Finland	1984–87	PMR/GCA	–	–	69.8
		1987–88		–	–	94.4[d]
[126]	Finland	1970–79	GCA	–	–	5
		1980–89		–	9	–
[127]	Iceland	1984–90	GCA	18	36	27
[1]	Norway	1987–94	PMR	83	138	112
			GCA	16	40	29
[102]	Scotland	1964–77	GCA	2.6	5.4	4.2
[10]	Sweden	7- year period	PMR	–	–	12.0
[5]	Sweden	1973–75	GCA	20.4	35.3	28.6
[9]	Sweden	1987	PMR/GCA	9.0	52.3	33.6
[128]	Sweden	1985–87	PMR	33	63	50
[37]	Sweden	1976–95	GCA	13	30	22
Mediterranean						
[40]	France	1970–79	GCA	–	–	9.4
[7]	Italy	1981–85	PMR	11.4	13.9	12.8
			GCA	5.0	11.7	8.8
[35]	Italy	1980–88	PMR	9.7	14.9	12.7
			GCA	5.8	7.8	6.9
[129]	Spain	1981–90	GCA	–	–	6.0
[23]	Spain	1986–91	GCA	11	6	–
		1991–95		12	9	10
[34]	Spain	1987–96	PMR	–	–	19 (14[e])
Other						
[39]	Israel	1960–78	GCA	–	–	0.5
[36]	Israel	1980–91	GCA	8 (5–11)	12 (9–15)	10 (8–12)

[a] All based on population of Olmsted Country.

[b] Rates are for age 65 and over.

[c] Figures are for whites only.

[d] Prospective.

[e] Excluding those with GCA.

Influence of age and gender

The influence of gender on the incidence of both PMR and GCA is illustrated by the data in Table 11.4. There is typically a female excess reported across all ages combined for both disorders, although for GCA, in some studies, for example [23], the increase is fairly modest. As females survive longer than males, then the all-ages excess might be explained by age rather than gender influences. Recent age-specific incidence data from the prospective Norwegian study for GCA are illustrated in Table 11.5. Small numbers limit the con-

Table 11.5   Age and sex specific-incidence rates of biopsy-proven GCA in Aust Agder County, South Norway 1987–94

Age	Incidence (number of cases) per 100 000		
	Males	Females	Both
50–54	0 (0)	0 (0)	0 (0)
55–59	6 (1)	12 (2)	9 (3)
60–64	27 (4)	27 (4)	27 (8)
65–69	21 (3)	72 (11)	48 (14)
70–74	37 (5)	80 (14)	61 (19)
75–79	28 (3)	71 (11)	53 (14)
80–84	15 (1)	27 (4)	27 (5)
85	0 (0)	31 (3)	21 (3)

Source: [1].

Table 11.7   Age and sex-specific incidence rates of PMR, 1970–1991, in Olmsted County, Minnesota, US

Age	Incidence (95% CI) per 100 000		
	Males	Females	Both
50–59	12 (6–22)	14 (7–24)	13 (8–19)
60–69	41 (26–61)	53 (37–73)	47 (36–61)
70–79	83 (55–121)	168 (135–225)	136 (112–163)
80+	85 (44–148)	102 (71–141)	97 (71–129)
All ages 50+[a]	40 (31–49)	62 (52–71)	53 (46–59)

[a] Age standardized to US 1970 age 50+ white population,
Source: [32].

clusions but the disorder rises in incidence in both males and females to reach a peak at age 70–74 and then declines. This pattern has been observed in other studies (Table 11.6). The most robust data (Table 11.7) on the influence of age on the incidence of PMR are from Olmsted County (Mayo Clinic), and these show a similar trend with a peak onset in the eighth decade with a subsequent decline [32]. Again, the same pattern was seen from European data (Table 11.6).

Time trends

There are a number of reports suggesting a changing occurrence over time, particularly in GCA. The most dramatic is a reported 20-fold increase between 1960–78 and 1980–91 in Jerusalem [36]. The role of greater case ascertainment is unclear. Recently published data over a 40-year period of the incidence of GCA in Olmsted County show a steady increase in incidence over time until 1984 with a recent decline (Table 11.8), occurring over a longer period in males. Possible explanations for this are complicated given the possible phenomenon of enhanced case finding as a

Table 11.8   Trends in incidence of GCA, 1950–1991, in Olmsted county, Minnesota, US

Period	Incidence/100 000		
	Males	Females	Both
1950–54	0 (–)	12 (0–25)	7 (0–16)
1953–59	4 (0–12)	6 (0–18)	5 (0–11)
1960–64	3 (0–10)	21 (6–35)	9 (13–22)
1965–69	6 (0–15)	20 (7–33)	15 (6–23)
1970–74	19 (4–33)	21 (4–34)	20 (10–29)
1975–79	11 (0–23)	28 (15–42)	22 (12–31)
1980–84	8 (0–16)	37 (22–52)	26 (16–35)
1985–91	8 (1–16)	27 (17–37)	19 (13–26)

Source: [31].

result of an increased use of temporal artery biopsy. Underlying these trends, however, is a possible cyclical phenomenon with peaks of incidence lasting about 3 years occurring every 7 years [31] (Fig. 11.1). The temporal artery biopsy rate did increase in the denominator population from 32 to 76/100 000 between 1965–69 and 1980–85, though interestingly the rate of positive biopsies did not change [30]. The male biopsy rate was approximately half that in the females. The

Table 11.6   Effect of age on incidence (rate/100 000) by disease category

Age	Incidence rate									
	Males					Females				
	GCA		GCA/PMR		PMR	GCA[a]		GCA/PMR		PMR
	(a)	(b)	(a)	(b)	(c)	(a)	(b)	(a)	(b)	(c)
50–59	4.6	2.1	6.8	6.3	17.7	3.2	4.8	6.4	5.7	21.8
60–69	16.8	7.2	19.8	7.2	43.0	19.1	7.5	34.3	14.0	52.0
70–79	31.8	10.7	40.4	17.8	74.1	42.3	11.8	78.8	29.9	134.6
80+	18.3	5.9	73.1	17.7	52.4	36.8	7.6	68.3	10.1	102.9

Sources: (a) [5]; (b) [35]; (c) [18].
[a] Biopsy proven.

Table 11.9 Trends in incidence of PMR, 1970–1991, in Olmsted County, Minnesota, US

Period	Incidence (95% CI) per 100 000		
	Males	Females	Both
1970–73	46 (21–71)	35 (17–52)	40 (25–55)
1974–76	40 (14–67)	66 (37–95)	54 (35–74)
1977–79	37 (14–65)	78 (49–107)	62 (42–82)
1980–82	42 (16–69)	56 (32–80)	50 (33–68)
1983–85	44 (18–70)	55 (32–78)	50 (33–67)
1986–88	43 (19–67)	62 (38–86)	54 (37–72)
1989–91	27 (8–45)	82 (54–110)	58 (40–76)

Source: [32].

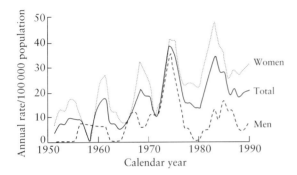

Fig. 11.1 Annual incidence rates of GCA in Olmsted County, Minnesota, per 100 000 persons 50 years of age or older. Reproduced with permission of ACP-ASIM from [31].

annual incidence has also been reported to have statistically significantly increased in time in Gothenburg [37]. Other recent studies suggest that cases are becoming less 'classical' in their presentation [23] suggesting, at least in part, an increased awareness of the less common presentations. Time trends in the incidence of PMR from Olmsted County are shown in Table 11.9. The incidence has shown little change between 1970

and 1991, in that population such differences that have emerged might be explained by sampling error. The trends in incidence and fluctuation of GCA have also been studied in the Lugo region of northwestern Spain [130]. This revealed an annual increase in incidence in men of 8% (95% CI 4–13%; p <0.0001) and an annual increase in women of 11% (95% CI 6–14%; p < 0.0001). No seasonal pattern of peaks in incidence were reported.

Prevalence

As stated above, there is a problem in estimating the point prevalence of this disorder. Estimates of prevalence based on calculating all living patients at a single point in time from retrospective studies of medical records are available (Table 11.10). Apart from the Danish [6] and UK studies [6,38], all the estimates are based solely on the Mayo data. Interestingly, the incidence to prevalence ratios for the various studies (which provide an estimate of disease duration) vary from less than 2 years [6] to over 10 years [29]. As it seems unlikely that there is such a disparity it suggests that the definition of an active case for prevalence estimation purposes is variable. The data from the UK are based on review of primary care records

Table 11.11 Prevalence of PMR/GCA by age and sex: rate per 100 000 population

Age group	Prevalence		
	Males	Females	All
50–59	9.0	46.7	27.3
60–69	64.1	226.0	146.7
70–79	219.6	315.6	373.6
80+	94.6	261.7	198.1

Source: [6].

Table 11.10 Prevalence per 1000 of PMR/GCA in populations aged 50+

Reference	Country	Year	Disease group	Prevalence		
				Males	Females	All
[28]	US	1968	GCA	0.1	0.4	0.2
[29]	US	1970	GCA			1.3
[6]	Denmark	1986	PMR/GCA	0.8	1.9	1.4
[18]	US	1980	PMR			5.5
[30]	US	1984	GCA			2.2
[32]	US	1992	PMR			6.3
[38]	UK	1999	PMR			10.9 (9.5–12.3)
			GCA			1.4 (0.9–1.9)

and might therefore be expected to have a higher as-certainment [38]. These data do suggest that the prevalence of PMR reported previously may indeed be underestimated. Prevalence rates from these studies show the same age and sex pattern as the incidence rates with a maximal prevalence in the eighth decade. The prevalence by gender are different with a marked female excess (Table 11.11) perhaps suggesting an enhanced female survival or greater ascertainment.

There have been some small-scale screening surveys of a 'normal' population suggesting that only a proportion of cases will be diagnosed and thus hospital-based prevalence estimates are inaccurate. A study of elderly residents in an old people's home revealed a prevalence of 12/1000 with two of the three cases detected being previously undiagnosed [21]. A similar study suggested a prevalence of 9 per cent for GCA in a group of elderly people aged 50–99 [20]. This perhaps seems unlikely given that careful post-mortem study (see above) only revealed a prevalence of less than 2 per cent.

Geographical and ethnic differences

Interestingly, many of the epidemiological studies have been from populations of the same ethnic origins. Thus of the 29 incidence studies listed in Table 11.4, 12 were from Scandinavia and a further six from the largely originally Scandinavian population in Olmsted County served by the Mayo Clinic. There are no consistent differences in GCA incidence between the populations studied in Scandinavia or the US. Differences in PMR might be explained by methodological differences. It has recently been confirmed that southern Norway has the highest known incidence of temporal arteritis worldwide [131]. The study from Israel [39] had the lowest recorded incidence of 0.5/100 000 and more recent studies from Israel [36] revealed an incidence of GCA very similar to Northern European/US rates.

Table 11.12   Racial differences in incidence of GCA (rate/100 000 age 50+)

Group	Incidence		
	Male	Females	Both
Blacks	0	0.61	0.36
Whites	0.65	3.38	2.24

Source: [41].

Similarly the studies from Southern Europe—France [40] and Italy [7]—yielded incidence estimates substantially lower than most of the major Northern European and United States studies (Table 11.4). The one exception to the latter is the study from the Southern US [41] which at 2.4/100 000 in whites had the lowest incidence rate for GCA (apart from the Israeli study of Friedman [39]).

There have been few studies in different ethnic groups within the same population using the same methodology. PMR is stated to be rare in black African populations [42] although there have been a number of cases series of GCA/PMR in black patients [43–45]. The epidemiological value of such case series is, however, negligible. The study from Tennessee [41] provides the only epidemiological data on the relative incidence in black and white groups (Table 11.12). The results show a substantial relative excess in both male and female whites, with the rates in blacks being extremely low. Although reports have suggested a similar incidence of visual loss due to arteritis in blacks and whites in a series from Washington, American blacks with GCA had a higher likelihood of visual loss [46]. The disease is rare in African populations [47] and, as an example, amongst over 34 000 patients attending a rheumatology/dermatology service in Lomé, Togo, there was only one patient with GCA [48]. The distribution of that population would be against finding many cases. The disease is rare in Asians [49] and Arab groups. Only 72 temporal artery biopsies were performed over a 15-year period in Saudi Arabia [50] although there have been substantial series of patients reported from Japan [17].

Non-genetic host factors

Co-morbidity

There has been considerable interest in the possible association between autoimmune thyroid disease and PMR/GCA. Case series and reports have suggested that there is an association with both hyperthyroidism [51] and hypothyroidism [52]. Further, prospective follow-up of 250 elderly women with hypothyroidism revealed that 10 per cent developed PMR/GCA [53]. Not all reports have been consistent with three series of PMR patients finding no association [54–56]. There remains the possibility that the symptoms of PMR overlap with those of hypothyroidism to explain some of the association. Further, in uncontrolled case series based on hospital patients there is likely to be a selective referral, especially in the elderly, of patients with multiple pathology. There were, however, no associations in the two controlled studies reported [57,58]. In the first study, thyroid disease was defined as any mention of thyroid disease in the medical record, but the latter study undertook intensive investigation of 285 cases and 222 controls for thyroid hormones and autoantibodies, with no evidence of increased hyperthyroidism.

The other co-morbid event linked to PMR/GCA is the presence of peripheral vascular disease, with two such reports suggesting a link [40,57]. In the latter study, which was controlled, there were increased risks, as measured by the odds ratio, for the presence of angina (OR = 2.0), peripheral vascular disease (OR = 1.5), and myocardial infarction (OR = 1.8). Only the ratio for angina, however, was statistically significant and could perhaps be explained by the link in the same study with previous smoking (OR = 2.3). This topic has been further investigated in a case–control study which yielded an OR of 5.5 for ever smoking and an OR of 14 for those who had smoked more than 10 pack-years [59]. That study also showed an increased likelihood of arterial disease and arterial murmurs but no increase in association with other cardiovascular risk factors such as raised cholesterol or hypertension. The authors hypothesized that vascular damage from cardiovascular disease exposes the arterial wall to an increased likelihood of immune attachment.

Pregnancy

Although a consistently higher occurrence of PMR/GCA has been reported in females, few investigations have focused on a possible aetiological role for pregnancy and hormonal factors. In a large case–control

Table 11.13 Familial clustering for PMR/GCA

Reference	Family cases	Disease
[61]	2 sisters	PMR
[10]	4 pairs of sibling	PMR
[62]	1 sibling pair	PMR
[63]	2 mother/daughter pairs	GCA/PMR
[64]	4 siblings—3 biopsy proven, 1? GCA	GCA
[65]	Concordant MZ twins	GCA
[66]	1 sibling pair	
[67]	2 sibling pairs	GCA

study [60] cases were twice as likely to be nulliparous (*p* = 0.002), an observation more pronounced in those with GCA compared to those with PMR.

Genetics

Evidence of clustering within families comes from a number of case reports (Table 11.13). In 93 consecutive cases, there were four probands with affected siblings [10]. In a similar series of approximately 250 patients, there were four instances of relative pairs (two mother/daughter and two sister/sister) [63]. In the latter study the timing of onset within three of the pairs was less than 1 year, perhaps suggesting a shared environmental influence, although the two sisters in one of the pairs lived 150 miles apart. There are only two reports from identical (monozygotic) twins. In the one [68] the twins were discordant for PMR and in the other [65] the twins were concordant for GCA with ophthalmic arteritis. It is impossible to separate out shared environment or genes in this report given their close geographical proximity and similarity in lifestyle, although there was a 5-year gap in disease onset. One line of evidence, however, suggesting a biological (genetic) link is the increased occurrence of low CD8 and T cell counts in unaffected siblings of GCA/PMR probands [69].

Immunogenetics

There have been a considerable number of studies of specific HLA alleles and PMR/GCA, with the more consistent association being with HLA-DRB1*4. Initial studies for class I antigens were largely negative. Two reports suggested an association with A10 and B8 [70,71]. Similar associations, but non-significant, were seen in a separate study [72] and a further report suggested a link with B14 [73]. Other reports have either been negative for any association with class I antigens or suggested other associations unconfirmed by others [74–81]. The results from investigating HLA class II have been interesting but no consistent finding has emerged despite several studies. One key source of confusion is whether there are separate associations between HLA class II with PMR from those with GCA, when it is not clear whether the two disorders have been sufficiently separated for analysis. Data from serological studies undertaken between 1980 and 1996 suggested that HLA-DR4 was associated with both PMR and GCA independently and in combination

Table 11.14　HLA-DR4 and PMR GCA

Reference	Disease	Cases		Controls	
		N	DR4 (%)	N	DR4 (%)
[82]	GCA	48	40	146	19
[83]	PMR/GCA	69	49	113	20
[84]	PMR/GCA	78	68	45	a
[85]	PMR	34	59	153	34
[79]	GCA	26	39	200	23
	PMR	37	27	–	–
[80]	GCA	21	29	243	30
	GCA/PMR	22	55	–	–
	PMR	16	50	–	–
[86]	GCA/PMR	34	59	200	20
	GCA	31	19	–	–
[87]	PMR	44	67	132	30
[35]	PMR	41	24	242	14
	GCA	14	36	–	–

Pooled odds ratios: GCA 1.8 (95% CI 1.2–2.6); PMR 2.4 (95% CI 1.7–3.4); PMR/GCA 4.0 (95% CI 2.6–6.2).
a Total not stated.

(Table 11.14). The recent interest has been in investigating alleles at the DNA level and comparing the findings from similar studies in relation to HLA-DR4 and rheumatoid arthritis (RA).

The results (Table 11.14) are not easy to reconcile. In studies of UK [88] and Spanish patients [88,89], there was strong evidence of an association with the same shared epitope on the third hypervariable region (3rd HVR) of the DRB1 gene that is associated with RA. However, in the UK patients, this association was clearly observed in patients with PMR, whereas in the Spanish patients such an association was restricted only to those patients with GCA. A recent Italian study [90], showed no relation with 3rd HVR alleles and PMR. Similar negative results were obtained with DQA1 and DQB1. An earlier US study confirmed a strong association with DRB1*04 but was not restricted to 3rd HVR bearing alleles and the hypothesis was raised of a shared sequence on the second HVR [91]. This may be difficult to prove given its presence in over 90 per cent of the normal population. A small French study [92] suggested other differences between PMR and GCA. The rather unsatisfactory conclusion is that there are associations between HLA class II and both PMR and GCA but whether these are the same, and whether the susceptibility alleles are the same as in RA, cannot be confirmed. There is, however, no suggestion that other class II alleles, that is DQ or DP, have revealed any new associations other than might be expected from their linkage with DR. HLA-DRB1 alleles might, however, influence disease severity [90], likelihood of

relapse [34], and resistance to corticosteroid therapy [93]. Others have investigated genes outside the MHC including the switch region of immunoglobulin μ and $\alpha 1$ heavy genes and T cell receptor genes, without an association being discovered [87]. A recent report suggested that a polymorphism within the interleukin-6 gene might be associated with GCA risk, which might explain the strong acute phase response [94].

Environmental factors

Clustering

The reporting of apparent clusters of cases in time and or space is evidence in support of an environmental influence. Sonnenblick [95] reported a cluster of five cases in Jerusalem in a 7-week period compared to their expected annual referral rate of one case. Studies in general practice in the UK were also suggestive of a cluster with six cases of PMR and two of GCA presenting in a 7-month period in a population of 4400 [96]. The role of increased awareness and changes in diagnostic sensitivity in producing such clusters is unknown. There are three reports of spouse pairs. In the first [97], the onset was within 1 month with the husband presenting with undoubted PMR and his wife with GCA. In the second [98], there was an 8-month delay between the wife presenting with PMR and the husband with GCA. In the most recent report, onset was simultaneous [99]. The chance occurrence of such events is likely to be small but cannot be ruled out.

Seasonality and climate

One of the most unusual aspects of the epidemiology of PMR/GCA is the suggestion of seasonality in incidence. However, the results are conflicting. Thus an initial report of clustering in summer [100] was followed by two reports of a definite winter peak [101,102,132], a further suggesting a summer peak [36], and one suggesting both a summer and a winter peak! [103]. Four more recent studies showed no such seasonality [18,37,104,105]. In a study comparing PMR with early-onset rheumatoid arthritis patients [106], a summer peak was observed as well as a correlation with outside temperature and hours of sunshine. This report is supported by a case report of two patients with actinic granuloma occurring concurrently with GCA [107]. The results from the positive studies, therefore, do suggest that clustering in time, and indeed in space, might be responsible for some of the incidence of this disease, but the disparity between studies makes it difficult to reach an overall conclusion [108].

Possible infectious agent exposure

The data suggests cyclic patterns of incidence [31], the possibility of a seasonal influence on occurrence, and the development of disease in spouse pairs all point to a possible infectious cause. Other epidemiological data supporting this is the increased incidence in areas with a high population density as reported from a large Danish study [109].

There are a number of possible candidate microbial agents. In a study comparing the incidence of GCA with reported disease outbreaks of five disease peaks between 1982 and 1989, two coincided with outbreaks of *Mycoplasma pneumoniae*, two with outbreaks of human parvovirus B19 (HPV B19), and one with *Chlamydiae pneumoniae* [109]. A recent case–control study [110] that used PCR techniques on temporal artery biopsy specimens found an eight-fold increased frequency of HPV B19 DNA in those with, compared to those without, histological evidence of arteritis [110]. By contrast, a serological study of antibodies directed against both structural and non-structural HPV B19 viral proteins showed no difference between 110 PMR cases (none of whom had GCA) and 135 controls [111]. A seroepidemiological study com-

paring 42 new onset PMR cases with 22 controls showed no association with recent chlamydial infection but evidence of recent enterovirus infection was observed in two patients [112]. In a similar small study, all 26 PMR cases had evidence of adenovirus infection compared to only 50 per cent of 26 controls; similar findings were observed in relation to respiratory syncitial virus (RSV) [113].

A study relying on only infections reported in medical records with the obvious scope for ascertainment bias, revealed a three-fold increase of prior infection in cases with GCA compared to hip fracture controls [114]. Other candidates include the hepatitis B virus following a report of HBsAb in 9/12 patients but only 1/12 age matched controls [115] and was supported by data from another study [116]. However, the absence of an increase in HBsAg in incident cases [115] and the failure to find an association with HBsAb in a third study [117] perhaps argue against an aetiological role.

Other infectious agents considered have included *Bedsoniae*, following the report of a high prevalence (46 per cent) of cases reporting contact with birds in the 5 years prior to disease onset compared to 26 per cent of controls [118]. A possible link with lymphogranuloma venereum was proposed given the fact that the latter is also a vasculitic disease and is caused by a *Bedsonia* organism. Other possibilities raised include hypersensitivity to bird droppings, feathers, etc. Other reports of PMR following contact with birds have been made [119,120]. One study also postulated a role for *Borrelia* with 12/19 patients with PMR/GCA having raised IgG to *B. Burgdorferi* [121], the agent responsible for Lyme disease. Other case reports have implicated HTLV1 [122] and parvovirus B19 [123].

A large recent study of 305 new cases of GCA compared serological responses to para-influenza virus (HPIV), RSV, measles virus, herpes virus Type 1 and Type 2, and Epstein–Barr virus, to age and sex-matched controls. Both IgM and IgG responses were investigated. IgM positivity to HPIV was twice as likely in the cases ($p = 5 \times 10^{-5}$), a result that was more prominent in the biopsy-positive group. No differences were seen in any of the viral responses tested [124].

Acknowledgement

The authors are very grateful to Dr Miguel Gonzàlez-Gay for his constructive comments on this chapter.

References

1. Gran JT, Myklebust G. The incidence of polymyalgia rheumatica and temporal arteritis in the county of Aust Agder, South Norway: A prospective study 1987–94. *J Rheumatol* 1997; 24: 1739–1743.

2. Proven A, Gabriel SE, O'Fallon WM, Hunder GG. Polymyalgia rheumatica with low erythrocyte sedimentation rate at diagnosis. *J Rheumatol* 1999; 26: 1333–1337.

3. Jones JG, Hazleman BL. Prognosis and management of polymyalgia rheumatica. *Ann Rheum Dis* 1981; 40: 1–5.

4. Calvo-Romero JM, Margo-Ledesma D, Ramos-Salado JL, Buereo-Dacal JC, Diaz-Rodriguez E, Perez-Miranda M. Polymyalgia rheumatica with and without giant cell arteritis. *Rev Esp Reumatol* 1999; 26: 108–112.

5. Bengtsson B, Malmvall B. The epidemiology of giant cell arteritis including temporal arteritis and polymyalgia rheumatica. *Arthritis Rheum* 1981; 24: 899–904.

6. Boesen P, Sörensen SF. Giant cell arteritis, temporal arteritis, and polymyalgia rheumatica in a Danish county. *Arthritis Rheum* 1987; 30: 294–299.

7. Salvarani C, Macchioni PL, Tartoni PL *et al.* Polymyalgia rheumatica and giant cell arteritis: a 5 year epidemiologic and clinical study in Reggio Emilia, Italy. *Clin Exp Rheumatol* 1987; 5: 205–215.

8. Healey LA. On the epidemiology of polymyalgia rheumatica and temporal arteritis. *J Rheumatol* 1993; 20: 1639–1640.

9. Noltorp S, Svensson B. High incidence of polymyalgia rheumatica and giant cell arteritis in a Swedish community. *Clin Exp Rheumatol* 1991; 9: 351–355.

10. Hamrin B. Polymyalgia arteritica. *Acta Med Scan* 1972; 533: 62–65.

11. Hunder GG, Bloch DA, Michel BA, Stevens MB, Arend WP. The American college of rheumatology 1990 criteria for the classification of giant cell arteritis. *Arthritis Rheum* 1990; 33: 1122–1128.

12. Armona J, Rodriguez-Valverde V, González-Gay MA *et al.* Giant cell arteritis. A study of 191 patients. *Med Clin Barc* 1995; 105: 734–737.

13. Rao JK, Allen NB, Pincus T. Limitations of the 1990 American college of rheumatology classification criteria in the diagnosis of vasculitis. *Ann Intern Med* 1998; 129: 345–352.

14. Duhaut P, Demolombe-Rague S, Pinede L *et al.* Giant-cell arteritis with negative biopsy—sensitivity of diagnostic criteria—the GRACG multicentric study. *Rev Med Interne* 1993; 14: 441.

15. Astion ML, Wener MH, Thomas RG, Hunder GG, Bloch DA. Application of neural networks to the classification of giant cell arteritis. *Arthritis Rheum* 1994; 37: 760–770.

16. Bird HA, Esselinckx W, Dixon AJ, Mowat AG, Wood PHN. An evaluation of criteria for polymyalgia rheumatica. *Ann Rheum Dis* 1979; 38: 434–439.

17. Nobunaga M, Yoshioka K, Yasuda M, Shingu M. Clinical studies of polymyalgia rheumatica: a proposal of diagnosis. *Jpn J Med* 1989; 28: 452–456.

18. Chuang TY, Hunder GG, Ilstrup DM, Kurland LT. Polymyalgia rheumatica: a 10-year epidemiologic and clinical study. *Ann Intern Med* 1982; 97: 672–680.

19. Arnold MH, Corrigall VM, Pitzalis C, Panayi GS. The sensitivity and specificity of reduced CD8 lymphocyte levels in the diagnosis of polymyalgia rheumatica/giant cell arteritis. *Clin Exp Rheumatol* 1993; 11: 629–634.

20. Nosenzo C, Dughera L, Macchioni P, Judica-Cordiglia A, Gelato D. L'Incidenza dell'arterite temporale nelle persone anziane: studio clinico su 100 ricoverati in Gerontocomio. *Acta Gerontol* 1967; 17: 238–245.

21. Silman AJ, Currey HLF. Polymyalgia rheumatica in a defined elderly community. *Rheumatol Rehabil* 1982; 21: 235–237.

22. Matteson EL, Gold KN, Bloch DA, Hunder GG. The American college of rheumatology giant cell arteritis classification criteria cohort. *Am J Med* 1996; 100: 193–196.

23. González-Gay MA, Blanco R, Sánchez-Andrade A, Vázquez-Caruncho M. Giant cell arteritis in Lugo, Spain: a more frequent disease with fewer classic features. *J Rheumatol* 1997; 24: 2166–2170.

24. Ostberg G. Temporal arteritis in a large necropsy series. *Ann Rheum Dis* 1971; 30: 224–235.

25. Cameron A. Temporal arteritis in general practice. *BMJ* 1959; 268: 1291–1296.

26. Alestig K, Barr J. Giant cell arteritis: a biopsy study of polymyalgia rheumatica. *Lancet* 1963; 1: 1228–1230.

27. Hamrin B, Jonsson N, Landberg T. Involvement of large vessels in polymyalgia arteritica. *Lancet* 1965; 1: 1193–1196.

28. Hauser WA, Ferguson RH, Holley KE, Kurland LT. Temporal arteritis in Rochester, Minnesota. *Mayo Clin Proc* 1971; 46: 597–602.

29. Huston KA, Hunder GG, Lie JT, Kennedy RH, Elveback LR. Temporal arteritis. A 25 year epidemiologic, clinical and pathologic study. *Ann Intern Med* 1978; 88: 162–167.

30. Machado EBV, Michet CJ, Ballard DJ *et al.* Trends in incidence and clinical presentation of temporal arteritis in Olmsted county, Minnesota, 1950–1985. *Arthritis Rheum* 1988; 31: 745–749.

31. Salvarani C, Gabriel SE, O'Fallon WM, Hunder GG. The incidence of giant cell arteritis in Olmsted County, Minnesota: apparent fluctuations in a cyclic pattern. *Ann Intern Med* 1995; 123: 192–194.

32. Salvarani C, Gabriel SE, O'Fallon WM, Hunder GG. Epidemiology of polymyalgia rheumatica in Olmsted County, Minnesota, 1970–1991. *Arthritis Rheum* 1995; 38: 369–373.

33. Franzen P, Sutinen S, von Knorring J. Giant cell arteritis and polymyalgia rheumatica in a region of Finland: an epidemiologic, clinical and pathologic study, 1984–1988. *J Rheumatol* 1992; 19: 273–276.

34. González-Gay MA, Garcia-Porrua C, Vázquez-Caruncho M, Dababneh A, Hajeer A, Ollier WE. The spectrum of polymyalgia rheumatica in northwestern Spain: incidence and analysis of variables associated with relapse in a 10 year study. *J Rheumatol* 1999; 26: 1326–1332.

35. Salvarani C, Macchioni P, Zizzi F, Mantovani W, Rossi F. Epidemiologic and immunogenetic aspects of poly-

myalgia rheumatica and giant cell arteritis in Northern Italy. *Arthritis Rheum* 1991; **34**: 351–356.

36. Sonnenblick M, Nesher G, Friedlander Y, Rubinow A. Giant cell arteritis in Jerusalem: a 12-year epidemiological study. *Br J Rheumatol* 1994; **33**: 938–941.

37. Petursdottir V, Johansson H, Nordborg E, Nordborg C. The epidemiology of biopsy-positive giant cell arteritis: special reference to cyclic fluctuations. *Rheumatology* 1999; **38**: 1208–1212.

38. Sen D, Scott DGI, Harvey I, Shepstone L. The epidemiology of polymyalgia rheumatica and giant cell arteritis: a community based study in the UK. *Arthritis Rheum* 1999; **42**: S300.

39. Friedman G, Friedman B, Benbassat J. Epidemiology of temporal arteritis in Israel. *Isr J Med Sci* 1982; **18**: 241–244.

40. Barrier J, Pion P, Massari R, Peltier P, Rojouan J, Grolleau JY. Approche epidemiologique de la maladie de Horton dans le departement de Loire-Atlantique 110 cas en 10 ans (1970–1979). *Rev Med Interne* 1982; **3**: 13–20.

41. Smith CA, Fidler WJ, Pinals RS. The epidemiology of giant cell arteritis. *Arthritis Rheum* 1983; **26**: 1214–1219.

42. Bell WR, Klinefelter HF. Polymyalgia rheumatica. *John Hopkins Med J* 1967; **121**: 175–187.

43. Sanford RG, Berney SN. Polymyalgia rheumatica and temporal arteritis in blacks—clinical features and HLA typing. *J Rheumatol* 1977; **4**: 435–442.

44. Kaufman RL. Polymyalgia rheumatica in blacks. *JAMA* 1978; **239**: 1612.

45. Love DC, Rapkin J, Lesser R *et al.* Temporal arteritis in blacks. *Ann Intern Med* 1986; **105**: 387–389.

46. Gilbert JL, Coe MD, Nam MH, Kolsky MP, Barth WF. Giant cell arteritis in African Americans. *J Clin Rheumatol* 1999; **5**: 116–120.

47. Emmerich J, Fiessinger JN. Epidemiologie et facteurs etiologiques des arterites a cellules geantes (maladie de Horton et maladie de Takayasu). *Ann Med Interne* 1998; **149**: 425–432.

48. Mijiyawa M, Amanga K, Oniankitan OI, Pitche P, Tchangai-Walla K. Les connectivites en consultation hospitaliere a Lome (Togo). *Rev Med Interne* 1999; **20**: 13–17.

49. Lie JT. Giant cell temporal arteritis in a Laotian Chinese. *J Rheumatol* 1992; **19**: 1651–1652.

50. Bosley TM, Riley FC. Giant cell arteritis in Saudi Arabia. *Int Ophthalmol* 1998; **22**: 59–60.

51. Thomas RD, Croft ND. Thyrotoxicosis and giant cell arteritis. *BMJ* 1974; **2**: 408–409.

52. Wiseman P, Stewart K, Rai GS. Hypothyroidism in polymyalgia rheumatica and giant cell arteritis. *BMJ* 1989; **298**: 647–648.

53. Dent RG, Edwards OM. Autoimmune thyroid disease and the polymyalgia rheumatica-giant cell arteritis syndrome. *Clin Endocrinol* 1978; **9**: 215–219.

54. Dasgupta B, Grundy E, Stainer E. Hypothyroidism in polymyalgia rheumatica and giant cell arteritis: lack of any association. *BMJ* 1990; **301**: 96–97.

55. Paice E, Smith C. Hypothyroidism in polymyalgia rheumatica and giant cell arteritis. *BMJ* 1990; **301**: 389.

56. Barrier JH, Abram M, Brisseau JM, Planchon B, Grolleau JY. Autoimmune thyroid disease, thyroid antibodies and giant cell arteritis: the supposed correlation appears fortuitous. *J Rheumatol* 1992; **19**: 1733–1734.

57. Machado EBV, Gabriel SE, Beard CM, Michet CJ, O'Fallon WM, Ballard DJ. A population-based case-control study of temporal arteritis: evidence for an association between temporal arteritis and degenerative vascular disease? *Int J Epidemiol* 1989; **18**: 836–841.

58. Duhaut P, Bornet H, Pinede L *et al.* Giant cell arteritis and thyroid dysfunction: multicentre case-control study. *BMJ* 1999; **318**: 434–435.

59. Duhaut P, Pinede L, Demolombe-Rague S. Giant cell arteritis and cardiovascular risk factors: a multicenter, prospective case-control study. *Arthritis Rheum* 1998; **41**: 1960–1965.

60. Duhaut P, Pinede L, Demolombe-Rague S *et al.* Giant cell arteritis and polymyalgia rheumatica: are pregnancies a protective factor? A prospective, multicentre case-control study. GRACG (Groupe de Recherche sur l'Arterite a Cellules Geantes). *Rheumatology* 1999; **38**: 118–123.

61. Barber HS. Myalgic syndrome with constitutional effects: polymyalgia rheumatica. *Ann Rheum Dis* 1957; **16**: 230–237.

62. Wadman B, Werner I. Observations on temporal arteritis. *Acta Med Scan* 1972; **192**: 377–383.

63. Liang GC, Simkin PA, Hunder GG, Wilske KR, Healey LA. Familial aggregation of polymyalgia rheumatica and giant cell arteritis. *Arthritis Rheum* 1974; **17**: 19–24.

64. Kvernebo K, Brath HK. Polymyalgia arteritica. *Scand J Rheumatol* 1980; **9**: 187–189.

65. Kemp A. Monozygotic twins with temporal arteritis and ophthalmic arteritis. *Acta Ophthalmol* 1977; **55**: 183–190.

66. Moss RR, Soukop M. Polymyalgia rheumatica in a sibling pair. two case reports and a brief review of the literature. *Scott Med J* 1988; **33**: 342–343.

67. Schwizer B, Pirovino M. Giant-cell arteritis—a genetically-determined disease. *Schweiz Med Wochenschr* 1994; **124**: 1959–1961.

68. Meyerhoff J, Hochberg MC. Monozygotic twins discordant for polymyalgia rheumatica. *J Rheumatol* 1982; **9**: 477–478.

69. Johansen M, Elling P, Elling H, Olsson A. A genetic approach to the aetiology of giant cell arteritis: depletion of the CD8+ T-lymphocyte subset in relatives of patients with polymyalgia rheumatica and arteritis temporalis. *Clin Exp Rheumatol* 1995; **13**: 6–8.

70. Rosenthal M, Muller W, Albert ED, Schattenkirchner M. HLA antigen in polymyalgia rheumatica. *N Engl J Med* 1975; **292**: 595.

71. Hazleman B, Goldstone A, Voak D. Association of polymyalgia rheumatica and giant-cell arteritis with HLA-B8. *BMJ* 1977; **2**: 989–990.

72. Hunder GG, Taswell HF, Pineda AA, Elveback LR. HLA antigens in patients with giant cell arteritis and polymyalgia rheumatica. *J Rheumatol* 1977; **4**: 321–323.

73. Seignalet J, Janbon C, Sany J *et al.* HLA in temporal arteritis. *Tissue Antigens* 1977; **9**: 69.

74. Armstrong RD, Behn A, Myles A, Panayi GS, Welsh KI. Histocompatibility antigens in polymyalgia rheumatica and giant cell arteritis. *J Rheumatol* 1983; **10**: 659–661.

75. Bridgeford PH, Lowenstein M, Bocanegra TS, Vasey FB, Germain BF, Espinoza LR. Polymyalgia rheumatica and giant cell arteritis: histocompatibility typing and hepatitis-B infection studies. *Arthritis Rheum* 1980; **23**: 516–518.

76. Hansen JA, Healey LA, Wilske KR. Association between giant cell (temporal) arteritis and HLA-CW3. *Hum Immunol* 1985; **13**: 193–198.

77. Malmvall BE, Bengtsson BA, Rydberg L. HLA antigens in patients with giant cell arteritis, compared with two control groups of different ages. *Scand J Rheumatol* 1980; **9**: 65–68.

78. Mattingly PC, Mowat AG, Gunson HH, Jackman C. HLA antigens in polymyalgia rheumatica. *BMJ* 1978; **1**: 989–990.

79. Ninet J, Gebuhrer L, Bonvoisin B *et al.* Groupage HLA DR dans les arterites a cellules geantes non apparentees. *Presse Med* 1987; **16**: 1725–1728.

80. Richardson JE, Dafna DG, Fam A, Keystone EC. HLA-DR4 in giant cell arteritis; association with polymyalgia rheumatica syndrome. *Arthritis Rheum* 1987; **30**: 1293–1297.

81. Terasaki PI, Healey LA, Wilske KR. Distribution of HLA haplotypes in polymyalgia rheumatica. *N Engl J Med* 1976; **295**: 905.

82. Barrier J, Bignon JD, Soulihollou JP, Grolleau J. Increased prevalence of HLA DR4 in giant cell arteritis. *N Engl J Med* 1981; **305**: 104–105.

83. Calamia KT, Moore SB, Elveback LR, Hunder GG. HLA-DR locus antigens in polymyalgia rheumatica and giant cell arteritis. *J Rheumatol* 1981; **8**: 993–996.

84. Lowenstein MB, Bridgeford PH, Vasey FB, Germain BF, Espinoza LR. Increased frequency of HLA-DR3 and DR4 in polymyalgia rheumatica-giant cell arteritis. *Arthritis Rheum* 1982; **25**: 31.

85. Armstrong RD, Panayi GS, Welsh KI. Polymyalgia rheumatica and rheumatoid arthritis; similarity of HLA antigen frequencies. *Arthritis Rheum* 1984; **27**: 1438–1439.

86. Cid MC, Ercilla G, Vilaseca J, Sanmarti R, Villalta J. Polymyalgia rheumatica: a syndrome associated with HLA-DR4 antigen. *Arthritis Rheum* 1988; **31**: 678–682.

87. Sakkas LI, Loqueman N, Panayi GS, Myles AB, Welsh KI. Immunogenetics of polymyalgia rheumatica. *Br J Rheumatol* 1990; **29**: 331–334.

88. Haworth S, Ridgeway J, Stewart I, Dyer PA, Pepper L, Ollier W. Polymyalgia rheumatica is associated with both HLA-DRB1*0401 and DRB1*0404. *Br J Rheumatol* 1996; **35**: 632–635.

89. Dababneh A, González-Gay MA, Garcia-Porrua C, Hajeer A, Thomson W, Ollier W. Giant cell arteritis and polymyalgia rheumatica can be differentiated by distinct patterns of HLA class II association. *J Rheumatol* 1998; **25**: 11–15.

90. Salvarani C, Boiardi L, Mantovani V *et al.* HLA-DRB1 alleles associated with polymyalgia rheumatica in northern Italy: correlation with disease severity. *Ann Rheum Dis* 1999; **58**: 303–308.

91. Weyand CM, Hunder NN, Hicok KC, Hunder GG, Goronzy JJ. HLA-DRB1 alleles in polymyalgia rheumatica, giant cell arteritis, and rheumatoid arthritis. *Arthritis Rheum* 1994; **37**: 4–20.

92. Labbe P, Flipo RM, Fajardy I *et al.* HLA DRB1 polymorphism in rhizomelic pseudo-polyarthritis and Horton disease. *Rev Med Interne* 1995; **16**: 10–81.

93. Rauzy O, Fort M, Nourhashemi F *et al.* Relation between HLA DRB1 alleles and corticosteroid resistance in giant cell arteritis. *Ann Rheum Dis* 1998; **57**: 6–2.

94. Weyand CM, Goehring BE, Ferrari G, Goronzy JJ. Polymorphisms of the interleukin-6 gene as disease risk factors in giant cell arteritis. *Arthritis Rheum* 1999; **42**: S209.

95. Sonnenblick M, Nesher B, Kramer MR, Gottschalk S. Increased frequency of temporal arteritis. *Harefuah* 1986; **110**: 556–558.

96. McCreary RD. 'Epidemic' of polymyalgia and temporal arteritis. *J Roy Coll Gen Pract* 1986; **36**: 523–524.

97. Nielsen JL. Polymyalgia rheumatica in a husband and wife. *Scand J Rheumatol* 1990; **9**: 177–178.

98. Garfinkel D, Bograd H, Salamon F *et al.* Polymyalgia rheumatica and temporal arteritis in a married couple. *Am J Med Sci* 1984; **287**: 48–49.

99. Faerk KK. Simultaneous occurrence of polymyalgia rheumatica in a married couple. *J Intern Med* 1992; **231**: 621–622.

100. Kinmont PC, McCallum DI. The aetiology, pathology and course of giant cell arteritis—the possible role of light sensitivity. *Br J Dermatol* 1965; **77**: 193.

101. Coomes EN, Ellis RM, Kay AG. A prospective study of 102 patients with the polymyalgia rheumatica syndrome. *Rheumatol Rehabil* 1976; **15**: 270–276.

102. Jonasson F, Cullen JF, Elton RA. Temporal arteritis. *Scott Med J* 1979; **24**: 111–117.

103. Mowat AG, Hazleman BL. A clinical study with particular reference to arterial disease. *J Rheumatol* 1974; **1**: 190–202.

104. Omland O, Sommer G, Elling H. Incidence of polymyalgia rheumatica/temporal arteritis in a Danish county. *Ugeskr Laeger* 1986; **148**: 981–983.

105. Raynauld JP, Bloch DA, Fries JF. Seasonal variation in the onset of Wegener's granulomatosis, polyarteritis nodosa and giant cell arteritis. *J Rheumatol* 1993; **20**: 1524–1526.

106. Cimmino MA, Caporali R, Montecucco CM, Rovida S, Baratelli E. A seasonal pattern in the onset of polymyalgia rheumatica. *Ann Rheum Dis* 1990; **49**: 521–523.

107. Lau H, Reid BJ, Weedon D. Actinic granuloma in association with giant cell arteritis: are both caused by sunlight? *Pathology* 1997; **29**: 260–262.

108. Liozon E, Loustaud V, Vidal E. Seasonal pattern in the incidence of giant cell arteritis: what can we conclude? *Rev Med Interne* 1999; **20**: 372–373.

109. Elling P, Olsson AT, Elling H. Synchronous variations of the incidence of temporal arteritis and polymyalgia rheumatica in different regions of Denmark: association with epidemics of mycoplasma pneumoniae infection. *J Rheumatol* 1996; **23**: 112–119.

110. Gabriel SE, Espy M, Erdman DD, Bjornsson J, Smith TF, Hunder GG. The role of parvovirus B19 in the pathogenesis of giant cell arteritis—a preliminary evaluation. *Arthritis Rheum* 1999; **42**: 1255–1258.

111. Hemauer A, Modrow S, Georgi J *et al*. There is no association between polymyalgia rheumatica and acute parvovirus B19 infection. *Ann Rheum Dis* 1999; **58**: 657–657.

112. Uddhammar A, Boman J, Juto P, Rantapaa-Dahlqvist S. Antibodies against Chlamydia pneumoniae, cytomegalovirus, enteroviruses and respiratory syncytial virus in patients with polymyalgia rheumatica. *Clin Exp Rheumatol* 1997; **15**: 299–302.

113. Cimmino MA, Grazi G, Balistreri M, Accardo S. Increased prevalence of antibodies to adenovirus and respiratory syncytial virus in polymyalgia rheumatica. *Clin Exp Rheumatol* 1993; **11**: 309–313.

114. Russo MG, Waxman J, Abdoh AA, Serebro LH. Correlation between infection and the onset of the giant cell (temporal) arteritis syndrome. *Arthritis Rheum* 1995; **38**: 374–380.

115. Bacon PA, Doherty SM. Hepatitis-B antibody in polymyalgia rheumatica. *Lancet* 1975; **2**: 476–478.

116. Elling H, Skinhoj P, Elling P. Hepatitis B virus and polymyalgia rheumatica; a search for HBsAg, HBsAb, HBeAg, and HBeAb. *Ann Rheum Dis* 1980; **39**: 511–513.

117. Liang M, Greenberg H, Pincus T, Robinson WS. Hepatitis B antibody in polymyalgia rheumatica. *Lancet* 1976; **1**: 43.

118. Fessel WJ. Polymyalgia rheumatica, temporal arteritis, and contact with birds. *Lancet* 1969; **2**: 1249–1250.

119. Ornilla E, Swannell AJ, Dixon AS. Myalgia and bird keeping. *Lancet* 1970; **1**: 96.

120. White AG, Innes EH. Polymyalgia rheumatica and contact with melopsittacus undulatus. *Rheum Phys Med* 1972; **11**: 380–384.

121. Vaith P, Rother E, Vogt A, Peter HH. Polymyalgia rheumatica nach Borrelieninfektion. *Immun Infekt* 1988; **16**: 71–73.

122. Shimamoto Y, Matsunaga C, Suga K, Fukushima N, Nomura K, Yamaguchi M. A human T-cell lymphotropic virus type I carrier with temporal arteritis terminating in acute myelogenous leukemia. *Scand J Rheumatol* 1994; **23**: 151–153.

123. Staud R, Corman LC. Association of parvovirus B19 infection with giant cell arteritis. *Clin Infect Dis* 1996; **22**: 6.

124. Duhaut P, Bosshard S, Calvet A *et al*. Giant cell arteritis, polymyalgia rheumatica, and viral hypotheses: a multicenter, prospective case-control study. Groupe de Recherche sur l'Arterite a Cellules Geantes. *J Rheumatol* 1999; **26**: 361–369.

125. Kyle V, Silverman B, Silman AJ, King RH, Reiss BB, Oswald NTA. Polymyalgia rheumatica/giant cell arteritis in a Cambridge general practice. *BMJ* 1985; **291**: 385–387.

126. Rajala SA, Ahvenainen JE, Mattila KJ, Saarni MI. Incidence and survival rate in cases of biopsy-proven temporal arteritis. *Scand J Rheumatol* 1993; **22**: 289–291.

127. Baldursson O, Steinsson K, Bjornsson J, Lie JT. Giant cell arteritis in Iceland. *Arthritis Rheum* 1994; **37**: 1007–1012.

128. Schaufelberger C, Bengtsson BA, Andersson R. Epidemiology and mortality in 220 patients with polymyalgia rheumatica. *Br J Rheumatol* 1995; **34**: 261–264.

129. González-Gay MA, Alonso MD, Aguero JJ, Bal M, Fernandez-Camblor B. Temporal arteritis in a Northwestern area of Spain: study of 57 biopsy proven patients. *J Rheumatol* 1992; **19**: 277–280.

130. Gonzalez-Gay MA, Garcia-Porrua C, Rivas MJ, Rodriguez-Ledo P, Llorca J. Epidemiology of biopsy proven giant cell arteritis in northwestern Spain: trend over a 18 year period. *Ann Rheum Dis* 2001; **60**: 367–371.

131. Haugeberg G, Paulsen PQ, Bie RB. Temporal arteritis in Vest Agder County in southern Norway: Incidence and clinical findings. *J Rheumatol* 2000; **27**: 2624–2627.

132. Liozon E, Loustaud V, Ly K, Vidal E. Association between infection and onset of giant cell arteritis: Can seasonal patterns provide the answer? *J Rheumatol* 2001; **28**: 1197–1198.

PART III

Degenerative and metabolic bone and joint diseases

12 | Osteoarthritis

Marc C. Hochberg

Osteoarthritis, also referred to as osteoarthrosis and degenerative joint disease, is the most common form of arthritis [1,2]. Prior to 1986, no standard definition of osteoarthritis existed; most authors described osteoarthritis as a disorder of unknown etiology in which articular cartilage and subchondral bone were primarily affected in contrast to rheumatoid arthritis, which primarily affects the synovial membrane. A standard definition of osteoarthritis, developed by the Subcommittee on Osteoarthritis of the American College of Rheumatology Diagnostic and Therapeutic Criteria Committee, was as follows [3]:

A heterogeneous group of conditions that lead to joint symptoms and signs which are associated with defective integrity of articular cartilage, in addition to related changes in the underlying bone at the joint margins.

A more comprehensive definition of osteoarthritis was developed by a National Institutes of Health sponsored conference on the Etiopathogenesis of Osteoarthritis and summarizes the clinical, pathophysiologic, biochemical, and biomechanical changes that characterize osteoarthritis [4]:

Clinically, the disease is characterized by joint pain, tenderness, limitation of movement, crepitus, occasional effusion, and variable degrees of local inflammation, but without systemic effects. Pathologically, the disease is characterized by irregularly distributed loss of cartilage more frequently in areas of increased load, sclerosis of subchondral bone, subchondral cysts, marginal osteophytes, increased metaphyseal blood flow, and variable synovial inflammation. Histologically, the disease is characterized early by fragmentation of the cartilage surface, cloning of chondrocytes, vertical clefts in the cartilage, variable crystal deposition, remodeling, and eventual violation of the tidemark by blood vessels. It is also characterized by evidence of repair, particularly in osteophytes, and later by total loss of cartilage, sclerosis, and focal osteonecrosis of the subchondral bone. Biomechanically, the disease is characterized by alteration of the tensile, compressive, and shear properties and hydraulic permeability of the cartilage, increased water, and excessive swelling. These cartilage changes are accompanied by increased stiffness of the subchondral bone. Biochemically, the disease is characterized

by reduction in the proteoglycan concentration, possible alterations in the size and aggregation of proteoglycans, alteration in collagen fibril size and weave, and increased synthesis and degradation of matrix macromolecules.

A more recent definition of osteoarthritis was developed in 1994 at a workshop entitled 'New Horizons in Osteoarthritis' sponsored by the American Academy of Orthopedic Surgeons, National Institute of Arthritis, Musculoskeletal and Skin Diseases, National Institute on Aging, Arthritis Foundation, and Orthopedic Research and Education Foundation [5]. This definition underscores the concept that osteoarthritis may not represent a single disease entity:

Osteoarthritis is a group of overlapping distinct diseases, which may have different etiologies but with similar biologic, morphologic, and clinical outcomes. The disease processes not only affect the articular cartilage, but involve the entire joint, including the subchondral bone, ligaments, capsule, synovial membrane, and periarticular muscles. Ultimately, the articular cartilage degenerates with fibrillation, fissures, ulceration, and full thickness loss of the joint surface.

This chapter will focus on issues of case definition of subjects with osteoarthritis in epidemiologic studies, morbidity and mortality of osteoarthritis, and risk factors for the development and progression of osteoarthritis by the joint group affected.

Classification

Osteoarthritis, as noted above, is a disorder of diverse etiologies which affects both small and large joints, either singly or in combination. A classification schema for osteoarthritis developed at the 'Workshop on Etiopathogenesis of Osteoarthritis' is shown in Table 12.1 [4]. Idiopathic osteoarthritis is divided into two forms: localized or generalized; the latter represents the form of osteoarthritis described by Kellgren and Moore [6] involving three or more joint groups. Hence, patients with osteoarthritis localized to the

Table 12.1   Classification of osteoarthritis

I. Idiopathic
  A. Localized
    1. Hands
    2. Feet
    3. Knee
    4. Hip
    5. Spine
    6. Other single sites
  B. Generalized
II. Secondary
  A. Traumatic
  B. Congenital or developmental diseases
  C. Metabolic diseases
    1. Ochronosis
    2. Haemochromatosis
    3. Wilson's disease
    4. Gaucher's disease
  D. Endocrine diseases
    1. Acromegaly
    2. Hyperparathyroidism
    3. Diabetes mellitus
    4. Hypothyroidism
  E. Calcium deposition disease
    1. Calcium pyrophosphate dihydrate deposition disease
    2. Apatite arthropathy
  F. Other bone and joint diseases
  G. Neuropathic (Charcot) arthropathy
  H. Endemic disorders
  I. Miscellaneous conditions

Modified from [4].

graphic changes described by Kellgren and Lawrence [8] and illustrated in the *Atlas of Standard Radiographs* [9]. These features include:

(1) formation of osteophytes on the joint margins or in ligamentous attachments, as on the tibial spines;

(2) periarticular ossicles, chiefly in relation to distal and proximal interphalangeal joints;

(3) narrowing of joint space associated with sclerosis of subchondral bone;

(4) cystic areas with sclerotic walls situated in the subchondral bone; and

(5) altered shape of the bone ends, particularly the head of the femur.

Combinations of these changes considered together led to the development of an ordinal grading scheme for severity: 0 = normal, 1 = doubtful, 2 = minimal, 3 = moderate, and 4 = severe. Different joints were graded using different characteristics; these differences are summarized for the small joints of the hands,

hands but involving three joint groups (i.e. distal and proximal interphalangeal joints and the thumb base) would be classified as having idiopathic generalized osteoarthritis. Furthermore, generalized osteoarthritis may occur either with or without Heberden's and Bouchard's nodes.

Patients with an underlying disease that appears to have caused their osteoarthritis are classified as having secondary osteoarthritis. Some forms of secondary osteoarthritis (e.g. that due to chronic trauma from leisure and/or occupation activities) may be considered as risk factors for idiopathic osteoarthritis; conversely, risk factors for idiopathic osteoarthritis (e.g. obesity) may be considered as causes of secondary osteoarthritis. A detailed discussion of the forms of secondary osteoarthritis can be found elsewhere [7].

Radiographic criteria

Classically, the diagnosis of osteoarthritis in epidemiologic studies has relied on the characteristic radio-

Table 12.2   Grades of severity of osteoarthritis in the small joints of the hands (*Atlas of Standard Radiographs*)

Distal interphalangeal joints
Grade 1: Normal joint except for one minimal osteophyte
Grade 2: Definite osteophytes at two points with minimal subchondral sclerosis and doubtful subchondral cysts, but good joint space and no deformity
Grade 3: Moderate osteophytes, some deformity of bone ends and narrowing of joint space
Grade 4: Large osteophytes and deformity of bone ends with loss of joint space, sclerosis and cysts

Proximal interphalangeal joints
Grade 1: Minimal osteophytosis at one point and possible cyst
Grade 2: Definite osteophytes at two points and possible narrowing of joint space at one point
Grade 3: Moderate osteophytes at many points, deformity of bone ends
Grade 4: Large osteophytes, marked narrowing of joint space, subchondral sclerosis and slight deformity

First carpometacarpal joint
Grade 1: Minimal osteophytosis and possible cyst formation
Grade 2: Definite osteophytes and possible cysts
Grade 3: Moderate osteophytes, narrowing of joint space and subchondral sclerosis and deformity of bone ends
Grade 4: Large osteophytes, severe sclerosis and narrowing of joint space

Modified from [5].

Table 12.3 Grades of severity of osteoarthritis of the knee (*Atlas of Standard Radiographs*)

Grade 1: Doubtful narrowing of joint space and possible osteophytic lipping
Grade 2: Definite osteophytes and possible narrowing of joint space
Grade 3: Moderate multiple osteophytes, definite narrowing of joint space and some sclerosis and possible deformity of bone ends
Grade 4: Large osteophytes, marked narrowing of joint space, severe sclerosis, and definite deformity of bone ends

Source: [5].

Table 12.4 Grades of severity of osteoarthritis of the hip (*Atlas of Standard Radiographs*)

Grade 1: Possible narrowing of joint space medially and possible osteophytes around femoral head.
Grade 2: Definite narrowing of joint space inferiorly, definite osteophytes and slight sclerosis.
Grade 3: Marked narrowing of joint space, slight osteophytes, some sclerosis and cyst formation and deformity of femoral head and acetabulum.
Grade 4: Gross loss of joint space with sclerosis and cysts, marked deformity of femoral head and acetabulum and large osteophytes.

Source: [5].

knees, and hips in Tables 12.2 to 12.4 and Figs 12.1 to 12.5, respectively.

Potential limitations of the use of the Kellgren–Lawrence grading schema, as illustrated in the *Atlas on Standard Radiographs* [9], have been noted [10–13]. In an attempt to address the limitations of a global grading scale, several groups developed radiographic grading schema which focus on individual radiographic features of osteoarthritis at specific joint groups; reliable grading scales have now been published for the hand [14], hip [15,16], knee [17,18], and all three peripheral joint groups [19]. Rating methods used in these scales for grading individual features are outlined in Tables 12.5–12.8, respectively. Using published atlases, trained readers have been shown to have excellent intra-reader and very good-to-excellent inter-reader reliability in measuring the presence and severity of osteoarthritis of the hand, hip, and knee; results of reproducibility studies were reviewed by Hart and Spector [12,13] and Lane and Kremer [20].

The validity of using individual radiographic features and a revised composite grading scale has been demonstrated in several studies. Croft *et al.* [15] examined the

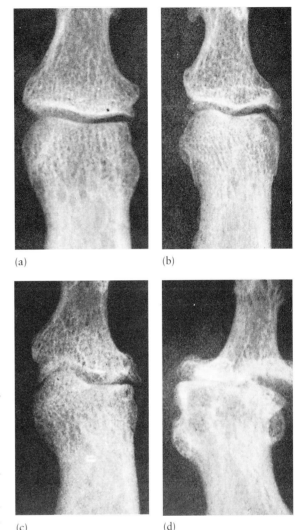

(a)   (b)

(c)   (d)

Fig. 12.1 Grades of severity of osteoarthritis of the distal interphalangeal joints. (a = Grade 1, b = Grade 2, c = Grade 3, d = Grade 4.)

association of individual radiographic features of osteoarthritis of the hip with reported hip pain in 759 men aged 60–75 years who had undergone intravenous urograms. The radiographic feature most strongly associated with reported hip pain was minimal joint space measured in millimeters; in addition, an overall qualitative grade of 3 or higher (see Table 12.7) was also strongly associated with reported hip pain. These findings were subsequently confirmed by Scott *et al.* [21] in a study of women aged 65 and above who had pelvic radiographs obtained on entry into a longitudinal study of risk factors for osteoporotic fractures.

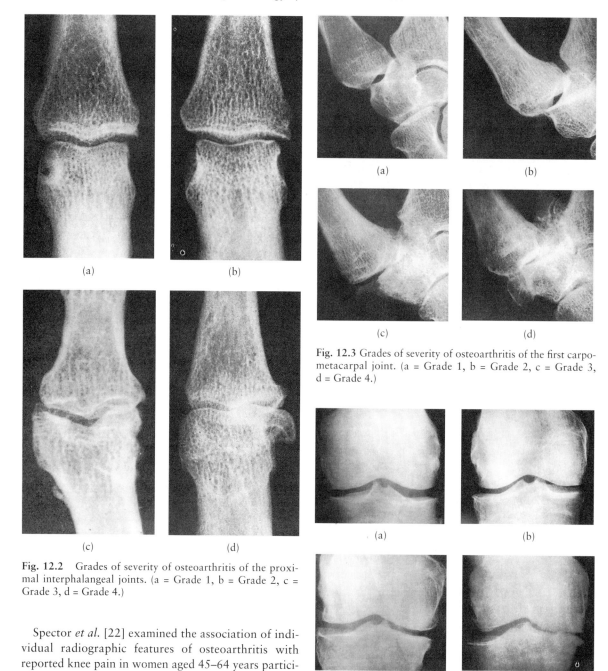

Fig. 12.2 Grades of severity of osteoarthritis of the proximal interphalangeal joints. (a = Grade 1, b = Grade 2, c = Grade 3, d = Grade 4.)

Fig. 12.3 Grades of severity of osteoarthritis of the first carpometacarpal joint. (a = Grade 1, b = Grade 2, c = Grade 3, d = Grade 4.)

Fig. 12.4 Grades of severity of osteoarthritis of the knee joints. (a = Grade 1, b = Grade 2, c = Grade 3, d = Grade 4.)

Spector *et al.* [22] examined the association of individual radiographic features of osteoarthritis with reported knee pain in women aged 45–64 years participating in the Chingford Study. They noted that the presence of definite osteophytes was the individual feature most strongly associated with reported knee pain. An analysis of data from the Baltimore Longitudinal Study on Aging [23] examined the association of both individual radiographic features and the global Kellgren–Lawrence grade with reported knee pain in 452 men and 223 women aged 18 and above. They

found that the strength of the association of definite osteophytosis with current knee pain was of a similar magnitude to that of grade 2 or higher osteoarthritis

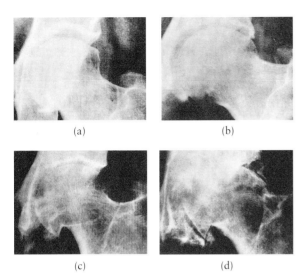

(a)   (b)

(c)   (d)

Fig. 12.5 Grades of severity of osteoarthritis of the hip joints. (a = Grade 1, b = Grade 2, c = Grade 3, d = Grade 4.)

Table 12.5 Baltimore Longitudinal Study of Aging grading scale for osteoarthritis of the hand

Feature	Grade	Definition
Osteophytes	0	None
	1	Small (definite) osteophyte
	2	Moderate osteophyte
	3	Large osteophyte
Joint space narrowing	0	None
	1	Mild definite narrowing
	2	Moderate-to-severe narrowing
	3	Bone-on-bone at ≥ 1 point
Subchondral sclerosis	0	Absent
	1	Present
Subchondral cysts	0	Absent
	1	Present
Lateral deformity	0	Absent
	1	Present
Collapse	0	Absent
	1	Present

Modified from [12].

using the Kellgren–Lawrence scale: OR of 4.4 (95% CI 2.6, 7.5) and 4.8 (95% CI 2.5, 8.5), respectively. This relationship was stronger and consistent among the more severe grades of osteoarthritis: osteophytes of grade 2 or higher were associated with current knee pain with an OR of 17.1 (95% CI 7.5, 38.7), while a Kellgren–Lawrence grade of 3 or higher was associated with current knee pain with an OR 20.8 (95% CI 8.6, 50.4). Thus, based on validity and reliability, future

Table 12.6 Baltimore Longitudinal Study of Aging grading scale for osteoarthritis of the knee

Feature	Grade	Definition
Osteophytes	0	None
	1	Small (definite) osteophyte
	2	Moderate osteophyte
	3	Large osteophyte
Joint space narrowing	0	None
	1	Mild definite narrowing
	2	Moderate narrowing
	3	Severe narrowing
Subchondral sclerosis	0	Absent
	1	Present
Sharpening of tibial spine	0	Absent
	1	Present
Chondrocalcinosis	0	Absent
	1	Present

Modified from [16].

Table 12.7 Croft's overall qualitative grade of osteoarthritis of the hip

Grade	Definition
0	No changes of osteoarthritis
1	Osteophytosis only
2	Joint space narrowing only
3	Two of osteophytosis, joint space narrowing, subchondral sclerosis, and cyst formation
4	Three of osteophytosis, joint space narrowing, subchondral sclerosis, and cyst formation
5	As in grade 4, but with deformity of femoral head

Modified from [13].

Table 12.8 Study of osteoporotic fractures grading scale for osteoarthritis of the hip

Grade	Definition
0	Normal film
1	Mild (grade 1) osteophyte and/or mild (grade 1) narrowing
2	Moderate (grade 2) narrowing and/or moderate-to-severe (grade 2–3) osteophyte
3	Severe (grade 3) narrowing and mild-severe (grade 1–3) osteophytes

Modified from [14].

population-based epidemiologic studies should consider relying on the presence of individual radiographic features of osteoarthritis for disease classification, and modified global scales, rather than on the Kellgren–Lawrence grading scale.

Clinical criteria

At the third International Symposium on population studies of the rheumatic diseases in 1966, the Subcommittee on Diagnostic Criteria for Osteoarthrosis recommended that future population-based studies should investigate the predictive value of certain historical, physical and laboratory findings for the typical radiographic features of osteoarthritis on a joint-by-joint basis [24]. Such historical features included pain on motion, pain at rest, nocturnal joint pain, and morning stiffness. Physical features included bony enlargement and expansion, limitation of motion, and crepitus. Laboratory features included erythrocyte sedimentation rate, tests for rheumatoid factor, serum uric acid, and appropriate analyses of synovial fluid.

In 1981, the Subcommittee on Osteoarthritis of the American College of Rheumatology's Diagnostic and Therapeutic Criteria Committee was established to develop clinical criteria for the classification of osteoarthritis [25]. The Subcommittee developed and validated criteria sets for the classification of osteoarthritis of the knee [3], hand [26], and hip [27]; these criteria sets have been amplified into algorithms for ease of use in clinical research and population-based studies [28]. It should be noted that these criteria sets identify subjects or patients with clinical osteoarthritis, as the major inclusion parameter is joint pain for most days of the prior month. This contrasts with the use of radiographic changes alone wherein many, if not most, subjects do not report joint pain. Thus, prevalence estimates using different case definitions will likely be systematically lower when based on the American College of Rheumatology criteria as opposed to traditional radiographic criteria: for example in a study of 400 women aged 45–65 years in Chingford, UK, Hart *et al.* [29] noted the prevalence of symptomatic knee osteoarthritis was only 2.3 per 100 compared to that of radiologically-defined knee osteoarthritis of 17 per 100. Readers, therefore, need to be aware of this when reviewing published studies.

The algorithms for classification of osteoarthritis of the knee (Table 12.9), hand (Table 12.10), and hip (Table 12.11) were all developed using patients with symptomatic osteoarthritis as cases and patients with site-specific joint pain due to other arthritic or musculoskeletal diseases as controls. For osteoarthritis of the knee, data on 85 historical, physical, laboratory, and radiographic features were collected in 130 patients with symptomatic osteoarthritis of the knee and 105 control patients with knee pain of other etiologies: 55 had rheumatoid arthritis [3]. For osteoarthritis of the

Table 12.9 Algorithm for classification of osteoarthritis of the knee, Subcommittee on Osteoarthritis, American College of Rheumatology Diagnostic and Therapeutic Criteria Committee

Clinical:
1 Knee pain for most days of prior month
2 Crepitus on active joint motion
3 Morning stiffness ≤ 30 min in duration
4 Age ≥ 38 years
5 Bony enlargement of the knee on examination
Osteoarthritis present if items 1, 2, 3, 4 *or* 1, 2, 5 *or* 1, 4, 5 are present

Clinical and radiographic:
1 Knee pain for most days of prior month
2 Osteophytes at joint margins (X-ray)
3 Synovial fluid typical of osteoarthritis (laboratory)
4 Age ≥ 40 years
5 Morning stiffness ≤ 30 min
6 Crepitus on active joint motion
Osteoarthritis present if items 1, 2 *or* 1, 3, 5, 6 *or* 1, 4, 5, 6 are present

Modified from [3,10].

Table 12.10 Algorithm for classification of osteoarthritis of the hand, Subcommittee on Osteoarthritis, American College of Rheumatology Diagnostic and Therapeutic Criteria Committee

Clinical:
1 Hand pain, aching, or stiffness for most days of prior month
2 Hard tissue enlargement of ≥2 of 10 selected hand joints[a]
3 MCP swelling in ≤2 joints.
4 Hard tissue enlargement of ≥2 DIP joints.
5 Deformity of ≥1 of 10 selected hand joints.
Osteoarthritis present if items 1, 2, 3, 4 *or* 1, 2, 3, 5 are present

Modified from [8,10].
Abbreviations: DIP = distal interphalangeal, PIP = proximal interphalangeal, MCP = metacarpophalangeal, CMC = carpometacarpal.
[a] Ten selected hand joints include bilateral 2nd and 3rd DIP joints, 2nd and 3rd PIP joints, and 1st CMC joints.

Table 12.11 Algorithm for classification of osteoarthritis of the hip, Subcommittee on Osteoarthritis, American College of Rheumatology Diagnostic and Therapeutic Criteria Committee

Clinical and radiographic:
1 Hip pain for most days of the prior month
2 Erythrocyte sedimentation rate <20 mm/h (laboratory)
3 Radiographic femoral and/or acetabular osteophytes
4 Radiographic hip joint space narrowing
Osteoarthritis present if items 1, 2, 3 *or* 1, 2, 4 *or* 1, 3, 4 are present

Modified from [9,10].

hand, data on 51 historical, physical, laboratory, and radiographic features were collected from 100 patients with symptomatic osteoarthritis of the hand and 99 control patients with hand pain of other etiologies: 74 had rheumatoid arthritis [26]. For osteoarthritis of the hip, data on 76 historical, physical, laboratory, and radiographic features were collected from 114 patients with symptomatic osteoarthritis of the hip and 87 control patients with hip pain of other etiologies: 37 had rheumatoid arthritis [27]. The sensitivity, specificity and accuracy of these algorithms approached or exceeded 90 per cent at all three sites; therefore, misclassification bias would probably not be a major problem in clinical research studies. Furthermore, Bellamy *et al.* [30], in a study of 85 twin pairs who were examined by three different rheumatologists blinded to one another's assessments, showed that the interrater agreement for the clinical criteria was excellent.

Morbidity

Prevalence

The prevalence of osteoarthritis using radiographic criteria has been studied world-wide [31–52]. Lawrence

[53] noted that estimates of prevalence in different populations by different investigators vary widely, in part due to the lack of reliability in the case definition attributed to observer variability in reading radiographs for changes of osteoarthritis. He suggested that in comparative studies, radiographs should be read by the same observer and must be read mixed [54]. This technique has been adopted in a study of the comparative epidemiology of knee and hip osteoarthritis in Beijing, China, and the United States that is currently in progress.

Kelsey [55], in reviewing data from several prevalence surveys, concluded that prevalence studies provided data on the magnitude of the problem, the demographic characteristics of those affected, the joints most frequently involved, the characteristics of generalized osteoarthritis, the correlation between symptomatology and radiographic changes and geographic differences in disease occurrence.

The largest prevalence surveys were those from the United States, the Health Examination Survey and First National Health and Nutrition Examination Survey (reviewed in [1,55]), and the Zoetermeer Survey in the Netherlands [44]. The National Arthritis Data Workgroup [1,56], a committee convened by the Arthritis Foundation, National Arthritis Advisory Board and National Institutes of Health, reviewed

Table 12.12   Prevalence per 100 of radiological changes of osteoarthritis in hands, feet, knees, and hips, by age and sex, US

Part of body	Ages (years)	Grades 2–4			Grades 3–4		
		Males	Females	Total	Males	Females	Total
Hands	25–74	32.0	33.0	32.5	5.4	0.2	7.9
	25–34	4.8	2.1	3.4	0.1	–	–
	35–44	17.5	11.3	14.3	0.6	1.1	0.9
	45–54	39.0	34.0	36.4	1.8	5.5	3.7
	55–64	56.6	68.8	63.0	12.6	21.5	17.3
	65–74	71.0	77.1	74.5	22.4	37.0	30.7
Knees	25–74	2.6	4.9	3.8	0.5	1.3	0.9
	25–34	−0.1	0.0	–	0.0	0.0	
	35–44	1.7	1.5	1.6	0.1	0.5	0.3
	45–54	2.3	3.6	3.0	0.2	0.5	0.4
	55–64	4.1	7.3	5.7	1.0	0.9	0.9
	65–74	8.3	18.0	13.8	2.0	6.6	4.6
Hips	25–74	1.3	–	–	0.5	–	–
	25–34	0.4	–	–	0.2	–	–
	35–44	0.1	–	–	–	–	–
	45–54	0.7	–	–	0.1	–	–
	50–54	–	0.8	–	–	0.1	–
	55–64	2.6	2.8	2.7	0.7	1.6	1.2
	65–74	4.6	2.7	3.5	2.3	1.2	1.7
	55–74	3.5	2.8	3.1	1.4	1.4	1.4

Modified from [27].

United States data on the prevalence of osteoarthritis by joint group from the Health Examination Survey, 1960–1962 [33] and the First National Health and Nutrition Examination Survey, 1971–1975 (NHANES-I) [39]. The case definition of osteoarthritis was based on radiographic changes in the hands and feet in the Health Examination Survey and on radiographic changes in knees and hips in NHANES-I. The prevalence of osteoarthritis among adults aged 25–74 in the United States was 32.5, 22.2, and 3.8 per 100 for the hands, feet and knees, respectively (Table 12.12). Prevalence increased with increasing age through the 65–74 year age group in both sexes; among persons aged 55–74 years of age, corresponding prevalence ratios were 70 per cent for the hands, 40 per cent for the feet, 10 per cent for the knees, and 3 per cent for the hips. Radiographs of the knees obtained in the NHANES-I were not taken in a weight-bearing position; hence, joint space narrowing may not have been present in subjects with cartilage loss, leading to an underestimate of the prevalence of moderate-to-severe grades of radiographic knee osteoarthritis. Population-based data from the Framingham Osteoarthritis Study, a prevalence survey of radiographic knee osteoarthritis in white elders aged 63 to 93 years in Framingham, Massachusetts, suggest that one-third of persons in this age group have evidence of definite radiographic osteoarthritis of the knees [42]. These results are similar to those from the Baltimore Longitudinal Study on Aging [46].

The pattern of age- and sex-specific prevalence of osteoarthritis found in the Zoetermeer survey (Table 12.13) [44] is similar to that noted in the studies conducted in the United States. Indeed, Van Saase *et al.* noted that the slopes of age-specific site-specific prevalence rates by gender were comparable between ten population surveys [44]. Thus, it appears that osteoarthritis increases in prevalence with increasing age suggesting the continued development of new or incident cases as the population ages. The gender difference, however, is markedly dependent on age and site (Fig. 12.6). At younger ages, below age 45, men tend to be affected more often than women, while at ages 55 and above women are affected more often than men. The major exception is the hip, which in the 45–64 year age group is more frequent in men, though this is less obvious with more severe disease. In addition, patterns of joint involvement also demonstrate gender differences with women having on average more joints involved and more frequent complaints of joint pain, morning stiffness, and joint swelling.

Table 12.13 Prevalence per 100 of radiologic changes in specific joint sites (Netherlands)

Joint	Age	Grades 2–4		Grades 3 and 4	
		Males	Females	Males	Females
Cervical spine	25–34	3.3	1.8	0.4	0.2
	35–44	18.0	13.1	4.3	3.8
	45–54	43.9	41.4	21.9	16.4
	55–64	64.3	63.0	36.6	34.3
	65–74	78.6	68.6	61.4	45.4
Lumber spine	25–34	–	–	–	–
	35–44	–	–	–	–
	45–54	42.9	52.0	15.8	18.9
	55–64	59.9	57.6	27.3	24.5
	65–74	71.6	64.0	36.7	35.9
Hand: DIP	25–34	1.2	0.4	–	–
	35–44	5.5	6.6	0.5	0.2
	45–54	18.7	30.6	2.2	2.4
	55–64	44.3	61.5	7.3	11.3
	65–74	54.7	75.5	9.5	22.3
Hand: CMCI	25–34	0.4	–	–	–
	35–44	2.3	3.7	–	0.1
	45–54	7.7	13.3	0.5	2.5
	55–64	17.9	29.0	3.7	6.3
	65–74	20.3	43.9	4.5	14.1
Knee: right	25–34	–	–	–	–
	35–44	–	–	–	–
	45–54	9.3	14.2	1.2	2.1
	55–64	16.8	18.6	3.3	2.4
	65–74	20.8	36.1	7.0	12.4
Knee: left	25–34	–	–	–	–
	35–44	–	–	–	–
	45–54	11.1	13.6	1.8	1.9
	55–64	14.3	18.3	2.5	3.6
	65–74	21.4	34.6	3.9	11.8
Hip: right	25–34	–	–	–	–
	35–44	–	–	–	–
	45–54	2.5	2.3	0.3	0.3
	55–64	7.8	3.1	1.5	1.4
	65–74	8.5	12.5	1.5	4.6
Hip: left	25–34	–	–	–	–
	35–44	–	–	–	–
	45–54	2.8	2.8	0.2	0.2
	55–64	8.3	2.6	2.0	0.7
	65–74	10.5	7.2	2.0	2.6

Source: [44]

Ethnic and geographic effects:

Racial differences have been noted in the distribution of joints affected by osteoarthritis. Some, but not all, studies found that African-American women have a higher age-adjusted prevalence of osteoarthritis of the knee than

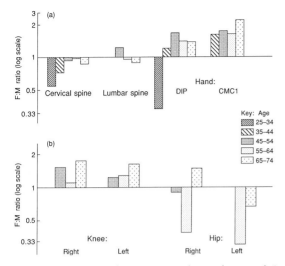

Fig. 12.6 Female to male ratio in prevalence of osteoarthritis (Grades 2–4) by age and site. (a) spine and hand joints; (b) hips and knees.

Caucasian women [52,57,58]. There are conflicting reports regarding differences in the age-adjusted prevalence of radiographic changes of osteoarthritis of the hand [33,52], but African-American women are less likely to have Heberden's nodes on physical examination than Caucasian women [59]. Studies among African blacks in Nigeria and Liberia and Jamaican blacks confirm the lower prevalence of Heberden's nodes [53]. There is no apparent difference between African-Americans and Caucasians [58,60] or between Native Americans and Caucasians [61] in the prevalence of radiographic changes of osteoarthritis of the hip. It has been suggested, however, that the prevalence of hip osteoarthritis is lower in Asian-Americans than in Caucasians; this inference is derived from comparative rates of total hip replacement for osteoarthritis in San Francisco, California, but may be subject to several limitations, including cultural and referral biases [62].

In contrast to the apparent lack of racial differences in prevalence of hip osteoarthritis between African-Americans and Caucasians in the United States, epidemiologic studies have found that Jamaican blacks [63], African and South African blacks [38,64], Chinese [65,66], and Asian Indians [67] all have lower prevalence rates of hip osteoarthritis than European Caucasians. This has been felt to be attributable to a lower rate of developmental hip disorders, one of the major risk factors for hip osteoarthritis [68], as well as the common use of the squatting posture, which forces the hip joint through an extreme range of motion [65].

Incidence

Several studies have examined the incidence of osteoarthritis of the hand. Plato and Norris [69] examined radiographs of the left hand of 478 male participants in the Baltimore Longitudinal Study of Aging who had two or more radiographs taken between 1958 and 1975. All films were read by one observer, blinded to time-sequence, using the Kellgren–Lawrence grading schema. These authors found that incidence of osteoarthritis at the distal interphalangeal joint increased with duration of follow-up and with advancing age given uniform duration of follow-up. In addition, these authors also found that existing osteoarthritis progressed with longer follow-up and the rate of progression increased at older ages.

Kallman *et al.* [70] analyzed data on 177 male participants from this dataset who were selected on the basis of having at least four hand radiographs taken over a 20-year follow-up interval. Herein, all films were also read by one observer, blinded to time-sequence, using both Kellgren–Lawrence scales and a new grading schema developed by the authors based on individual radiographic features [14]. They found that the incidence of osteoarthritis, defined by either Kellgren–Lawrence or individual features scales, was greatest at the distal interphalangeal joints and was significantly highest in the oldest age group, exceeding a rate of 100 per 1000 person-years at risk. Indeed, the relative risk of developing osteoarthritis in these men was 4 per cent per year. Thus, in men, the incidence of hand osteoarthritis increases with advancing age.

Sowers *et al.* [71] and Carman *et al.* [72] reported the 23-year cumulative incidence of hand osteoarthritis among women participants in the Tecumseh Community Health Study. They obtained radiographs of the hands and wrists of 588 men and 688 women who were aged 50 to 74 years old in 1985 and who had participated in the survey from 1962–65 when baseline radiographs were obtained. Age at baseline radiograph and greater baseline relative weight both predicted the grade of the following radiograph in a significant dose–response relationship. Thus, in both men and women, the development of hand osteoarthritis in females is directly related to age.

The incidence of radiographic osteoarthritis of the hand was also examined in 751 surviving members of the Framingham Osteoarthritis Study who underwent repeat hand radiographs in 1992–1993; these individuals had a mean age of 55 years at time of their baseline radiographs in 1967–1969 [73]. In those without hand osteoarthritis at baseline, the cumulative incidence of radiographic hand osteoarthritis was higher in women than men; the most common joints affected were the distal and proximal interphalangeal joints and joints at the thumb base. For those of both genders, with prevalent hand osteoarthritis at baseline, involvement of one joint in a row predicted an increased risk for incident osteoarthritis in another joint in that row. Similarly, involvement of one joint in a ray also increased the risk for incident osteoarthritis in another joint in that ray. Finally, prevalent osteoarthritis in the interphalangeal joints was a stronger predictor for incident osteoarthritis than prevalent disease in the joints of the thumb base.

The incidence of radiographic osteoarthritis of the knee was examined in 869 surviving members of the Framingham Osteoarthritis Study who underwent repeat standing knee radiographs in 1992–1993; these individuals had a mean age of 71 years at time of baseline knee radiographs in 1983–1985 [74]. The cumulative incidence of radiographic knee osteoarthritis was 18.1 per cent in women; the incidence was 1.7 times higher in women than men (95 % CI 1.0, 2.7). The cumulative incidence of symptomatic knee osteoarthritis was 8.1 per cent in women. These rates did not differ by age (persons below age 70 or age 70 and above); as noted above, rates were 80 to 100 per cent higher in women than men, after adjusting for age. The incidence of radiographic knee osteoarthritis was also examined in 715 middle-aged women from the Chingford Study who underwent repeat standing knee radiographs at baseline and 4 years later [75]. The paired films were read for the individual radiographic features of osteophytes and joint space narrowing using an atlas. Incident knee osteophytes developed in 13.3 per cent of women, equating to an incidence rate of 3.3 per 100 per year.

The incidence of clinically diagnosed, symptomatic osteoarthritis of the hand, hip, and knee has been estimated in two studies [76,77]. Wilson *et al.* [76] identified all residents of Rochester, Minnesota who sought medical care for the first time in 1985 for symptomatic osteoarthritis of a lower limb joint. They estimated age- and sex-adjusted incidence rates of 205 cases of symptomatic lower limb osteoarthritis per 100 000 person-years. Incidence was greater for knee than hip osteoarthritis, was greater in women than in men, and increased with increasing age in both sexes. The more recent data, based on persons who were members of the Fallon Community Health Plan in Massachusetts between 1988 and 1992, showed that the age- and sex-standardized incidence of symptomatic hand, hip, and knee osteoarthritis, defined by

joint symptoms with radiographic confirmation of disease, was 100 (95% CI 86, 115) per 100 000 person-years, 88 (95% CI 75, 101) per 100 000 person-years, and 240 (95% CI 218, 262) per 100 000 person-years, respectively [77]. Incidence rates increased with increasing age in both sexes, and rates were higher in women than in men, especially after age 50. Maximal incidence rates in women were 529, 583, and 1082 cases per 100 000 person-years in the 70–79 year age group, respectively. Incidence rates remained steady or declined slightly in persons aged 80 to 89 years. No cases of symptomatic osteoarthritis occurred in women below age 30, while only five cases occurred in women below age 40 years.

Mortality

Few data are available on mortality with osteoarthritis [78]. Osteoarthritis is not a disorder that, by itself, causes death. However, treatments administered to patients with osteoarthritis, particularly non-steroidal anti-inflammatory drugs, and factors associated with osteoarthritis, for example obesity, may contribute to excess mortality and/or decreased survival among patients with osteoarthritis.

Manson and Hall [79] studied mortality among 617 patients with osteoarthritis admitted to the Robert Breck Brigham Hospital in Boston, Massachusetts between 1930 and 1960. They determined vital status as of 1972 and compared the observed results to those expected using the age-sex-specific mortality rates for the State of Massachusetts and the United States. The relative survival rates remained near 100 for at least 10 years after admission in both males and females. The standardized mortality ratio, based on 338 observed deaths, was 111; for individual causes of death, this ratio exceeded 200 for gastrointestinal disorders. Indeed, gastrointestinal disorders comprised 6 per cent of observed deaths compared to only 3 per cent of expected deaths. This is probably attributed to the use of regular doses of aspirin by these patients, since aspirin and related non-steroidal anti-inflammatory drugs have been shown to be associated with both the development of and death from peptic ulcer disease and upper gastrointestinal bleeding [80–82].

The excess mortality and decreased survival of persons with osteoarthritis was confirmed in a secondary analysis of data from the First National Health and Nutrition Examination Survey and the National Health and Nutrition Examination-I Followup

Epidemiologic Survey [83]. Survival rates, adjusted for age and duration of follow-up in proportional hazards models, were significantly lower in women with knee osteoarthritis than in women with normal knee radiographs, no differences were found among men. Too few subjects with hip osteoarthritis were identified for performing reliable survival analysis. Causes of death and proportionate mortality ratios have not been reported for these subjects.

The relationship between radiographically defined osteoarthritis and survival was examined in a cohort of 296 women who underwent full-body radiographs when first employed in the radium dial-painting industry [84]. Women with an increasing number of joints affected with osteoarthritis had decreased survival; the age-adjusted hazard ratio was 1.45 for each 3-unit increase in the number of joints involved. These results were largely unchanged after adjustment for body mass index, smoking, and comorbid conditions.

Risk factors

The approach to considering risk factors for the development of osteoarthritis is related to considerations of idiopathic/primary osteoarthritis or secondary osteoarthritis. As noted in Table 12.1, for purposes of classification, when a particular factor is identified as causing osteoarthritis, for example congenital or developmental hip disease and hip osteoarthritis, then the subject is classified as having secondary osteoarthritis. Despite this somewhat artificial classification, studies of risk factors for osteoarthritis are best approached by considering the disease on a joint-specific basis. Furthermore, risk factors can be broadly categorized as genetic and non-genetic host factors, and environmental factors. Thus, we will first examine the role of genetic factors followed by the association of other host factors and environmental factors by joint-group affected.

Genetic factors

Family studies

The subset of osteoarthritis in which genetic factors appear to be most important is generalized osteoarthritis accompanied by Heberden's nodes. Stecher [85] first presented evidence that the occurrence of Heberden's nodes was strongly influenced by heredity. Family his-

tories of Heberden's nodes were determined from 66 Caucasian female probands; Heberden's nodes were reported in 21 of 66 mothers and 33 of 129 sisters. In a control series of 43 non-arthritic women, none of the mothers and only five of 109 sisters had Heberden's nodes. Furthermore, there was a two-fold excess of Heberden's nodes among mothers and three-fold excess among sisters when compared with expected values. Subsequently, Stecher and Hersh [86] examined the mode of inheritance of Heberden's nodes in multicase families. Analysis based on 74 pedigrees containing 72 female and two male probands, and 143 sisters and 125 brothers, suggested autosomal dominant inheritance in women (108 of 215 affected), and autosomal recessive inheritance in men (only four of 127 affected). Gene frequency analysis, using a phenotypic frequency of 30 per cent in women age 70 and above, revealed a frequency of 0.163 for the dominant allele and 0.837 for the recessive normal allele. Further studies, correcting for small family size and analyzing types of parental matings, were consistent with the single gene model [87,88].

Further studies of the genetic factors in generalized osteoarthritis were conducted by Kellgren and colleagues in England in the 1950s [53,89]. They studied families of probands with generalized osteoarthritis involving six or more joint groups and found a two-fold excess in relatives aged 45 and above compared with expected prevalence: 36 per cent versus 17 per cent in males and 49 per cent versus 26 per cent in females [89]. Analysis of the subset of probands with Heberden's nodes revealed a striking familial aggregation with a 4.5-fold excess in female relatives of female probands and an 8.5-fold excess in female relatives of male probands. The authors concluded that there is an hereditary predisposition to this form of osteoarthritis in females. Further analysis of these family data demonstrated that they were more consistent with a polygenic rather than a single gene autosomal dominant model in families with female probands [52].

Recent analyses of data from the Baltimore Longitudinal Study on Aging confirmed familial aggregation of osteoarthritis at each of the three commonly affected joint groups in the hands, as well as polyarticular osteoarthritis, in sib pairs [90]. Similar results were noted in the Framingham Study where a formal segregation analysis suggested that the best-fit models were mixed models with a Mendelian mode of inheritance and a residual multifactorial component, representing either polygenic or environmental factors [91].

Family studies have also demonstrated familial aggregation of severe hip osteoarthritis resulting in total hip arthroplasty [92]. The authors studies 1171 sibs and 376 spouses of 402 probands who underwent total joint arthroplasty for idiopathic osteoarthritis. They reported an increased risk for both total hip and total knee arthroplasty among sibs using the spouses as controls: RR of 1.86 (95% CI 0.93, 3.69) and 4.8 (95% CI 0.64, 36.4), respectively. Combining the outcome to any lower limb total joint arthroplasty and limiting the analysis to sibs and spouses aged 65 and above gave a significant increased RR of 2.32 (95% CI 1.22, 4.43). Although shared environmental factors in early life could account for these findings, they do support a role for genetic factors in the development of severe lower limb osteoarthritis.

Twin studies

The original twin studies conducted by the Arthritis and Rheumatism Council in the UK confirmed a hereditary nature for nodal generalized osteoarthritis involving three or more joint groups [53]. More recently, classic twin studies of twin pairs identified from twin registries have been used to examine the genetic influences on osteoarthritis [93,94]. Spector *et al.* [93] studied 130 monozygotic and 120 dizygotic female twin pairs aged 44–77 years for the heritability of radiographic features of osteoarthritis of the hands and knees. They found that the intra-class correlation of total radiographic osteoarthritis, including osteophytes and joint space narrowing, was greater in identical than in non-identical twins, with an estimated heritability of 54 per cent (95% CI 43, 65) after adjustment for age and weight. Of interest, estimated heritability was greater for osteoarthritis of the knees than osteoarthritis of the hands. They concluded that there was a clear genetic influence on radiographic features of osteoarthritis of both the hand and knee in women, independent of other major risk factors for osteoarthritis in women. Recently, these findings have been extended to osteoarthritis of the hip by the same investigative group [95]. In this study of 135 monozygotic and 277 dizygotic female twin pairs aged 50 and above, the estimated heritability for osteoarthritis of the hip was 58 per cent.

Genetic markers

Many studies have been conducted to explore the molecular basis for the genetic predisposition to generalized osteoarthritis in multiplex families [96–99]. The earliest interest focused on the gene for type II collagen, COL2A1. Pelotie *et al.* [96] reported the cosegregation of a polymorphism of COL2A1 with generalized osteoarthritis in two families, while Knowlton *et al.* [98] reported cosegregation of a polymorphism of COL2A1 with disease in a family with 'primary osteoarthritis and a mild chondrodysplasia'. Subsequent studies by the latter group demonstrated a single base mutation converting a codon for arginine at position 519 to one for cysteine [97]. However, in a study of 61 patients with nodal generalized osteoarthritis, there was no significant difference in the allelic frequencies of COL2A1 compared to expectations based on data from 37 health unrelated controls [100]. Two additional studies failed to confirm an association between loci encoding COL2A1 and either generalized osteoarthritis [101,102]. Analysis of data from the Rotterdam Study, on the other hand, did demonstrate an association between both a Hind III and a VNTR polymorphism of the COL2A1 gene and generalized osteoarthritis [103]; more recent analyses from this data set showed that the VNTR polymorphism was associated with joint space narrowing rather than osteophyte formation [104].

These data raise the possibility that polymorphisms of other genes encoding other cartilage components such as types IX and XI collagen, proteoglycans, or link proteins may lead to a syndrome which phenotypically resembles generalized osteoarthritis. Horton *et al.* [105] studied the relationship between polymorphisms of the human aggrecan proteoglycan gene and hand osteoarthritis in older Caucasian men from the Baltimore Longitudinal Study on Aging. They identified an association between the presence of the VNTR allele 27 with bilateral hand osteoarthritis (OR 3.23; 95% CI 1.24, 8.41); the association of this allele with bilateral knee osteoarthritis was not significant.

Other attention has focused on the relationship between the vitamin D receptor (VDR) gene and osteoarthritis. Of five published studies, two noted an association between a VDR polymorphism and radiographic osteoarthritis of the knee, characterized by osteophytosis [104,106,107], while three studies, which included cases of osteoarthritis at the hand, hip, knee and other sites, failed to demonstrate an association [102,108,109]. It is possible that the association between VDR polymorphisms and radiographic osteoarthritis may differ by site of osteoarthritis, may be confounded by bone mineral density, or may vary by ethnic group studied.

Finally, one study has noted an association between a polymorphism in the promoter region of the gene for insulin-like growth factor 1 (IGF-1) and the presence of radiographic osteoarthritis with a dose–response relationship: for heterozygous subjects OR = 1.9 (95% CI 1.2, 3.1) and homozygous subjects OR = 3.6 (95% CI 0.8, 16.2) [110].

Obviously, further studies of genetic markers of osteoarthritis will continue with the hope of identifying genes not only associated with disease in population samples, but also linked to disease in multiplex families.

Non-genetic host factors

Overweight

Overweight is clearly the most important, modifiable risk factor for the development of knee osteoarthritis in both sexes; however, its association with hand and hip osteoarthritis remains somewhat controversial.

Many epidemiologic studies have found a cross-sectional association between obesity and radiographic knee osteoarthritis [53,57,111–122]. In both sexes, mean body mass index is significantly higher among subjects with knee osteoarthritis than without, and body mass index is associated with knee osteoarthritis in a dose–response relationship [57]. In addition, high body mass index is more strongly associated with bilateral than unilateral knee osteoarthritis [116]. Furthermore, the strength of the association between body mass index and knee osteoarthritis is not diminished by adjustment for fat distribution and per cent body fat [117,120], nor is it diminished by adjustment for potential confounding variables including age, race, blood pressure, serum cholesterol, serum uric acid, body fat distribution, and history of diabetes [115,123,124].

These cross-sectional data have been confirmed in analyses of longitudinal data reported from the Framingham Study [113,125], the Chingford Study [126], the Baltimore Longitudinal Study of Aging [127], the Matsudai Knee Osteoarthritis Survey [128], the Johns Hopkins Precursors Study [129], and a longitudinal study conducted in Bristol, UK [130].

In persons who are overweight, data from the Framingham Study suggest that weight loss results in a decreased risk of developing knee osteoarthritis [125,131]. In the Framingham Osteoarthritis Study, persons who lost weight in the 10-year period prior to their baseline radiograph had 50 per cent reduced odds

of having radiographic knee osteoarthritis for every 2 kg/m^2 decrease in body mass index [131]. In the prospective component of the Framingham Osteoarthritis Study, persons who lost 5 pounds or more between the baseline and follow-up radiographs had a reduced risk of developing knee osteoarthritis compared to persons who weight remained stable: RR = 0.5 (95% CI 0.2, 1.1) [125]. In the Matsudai Knee Osteoarthritis Survey, overweight women who lost 2 or more body mass index units during the 14 years of follow-up had a lower risk of progression of their knee osteoarthritis [128].

The association of obesity with radiographic hand osteoarthritis remains controversial [49,53,72,111, 117–119,121,132–134]. A secondary analysis of data from the US Health Examination Survey failed to demonstrate a significant association between body mass index and hand osteoarthritis in either males or females after adjustment for age and body fat distribution [117]. Analyses of data from the Baltimore Longitudinal Study of Aging also failed to demonstrate a significant association between body mass index and hand osteoarthritis in men or women after adjustment for age [133,134]. However, these results were derived from cross-sectional analyses. Carman *et al.* [72] analyzed prospective data from the Tecumseh Community Health Study and found that baseline obesity, as measured by an index of relative weight, was a significant independent predictor of both the incidence and severity of hand osteoarthritis. Hochberg and colleagues, in an analysis of data from the Baltimore Longitudinal Study of Aging, did not find an association between increased body weight and incidence or progression of hand osteoarthritis in men [135].

The results of cross-sectional studies examining the association of obesity with radiographic hip osteoarthritis suggest that the relationship is of lower strength that that with osteoarthritis of the knee [60,112,118,136–139]. Several of these studies have demonstrated that the association with overweight is stronger for bilateral hip osteoarthritis than unilateral hip osteoarthritis [60,136,139]. Finally, obesity has also been shown to be a risk factor for symptomatic incident osteoarthritis involving the hands, hips, and knees [140], and incident symptomatic arthritis [141].

Sex hormones

The recognized gender differences in the prevalence of site-specific osteoarthritis (see above) have led several investigators to examine the role of female reproductive variables and gynecologic disorders and procedures as risk factors for osteoarthritis [142–144]. Spector *et al.* [142] found that patients with osteoarthritis were more likely to have undergone a hysterectomy than patients with rheumatoid arthritis and non-arthritis controls. Hannan *et al.* [143], analyzing data from the Framingham study, failed to confirm this association. Dennison *et al.* [144] were also unable to find an association of hysterectomy with hip osteoarthritis, although they did note an association between oophorectomy and hip osteoarthritis (OR = 1.9; 95% CI 1.0, 3.7). Given the lack of consistent findings across these studies, it is unlikely that a specific gynecologic procedure is itself a risk factor for osteoarthritis.

The role of estrogen replacement therapy as a protective factor has been examined by several groups. Hannan *et al.* [143] reported that postmenopausal women who were current users of hormone replacement therapy had reduced odds of radiographic knee osteoarthritis; this association, however, failed to achieve statistical significance. Some, but not all, subsequent studies provided supporting data for a protective association between current use of hormone replacement therapy and radiographic changes of lower limb osteoarthritis [137,138,144–147]. Indeed, a meta-analysis of these observational studies supports such a protective association [148]. Two recent prospective epidemiologic studies both reported a reduction in the relative risk for incident radiographic knee osteoarthritis among postmenopausal women who were current users of estrogen replacement therapy; however, in neither study was the association statistically significant [75,149]. In the Framingham Study, the RR among current users compared to never users was 0.4 (95% CI 0.1, 3.0) [149], while in the Chingford Study, the RR among current users compared to never users was 0.4 (95% CI 0.1, 1.4) [75]. These recent data were reviewed by Wluka and colleagues [150] in the context of an overview of the relationship between menopause, hormone replacement therapy, and musculoskeletal disease in general.

It is unclear, however, whether the association described above is clinically relevant. Sahyoun and colleagues [151] noted that postmenopausal women who were participants in the NHANES-I Epidemiologic Followup Survey and took hormone replacement therapy had a greater risk of developing symptomatic arthritis than women who did not use hormone replacement therapy. Sandmark *et al.* [152] noted that postmenopausal women who underwent total knee arthroplasty had a greater odds of having taken hormone replacement therapy (OR = 1.8; 95% CI 1.2– 2.6). Finally, estrogen replacement therapy was not associated with the patterns of joint involvement in a cohort of 475 women who underwent total joint arthroplasty for severe lower limb osteoarthritis [153]. It is likely that a definitive resolution of this issue will not be available until final results from placebo-controlled, long-term trials of hormone replacement therapy (e.g. the Women's Health Initiative) are available later this decade.

The relationship between serum levels of gonadal sex hormones and osteoarthritis has been examined in several studies [154–156]. Sowers *et al.* [156] reported that women with more severe hand osteoarthritis had lower mean testosterone levels, while women with knee osteoarthritis had higher mean estradiol levels. Neither of the other studies found significant differences in hormone levels between cases with osteoarthritis and controls.

Bone mineral density

The relationship between bone mineral density and osteoarthritis has been studied for almost 30 years, since the initial observations of Foss and Byers [157] that the per cent cortical area of the second metacarpal was greater in patients who had femoral head resections for hip osteoarthritis compared to those who had femoral head resections for hip fracture. Many cross-sectional studies which utilized radiogrammetry and single photon absorptiometry confirmed the association between higher bone mineral density and osteoarthritis of the hip, but provided conflicting data on such an association with osteoarthritis of the hand and generalized osteoarthritis; these studies were reviewed by Star and Hochberg [158].

The advent of dual X-ray absorptiometry and the recruitment of cohorts of patients with osteoarthritis for longitudinal studies spurred investigation in this area. Several cross-sectional studies have reported associations between higher mean levels of bone mineral density measured at the lumbar spine and/or hip and presence of radiographic osteoarthritis at multiple sites including the hand, hip, knee, and lumbar spine [159–163]; these studies were reviewed by Sambrook and Naganathan [164] and Stewart and Black [165]. Higher levels of bone mineral density are also associated with increased risk of developing radiographic osteoarthritis of the knee [166].

While patients with osteoarthritis have higher adjusted levels of bone mineral density, there appears to be no difference in the rate of fractures, possibly due to differences in muscle strength and body sway, which might contribute to the risk of falling [167–169].

Possible explanations for the relationship between higher bone mineral density and radiographic osteoarthritis include shared genetic factors, particularly common genetic markers such as the VDR polymorphism (see above), as well as non-genetic factors related to rates of bone turnover [170,171] and use of non-steroidal anti-inflammatory drugs [172,173].

Acetabular dysplasia and hip osteoarthritis

One prospective study has demonstrated an association between acetabular dysplasia, defined as an abnormal center-edge angle or decreased acetabular depth, with an increased incidence of radiographic hip osteoarthritis: the RR, adjusted for age and body mass index, was 2.8 (95% CI 1.0, 7.9) [174].

Chondrocalcinosis and knee osteoarthritis

Two population-based studies have both demonstrated a significant association between radiographic articular chondrocalcinosis in the knees and knee osteoarthritis [175,176]. In data from the First Health and Nutrition Examination Survey limited to subjects age 55 to 74 years, chondrocalcinosis was associated with knee osteoarthritis with an odds ratio of 2.7 [175]. In the Framingham Osteoarthritis Study, the age-adjusted odds ratio was 1.5 in both sexes [176]. The epidemiology of calcium pyrophosphate dihydrate crystal deposition disease is reviewed in Chapter 14.

Other factors

Serum uric acid levels were reported to be associated with non-nodal generalized osteoarthritis in data from the New Haven Survey of Joint Diseases [111]; however, there was no association of serum acid levels and knee osteoarthritis in the Framingham study [177], the First National Health and Nutrition Examination Survey [57], or the Chingford Study [123]. In the latter study, the authors did note an association between elevated blood glucose levels and knee osteoarthritis independent of body mass index [123]. However, Frey *et al.* [178] were unable to demonstrate an association between either impaired glucose tolerance or non-insulin dependent diabetes mellitus and the presence of clinical osteoarthritis.

Environmental factors

Occupation

Certain occupations which require repetitive use of particular joints over long periods of time have been associated with the development of site-specific osteoarthritis. Specific occupational groups with increased risks include: miners, who have an excess of knee and lumbar spine disease [179]; dockers and shipyard laborers, who have an excess of hand and knee osteoarthritis [180,181]; cotton and mill workers, who have an excess of hand osteoarthritis involving specific finger joints [182,183]; pneumatic drill operators, who have an excess of elbow and wrist osteoarthritis [184]; and farmers, who have an excess of hip osteoarthritis [185–190]. A systematic review and meta-analysis of the relationship between occupational physical activity and lower limb osteoarthritis was published by Maetzel and colleagues [191].

Data from two large United States population surveys have also been analyzed to study this association in unselected groups. Engel and Burch [132] reported that the prevalence of hand osteoarthritis was higher than expected in men employed as craftsmen and/or foremen, and lower than expected in men employed as either clerical or sales workers or private household or service workers. Anderson and Felson [57] found that occupations requiring high knee-bending demands and physically demanding labor were significantly associated with knee osteoarthritis in men and women aged 55 to 64 years after adjustment for race, body mass index, and educational level.

The association between occupational knee bending and physically demanding work was confirmed in men in the Framingham cohort [192]. Men who were employed in jobs requiring knee-bending and medium, heavy, or very heavy physical demands had a two-fold greater risk of developing radiographic knee osteoarthritis than men employed in jobs not requiring knee bending and with only sedentary or light physical demands. Cooper *et al.* [193] also tested the hypothesis that specific occupational physical activities were risk factors for knee osteoarthritis in a population-based, case–control study in Bristol, England. Subjects with moderate-to-severe knee osteoarthritis were significantly more likely than controls to report occupations which required 30 min per day or more of squatting or kneeling, or climbing more than 10 flights of stairs.

Occupational physical activity has also been shown to be associated with hip osteoarthritis [194–196].

Roach *et al.* [194] compared work load, based on estimated joint compression forces produced by an occupational activity, in 99 men with idiopathic hip osteoarthritis and 233 controls known to be free of hip osteoarthritis. After adjustment for overweight and history of sports activities, men with hip osteoarthritis had a 2.5-fold greater odds of having performed heavy workload than controls. Furthermore, there was a dose–response relationship between a greater duration of work requiring heavy workload and greater odds of hip osteoarthritis. Vingard *et al.* [195,196] performed a register-based cohort study to investigate the relationship between occupational exposure with the risk of symptomatic knee and hip osteoarthritis requiring hospitalization. Several associations were identified between specific blue-collar occupations and an increased risk of hospitalization for both symptomatic knee and hip osteoarthritis in both men and women. These occupations shared a common feature of requiring heavy physical work load. However, a recent case–control study conducted in England failed to demonstrate an association between occupational lifting and hip osteoarthritis in women [139]. In this study, only 15 per cent of the 401 women studied had been in paid employment for 90 per cent or more of their working lives [139].

Thus, certain occupations that repetitively stress apparently normal joints through repeated use appear to predispose to the development of lower limb osteoarthritis.

Sports, leisure-time activity, and joint injury

Most data suggest that individuals who participate in sports at a highly competitive level (i.e. elite athletes) or who have abnormal or injured joints are at increased risk of developing osteoarthritis [197–204]. In contrast, individuals who have normal joints and participate in low-impact sports as a recreational activity do not appear to be at an increased risk of developing osteoarthritis, unless they have extremely high levels of leisure-time physical activity [205–207]. Clearly, joint injury plays a major role, probably as an effect modifier of the relationship between both sports activity and leisure-time physical activity in osteoarthritis.

In an analysis of data from the First National Health and Nutritional Examination Survey, Davis and colleagues [116] found that a history of knee injury was significantly associated with both ipsilateral and bilateral knee osteoarthritis, but not contralateral knee osteoarthritis. Overall, a history of right knee injury

was present in 5.8 per cent of subjects with bilateral knee osteoarthritis, 15.8 per cent of 37 subjects with right knee osteoarthritis and 1.5 per cent of controls, while a history of left knee injury was present in 4.6 per cent of those with bilateral knee osteoarthritis, 27.0 per cent of subjects with left knee osteoarthritis, and 1.8 per cent of controls. In multiple polychotomous logistic regression analysis adjusting for age, sex, and body mass index, the OR for the association of knee injury with bilateral knee osteoarthritis was 3.51 (95% CI 1.80, 6.83) as compared with right knee osteoarthritis and left knee osteoarthritis of 16.30 (95% CI 6.50, 40.9) and 10.90 (95% CI 3.72, 31.93), respectively. The association between lower limb injury during young adulthood and an increased risk for knee osteoarthritis has recently been confirmed in a longitudinal study of male physicians [208]. In this study, the RR for developing knee osteoarthritis was 2.95 (95% CI 1.35, 6.45) for a history of knee injury during adolescence and young adulthood.

An association between a history of hip injury and ipsilateral and bilateral hip osteoarthritis, but not contralateral hip osteoarthritis, was also found in data from the First National Health and Nutrition Examination Survey [60]. In multiple logistic regression models adjusted for age, sex, race, and education, a history of hip injury was significantly associated with higher odds of hip osteoarthritis: (OR = 7.84, 95% CI 2.11–29.10). When the analysis was performed examining the relationship between hip injury and either unilateral or bilateral hip osteoarthritis, however, the OR for the association of hip injury with unilateral hip osteoarthritis was 24.2 (95% CI 3.84, 153) as compared with bilateral hip osteoarthritis of 4.17 (95% CI 0.50, 34.7). Heliovaara *et al.* [136] studied the relation between history of lower limb injury and clinically diagnosed hip osteoarthritis in a population study in Finland. In multiple logistic regression models adjusted for age, gender, body mass index, and physical stress at work, a history of lower limb injury was associated with osteoarthritis in both sexes. As in the NHANES-I data set, the association was stronger with unilateral than bilateral hip osteoarthritis. These results were confirmed in a case-control study of 210 men and 401 women undergoing total hip arthroplasty for hip osteoarthritis in England; previous hip injury was more strongly associated with unilateral as compared to bilateral hip osteoarthritis [209]. In the Johns Hopkins Precursors Study, the RR for hip osteoarthritis was 3.5 (95% CI 0.8–14.7) for a history of hip injury during adolescence, young adulthood, or during follow-up.

Smoking

Most but not all studies suggest that current smoking may protect against the development of knee osteoarthritis [56,145,152,210,211]. However, smoking is more common in symptomatic women with knee osteoarthritis than in women with radiographic knee osteoarthritis who don't report knee pain [59]. The relationship between smoking and osteoarthritis, if it exists, may warrant further investigation as smoking influences hepatic metabolism of female sex hormones and is an independent risk factor for osteoporosis and hip fracture.

Antioxidant nutrients

Data from the Framingham Study failed to demonstrate an association between dietary intake of vitamin C, vitamin D, or vitamin E with incidence of radiographic knee osteoarthritis [212,213]. Data from the Study of Osteoporotic Fractures did demonstrate a three-fold increased risk for the development of radiographic hip osteoarthritis, characterized by severe joint space narrowing, and serum levels of 25-hydroxy-vitamin D in the middle and lowest tertiles compared to those with levels in the highest tertile [214]. Data from the Framingham Study also showed a three-fold increased risk for progression of radiographic knee osteoarthritis among subjects in the middle and lowest tertiles compared to those with levels in the highest tertile [212].

Prognosis

The survival of persons with osteoarthritis has been discussed earlier. The remainder of this section will focus on results of epidemiologic studies of radiographic progression of osteoarthritis.

Radiographic changes of osteoarthritis appear to inexorably progress, albeit at a slow rate, in the hands [69,70,215], the knees [74,129,217–220], and the hips [221,222], although isolated reports of improvement in the radiographic features of hip osteoarthritis have been noted [221]. In the hand, radiographic changes progress at a greater rate with increasing age [215]; the rate of progression does not appear to be associated with body mass index, bone mineral density, body fat distribution, grip strength, or forearm circumference [216].

Factors associated with radiographic progression in the knee include: female sex [74], obesity [126], presence of nodal generalized osteoarthritis [223], presence of knee effusion and calcium pyrophosphate dihydrate crystals in the synovial fluid [223], higher serum levels of insulin-like growth factor I [224], higher baseline serum levels of hyaluronic acid [225], increasing levels of serum cartilage oligomeric matrix protein [226], use of indomethacin as a non-steroidal anti-inflammatory drug [227], low levels of dietary intake of vitamin C [213], low levels of dietary intake and low serum levels of vitamin D [212], increased serum levels of C-reactive protein [228,229], and lower bone mineral density at the femoral neck [166].

Osteoarthritis of the hip has been characterized by a slowly progressive and a rapidly progressive form, the latter often leading to total joint arthroplasty within 1 year from time of presentation [222,230]. In a secondary analysis of 506 patients with hip osteoarthritis recruited for participation in a clinical trial, rapidly progressive hip osteoarthritis occurred in 22 per cent; factors associated with rapidly progressive disease included female gender and age of 65 and above. In a study of 136 hospital-referred patients with hip osteoarthritis, Ledingham *et al.* [231] noted that women were more likely than men to have rapidly progressive hip osteoarthritis. Age at presentation, body mass index, presence of radiographic chondrocalcinosis, and hand osteoarthritis did not influence rate of progression in this study. Serum levels of C-reactive protein were related to progression of hip osteoarthritis [232,233] but neither serum levels of cartilage oligomeric matrix protein nor bone sialoprotein were related to progression of hip osteoarthritis [232,233].

The prognosis of a cohort of 500 clinically diagnosed patients with lower limb osteoarthritis has also been examined. After 3 years, 415 patients with a mean age of 66 years were assessed [234]. The majority reported a worsening of their condition, with an increase in disability and use of walking aids. No correlation was found between indices of radiographic progression and change in clinical status. After 8 years, 349 patients with a mean age of 71 years were assessed [235]. Although the outcomes were heterogeneous, the authors concluded that lower limb osteoarthritis generally results in high levels of physical disability with a high level of utilization of health care resources, including joint replacement surgery. No baseline variables emerged as strong predictors of clinical outcomes.

References

1. Lawrence RC, Helmick CG, Arnett FC, *et al.* Estimates of the prevalence of arthritis and selected musculo-skeletal diseases in the United States. *Arthritis Rheum* 1998; **41**: 778–99.

2. Felson DT, conference chair: Osteoarthritis: new insights. Part I: The disease and its risk factors. *Ann Intern Med* 2000; **133**: 637–46.

3. Altman R, Asch E, Bloch D, *et al.* Development of criteria for the classification and reporting of osteo-arthritis: classification of osteoarthritis of the knee. *Arthritis Rheum* 1986; **29**: 1039–49.

4. Brandt KD, Mankin HJ, Shulman LE, eds. Workshop on etiopathogenesis of osteoarthritis. *J Rheumatol* 1986; **13**: 1126–60.

5. Keuttner K, Goldberg VM, eds.. *Osteoarthritic disorders.* Rosemont: American Academy of Orthopaedic Surgeons, 1995: xxi–v.

6. Kellgren JH, Moore R. Generalized osteoarthritis and Heberden's nodes. *Br Med J* 1952; **1**: 181–7.

7. Schumacher HR Jr. Secondary osteoarthritis. In: RW Moskowitz, DS Howell, VM Goldberg, HJ Mankin, eds. *Osteoarthritis: diagnosis and surgical management,* 2nd edn. Philadelphia: W.B. Saunders Company, 1993: 367–98.

8. Kellgren JH, Lawrence JS. Radiologic assessment of osteoarthrosis. *Ann Rheum Dis* 1957; **16**: 494–501.

9. Department of Rheumatology and Medical Illustration, University of Manchester. *The Epidemiology of Chronic Rheumatism*: Vol. II. *Atlas of Standard Radiographs of Arthritis.* Philadelphia: F. A. Davis Company, 1973: 1–15.

10. Spector TD, Cooper C. Radiographic assessment of osteoarthritis inpopulation studies: whither Kellgren and Lawrence? *Osteoarthritis and Cartilage* 1993; **1**: 203–6.

11. Spector TD, Hochberg MC. Methodological problems in the epidemiological study of osteoarthritis. *Ann Rheum Dis* 1994; **53**: 143–6.

12. Hart DJ, Spector TD. Radiographic criteria for epidemiologic studies of osteoarthritis. *J Rheumatol* 1995; **43** (Suppl): 46–8.

13. Hart DJ, Spector TD. The classification and assessment of osteoarthritis. *Bailliere's Clinical Rheumatol* 1995; **9**: 407–32.

14. Kallman DA, Wigley FM, Scott WW Jr, Hochberg MC, Tobin JD. New radiographic grading scales for osteoarthritis of the hand: reliability for determining prevalence and progression. *Arthritis Rheum* 1989; **32**: 1584–91.

15. Croft P, Cooper C, Wickham C, Coggon D. Defining osteoarthritis of the hip for epidemiologic studies. *Am J Epidemiol* 1990; **132**: 514–22.

16. Lane NE, Nevitt MC, Genant HK, Hochberg MC. Reliability of new indices of radiographic osteoarthritis of the hand and hip and lumbar disc degeneration. *J Rheumatol* 1993; **20**: 1911–8.

17. Spector TD, Cooper C, Cushnaghan J, Hart DJ, Dieppe PA. *A radiographic atlas of knee osteoarthritis.* Springer-Verlag: London, 1992.

18. Scott WW Jr, Lethbridge-Cejku M, Reichle R, Wigley FM, Tobin JD, Hochberg MC. Reliability of grading scales for individual radiographic features of osteo-arthritis of the knee: the Baltimore Longitudinal Study of Aging atlas of knee osteoarthritis. *Investigative Radiology* 1993; **28**: 497–501.

19. Altman RD, Hochberg MC, Murphy WA Jr, Wolfe F, Lequesne M. Atlas of individual radiographic features in osteoarthritis. *Osteoarthritis and Cartilage* 1995; **3**(Suppl A): 3–70.

20. Lane NE, Kremer LB. Radiographic indices for osteoarthritis. *Rheum Dis Clin N Am* 1995; **21**: 379–94.

21. Scott JC, Nevitt MC, Lane NE, Genant HK, Hochberg MC. Association of individual radiographic features of hip osteoarthritis with pain. *Arthritis Rheum* 1992; **35**(Suppl 9): S81.

22. Spector TD, Hart DJ, Byrne J, Harris PA, Dacre JE, Doyle DV. Defining the presence of osteoarthritis of the knee in epidemiologic studies. *Ann Rheum Dis* 1993; **52**: 790–4.

23. Lethbridge-Cejku M, Scott WW Jr, Reichle R, *et al.* Association of radiographic features of osteoarthritis of the knee with knee pain: Data from the Baltimore Longitudinal Study of Aging. *Arthritis Care Res* 1995; **9**: 182–8.

24. Bennett PH, Wood PHN. *Population studies of the rheumatic diseases.* International congress series No. 148. Excereta Medica Foundation: Amsterdam, 1968: 417–19.

25. Altman RD, Meenan RF, Hochberg MC, *et al.* An approach to developing criteria for the clinical diagnosis and classification of osteoarthritis. *J Rheumatol* 1983; **10**: 180–83.

26. Altman R, Alarcon G, Appelrough D, *et al.* The American College of Rheumatology criteria for the classification and reporting of osteoarthritis of the hand. *Arthritis Rheum* 1990; **33**: 1601–10.

27. Altman R, Alarcon G, Appelrough D, *et al.* The American College of Rheumatology criteria for the classification and reporting of osteoarthritis of the hip. *Arthritis Rheum* 1991; **34**: 505–14.

28. Altman R. Classification of disease: osteoarthritis. *Semin Arthritis Rheum* 1991; **20**(Suppl 2): 40–47.

29. Hart DJ, Leedham-Green M, Spector TD. The prevalence of knee osteoarthritis in the general population using different clinical criteria: the Chingford Study. *Br J Rheum* 1991; **30**(S2): 72.

30. Bellamy N, Klestov A, Muirden K, *et al.* Perceptual variation in categorizing individuals according to American College of Rheumatology classification criteria for hand, knee, and hip osteoarthritis OA.: observations based on an Australian Twin Registry study of OA. *J Rheum* 1999; **26**: 2654–8.

31. Kellgren JH, Lawrence JS. Osteoarthritis and disk degeneration in an urban population. *Ann Rheum Dis* 1958; **17**: 388–97.

32. Lawrence JS, Bremner JM, Bier F: Osteoarthrosis: prevalence in the population and relationship between symptoms and x-ray changes. *Ann Rheum Dis* 1966; **25**: 1–24.

33. Roberts J, Burch TA. *Prevalence of osteoarthritis in adults by age, sex, race and geographic area: United*

States, 1960–1962. Vital and Health Statistics. Series 11, Number 15. PHS Pub. No. 1000. Washington D.C., National Center for Health Statistics, 1966.

34. Mikkelsen WM, Dodge HJ, Duff IF, *et al*. Estimates of the prevalence of rheumatic diseases in the population of Tecumseh, Michigan, 1959–60. *J Chron Dis* 1967; **20**: 351–69.

35. Mikkelsen WM, Duff IF, Dodge HJ. Age-sex specific prevalence of radiographic abnormalities of the joints of the hands, wrists and cervical spine of adult residents of the Tecumseh, Michigan Community Health Study area, 1962–1965. *J Chron Dis* 1970; **23**: 151–59.

36. Bennett PH, Burch TA. Osteoarthrosis in the Blackfeet and Pima Indians. In: Bennett PH, Wood PHN, eds. *Population studies of the rheumatic diseases*. Exerpta Medica Foundation: Amsterdam, 1968: 407–12.

37. Tzonchev VT, Pilossoff T, Kanev K. Prevalence of osteoarthrosis in Bulgaria. In: Bennett PH, Wood PHN, eds. *Population studies of the rheumatic diseases*. Exerpta Medica Foundation: Amsterdam, 1968: 413–16.

38. Solomon L, Beighton P, Lawrence JS.Osteoarthritis in a rural South African negro population. *Ann Rheum Dis* 1976; **35**: 274–78.

39. Maurer K. *Basic data on arthritis knee, hip and sacro-iliac joints in adults ages 25–74 years, United States, 1971–1975*. Vital and Health Statistics. Series 11, Number 213. USDHEW, 1979.

40. Beighton SW, DeLa Harpe AL, VanStaden DA. The prevalence of osteoarthritis in a rural African community. *Br J Rheumatol* 1985; **24**: 321–25.

41. Bergstrom G, Bjelle A, Sorensen LB, Sundh V, Svanborg A. Prevalence of rheumatoid arthritis, osteoarthritis, and gouty arthritis at age 79. *J Rheumatol* 1986; **13**: 527–34.

42. Felson DT, Naimark A, Anderson J, Kazis L, Castellani W, Meenan RF. The prevalence of knee osteoarthritis in the elderly. *Arthritis Rheum* 1987; **30**: 914–18.

43. Butler WJ, Hawthorne VM, Mikklesen WM, *et al*. Prevalence of radiologically defined osteoarthritis in the finger and wrist joints of adult residents of Tecumseh, Michigan, 1962–65. *J Clin Epidemiol* 1988; **41**: 467–73.

44. Van Sasse JLCM, Van Romunde LKJ, Cats A, Vandenbroucke JP,Valkenburg HA. Epidemiology of osteoarthritis: Zoertermeer survey. Comparison of radiologic osteoarthritis in a Dutch population with that in 10 other populations. *Ann Rheum Dis* 1989; **48**: 271–80.

45. Bagge E, Bjelle A, Eden S, Svanborg A. Factors associated with radiographic osteoarthritis: results from a population study 70-year-old people in Goteborg. *J Rheumatol* 1991; **18**: 1218–22.

46. Lethbridge-Cejku M, Tobin JD, Scott WW Jr, Reichle R, Plato CC, Hochberg MC. The relationship of age and gender to prevalence and pattern of radiographic changes of osteoarthritis of the knee: data from the Baltimore Longitudinal Study of Aging. *Aging Clin Exp Res* 1994; **6**: 353–7.

47. Aspelund G, Gunnarsdottir S, Jonsson P, *et al*. Hand osteoarthritis in the elderly: application of clinical criteria. *Scand J Rheumatol* 1996; **25**: 34–6.

48. Hirsch R, Fernandes RJ, Pillemer SR, *et al*. Hip osteoarthritis prevalence estimates by three radiographic scoring systems. *Arthritis Rheum* 1998; **41**: 361–8.

49. Sowers MF, Hochberg M, Crabbe JP, Muhich A, Crutchfield M, Updike S. Association of bone mineral density and sex hormone levels with osteoarthritis of the hand and knee in premenopausal women. *Am J Epidemiol* 1996; **143**: 38–47.

50. Ingvarrson T, Hagglund G, Lohmander LS. Prevalence of hip osteoarthritis in Iceland. *Ann Rheum Dis* 1999; **58**: 201–7.

51. Inoue K, Shichikawa K, Ota H. Prevalence of hip osteoarthritis and acetabular dysplasia in Kamitonda: from a longitudinal population-based epidemiological study of rheumatic diseases in Japan. *Rheumatol* 1999; **38**: 793–4.

52. Sowers M, Lachance L, Hochberg M, Jamadar D. Radiographically defined osteoarthritis of the hand and knee in young and middle-aged African American and Caucasian women. *Osteoarthritis Cart* 2000; **8**: 69–77.

53. Lawrence JS. *Rheumatism in populations*. William Heinemann Medical Books: London, 1977: 98–155.

54. Lawrence JS, Sebo M. The geography of osteoarthritis. In: Nuki G, ed. *The aetiopathogenesis of osteoarthritis*. University Park Press: Baltimore, 1980: 155–83.

55. Kelsey JL. Prevalence studies of the epidemiology of osteoarthritis. In: Lawrence RC, Shulman LE, eds. *Epidemiology of the rheumatic diseases*.Gower Medical Publishing: New York, 1984: 282–88.

56. Lawrence RC, Hochberg MC, Kelsey JL, *et al*. Estimates of the prevalence of selected arthritis and musculoskeletal diseases in the United States. *J Rheumatol* 1989; **16**: 427–41.

57. Anderson JJ, Felson DT. Factors associated with osteoarthritis of the knee in the First National Health and Nutrition Examination Survey HANES I.: evidence for an association with overweight, race and physical demands of work. *Am J Epidemiol* 1988; **128**: 179–89.

58. Jordan JM, Linder GF, Renner JB, Fryer JG. The impact of arthritis in rural populations. *Arthritis Care Res* 1995; **8**: 242–50.

59. Hochberg MC, Lawrence RC, Everett DF, Cornoni-Huntley J. Epidemiologic associations of pain in osteoarthritis of the knee: data from the National Health and Nutrition Examination Survey and the National Health and Nutrition Examination—I Epidemiologic Followup Survey. *Semin Arthritis Rheum* 1989; **18** (suppl 2): 4–9.

60. Tepper S, Hochberg MC. Factors associated with hip osteoarthritis: data from the First National Health and Nutrition Examination Survey. *Am J Epidemiol* 1993; **137**: 1081–8.

61. Hirsch R, Fernandes RJ, Pillemer SR, *et al*. Hip osteoarthritis prevalence estimates by three radiographic scoring systems. *Arthritis Rheum* 1998; **41**: 361–8.

62. Hoaglund FT, Oishi CS, Gialamas GG. Extreme variations in racial rates of total hip arthroplasty for primary coxarthrosis: a population-based study in San Francisco. *Ann Rheum Dis* 1995; **54**: 107–10.

63. Bremner JM, Lawrence JS, Miall WE. Degenerative joint disease in a Jamaican rural population. *Ann Rheum Dis* 1968; **27**: 326–32.

64. Solomon L, Beighton P, Lawrence JS. Rheumatic disorders in the South African Negro. II. Osteoarthritis. *South Afr Med J* 1975; **49**: 1737–40.

65. Hoaglund FT. Osteoarthritis of the hip and other joints in Southern Chinese in Hong Kong. *J Bone Joint Surg* 1973; **55**: 545–57.

66. Lau EM, Symmons DP, Croft P. The epidemiology of hip osteoarthritis and rheumatoid arthritis in the Orient. *Clin Orthop* 1996; **323**: 81–90.

67. Mukhopadhaya B, Barooah B. Osteoarthritis of the hip in Indians: an anatomical and clinical study. *Indian J Orthop* 1967; **1**: 55–63.

68. Scott JC, Hochberg MC. Epidemiologic insights into the pathogenesis of hip osteoarthritis. In: Hadler NM, ed. *Clinical concepts in regional musculoskeletal illness*. Greene and Stratton: Orlando, 1987: 89–107.

69. Plato CC, Norris AH. Osteoarthritis of the hand: longitudinal studies. *Am J Epidemiol* 1979; **110**: 740–46.

70. Kallman DA, Wigley FM, Scott WW Jr, Hochberg MC, Tobin JD. The longitudinal course of hand osteoarthritis in a male population. *Arthritis Rheum* 1990; **33**: 1323–32.

71. Sowers M, Zobel D, Weissfeld L, Hawthorne VM, Carman W. Progression of osteoarthritis of the hand and metacarpal bone loss: a twenty-year following of incident cases. *Arthritis Rheum* 1991; **34**: 36–42.

72. Carman WJ, Sowers M, Hawthorne VM, Weissfield LA. Obesity as a risk for osteoarthritis of the hand and wrist: a prospective study. *Am J Epidemiol* 1994; **139**: 119–29.

73. Chaisson CE, Zhang Y, McAlindon TE, *et al*. Radiographic hand osteoarthritis: incidence, patterns, and influence of pre-existing disease in a population based sample. *J Rheumatol* 1997; **24**: 1337–43.

74. Felson DT, Zhang Y, Hannan MT, *et al*. The incidence and natural history of knee osteoarthritis in the elderly. *Arthritis Rheum* 1995; **38**: 1500–5.

75. Hart DJ, Doyle DV, Spector TD. Incidence and risk factors for radiographic knee osteoarthritis in middle-aged women: the Chingford Study. *Arthritis Rheum* 1999 **42**: 17–24.

76. Wilson MG, Michet CJ, Ilstrup DM, Melton III LJ. Idiopathic symptomatic osteoarthritis of the hip and knee: a population-based incidence study. *Mayo Clin Proc* 1990; **65**: 1214–21.

77. Oliveria SA, Felson DT, Reed JI, Cirillo PA, Walker AM. Incidence of symptomatic hand, hip, and knee osteoarthritis among patients in a health maintenance organization. *Arthritis Rheum* 1995; **38**: 1134–41.

78. Callahan LF, Pincus T. Mortality in the rheumatic diseases. *Arthritis Care Res* 1995; **8**: 229–41.

79. Manson RR, Hall AP. Mortality among arthritis. *J Chron Dis* 1976; **29**: 459–67.

80. Griffin MR, Ray WA, Schaffner W. Nonsteroidal anti-inflammatory drug use and death from peptic ulcer in elderly persons. *Ann Intern Med* 1988; **109**: 359–63.

81. Guess HA, West R, Strand LM, *et al*. Fatal upper gastrointestinal hemorrhage or perforation among users and nonusers of nonsteroidal anti-inflammatory drugs in Saskatchewan, Canada, 1983. *J Clin Epidemiol* 1988; **41**: 35–45.

82. Hochberg MC. Association of nonsteroidal anti-inflammatory drugs with upper gastrointestinal disease: epidemiologic and economic considerations. *J Rheumatol* 1992; **19**(Suppl 36): 63–7.

83. Lawrence RC, Everett DF, Hochberg MC. Arthritis. In: Huntley R, Cornoni-Huntley J, eds. health status and well being of the elderly: national health and nutrition examination—I Epidemiologic followup survey. Oxford University Press: New York, 1990: 133–51.

84. Cerhan JR, Wallace RB, el-Khoury GY, Moore TE, Long CR. Decreased survival with increasing prevalence of full-body, radiographically defined osteoarthritis in women. *Am J Epidemiol* 1995; **141**: 225–34.

85. Stecher RM. Heberden's nodes: heredity in hypertrophic arthritis of the finger joints. *Am J Med Sci* 1941; **210**: 801–9.

86. Stecher RM, Hersh AH. Heberden's nodes: mechanism of inheritance in hypertrophic arthritis of the fingers. *J Clin Invest* 1944; **23**: 699.

87. Stecher RM, Hersh AH, Hauser H. Heberden's nodes: the family history and radiographic appearance of a large family. *Am J Hum Genet* 1953; **5**: 46–60.

88. Stecher RM. Heberden's nodes: a clinical description of osteoarthritis of the finger joints. *Ann Rheum Dis* 1955; **14**: 1–10.

89. Kellgren JH, Lawrence JS, Bier F. Genetic factors in generalized osteoarthritis. *Ann Rheum Dis* 1963; **22**: 237–55.

90. Hirsch R, Lethbridge-Cejku M, Hanson R, *et al*. Familial aggregation of osteoarthritis. *Arthritis Rheum* 1998; **41**: 1227–32.

91. Felson DT, Couropmitree NN, Chaisson CE, *et al*. Evidence for a Mendelian gene in a segretation analysis of generalized radiographic osteoarthritis. *Arthritis Rheum* 1998; **41**: 1064–71.

92. Chitnavis J, Sinsheimer JS, Clipsham K, *et al*. Genetic influences in end-stage osteoarthritis. Sibling risks of hip and knee replacement for idiopathic osteoarthritis. *J Bone Joint Surg* 1997; **79B**: 660–4.

93. Spector RD, Cicuttini F, Baker J, *et al*. Genetic influences on osteoarthritis in women: a twin study. *Br Med J* 1996; **312**: 940–3.

94. MacGregor AJ, Spector TD. Twins and the genetic architecture of osteoarthritis. *Rheumatol* 1999; **38**: 583–90.

95. MacGregor AJ, Antoniades L, Matson M, Andrew T, Spector TD. The genetic contribution to radiographic hip osteoarthritis in women: results of a classic twin study. *Arthritis Rheum* 2000; **43**: 2410–6.

96. Pelotie A, Vaisaner P, Ott J, *et al*. Predisposition to familial osteoarthrosis is linked to type II collage gene. *Lancet* 1989; **1**: 924–27.

97. Ala-Konno L, Baldwin CT, Moskowitz RW, Prockop DJ. Single base mutation in the type II procollagen gene COL2A1. As a cause of primary osteoarthritis associated with a mild chondrodysplasia. *Proc Natl Acad Sci USA* 1990; **87**: 6565–68.

98. Knowlton RG, Katzenstein PL, Moskowitz RW, *et al*. Demonstration of genetic linkage of the type II pro-

collagen gene COL2A1. To primary osteoarthritis associated with a mild chondrodysplasia. *N Eng J Med* 1990; **322**: 526–30.

99. Jimenez SA. Molecular biological approaches to the study of heritable osteoarthritis. *J Rheumatol* 1991; **18** (Suppl. 27): 7–9.

100. Priestley L, Fergusson C, Ogilvie D, *et al*. A limited association of generalised osteoarthritis with alleles at the Type II collagen locus COL2A1. *Br J Rheumatol* 1991; **30**: 272–5.

101. Loughlin J, Irven C. Ferguson C, Sykes B. Sibling pair analysis shows no linkage of generalized osteoarthritis to the loci encoding type II collagen, cartilage link protein or cartilage matrix protein. *Br J Rheumatol* 1994; **33**: 1103–6.

102. Aerssens J, Dequeker J, Peeters J, Breemans S, Boonen S. Lack of association between osteoarthritis of the hip and gene polymorphisms of VDR, COLIAI, and COL2A1 in postmenopausal women. *Arthritis Rheum* 1998; **41**: 1946–50.

103. Meulenbelt I, Bijkerk C, De Wildt SC, *et al*. Haplotype analysis of three polymorphisms of the COL2AI gene and associations with generalised radiological osteoarthritis. *Ann Hum Genet* 1999; **63**: 393–400.

104. Uitterlinden AG, Burger H, van Duijn CM, *et al*. Adjacent genes, for COL2A1 and the vitamin D receptor, are associated with separate features of radiographic osteoarthritis of the knee. *Arthritis Rheum* 2000; **43**: 1456–64.

105. Horton WE Jr, Lethbridge-Cejky M, Hochberg MC, *et al*. An association between an aggrecan polymorhic allele and bilateral hand osteoarthritis in elderly white men. *Osteoarthritis Cartilage* 1998; **6**: 245–51.

106. Uitterlinden AG, Burger H, Huang Q, *et al*. Vitamin D receptor genotype is associated with radiographic osteoarthritis at the knee. *J Clin Invest* 1997; **15**: 259–63.

107. Keen RW, Hart DJ, Lanchbury JS, Spector TD. Association of early osteoarthritis of the knee with a Taq I polymorphism of the vitamin D receptor gene. *Arthritis Rheum* 1997; **40**: 1444–9.

108. Huang J, Ushiyama T, Inoue K, Kawasaki T, Hukuda S. Vitamin D receptor gene polymorphisms and osteoarthritis of the hand, hip, and knee: a case-control study in Japan. *Rheumatol* 2000; **39**: 79–84.

109. Loughlin J, Sinsheimer JS, Mustafa Z, *et al*. Association analysis of the vitamin D receptor gene, the type I collagen gene COLIAI, and the estrogen receptor gene in idiopathic osteoarthritis. *J Rheumatol* 2000; **27**: 779–84.

110. Meulenbelt I, Bijkerk C, Miedema HS, *et al*. A genetic association study of the IGF-1 gene and radiological osteoarthritis in a population-based cohort study the Rotterdam Study. *Ann Rheum Dis* 1998; **57**: 371–4.

111. Acheson R, Collart AB. New Haven survey of joint diseases. XVII. Relationship between some systemic characteristics and osteoarthrosis in a general population. *Ann Rheum Dis* 1975; **34**: 379–87.

112. Hartz AJ, Fischer ME, Brill G, *et al* . The association of obesity with joint pain and osteoarthritis in the HANES data. *J Chron Dis* 1986; **39**: 311–19.

113. Felson DT, Anderson JJ, Naimark AA, *et al*. Obesity and knee osteoarthritis. *Ann Intern Med* 1988; **109**: 18–24.

114. Davis MA, Ettinger WH, Neuhaus JM, Hauck WW. Sex differences in osteoarthritis of the knee: the role of obesity. *Am J Epidemiol* 1988; **127**: 1019–30.

115. Davis MA, Ettinger WH, Neuhaus JM. The role of metabolic factors and blood pressure in the association of obesity with osteoarthritis of the knee. *J Rheumatol* 1988; **15**: 1827–32.

116. Davis MA, Ettinger WH, Neuhaus JM, Cho SA, Houck WW. The association of knee injury and obesity with unilateral and bilateral osteoarthritis of the knee. *Am J Epidemiol* 1989; **130**: 278–88.

117. Davis MA, Neuhaus, JM, Ettinger WH, Muller WH. Body fat distribution and osteoarthritis. *Am J Epidemiol* 1990; **132**: 701–7.

118. Van Saase JLCM, Vandenbroucke JP, van Romunde LKJ, Valkenburg HA. Osteoarthritis and obesity in the general population: a relationship calling for an explanation. *J Rheumatol* 1988; **15**: 1152–58.

119. Hart DJ, Spector TD. The relationship of obesity, fat distribution and osteoarthritis in women in the general population: the Chingford study. *J Rheumatol* 1993; **20**: 331–5.

120. Hochberg MC, Lethbridge-Cejku M, Scott WW Jr, Reichle R, Plato CC, Tobin JD. The association of body weight, body fatness and body fat distribution with osteoarthritis of the knee: data from the Baltimore Longitudinal Study of Aging. *J Rheumatol* 1995; **22**: 488–493.

121. Cicuttini FM, Baker JR, Spector TD. The association of obesity with osteoarthritis of the hand and knee in women: a twin study. *J Rheumatol* 1996; **23**: 1221–6.

122. Jordan JM, Luta G, Renner JB, *et al*. Self-reported functional status in osteoarthritis of the knee in a rural southern community: the role of sociodemographic factors, obesity, and knee pain. *Arthritis Care Res* 1996; **9**: 273–8.

123. Hart DJ, Doyle DV, Spector TD. Association between metabolic factors and knee osteoarthritis in women: the Chingford Study. *J Rheumatol* 1995; **22**: 1118–23.

124. Martin K, Lethbridge-Cejku M, Muller DC, *et al*. Metabolic correlates of obesity and radiographic features of knee osteoarthritis. *J Rheumatol* 1997; **24**: 702–7.

125. Felson DT, Zhang Y, Hannan MT, *et al*. Risk factors for incident radiographic knee osteoarthritis in the elderly: The Framingham Study. *Arthritis Rheum* 1997; **40**: 728–33.

126. Spector TD, Hart DJ, Doyle DV. Incidence and progression of osteoarthritis in women with unilateral knee disease in the general population: the effect of obesity. *Ann Rheum Dis* 1994; **53**: 565–8.

127. Lethbridge-Cejku M, Creamer P, Wilson PD, *et al*. Risk factors for incident knee osteoarthritis: data from the Baltimore Longitudinal Study on Aging. *Arthritis Rheum* 1998; **419** (Suppl.): S182.

128. Shiozaki H, Koga Y, Omori G, *et al*. Obesity and osteoarthritis of the knee in women: results from the Matsudai Knee Osteoarthritis Survey. *Knee* 1999; **6**: 189–92.

129. Gelber AC, Hochberg MC, Mead LA, Want NY, Wigley FM, Klag MJ. Body mass index in young men

and the risk of subsequent knee and hip osteoarthritis. *Am J Med* 1999; **107**: 542–8.

130. Cooper C, Snow S, McAlindon TE, Kellingray S, Stuart D, Dieppe PA. Risk factors for the incidence and progression of radiographic knee osteoarthritis. *Arthritis Rheum* 2000; **43**: 995–1000.

131. Felson DT, Zhang Y, Anthony JM, Naimark A, Andeson JJ. Weight loss reduces the risk for symptomatic knee osteoarthritis in women. *Ann Intern Med* 1992; **116**: 535–9.

132. Engel A, Burch TA. *Osteoarthritis in adults by selected demographic characteristics*. Vital and Health Statistics. Series 11, No. 20. Washington, D.C., USDHEW, 1966.

133. Hochberg MC, Lethbridge-Cejku M, Plato CC, Wigley FM, Tobin JD. Factors associated with osteoarthritis of the hand in males: data from the Baltimore Longitudinal Study of Aging. *Am J Epidemiol* 1991; **143**: 1121–7.

134. Hochberg MC, Lethbridge-Cejku M, Scott WW Jr, Plato CC, Tobin JD. Obesity and osteoarthritis of the hands in women. *Osteoarthritis Cart* 1993; **1**: 129–35.

135. Hochberg MC, Lethbridge M, Wigley F, Plato C, Tobin JD. Factors predicting progression of hand osteoarthritis in males: data from the Baltimore Longitudinal Study of Aging. *Arthritis Rheum* 1991; **34** (Suppl. 9): S34.

136. Heliovaara M, Makela M, Imprivaara O, Knekt P, Aromaa A, Sievers K. Association of overweight, trauma and workload with coxarthrosis: a health study of 7.217 persons. *Acta Orthop Scand* 1993; **64**: 513–8.

137. Nevitt MC, Cummings SR, Lane NE, *et al.*, for the Study of Osteoporotic Fractures Research Group. Association of estrogen replacement therapy with the risk of osteoarthritis of the hip in elderly white women. *Arch Intern Med* 1996; **156**: 2073–80.

138. Vingard E, Alfredsson L, Malchau H. Lifestyle factors and hip arthrosis. A case referent study of body mass index, smoking and hormone therapy in 503 Swedish women. *Acta Orthop Scand* 1997; **68**: 216–20.

139. Cooper C, Inskip H, Croft P, *et al.* Individual risk factors for hip osteoarthritis: obesity, hip injury, and physical activity. *Am J Epidemiol* 1998; **147**: 516–22.

140. Oliveria SA, Felson DT, Cirillo PA, Reed JI, Walker AM. Body weight, body mass index, and incident symptomatic osteoarthritis of the hand, hip, and knee. *Epidemiol* 1999; **10**: 161–6.

141. Sahyoun NR, Hochberg MC, Helmick CG, Harris T, Pamuk ER. Body mass index, weight change, and incidence of self-reported physician-diagnosed arthritis among women. *Am J Public Health* 1999; **89**: 391–4.

142. Spector TD, Brown GC, Silman A. Increased rates of previous hysterectomy and gynecological operations in women with osteoarthritis. *Br Med J* 1988; **297**: 899–900.

143. Hannan MT, Felson DT, Anderson JJ, Naimark A, Kannel WB. Estrogen use and radiographic osteoarthritis of the knee in women. *Arthritis Rheum* 1990; **33**: 525–32.

144. Dennison EM, Arden NK, Kellingray S, *et al*. Hormone replacement therapy, other reproductive variables and symptomatic hip osteoarthritis in elderly white women: a case-control study. *Br J Rheumatol* 1998; **37**: 1198–202.

145. Samanta A, Jones A, Regan M, Wilson S, Doherty M. Is osteoarthritis in women afected by hormonal changes or smoking. *Br J Rheumatol* 1993; **32**: 366–70.

146. Oliveria SA, Felson DT, Klein RA, Reed JI, Walker AM. Estrogen replacement and the development of osteoarthritis. *Epidemiol* 1996; **7**: 415–9.

147. Spector TD, Nandra D, Hart DJ, Doyle DV. Is hormone replacement therapy protective for hand and knee osteoarthritis in women? The Chingford Study. *Ann Rheum Dis* 1997; **56**: 432–2.

148. Nevitt MC, Felson DT. Sex hormones and the risk of osteoarthritis in women: epidemiological evidence. *Ann Rheum Dis* 1996; **55**: 673–6.

149. Zhang Y, McAlindon TE: Hannan MT, *et al.* Estrogen replacement therapy and worsening of radiographic knee osteoarthritis: the Framingham Study. *Arthritis Rheum* 1998; **41**: 1867–73.

150. Wluka AE, Cicuttini FM, Spector TD. Menopause, oestrogens and arthritis. *Maturitas* 2000; **30**: 183–99.

151. Sahyoun N, Brett KM, Hochberg MC, Pamuk ER. Estrogen replacement therapy and incidence of self-reported physician-diagnosed arthritis. *Prev Med* 1999; **28**: 458–64.

152. Sandmark H, Hogstedt C, Lewold S, Vingard E. Osteoarthritis of the knee in men and women in association with overweight, smoking, and hormone therapy. *Ann Rheum Dis* 1999; **58**: 151–5.

153. Erb A, Brenner H, Gunther KP, Sturmer T. Hormone replacement therapy and patterns of osteoarthritis: baseline data from the Ulm Osteoarthritis Study. *Ann Rheum Dis* 2000; **59**: 105–9.

154. Spector TD, Perry LA, Jubb RW. Endogenous sex steroid levels in women with generalised osteoarthritis. *Clin Rheumatol* 1991; **10**: 316–9.

155. Cauley JA, Kwoh CK, Egeland G, *et al.* Serum sex hormones and severity of osteoarthritis of the hand. *J Rheumatol* 1993; **20**: 1170–5.

156. Sowers M, Hochberg M, Crabbe JP, Muhich A, Crutchfield M, Updike S. Association of bone mineral density and sex hormone levels with osteoarthritis of the hand and knee in premenopausal women. *Am J Epidemiol* 1996; **143**: 38–47.

157. Foss MVL, Byers PD. Bone density, osteoarthritis of the hip, and fracture of the upper end of the femur. *Ann Rheum Dis* 1972; **31**: 259.

158. Star VL, Hochberg MC. Osteoporosis in patients with rheumatic diseases. *Rheum Dis Clinic North Am* 1994; **20**: 561–76.

159. Hannan MT, Anderson JJ, Zhang Y, Levy D, Felson DT. Bone mineral density and knee osteoarthritis in elderly men and women. The Framingham Study. *Arthritis Rheum* 1993; **36**: 1671–80.

160. Hart DJ, Mootoosamy I, Doyle DV, Spector TD. The relationship between osteoarthritis and osteoporosis in the general population: the Chingford Study. *Ann Rheum Dis* 1994; **53**: 158–62.

161. Nevitt MC, Lane NE, Scott JC, *et al.* Radiographic osteoarthritis of the hip and bone mineral density. *Arthritis Rheum* 1995; **38**: 907–16.

162. Burger H, van Daele PL, Odding E, *et al.* Association of radiographically evident osteoarthritis with higher bone mineral density and increased bone loss with age. The Rotterdam Study. *Arthritis Rheum* 1996; **39**: 81–6.

163. Lethbridge-Cejku M, Tobin JD, Scott WW Jr, *et al.* Axial and hip bone mineral density and radiographic changes of osteoarthritis of the knee: data from the Baltimore Longitudinal Study of Aging. *J Rheumatol* 1996; **23**: 1943–7.

164. Sambrook P, Naganathan V. What is the relationship between osteoarthritis and osteoporosis? *Baillieres Clin Rheumatol* 1997; **11**: 695–710.

165. Stewart A, Black AJ. Bone mineral density in osteoarthritis. *Curr Opin Rheumatol* 2000; **12**: 464–7.

166. Zhang Y, Hannan MT, Chaisson CE, *et al.* Bone mineral density and risk of incident and progressive radiographic knee osteoarthritis in women. *J Rheumatol* 2000; **27**: 1032–7.

167. Jones G, Nguyen T, Sambrook PN, Lord SR, Kelly PJ, Eisman JA. Osteoarthritis, bone density, postural stability, and osteoporotic fractures: a population based study. *J Rheumatol* 1995; **22**: 921–5.

168. Arden NK, Griffiths CO, Hart DJ, Doyle DV, Spector TD. The association between osteoarthritis and osteoporotic fracture: the Chingford Study. *Br J Rheumatol* 1996; **35**: 1299–304.

169. Arden NK, Nevitt MC, Lane NE, *et al.* Osteoarthritis and risk of falls, rates of bone loss, and osteoporotic fractures. Study of Osteoporotic Fractures Research Group. *Arthritis Rheum* 1999; **42**: 1378–85.

170. Stewart A, Black A, Robins SP, Reid DM. Bone density and bone turnover in patients with osteoarthritis and osteoporosis. *J Rheumatol* 1999; **26**: 622–6.

171. Sowers M, Lachance L, Jamadar D, *et al.* The association of bone mineral density and turnover markers with osteoarthritis of the hand and knee in pre-and-perimenopausal women. *Arthritis Rheum* 1999; **42**: 483–9.

172. Bauer DC, Orwoll ES, Fox KM, *et al.* Aspirin and NSAID use in older women: effect on bone mineral density and fracture risk, Study of Osteoporotic Fractures Research Group. *J Bone Miner Res* 1996; **11**: 29–35.

173. Morton DJ, Barrett-Connor EL, Schneider DL. Nonsteroidal anti-inflammatory drugs and bone mineral density in older women. *J Bone Miner Res* 1998, **13**: 1924–31.

174. Lane NE, Lin P, Christiansen L, Gore LR, *et al.* Association of mild acetabular dysplasia with an increased risk of incident hip osteoarthritis in elderly white women: the study of osteoporotic fractures. *Arthritis Rheum* 2000; **43**: 400–4.

175. Hochberg MC. Chondrocalcinosis articularis of the knee: prevalence and association with osteoarthritis of the knee. *Arthritis Rheum* 1984; **27**(Suppl.): S49.

176. Felson DT, Anderson JJ, Naimark AA, *et al.* The prevalence of chondrocalcinosis in the elderly and its association with knee osteoarthritis. *J Rheumatol* 1989; **16**: 1241–45.

177. Felson DT. The epidemiology of knee osteoarthritis: results from the Framingham Osteoarthritis Study. *Semin Arthritis Rheum* 1990; **20**(Suppl. 1): 42–50.

178. Frey MI, Barrett Connor E, Sledge PA, *et al.* The effect of noninsulin dependent diabetes mellitus on the prevalence of clinical osteoarthritis: a population based study. *J Rheumatol* 1996; **23**: 716–22.

179. Kellgren JH, Lawrence JS. Rheumatism in coal miners II: x-ray study. *Br J Ind Med* 1952; **9**: 197–207.

180. Partridge REH, Duthie JJR. Rheumatism in dockers and civil servants: a comparison of heavy manual and sedentary workers. *Am Rheum Dis* 1968; **27**: 559–68.

181. Lindberg H, Montgomery F. Heavy labor and the occurrence of gonarthrosis. *Clin Orthop* 1987; **214**: 235–36.

182. Lawrence JS. Rheumatism in cotton operatives. *Br J Ind Med* 1961; **18**: 270–76.

183. Hadler NM, Gillings DB, Imbus HR, *et al.* Hand-structure and function in an industrial setting. *Arthritis Rheum* 1978; **21**: 210–20.

184. Copeman W. The arthritis sequelae of pneumatic drilling. *Ann Rheum Dis* 1940; **2**: 141–46.

185. Lougot P, Savin R. La coxarthrose chez l'agriculture. *Rev Rheum Mal Osteoartic* 1966; **33**: 625–32.

186. Typpo T. Osteoarthritis of the hip: radiologic findings and etiology. *Ann Chir Gynaecol* 1985; **74**: 5–38.

187. Jacobsson B, Dalen N, Tjornstrand B. Coxarthrosis and labour. *Int J Orthop* 1987; **11**: 311–3.

188. Axmacher B, Lindberg H. Coxarthrosis in farmers as appearing on colon radiograms and urograms. In: Hogstedt C, Reuterwall C, eds. *Progress in occupational epidemiology*. Excerpta Medica: Amsterdam, 1988: 203–6.

189. Thelin A. Hip joint arthrosis: an occupational disorder among farmers. *Am J Ind Med* 1990; **18**: 339–43.

190. Croft P, Coggon D, Cruddas M, Cooper C. Osteoarthritis of the hip: an occupational disease in farmers. *Br Med J* 1992; **304**: 1269–72.

191. Maetzel A, Makela M, Hawker G, Bombardier C. Osteoarthritis of the hip and knee and mechanical occupational exposure: a systematic review of the evidence. *J Rheumatol* 1997; **24**: 1599–607.

192. Felson DT, Hannan MT, Naimark A, *et al.* Occupational physical demands, knee bending, and knee osteoarthritis: results from the Framingham study. *J Rheumatol* 1991; **18**: 1587–92.

193. Cooper C, McAlindon T, Coggon D, Egger P, Dieppe P. Occupational activity and osteoarthritis of the knee. *Ann Rheum Dis* 1994; **53**: 90–3.

194. Roach KE, Persky V, Miles T, Budiman-Mak E. Biomechanical aspects of occupation and osteoarthritis of the hip: a case-control study. *J Rheumatol* 1994; **21**: 2334–40.

195. Vingard E, Alfredsson L, Goldie I, *et al.* Occupation and osteoarthrosis of the hip and knee: a register-based cohort study. *Int J Epidemiol* 1991; **20**: 1025–31.

196. Vingard E, Hogstedt C, Alfredsson L, *et al.* Coxarthrosis and physical work load. *Scand J Work Env Health* 1991; **17**: 104–9.

197. Puranen J, Ala-Ketola L, Peltokallio P, *et al.* Running and primary osteoarthritis of the hip. *Br Med J* 1975; **1**: 424–35.

198. Sohn RS, Micheli LJ. The effect of running on the pathogenesis of osteoarthritis of the hips and knees. *Clin Orthop* 1985; **198**: 106–9.

199. Lane NE, Bloch DA, Jones HH, *et al.* Long distance running, bone density and osteoarthritis. *J Am Med Assoc* 1986; **255**: 1147–51.

200. Panush RS, Schmidt C, Caldwell JR, *et al.* Is running associated with degenerative joint disease? *J Am Med Assoc* 1986; **255**: 1152–55.

201. Lane NE, Bloch DA, Hubert HB, *et al.* Running, osteoarthritis, and bone density: initial 2-year longitudinal study. *Am J Med* 1990; **88**: 452–59.

202. Lane NE, Michel B, Bjorkengren A, *et al.* The risk of osteoarthritis with running and aging: a 5-year longitudinal study. *J Rheumatol* 1993; **20**: 461–8.

203. Spector TD, Harris PA, Hart DJ, *et al.* Risk of osteoarthritis associated with long-term weight-bearing sports: a radiologic survey of the hips and knees in female ex-athletes and population controls. *Arthritis Rheum* 1996; **39**: 988–95.

204. Lane NE, Oehlert JW, Bloch DA, Fries JF. The relationship of running to osteoarthritis of the knee and hip and bone mineral density of the lumbar spine: a 9 year longitudinal study. *J Rheumatol* 1998; **25**: 334–41.

205. Hannan MT, Felson DT, Anderson JJ, Naimark A. Habitual physical activity is not associated with knee osteoarthritis. *J Rheumatol* 1993; **20**: 704–9.

206. Lane NE, Hochberg MC, Pressman A, Scott JC, Nevitt MC. Recreational physical activity and the risk of osteoarthritis of the hip in elderly women. *J Rheumatol* 1999; **26**: 849–54.

207. McAlindon TE, Wilson PW, Aliabadi P, Weissman B, Felson DT. Level of physical activity and the risk of radiographic and symptomatic knee osteoarthritis in the elderly. *Am J Med* 1999; **106**: 151–7.

208. Gelber AC, Hochberg MC, Mead LA, Wang NY, Wigley FM, Klag MJ. Joint injury in young adults and risk for subsequent knee and hip osteoarthritis. *Ann Intern Med* 2000; **133**: 321–8.

209. Coggon D, Kelingray S, Inskip H, Croft P, Campbell L, Cooper C. Osteoarthritis of the hip and occupational lifting. *Am J Epidemiol* 1998; **147**: 523–8.

210. Felson DT, Anderson JJ, Naimark AA, *et al.* Does smoking protect against osteoarthritis? *Arthritis Rheum* 1989; **32**: 166–72.

211. Hart DJ, Spector TD. Cigarette smoking and risk of osteoarthritis in women in the general population: the Chingford study. *Ann Rheum Dis* 1003; **52**: 93–6.

212. McAlindon RE, Felson DT, Zhang Y, *et al.* Relation of dietary intake and serum levels of vitamin D to progression of osteoarthritis of the knee among participants in the Framingham study. *Ann Intern Med* 1996; **125**: 353–9.

213. McAlindon RE, Jacques P, Zhang Y, *et al.* Do antioxidant micronutrients protect against the development and progression of knee osteoarthritis? *Arthritis Rheum* 1996; **39**: 648–56.

214. Lane NE, Gore LR, Cumings SR, *et al.* Serum vitamin D levels and incident changes of radiographic hip osteoarthritis: a longitudinal study. *Arthritis Rheum* 1999; **42**: 854–60.

215. Busby J, Tobin J, Ettinger W, Roadarmel K, Plato CC. A longitudinal study of osteoarthritis of the hand: the effect of age. *Ann Hum Biol* 1991; **18**: 417–24.

216. Hochberg MC, Lethbridge-Cejku M, Scott WW Jr, Plato CC, Tobin JD. Age predicts progression of hand osteoarthritis in women: data from the Baltimore Longitudinal Study of Aging. *Arthritis Rheum* 1993; **36** (Suppl): R115.

217. Hernborg JS, Nilsson BE. The natural course of untreated osteoarthritis of the knee. *Clin Orthop* 1977; **123**: 130–37.

218. Massardo L, Watt I, Cushnaghan J, Dieppe P. Osteoarthritis of the knee joint: an eight year prospective study. *Ann Rheum Dis* 1989; **48**: 893–97.

219. Spector RD, Dacre JE, Harris PA, Huskisson EC. Radiological progression of osteoarthritis: an 11-year follow-up study of the knee. *Ann Rheum Dis* 1992; **51**: 1107–10.

220. Pavelka K, Gatterova J, Altman RD. Radiographic progression of knee osteoarthritis in a Czech cohort. *Clin Exp Rheumatol* 2000; **18**: 473–7.

221. Danielsson LG. Incidence and prognosis of coxarthrosis. *Acta Orthop Scand* 1964; **66**: 1–114.

222. Dougados M, Gueguen A, Nguyen M, *et al.* Radiological progression of hip osteoarthritis: definition, risk factors and correlations with clinical status. *Ann Rheum Dis* 1996; **55**: 356–62.

223. Ledingham J, Regan M, Jones A, Doherty M. Factors affecting radiographic progression of knee osteoarthritis. *Ann Rheum Dis* 1995; **54**: 53–8.

224. Schouten JS, Van den Ouweland FA, Valkenburg HA, Lamberts SW. Insulin-like growth factor-1: a prognostic factor of knee osteoarthritis. *Br J Rheumatol* 1993; **32**: 274–80.

225. Sharif M, George E, Shepstone L, *et al.* Serum hyaluronic acid level as a predictor of disease progression in osteoarthritis of the knee. *Arthritis Rheum* 1995; **38**: 760–7.

226. Sharif M, Saxne T, Shepstone L, *et al.* Relationship between serum cartilage oliomeric matrix protein levels and disease progression in osteoarthritis of the knee joint. *Br J Rheumatol* 1995; **34**: 306–10.

227. Huskisson EC, Berry H, Gishen P, Jubb RW, Whitehead J. Effects of antiinflammatory drugs on the progression of osteoarthritis of the knee: LINK Study Group. Longitudinal Investigation of Nonsteroidal Antiinflammatory Drugs in Knee Osteoarthritis. *J Rheumatol* 1995; **22**: 1941–6.

228. Spector TD, Hart DJ, Nandra D, *et al.* Low-level increases in serum C-reactive protein are present in early osteoarthritis of the knee and predict progressive disease. *Arthritis Rheum* 1997; **40**: 723–7.

229. Sharif M, Shepstone L, Elson CJ, Dieppe PA, Kirwan RJ. Increased serum C reactive protein may reflect events that precede radiographic progression in osteoarthritis of the knee. *Ann Rheum Dis* 2000; **59**: 71–4.

230. Dougados M, Gueguen A, Nguyen M, *et al.* Radiographic features predictive of radiographic progression of hip osteoarthritis. *Rev Rhum Engl Ed* 1997; **64**: 795–803.

231. Ledingham J, Dawson S, Preston B, Milligan G, Doherty M. Radiographic progression of hospital referred osteoarthritis of the hip. *Ann Rheum Dis* 1993; **52**: 263–7.

232. Conrozier T, Chappuis-Cellier C, Richard M, Mathieu P, Richard S, Vignon E. Increased serum C-reactive protein levels by immunonephelometry in patients with rapidly destructive hiposteoarthritis. *Rev Rhum Engl Ed* 1998; **65**: 759–65.

233. Conrozier T, Saxne T, Fan CS, *et al.* Serum concentrations of cartilage oligomeric matrix protein and bone sialoprotein in hip osteoarthritis: a one year prospective study. *Ann Rheum Dis* 1998; **57**: 527–32.

234. Dieppe P, Cushnaghan J, Shepstone L. The Bristol OA500 study: progression of osteoarthritis OA. over 3 years and the relationship between clinical and radiographic changes at the knee joint. *Osteoarthritis Cartilage* 1997; **5**: 87–97.

235. Dieppe P, Cushnaghan J, Tucker M, Browning S, Shepstone L. The Bristol OA500 Study: progression and impact of the disease after 8 years. *Osteoarthritis Cartilage* 2000; **8**: 63–8.

13 | Gout

Marc C. Hochberg

Gout is an ancient disease with a great deal known of both its pathophysiology and treatment. Clinically, it is characterized by: (1) recurrent attacks of acute arthritis involving one or more joints; (2) deposits of mono-sodium urate crystals in articular cartilage and/or synovial membrane which, when released into synovial fluid, provoke an acute inflammatory response; (3) elevation of serum and plasma concentrations of uric acid; and (4) the variable presence of renal disease including uric acid nephrolithiasis.

This chapter will focus on the areas of disease classification, morbidity rates, factors associated with the development of gout, and the relationship of gout and hyperuricemia with all-cause mortality and the development of coronary artery disease.

Classification criteria

The first criteria for the classification of gout were proposed at the Rome Symposium on Population Studies in the Rheumatic Diseases [1]; for a person to have gout, two of the following four criterion items had to be present: (1) a serum uric acid level above 7.0 mg/dl in males or 6.0 mg/dl in females; (2) tophi; (3) uric acid crystals in synovial fluid or tissues; and (4) a history of attacks of painful joint swelling of abrupt onset with remission within 2 weeks. These criteria were subsequently modified at the Third International Symposium in New York in 1966; the major changes being the addition of a response to colchicine and the removal of serum uric acid levels (Table 13.1) [2]. Rigby and Wood (1994) [3] compared the New York and Rome criteria in 59 patients with gout and 761 patients with other arthropathies. The best performing individual criterion was one or more attacks of podagra (see Table 13.1). Overall, the New York criteria were more sensitive and more specific than the Rome criteria.

Table 13.1 New York Criteria for the classification of gout

A. The presence of uric acid crystals in synovial fluid or of urate deposition in the tissues, demonstrated by chemical or microscopic examination. The demonstration of urate urinary calculi does not satisfy this criterion.

OR

B. The presence of two or more of the following criteria:
1. A clear history and/or observation of at least two attacks of painful limb joint swelling. The attacks, at least in the early stages, must exhibit an abrupt onset of severe pain and complete clinical remission within a week or two.
2. A clear history and/or observation of podagra—an attack as described in Criterion 1 involving the great toe.
3. The presence of a tophus, observed clinically.
4. A clear history and/or observation of a good response to colchicine, defined as a major reduction in objective signs of inflammation within 48 h of the onset of the therapy.

Modified from [2].

In 1977, the American College of Rheumatology (formerly the American Rheumatism Association) published preliminary criteria for the classification of gout for use in either clinical settings or in population-based epidemiologic surveys (Table 13.2) [4]. Subjects were classified as having gout with (1) the presence of urate crystals in joint fluid, (2) the presence of a proven tophus, or (3) the presence of at least six of the 12 clinical, laboratory, or radiographic features listed in Table 13.2A. This combination had a sensitivity of 97.8 per cent in 178 patients with gout while the specificity was 89.1 per cent in 110 patients with pseudogout and 98 per cent in 299 patients with rheumatoid arthritis. Recognizing that, in surveys, data on joint fluid analysis will not be available, the subcommittee recommended that subjects in population surveys be classified as having gout with the presence of at least six of the 11 criteria (Table 13.2B); this had a sensitivity of only 84.8 per cent but a

Table 13.2   ARA criteria for acute arthritis of primary gout

A. Clinical setting:
　　1. More than one attack of acute arthritis
　　2. Maximum inflammation developed within 1 day
　　3. Monoarthritis attack
　　4. Redness observed over joints
　　5. First MTP joint painful or swollen
　　6. Unilateral first MTP joint attack
　　7. Unilateral tarsal joint attack
　　8. Tophus (suspected)
　　9. Hyperuricemia
　　10. Asymmetric swelling within a joint on X-ray[a]
　　11. Subcortical cysts without erosions on X-ray
　　12. Joint fluid culture negative for organisms during attack
B. Survey setting:
　　1. More than one attack of acute arthritis
　　2. Maximum inflammation developed within 1 day
　　3. Oligoarthritis attack
　　4. Redness observed over joints
　　5. First MTP joint painful or swollen
　　6. Unilateral first MTP joint attack
　　7. Unilateral tarsal joint attack
　　8. Tophus (proven or suspected)
　　9. Hyperuricemia
　　10. Asymmetric swelling within a joint on X-ray[a]
　　11. Complete termination of an attack

[a] This criterion could logically be found on examination as well as on X-ray. However, the protocol did not request this information in regard to examination.
Modified from [4].

specificity of 92.7 per cent in patients with pseudo-gout and 98.3 per cent in patients with rheumatoid arthritis.

Occurrence

Measurement

The occurrence of gout is classically described in terms of prevalence, but examination of the available literature from population surveys suggests considerable variation in methodology. The most common method is to use a historical survey asking for a history of acute attacks of arthritis, particularly involving the first metatarsophalangeal joint (i.e. podagra). This method will, if recall is accurate, determine the cumulative prevalence to the age at survey. If the attack was at some distance in time, then the measure approximates to a period prevalence during the period of recall. In some surveys, cases over-report the occurrence of acute gout as validated by inspection of medical reports [5].

Other surveys have combined this period prevalence with current disease features including tophi, hyperuricemia, and, if performed, radiological change. Studies relying on current disease features will obviously underestimate lifetime or even period prevalence. It is, in practice, virtually impossible to determine from the available literature exactly the measure obtained and thus comparisons between studies are fraught with difficulties.

Prevalence

Gout is a common disease with a world-wide distribution. The results from a large number of surveys are summarized in Table 13.3. Currie [6] estimated the prevalence of gout in the United Kingdom using data from a sample of general practices; the overall prevalence was 2.6 per 1000 in both sexes combined for persons above age 15. Prevalence was greater in males than females and increased with increasing age in both sexes. More recent data, from 40 United Kingdom general practices with over 300 000 patients, show that the overall prevalence has risen to almost 10 per 1000 while the male-to-female ratio and the age gradient remain unchanged (Table 13.4) [7].

In the United States, data on the prevalence of gout come from the 1992 National Health Interview Survey and are based on self-report in response to the question 'Have you, or any member of your household, had gout within the past year?' [8,9]. Overall prevalence in respondents of all ages, both sexes, and all races combined was 8.4 per 1000. Prevalence was greater at all ages in males than females and increased with increasing age in both sexes, approaching 3 per 100 in persons aged 65 and above (Table 13.5). Of interest, prevalence among African-Americans was higher than among Caucasians at ages 45 and above in both sexes.

Geographic and ethnic variation

Low rates of gout were noted in early studies among Europeans living in rural as opposed to urban areas [10–12]. Native American populations, such as the Blackfeet and Pima, had low rates of gout compared to Caucasians [13]. The majority of studies that have identified geographic and ethnic variations in occurrence have been performed in Asian/Polynesian populations and in Africa.

Table 13.3 Prevalence rates of gout per 1000 population by age and sex

				Disease		Prevalence/1000	
Reference	Country	Population	N	Definition[a]	Age	Males	Females
(a) European							
[10]	Netherlands	Rural north	3378	H	15+	0	0
[11]	UK	Wensleydale	891	H,E,T	15+		
		Leigh	380	H,E,T	55–64		14.4
[105]	Bulgaria	Sofia	420	H,E,U	15+		
[12]	Finland	Rural	1785	H	16+	1	0
[62]	France	Paris (mainly police)	4321	H,E,U	20+	34.8	N/A
[106]	Denmark	Copenhagen-males	5249	H	40–59	16.6	N/A
[5]	UK	Cotswolds	3892	H[b]	35+	16.8	2.8
[6]	UK	General practices:			15+		
		England	259000			7.3	1.3
		Wales	40500			5.2	0.5
		Scotland	75000			2.8	0.7
[107]	UK	3 towns (males)	10539	H	45+	43.3	N/A
[7]	UK	42 GPs	300376	GPs		16.44	2.93
[108]	UK	Scottish Highlands	35251	GPs		5.3	1.5
(b) American							
[43]	US	New Haven	2060	H	15+	+16.9[c]	4.8
[109]	US	Tecumseh Michigan	4105	H,E,U	20+	7.2	0
[26]	Jamaica	Rural	522	H,E,U	35–64	8	0
[35]	US	Framingham	5127	H,U	32+	28.5	3.9
[13]	US	Pima Indians	948	H,U	30+	4.3	0
			1022			0	0
[110]	US	Sudbury	4626	Rome/New York	15+	6.6	1.0
(c) Asian/Pacific							
[111]	New Zealand	European				42[c]	Detailed data
		Maoris				33	not given
[112]	Mariana Islands	Chamorros	335	U,E	40+	High	
		Carolinians	55				
[113]	Japan	Akegawa	1053	H,U,X,T	40–64	3.0	1.2
		Onchi	1120				
		Minami-Takayasu	884				
[114]	New Zealand	European	430	H,U	20+	19.8	0
		Maoris	747			104.1	18.3
	Cook Island	Pukapuka	379			53.2	0
		Rarotonga	471			24.7	0
[115]	Japan	Hiroshima Nagasaki	17300	H,U	20+	1.3	0
[116]	Australia	Sydney (working males)	500	H	19–59	14	N/A
[117]	New Zealand	Maoris	766	H	15+	88	8

Table 13.3 *(continued)*

Reference	Country	Population	N	Disease Definition[a]	Age	Prevalence/1000 Males	Prevalence/1000 Females
[118]	Nauru	Micronesians	455	H,U	20+	69	4
[119]	Japan	Nagano	34000	ARA	20+	2.7	0.3
[48]	New Zealand	Maoris	115	H	N/S	86.9	N/S
[15]	Tokelau	Islanders migrant to New Zealand 1968–1974	903	H	15+	22.6	0
			998			17.9	0
	Tokelau	Islanders migrant to New Zealand 1980–1982	792	H	15+	18.8	0
			1318			46.5	6.5
[20]	China	Huangpu district (Shanghai)	2037	Questionnaire		7.7	3.4[c]
[22]	Taiwan	Atayal aborigines	342	Clinical presentation	18+	262	10
[24]	Java	Rural	4683	NY criteria 2+ ARA criteria 6+	15+	17	1
[33]	New Zealand	Maori (≥ 25% ancestry)	342	ARA criteria 6+	15+	139	19
		Europeans	315		15+	58	6
[19]	Taiwan	Aborigines	396	Wallace criteria	40+	152	48
		Non-aborigines	648		40+	34	28
(d) Africans							
[120]	Namibia	Hottentot	409	H,E,X	15+	0	0
[121]	South Africa	Tswana	370	H,E,X	14+	0	0
[122]	Xhosa	Xhosa	479	H,E,X,U	15+	0	0
[123]	Nigeria/Liberia	3 populations	831	H,E,X	15+	0	0

[a] H = History (normally of acute attack), E = Examination, T = Tophi, U = raised uric acid, X = X-ray, GP = General Practice diagnosis
[b] Checked with general practice records
[c] Both sexes combined

Table 13.4 Prevalence rates of gout per 1000 population of United Kingdom age 15 or over, by age and sex

Age range (years)	Males	Females
<35	0.96	0.09
35–44	12.86	0.54
45–54	23.42	1.70
55–64	35.48	3.84
65–74	49.91	8.80
≥75	53.08	14.31

Source: [7]

Table 13.5 Prevalence of gout per 1000 by sex and race in three age groups in the United States, 1992

	< 44	45–64	65+
Sex			
Males	4.4	26.3	44.1
Females	0.3	8.1	18.2
Race			
Black	1.4	38.5	54.5
White	2.5	14.7	26.7
Overall	1.8	16.8	29.0

Source: [8].

Asian/Polynesian populations

New Zealand Maoris [14], Polynesians from the Cook Islands, and the Marianas and Micronesians from Naura have the highest rates of gout in the world, approaching cumulative prevalence rates of 10 per 100 in men. Even in these populations, the prevalence in women is substantially less. Studies of the Tokelau Islanders are of particular interest [15–17]. Tokelau consists of three small islands north of New Zealand. The indigenous population was less than 5000, of whom over half had migrated to New Zealand by 1982. This migration has enabled a natural experiment on the effect of urbanization on the high occurrence of gout in the non-migrants. Undoubtedly, this population has a predisposition to hyperuricemia and on migration their increased predisposition to gout is not lost. Indeed, the increased exposure to alcohol and perhaps a 'western' diet enhances the risk in this already at-risk group [15].

The other classic migrant study of gout is that of Filipinos who had migrated to Hawaii and the continental United States who both have substantially increased rates of gout compared to the 'native' population in these areas. What is of considerable interest is that racially identical Filipinos, who have not migrated,

have low rates of gout and of hyperuricemia [18]. In summary, therefore, Polynesian groups do have a particular tendency to gout and this is enhanced by migration to westernized societies.

Studies in the past decade have focused on the prevalence of gout in Chinese and Taiwanese [19–23], Indonesians [24], and Thais [25]. A high prevalence has been noted in Aboriginal Taiwanese and Indonesian populations, but not in Chinese and those living in rural Thailand; this has been attributed to ethnic/genetic and dietary factors.

African populations

In contrast to the Polynesian story, there is almost a complete absence of gout in population surveys in African groups. The samples studied, however, were small and it might be postulated that there would be differences in recall of acute gout between European and African populations. Nonetheless, this broad ethnic group does seem protected against gout in contrast to the African-American populations. Furthermore, the prevalence of gout in Afro-Caribbeans living in Jamaica is comparable to European rates [26]. Gout has been described in clinical series from Africa [27–31].

Temporal trends in prevalence

Data on self-reported prevalence of gout from the United States National Health Interview Survey are available from 1969 through 1992 [9,32]. These data suggest that the overall prevalence of self-reported gout doubled during the period from 1969 through 1985, but has slightly declined or remained stable over the last 10 years with a ratio of approximately 8.5 cases per 1000 for age 18 and above, both sexes and all races combined.

Klemp *et al.* [33] compared results of a prevalence survey in New Zealand with earlier data and concluded that the prevalence of gout had increased in both Maori and Europeans, particularly in men. The increase in prevalence has also been noted in the United Kingdom when the data from Harris *et al.* [7] are compared to those of Currie *et al.* [6].

Incidence

The incidence of gout has been examined in both the United Kingdom [34] and the United States [35–39]. Using data from the Second and Third National Studies

Table 13.6 Annual incidence of gout per 1000 from the Second and Third National Studies of Morbidity in General Practice

Age (years)	Males		Females	
	1971	1981	1971	1981
25–44	1.4	1.7	0.4	0.4
45–64	3.7	4.5	0.8	1.2
65–74	3.1	4.7	0.9	1.7
75 +	4.1	7.6	0.6	2.5
All ages	1.6	2.1	0.4	0.7

Modified from [34].

of Morbidity in General Practice, Stewart and Silman [34] reported an overall incidence of 1.4 per 1000 in all ages and both sexes combined in 1981–82. Incidence was greater in males than females and increased with increasing age; of further interest was the apparent temporal increase from 1971–75 to 1981–82 (Table 13.6).

Hall *et al.* [35] studied the 14-year cumulative incidence of gout in subjects in the Framingham Study and noted that gout developed in 2.8 per cent of 2283 men and 0.4 per cent of 2844 females. More recent data from the Framingham Study show that 3.7 per cent of men and 0.6 per cent of women have developed gout [37]. As this study is constructed of biennial examinations, Abbott *et al.* [37] estimated the age- and sex-specific 2-year average incidence rate of gout; herein, gout incidence was 1.7 per 1000 per 2-years overall in both sexes combined, in persons aged 30 and above. Incidence was greater in males than females and peaked in the 50–59 year age group in males (Table 13.7).

The incidence of gout has also been estimated among 2046 initially 'healthy' men in the Veterans Administrations Normative Aging Study [36]. A total

Table 13.7 Average annual incidence of gout per 1000 by age and gender, the Framingham Study

Age range (years)	Annualized rate (per thousand)	
	Males	Females
30–39	1.3 (6/2345)[a]	0.2 (1/2845)
40–49	1.7 (22/6348)	0.1 (1/7922)
50–59	2.1 (38/8777)	0.3 (7/10997)
60–69	1.1 (14/6456)	0.2 (3/8562)
70 +	1.1 (6/2598)	0.5 (4/3804)
Total	1.6 (86/26524)	0.2 (16/34130)

Source: [37].
[a] Number of new cases/person-bienniums at risk.

of 84 new cases of gout occurred over a 15-year follow-up interval corresponding to an incidence rate of 2.8 per 1000 person-years of observation.

Roubenoff *et al.* [38] reported the incidence of gout among members of the Johns Hopkins Precursors Study, a prospective cohort study of medical students enrolled in the Johns Hopkins University School of Medicine between 1948 and 1964. During follow-up through 1988, gout developed in 60 of 1215 males but in none of the 121 females ($P < 0.01$); the average incidence of gout among males was 1.73 per 1000 person-years of follow-up, and the cumulative incidence was 8.6 per cent. Hochberg *et al.* [39] compared the incidence of gout between a subset of predominantly Caucasian men in the Johns Hopkins Precursors Study and male members of the Meharry Cohort Study, a prospective cohort study of African-American medical students enrolled in Meharry Medical College. The incidence of gout, based on self-report, was 3.11 per 1000 person-years in the Meharry men and 1.82 per 1000 person-years in the Hopkins men. The cumulative incidence was 10.9 and 5.8 per cent, respectively, corresponding to a relative risk (95 per cent confidence interval) of 1.7 (1.0, 2.8). Thus, not only prevalence but also incidence of gout was higher in African-American compared to Caucasian men.

Risk factors

Hyperuricemia

The primary risk factor for gout is sustained hyperuricemia. In the United States Caucasian population, serum uric acid levels follow a normal distribution with a skew towards higher levels, especially in males (Fig. 13.1) [40]. Mean serum uric acid levels increase during adolescence and remain stable throughout adulthood in men, while in females there is an increase during adolescence, a plateau during the reproductive years, a second increase concurrent with the menopausal years, and a second plateau in the postmenopausal years (Fig. 13.2) [40]. The higher mean serum uric acid level in postmenopausal compared to premenopausal women was studied by Wingrove *et al.* [41], who felt that this was related to metabolic changes as a consequence of the menopause.

Hyperuricemia can either be defined statistically, that is values greater than two standard deviations above the group mean, or physiologically; the latter corresponds to a level of 7.0 mg/dl or above where plasma

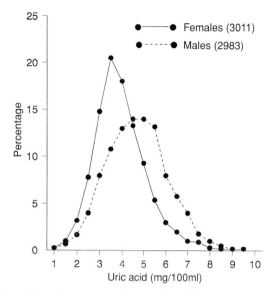

Fig. 13.1　Distribution of serum uric acid levels by gender.

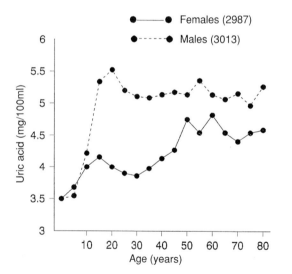

Fig. 13.2　Distribution of serum uric acid levels by age for males and females.

Table 13.8　Cumulative incidence per 100 of gout by baseline serum uric acid level and gender, the Framingham Study

Baseline SUA	Males		Females	
	No. at risk	Rate	No. at risk	Rate
< 6.0	1615	1.1	2405	0.1
6.0–6.9	354	7.3	71	7.0
7.0–7.9	78	14.2	11	27.2
≥ 8.0	22	36.7	1	0

Modified from 35].
SUA = serum uric acid in mg/100 ml.

Table 13.9　Cumulative incidence per 100 and incidence rate per 1000 person-years by baseline serum uric acid level in male subjects, Boston Veteran Administration Normative Aging Study

Baseline SUA	Incidence rate per 1000	Cumulative incidence
< 6.0	0.8	0.5
6.0–6.9	0.9	0.6
7.0–7.9	4.1	2.0
8.0–8.9	8.4	4.1
9.0–9.9	43.2	19.8
≥ 10.0	70.2	30.5

Modified from [36]
SUA = serum uric acid level in mg/dl.

years (Tables 13.8 and 13.9). Indeed, even among men with asymptomatic hyperuricemia, there is a dose–response relationship between higher serum uric acid levels and greater cumulative incidence of gout [42].

Hyperuricemia in different populations

It is obviously of interest to compare the population levels of uric acid with the rates of gout in the same populations. There have been a substantial number of population surveys examining levels of uric acid. A summary of the major surveys is shown in Table 13.10 for European, American, Asian/Pacific, and African populations. Not all the surveys are random population studies, many are surveys of occupational and other selected groups. The surveys presented cover very different age groups but in adult life, in cross-sectional studies, age has only a limited effect on serum uric acid levels in men. Indeed, within westernized societies, there seems to be little effect of social class [43], so that it may be reasonable to compare the results from different populations.

proteins become supersaturated with uric acid and tissue deposition of sodium urate occurs. The role of hyperuricemia as a risk factor for gout was established in population-based prospective cohort studies. In both the Framingham study [35] and the Veterans Administration Normative Aging Study [36], there was a dose–response relationship between serum uric acid levels and risk of developing gout measured as either cumulative incidence or incidence per 1000 person-

Table 13.10 Mean serum uric acid levels in different population surveys

Reference	Country	Population	N	Age	Mean uric acid (mg/100 ml) Males	Females
(a) European						
[11]	UK	Leigh (urban)	288	55–64	4.9	4.3
		Wensleydale (rural)	911	15+	4.5	3.7
[105]	Bulgaria	Sofia	420	15+	4.9	4.3
[62]	France	Paris	6182	20+	6.0	N/A
[124]	UK	Dorset	393	N/S	5.5	4.1
		Birmingham	373		5.5	3.9
[101]	Italy		181	38	348 ± 59 µM	277 ± 59 µM
[125]	German	North	3584	Adult	5.71 ±1.62	4.22 ± 1.06 µM
[72]	The Netherlands	Caucasian	460	65–79	341 ± 79 µM	305 ± 71 µM
(b) American						
[126]	US	Executives	339	25–64	5.8	N/A
		Craftsman	532		4.7	N/A
[40]	US	Tecumseh	6000	4+	4.9	42
[127]	US	New Haven	1213	15+	6.4	4.7
[26]	Jamaica	Blacks	522	35–64	5 (mode)	4 (mode)
[35]	US	Framingham	5172	32–64	5.1	4.0
[13]	US	Pima Indians	948	30+	4.6	4.5
		Blackfeet Indians	1022	30+	5.2	3.9
[110]	US	Sudbury	6000	15+	5.9	4.2
[128]	Canada	Sherbrooke	1191	10+	5.8	4.7
[44]	US	Bogalusa, Louisiana White	3983	19–26	6.49	4.2
(c) Asian/Pacific						
[50]	Alaska	Filipinos	113	40–67	6.3	N/A
		Caucasians	88	40–49	5.0	N/A
[129]	Hawaii	Pure Hawaiian	49	22–72	5.4	5.8
[46]	New Zealand	Maoris	755	20+	7.1	6.0
	Cook Island	Rarotonga	471		7.0	
		Pukapuka	379		7.0	6.2
[51]	Philippines	Filipino	483	21–87	5.2	
[113]	Japan	Akasaka	382	20+	4.9	3.9
		Shindo	430	20+	4.2	3.4
[22]	Central Taiwan	Atayal aborigines	342	18+	7.9	5.7
[24]	Indonesia	Java	4683	15+	6.2	5.2
[54]	China	Urban	2013	40.58	5.75	4.67
		Rural	1507	40.58	5.58	4.48
[71]	Japan		2686	48.56	5.74	–
[131]	Taiwan	Aborigines	396	40+	8.0	7.0
		Non-aborigines	648	40+	6.6	5.5

In all studies shown, there is a higher mean level of serum uric acid in men compared to women mirroring the excess male prevalence of gout. However, there is an imperfect association between mean population uric acid levels and the prevalence rates shown in Table 13.3. In part, this might reflect the lack of consistency in the disease prevalence surveys mentioned above.

Serum uric acid levels in European and North American Caucasian populations are similar. Studies in mixed racial populations in the United States show higher mean serum levels among young adult Caucasian than African-American subjects and a greater prevalence of hyperuricemia [44]. No such differences were found in a study comparing Caucasian and non-Caucasians in Brazil [45].

Studies in Asian/Pacific populations, particularly the Polynesians, provide the most interest. Polynesian populations, including New Zealand Maoris, Cook Islanders, and Micronesians, that have high rates of gout also have high serum uric acid levels [14,15,46,47]. The Tokelau Island migrant studies [15], as well as the studies of Cook Islanders who migrated from Pukapuka to Rarotanga and then to New Zealand [46], were very informative in separating out the effects of ethnicity and environment on serum uric acid levels. In brief, the differences in prevalence of gout was not apparently explained by differences in serum uric acid levels, and is probably related to environmental changes in a group already genetically susceptible. The high uric acid levels in the Maori men seem to be due to problems in renal urate clearance [48]. These conclusions have been extended to Polynesian women by Simmonds *et al.* [49], who found a reduced fractional clearance of uric acid in Polynesian women compared with healthy Caucasian women.

The other Asian migrant group studied in detail is the Filipinos. In Alaskan populations, the Filipinos have higher uric acid levels than Caucasians [50] which is not the case for Filipinos living in the Philippines [51]. Similarly, gout itself is substantially rarer in Filipinos in the Philippines than in those living in Hawaii [51]. The authors of that study also suggested that Filipinos have an inherited tendency to poor renal handling of uric acid that under western lifestyle influences leads to hyperuricemia and gout.

Japanese and Chinese populations have 'normal' uric acid levels [20,42,52–55], although Suomo wrestlers, of whom 11 per cent develop gout, have high levels, probably related to body weight [56]. Other Asian populations with high uric acid levels include Malays [57] and Samoans [58].

Time trends in uric acid levels

Glynn *et al.* [59] studied temporal trends in serum uric acid levels and examined factors predictive of a longitudinal increase in uric acid levels between baseline and third examination in 1141 men in the Veterans Administration Normative Aging Study. Using multiple regression analysis to predict serum uric acid at the third examination, the authors identified serum uric acid, serum triglyceride level, body mass index, and number of alcoholic drinks per day measured at baseline, as well as an increase in body mass index, to all contribute significantly. Indeed, after controlling for baseline serum uric acid level, the best predictor of the subsequent uric acid level was an increase in body mass index. Age, socioeconomic status, cigarette consumption, and blood urea nitrogen level failed to enter the regression model as significant variables.

Nakanishi *et al.* [60] examined risk factors for the development of hyperuricemia among 1445 Japanese male office workers aged 30 to 54 years. The incidence of hyperuricemia was significantly related to higher body mass index, higher mean blood pressure, alcohol intake, higher serum triglyceride levels, and not smoking. Both these studies provide important data as they identify variables that can be targeted for primary prevention if they are confirmed to be associated with incidence of gout in analytic epidemiologic studies.

Body weight

Several clinical and population-based cross-sectional studies of patients with gout have demonstrated an association with obesity, defined as either per cent above ideal body weight or body mass index [35,37,61–65]. Three prospective studies have confirmed the association between higher body mass index and a higher risk for the development of gout [36,38,42]. These data extended the observation that an increase in body mass index, shown to predict an increase in serum uric acid [55,59], also independently predicts the development of gout [38,42].

In the Veterans Administration Normative Aging Study, baseline body mass index was associated with the development of gout after adjustment for age, hypertension, cholesterol level, alcohol intake, glucose level, and socioeconomic status; in a Cox proportional hazards model, the relative risk was 1.11 (95 per cent confidence intervals 1.04, 1.19) [36].

In the Johns Hopkins Precursor Study, body mass index at age 35 predicted the development of gout with

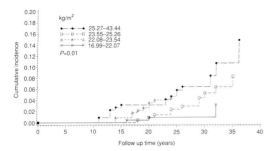

Fig. 13.3 Incidence of gout by body mass index at age 35, The Johns Hopkins Precursors Study.

a dose–response relationship; the cumulative incidence of gout rose from 3.2 to 14.8 per 100 from the lower quartile of body mass index (17–22 kg/m^2) to the highest quartile (>25 kg/m^2), P = 0.01 for trend (Fig. 13.3) [38]. Furthermore, increase in body mass index between cohort entry (median age 22) and age 35 also predicted the development of gout; subjects whose body mass index increased more than 1.88 kg/m^2 had a two-fold greater risk of gout even after adjustment for hypertension, P = 0.02. In a recent prospective study of 223 middle-aged Taiwanese men with asymptomatic hyperuricemia living on Kinmen Island, baseline obesity, defined as a body mass index of 27 or above, was associated with an increased risk of developing gout (OR = 1.91, 95% CI 0.98, 4.01), as was an increase in body mass index associated with an increased risk of developing gout (relative hazard = 1.51; 95% CI 1.12–2.19, per unit increase) [23].

Thus, both overweight and an increase in body weight during young adulthood and middle age are potentially modifiable risk factors for the development of gout. Data in 15 overweight subjects, six with gout [66], which was subsequently extended to 35 overweight subjects [67], showed that a mean weight loss of 7 kg was associated with a significant fall in both serum uric acid and urinary uric acid excretion, consistent with a decrease in production of uric acid via either a fall in *de novo* purine synthesis or decreased protein intake.

Hypertension

Hypertension is also an independent risk factor for the development of gout [36,38,39,68], confirming cross-sectional data from case–control studies [31,37,65]. In the Normative Aging Study, the presence of hypertension was associated with a three-fold excess risk of gout after adjustment for age [36]. Of interest, among

hypertensives, the incidence of gout increases with increasing age from 4.6 to 5.9 and 9.5 per 1000 person-years in the age groups 20–39 years, 40–59 years, and 60 and above, respectively. In a Cox proportional hazards model adjusting for other potential risk factors, hypertension remained a significantly independent predictor of gout with a RR = 1.99 (95% CI 1.15–3.42).

In the Johns Hopkins Precursors Study, the role of hypertension developing before gout was examined in Cox proportional hazard models using time-dependent covariates; again, hypertension was a significant predictor of gout with a RR = 2.7; 95% CI 1.5–5.1 [38]. When data from this cohort were analyzed in conjunction with those from the Meharry Cohort Study, incident hypertension was also independently associated with the development of gout with a RR = 3.8; 95% CI 2.2–6.6 [39]. Furthermore, the excess incidence of hypertension among African-American male physicians explained their greater risk of developing gout compared to Caucasian male physicians [39].

Grodzicki *et al.* [68] examined the incidence of gout in patients with hypertension and controls followed as part of the General Practice Hypertension Study Group. After 8 years of follow-up, gout developed in 3.1 per cent of 1190 hypertensive patients and 0.9 per cent of controls; the excess risk for gout in men with hypertension was present in those treated with diuretics (RR = 6.25, 95% CI 2.4–16.7) and those not treated with diuretics (RR = 3.93; 95% CI 1.6– 9.7).

Thus, hypertension, independent of body weight, is also a potentially modifiable risk factor for gout. It is unclear whether diuretic treatment for hypertension carries its own increased risk independent of the presence of hypertension alone [42]. Finally, it is also of note that higher serum uric acid levels are independently associated with an increased risk of developing hypertension among men initially free of hypertension even after adjusting for age, body mass index, and serum levels of cholesterol and triglycerides [69]. Thus, the relationship between serum uric acid levels, blood pressure and the development of gout is quite complex.

Alcohol intake

Alcohol intake has been shown to be associated with higher serum uric acid levels in both cross-sectional [55,70–72] and longitudinal studies [59]. However, the association of alcohol consumption with gout has not been firmly established as most published case studies have methodological flaws.

In a case–control study of risk factors for gout, Richter [65] and Hochberg *et al.* [39] confirmed an association between consumption of 'moonshine' whiskey and gout (OR = 2.8, 95% CI 1.6–5.0) but failed to demonstrate significant associations between either beer or wine consumption and gout. Moonshine whiskey has a high lead content as it is distilled using car radiators and the alcohol vapor leaches lead from solder as it cools. This form of gout has been referred to as 'saturnine' gout, and probably dates back in history to Roman times, drawing its name from Saturn, the Roman god of agriculture and civilization [73].

In a case–control study of 90 black South African patients with gout, alcohol consumption was associated with increased odds of gout in both men and women [31]. It is unclear whether this alcohol was commercially or individually produced.

Alcohol intake, although directly associated with serum uric acid levels [59], was not independently associated with gout in the Normative Aging Study [36]. Thus, while alcohol consumption has not been definitely shown to be an independent risk factor for gout, moonshine whiskey and alcohol, especially wines stored in lead crystal containers, should be avoided.

Lead exposure

As noted above, the role of lead exposure in the development of gout has been recognized since Roman times. Although saturnine gout is most often associated with consumption of moonshine whiskey in the United States, other sources of lead, including occupational and environmental exposures, should be considered.

Richter [65] performed a case–control study to assess the role of occupational and environmental exposure to lead as risk factors for gout in men. She obtained a lifetime occupational history from 100 cases and an equal number of age- and race-matched controls and a team of industrial hygienists, blinded to case status, classified all occupations as being at either no, low, medium, or high risk of lead exposure. Men who worked in jobs with either medium or high lead exposure were at a significantly greater risk of having gout, RR of 1.03 per year of exposure, even after adjustment for obesity, hypertension, socioeconomic status, and alcohol consumption. Furthermore, men employed in several industries or occupations known to carry a medium or high risk of lead exposure were also more likely to

have gout; examples include plumbers or pipefitters (OR = 5.3), shipbuilders (OR = 4.9), painters (OR = 3.3), or steelworkers (OR = 1.7). Other high-risk occupations, not sufficiently represented in this study, include battery and automotive radiator workers. Indeed, in a study of 105 storage battery workers in Hungary, Poor and Mituszova found significantly higher serum uric acid levels than in controls; this was felt to be due to decreased renal uric acid excretion secondary to lead nephrotoxicity [74]. Thus, occupational lead exposure is also a potentially modifiable risk factor for gout.

Genetic factors

The observation that there might be a genetic component to gout dates back over 350 years to the observation by Sydenham that gout sometimes 'invades those ... when they have received the ill seeds of this disease from their parents by inheritance' [75]. Much of the work on the genetics of gout has been based on family studies of hyperuricemia in first degree relatives of affected gouty probands. The demonstration of any clustering within families would be consistent both with the effects of a shared environment or shared genes in raising uric acid levels. Apart from rare diseases such as the X-linked hypoxanthine guanine phosphoribosyl transferase (HGPRT) deficiency, no genetic defects have currently been elucidated to explain the occurrence of hyperuricemia. One study of renal uric acid clearance in families taking a low purine diet showed a correlation between relatives and their gouty probands, suggestive of an inherited trait [76].

Population studies

There have been few studies of the familial aggregation of hyperuricemia or gout based on probands ascertained from a population survey. In a study of the Blackfeet and Pima Indians in North America, the uric acid levels of relatives of hyperuricemic probands were only marginally elevated above the population means [77]. In an analysis of population data from the Tecumseh survey in the state of Michigan, there were only very weak genetic associations between family members in uric acid levels [78]. Of interest, the associations in uric acid levels were strong and significant among sibs living in the same household, while those among sibs living in different households were not significant.

More recently, data from 2146 subjects in 685 nuclear families living in five North American communities participating in the Lipid Research Clinics Study have been analyzed to examine familial aggregation and segregation patterns of serum uric acid levels [79,80]. Familial resemblance of uric acid levels was detected with higher genetic heritability in offspring than parent pairs [79]. Segregation analysis detected a major effect not compatible with Mendelian transmission, with a remaining multifactorial component that accounted for more of the variation in uric acid levels in offspring than in parents [80].

Family studies

The available data should be interpreted with care. Many case reports or series of families are selected on the basis of a strong family history of gout, and, as a consequence, the attributable risk of shared familial factors in explaining the population occurrence of gout is impossible to determine. Results of some of the classical studies are shown in Table 13.11. Earlier studies suggested a Mendelian inheritance based on the observation that the distribution of uric acid levels in relative followed a bimodal distribution [81,82]; this was not confirmed in subsequent studies [78,83]. The Arthritis and Rheumatism Council Family Survey demonstrated an excess of clinical gout among 283 first-degree relatives of 124 hyperuricemic probands, 54 of whom had gout; it is unclear whether the familial cases occurred in relatives of probands with gout or asymptomatic hyperuricemia [84]. Statistical analysis of these family data was consistent with a polygenic mode of inheritance of gout; however, analysis of data regarding patterns of inheritance of hyperuricemia was not consistent with this model.

Twin studies

There is some similarity in uric acid levels in twins. In twins with normal levels, there was a greater similarity in monozygotic compared to dizygotic twins [85,86], though the similarity was less marked in male monozygotic twins suggesting perhaps a greater environmental component in men. In the Arthritis and Rheumatism Council's twin survey of 53 monozygotic and 192 dizygotic twins, unselected in relation to their uric acid level, there were no monozygotic twins with gout and only six dizygotic twin pairs discordant for gout. Similarly, hyperuricemia was present in eight index twins but all eight cotwins had normal serum uric acid levels.

In summary, while there is some evidence of genetic influence on uric acid levels, the data are conflicting and do not support a single model of inheritance. Furthermore, the role of genetic factors seems, at least in Caucasian populations, substantially less than the role of male sex, body weight, and environmental factors.

Prognosis

Gout, by itself, is not a fatal disease. Lawrence [84], however, noted that 'though life expectancy is not ... reduced in gout, there is nevertheless an appreciable mortality in this disease mainly from ... myocardial infarction'.

Talbott and Lilienfeld [87] studied 168 patients with gout followed for almost 1800 person-years and estimated a standardized mortality ratio of 87, not significantly different from 100. Of the 37 deaths, 16, or 44 per cent, were attributed to heart or coronary disease. Darlington *et al.* [88] also failed to find an

Table 13.11 Gout and hyperuricemia in relatives of gout probands

Reference	No. of probands	No. of relatives	Results
[130]	27	136	25% raised uric acid mainly raised to males
[82]	44	137	12% raised uric acid 'lower penetrance' in females? bimodal values
[81]	19	87	24% raised uric strong bimodality
[83]	32	261	7% gout. Raised uric acid compared to controls series'. No bimodality
[78]	19	251	Based on the same families as [81]. No bimodality
[84]	124	283	Prevalence of gout 3.4% relatives, 2.2% spouses (c.f. 0.1% population) SUA > 6 mg/100 ml in 30% male relatives. No increase in females
[74]	22	105	8.6% of relatives suffered from gout (15% in males and 1.9% in females) where 23.8% of relatives were hyperuricemic (30.3% of males and 17.3% of females)

excess number of total deaths or deaths attributed to coronary artery disease among 180 patients with gout or their first-degree relatives.

Abbott *et al.* [37], however, did note an excess incidence of coronary heart disease among men with gout in the Framingham Study. After adjustment for age, blood pressure, cholesterol, alcohol intake, body mass index, and diabetes, the relative risk for coronary heart disease in men with gout was 1.6 ($P < 0.05$); however, the RR for definite myocardial infarction of 1.4 was not significantly different from unity. No excess risk for coronary heart disease was found in women with gout.

Gelber *et al.* [89], however, failed to demonstrate an increased incidence of coronary heart disease events in Caucasian and African-American male physicians with gout compared to those without gout. Among 1552 male physicians, there were 106 cases of gout that developed and 182 coronary heart disease events that occurred over a median follow-up of 30 years. Using Cox proportional hazard models, with the development of gout as a time-dependent covariate, gout was not associated with an increased risk of having a coronary event in either physician group independent of known coronary heart disease risk factors.

Epidemiologic studies have demonstrated a consistent relationship between serum uric acid levels and an increased risk of all-cause and cardiovascular mortality, particularly in women [90–95]. Serum uric acid levels are related to an increased risk for cardiovascular events in some [94,96] but not all studies independent of body mass index, hypertension, and other confounders [90,93,97–100]. The relationship between serum uric acid levels and increased mortality from cardiovascular disease and other causes may be mediated by the relationship of uric acid as a marker for the insulin resistance syndrome [54,101–104].

References

1. Kellgren JH, Jeffrey MR, Ball J (eds). *The epidemiology of chronic rheumatism.* Oxford: Blackwell, 1963: 327.
2. Bennett PH, Wood PHN (eds). *Population studies of the rheumatic diseases: proceedings of the third international symposium, New York, June 5th–10th, 1966.* Amsterdam: Excerpta Medica Foundation, 1968: 457–458.
3. Rigby AS, Wood PHN. Serum uric acid levels and gout: what does this herald for the population? *Clin Exp Rheumatol* 1994; **12**: 395–400.
4. Wallace SL, Robinson H, Masi AT, Decker JL, McCarty DJ, Yu TF. Preliminary criteria for the classification of the acute arthritis of primary gout. *Arthritis Rheum* 1977; **20**: 895–900.
5. Badley EM, Meyrick JS, Wood PHN. Gout and serum uric acid levels in the Cotswolds. *Rheumatol Rehabil* 1978; **17**: 133–142.
6. Currie WJ. Prevalence and incidence of the diagnosis of gout in Great Britain. *Ann Rheum Dis* 1979; **38**: 101–106.
7. Harris CM, Lloyd DC, Lewis J. The prevalence and prophylaxis of gout in England. *J Clin Epidemiol* 1995; **48**: 1153–1158.
8. Benson V, Marano MA. Current estimates from the National Health Interview Survey, 1992. *Vital Health Stat* 1994; **189**: 1–269.
9. Lawrence RC, Helmick CG, Arnett FC, *et al.* Estimates of the prevalence of arthritis and selected musculoskeletal disorders in the United States. *Arthritis Rheum* 1998; **41**: 778–799.
10. De Blecourt JJ. Screening of the population for rheumatic diseases. *Ann Rheum Dis* 1954; **13**: 338–340.
11. Popert AJ, Hewitt JV. Gout and hyperuricemia in rural and urban populations. *Ann Rheum Dis* 1962; **21**: 154–163.
12. Isomaki HA, Takkunen H. Gout and hyperuricemia in a Finnish rural population. *Acta Rheumatol Scand* 1969; **15**: 112–120.
13. Bennett PH, Burch TA. Serum uric acid and gout in Blackfeet and Pima Indians. In: Bennett PH, Wood PHN, eds. *Population studies of the rheumatic diseases: proceedings of the third international symposium, New York, June 5th–10th, 1966.* Amsterdam: Excerpta Medica Foundation, 1968: 358–364.
14. Rose BS. Gout in Maoris. *Semin Arthritis Rheum* 1975; **5**: 121–145.
15. Prior IA, Welby TJ, Ostbye T, Salmond CE, Stokes YM. Migration and gout: the Tokelau Island migrant study. *Br Med J* 1987; **295**: 457–461.
16. Wigley RD, Prior IA, Salmond C, Stanley D, Pinfold B. Rheumatic complaints in Tokelau. I. Migrants resident in New Zealand. The Tokelau Island migrant study. *Rheumatol Int* 1987; **7**: 53–59.
17. Wigley RD, Prior IA, Salmond C, Stanley D, Pinfold B. Rheumatic complaints in Tokelau. II. A comparison of migrants in New Zealand and non-migrants. The Tokelau Island migrant study. *Rheumatol Int* 1987; **7**: 61–65.
18. Decker JL, Healey LA, Skeith MD. Ethnic variations in serum uric acid: Filipino hyperuricemia, the result of hereditary and environmental factors. In: Bennett PH, Wood PHN, eds. *Population studies of the rheumatic diseases: proceedings of the third international symposium, New York, June 5th–10th, 1966.* Amsterdam: Excerpta Medica Foundation, 1968: 336–343.
19. Chang SJ, Ko YC, Wang TN, Chang FT, Cinkotai FF, Chen CJ. High prevalence of gout and related risk factors in Taiwan's Aborigines. *J Rheumatol* 1997; **24**: 1364–1369.
20. Chen SL, Du H, Wang Y, Xu LQ. The epidemiology study of hyperuricemia and gout in a community population of Huangpu District in Shanghai. *Chin Med J* 1998; **111**: 228–230.

21. Chou CT, Pei L, Chang DM, Lee CF, Schumacher HR, Liang MH. Prevalence of rheumatic diseases in Taiwan: a population study of urban, suburban, rural differences. *J Rheumatol* 1994; **21**: 302–306.

22. Chou CT, Lai JS. The epidemiology of hyperuricaemia and gout in Taiwan aborigines. *Br J Rheumatol* 1998; **37**: 258–262.

23. Lin KC, Lin HY, Chou P. Community based epidemiological study on hyperuricemia and gout in Kin-Hu, Kinmen. *J Rheumatol* 2000; **27**: 1045–1050.

24. Darmawan J, Valkenburg HA, Muirden KD, Wigley RD. The epidemiology of gout and hyperuricemia in a rural population of Java. *J Rheumatol* 1992; **19**: 1595–1599.

25. Chaiamnuay P, Darmawan J, Muirden KD, Assawatanabodee P. Epidemiology of rheumatic disease in rural Thailand: a WHO-ILAR COPCORD study. Community Oriented Programme for the Control of Rheumatic Disease. *J Rheumatol* 1998; **25**: 1382–1387.

26. Bremner JM, Lawrence JS. Population studies of serum uric acid. *Proc R Soc Med* 1966; **59**: 319–325.

27. Beighton P, Solomon L, Soskolne CL, Sweet MB. Rheumatic disorders in the South African Negro. Part IV. Gout and hyperuricaemia. *S Afr Med J* 1977; **51**: 969–972.

28. Cassim B, Mody GM, Deenadayalu VK, Hammond MG. Gout in black South Africans: a clinical and genetic study. *Ann Rheum Dis* 1994; **53**: 759–762.

29. Lutalo SK. Gout: an experience from Zimbabwe. *Cent Afr J Med* 1993; **39**: 60–62.

30. Mody GM, Naidoo PD. Gout in South African blacks. *Ann Rheum Dis* 1984; **43**: 394–397.

31. Tikly M, Bellingan A, Lincoln D, Russell A. Risk factors for gout: a hospital-based study in urban black South Africans. *Rev Rhum Engl Ed* 1998; **65**: 225–231.

32. Lawrence RC, Hochberg MC, Kelsey JL, *et al.* Estimates of the prevalence of selected arthritic and musculoskeletal diseases in the United States. *J Rheumatol* 1989; **16**: 427–441.

33. Klemp P, Stansfield SA, Castle B, Robertson MC. Gout is on the increase in New Zealand. *Ann Rheum Dis* 1997; **56**: 22–26.

34. Stewart OJ, Silman AJ. Review of UK data on the rheumatic diseases–4. Gout. *Br J Rheumatol* 1990; **29**: 485–488.

35. Hall AP, Barry PE, Dawber TR, McNamara PM. Epidemiology of gout and hyperuricemia: a long-term population study. *Am J Med* 1967; **42**: 27–37.

36. Campion EW, Glynn RJ, DeLabry LO. Asymptomatic hyperuricemia. Risks and consequences in the Normative Aging Study. *Am J Med* 1987; **82**: 421–426.

37. Abbott RD, Brand FN, Kannel WB, Castelli WP. Gout and coronary heart disease: the Framingham Study. *J Clin Epidemiol* 1988; **41**: 237–242.

38. Roubenoff R, Klag MJ, Mead LA, Liang KY, Seidler AJ, Hochberg MC. Incidence and risk factors for gout in white men. *JAMA* 1991; **266**: 3004–3007.

39. Hochberg MC, Thomas J, Thomas DJ, Mead L, Levine DM, Klag MJ. Racial differences in the incidence of gout: the role of hypertension. *Arthritis Rheum* 1995; **38**: 628–632.

40. Mikkelsen WM, Dodge HJ, Valkenburg H. The distribution of serum uric acid values in a population unselected as to gout or hyperuricemia, Tecumseh, Michigan 1959–1960. *Am J Med* 1965; **39**: 242–251.

41. Wingrove CS, Walton C, Stevenson JC. The effect of menopause on serum uric acid levels in non-obese healthy women. *Metab Clin Exp* 1998; **47**: 435–438.

42. Lin KC, Lin HY, Chou P. The interaction between uric acid level and other risk factors on the development of gout among asymptomatic hyperuricemic men in a prospective study. *J Rheumatol* 2000; **27**: 1501–1505.

43. Acheson RM, O'Brien WM. Dependence of serum uric-acid on haemoglobin and other factors in the general population. *Lancet* 1966; **2**: 777–778.

44. Agamah ES, Srinivasan SR, Webber LS, Berenson GS. Serum uric acid and its relation to cardiovascular disease risk factors in children and young adults from a biracial community: the Bogalusa Heart Study. *J Lab Clin Med* 1991; **118**: 241–249.

45. Baaklini CE, Ferrari AJL, Goldenberg J, Atra E, Andrade LEC. Serum uric acid levels in a populational sample in Marilia county, Sao Paulo State and correlation with some biochemical and demographic parameters. *Rev Bras Reumatol* 1998; **38**: 65–70.

46. Prior IAM, Rose BS. Uric acid, gout and public health in the South Pacific. *N Z Med J* 1966; **65**: 295–300.

47. Reed D, Labarthe D, Stallones R, O'Sullivan JB. Epidemiologic studies of serum uric acid levels among Micronesians. *Arthritis Rheum* 1972; **15**: 381–390.

48. Gibson T, Waterworth R, Hatfield P, Robinson G, Bremner K. Hyperuricaemia, gout and kidney function in New Zealand Maori men. *Br J Rheumatol* 1984; **23**: 276–282.

49. Simmonds HA, McBride MB, Hatfield PJ, Graham R, McCaskey J, Jackson M. Polynesian women are also at risk for hyperuricaemia and gout because of a genetic defect in renal urate handling. *Br J Rheumatol* 1994; **33**: 932–937.

50. Decker JL, Lane JJ, Reynolds WE. Hyperuricemia in a male Filipino population. *Arthritis Rheum* 1962; **5**: 144–155.

51. Healey LA, Skeith MD, Decker JL, Bayani-Sioson PS. Hyperuricemia in Filipinos: interaction of heredity and environment. *Am J Hum Genet* 1967; **19**: 81–85.

52. Chou P, Soong LN, Lin HY. Community-based epidemiological study on hyperuricemia in Pu-Li, Taiwan. *J Formos Med Assoc* 1993; **92**: 597–602.

53. Woo J, Swaminathan R, Cockram C, Lau E, Chan A. Association between serum uric acid and some cardiovascular risk factors in a Chinese population. *Postgrad Med J* 1994; **70**: 486–491.

54. Li Y, Stamler J, Xiao Z, Folsom A, Tao S, Zhang H. Serum uric acid and its correlates in Chinese adult populations, urban and rural, of Beijing. The PRC-USA Collaborative Study in Cardiovascular and Cardiopulmonary Epidemiology. *Int J Epidemiol* 1997; **26**: 288–296.

55. Nakanishi N, Suzuki K, Kawashimo H, Nakamura K, Tatara K. Serum uric acid: correlation with biological, clinical and behavioral factors in Japanese men. *J Epidemiol* 1999; **9**: 99–106.

56. Hayashi E. A study on the incidence of gout in a particular professional group: Japanese wrestler, Sumo. *Ryumachi* 1971; **11**: 140.

57. Duff IF, Mikkelsen WM, Dodge HJ, Himes DS. Comparison of uric acid levels in some Oriental and Caucasian groups unselected as to gout or hyperuricemia. *Arthritis Rheum* 1968; **11**: 184–190.

58. Healey LA, Jones KW. Hyperuricemia in American Samoans. *Arthritis Rheum* 1971; **14**: 283–285.

59. Glynn RJ, Campion EW, Silbert JE. Trends in serum uric acid levels 1961–1980. *Arthritis Rheum* 1983; **26**: 87–93.

60. Nakanishi N, Tatara K, Nakamura K, Suzuki K. Risk factors for the incidence of hyperuricaemia: a 6-year longitudinal study of middle-aged Japanese men. *Int J Epidemiol* 1999; **28**: 888–893.

61. Grahame R, Scott JT. Clinical survey of 354 patients with gout. *Ann Rheum Dis* 1970; **29**: 461–468.

62. Zalokar J, Lellouch J, Claude JR, Kuntz D. Epidemiology of serum uric acid and gout in Frenchmen. *J Chronic Dis* 1974; **27**: 59–75.

63. Zalokar J, Lellouch J, Claude JR. [Serum urate and gout in 4663 young male workers (author's transl)]. *Sem Hop* 1981; **57**: 664–670.

64. Prior I. Epidemiology of rheumatic disorders in the Pacific with particular emphasis on hyperuricemia and gout. *Semin Arthritis Rheum* 1981; **11**: 213–229.

65. Richter BS. *A case-control study of lead exposure and other risk factors for gouty arthritis*. The Johns Hopkins University, 1987.

66. Nicholls A, Scott JT. Effect of weight-loss on plasma and urinary levels of uric acid. *Lancet* 1972; **2**: 1223–1224.

67. Scott JT, Sturge RA. The effect of weight loss on plasma and urinary uric acid and lipid levels. *J Clin Chem Clin Biochem* 1976; **14**: 319.

68. Grodzicki T, Palmer A, Bulpitt CJ. Incidence of diabetes and gout in hypertensive patients during 8 years of follow-up. The General Practice Hypertension Study Group. *J Hum Hypertens* 1997; **11**: 583–585.

69. Jossa F, Farinaro E, Panico S, Krogh V, Celentano E, Galasso R *et al*. Serum uric acid and hypertension: the Olivetti heart study. *J Hum Hypertens* 1994; **8**: 677–681.

70. Gordon T, Kannel WB. Drinking and its relation to smoking, BP, blood lipids, and uric acid: the Framingham study. *Arch Intern Med* 1983; **143**: 1366–1374.

71. Kono S, Shinchi K, Imanishi K, Honjo S, Todoroki I. Behavioural and biological correlates of serum uric acid: a study of self-defence officials in Japan. *Int J Epidemiol* 1994; **23**: 517–522.

72. Loenen HMJA, Eshuis H, Lowik MRH, *et al*. Serum uric acid correlates in elderly men and women with special refer-ence to body composition and dietary intake (Dutch Nutrition Surveillance System). *J Clin Epidemiol* 1990; **43**: 1297–1303.

73. Poor G, Mituszova M. Saturnine gout. *Baillieres Clin Rheumatol* 1989; **3**: 51–61.

74. Mituszova M, Judak A, Poor G, Gyodi E, Stenszky V. Clinical and family studies in Hungarian patients with gout. *Rheumatol Int* 1992; **12**: 165–168.

75. Sydenham T. *The whole works of that excellent practical physician, Dr. Thomas Sydenham*, 7th edn., (translated by J Peehey). London, 1977.

76. Scott JT, Pollard AC. Uric acid excretion in the relatives of patients with gout. *Ann Rheum Dis* 1970; **29**: 397–400.

77. O'Brien WM, Burch TA, Bunim JJ. Genetics of hyperuricaemia in Blackfeet and Pima Indians. *Ann Rheum Dis* 1966; **25**: 117–119.

78. Neel JV, Rakic MT, Davidson RT, Valkenburg HA, Mikkelsen WM. Studies in hyperuricemia. 2. A reconsideration of the distribution of serum uric acid values in the families of Smyth, Cotterman and Freyberg. *Am J Hum Genet* 1965; **17**: 14–22.

79. Rice T, Vogler GP, Perry TS, Laskarzewski PM, Province MA, Rao DC. Heterogeneity in the familial aggregation of fasting serum uric acid level in five North American populations: The Lipid Research Clinics family study. *Am J Med Genet* 1990; **36**: 219–225.

80. Rice T, Laskarzewski PM, Perry TS, Rao DC. Commingling and segregation analysis of serum uric acid in five North American populations: the Lipid Research Clinics family study. *Hum Genet* 1992; **90**: 133–138.

81. Smyth CJ, Cotterman CW, Freyberg RH. The genetics of gout and hyperuricemia: an analysis of nineteen families. *J Clin Invest* 1948; **27**: 749–759.

82. Stecher RM, Hersh AH, Solomon WM. The heredity of gout and its relationship to familial hyperuricemia. *Ann Intern Med* 1949; **51**: 595–614.

83. Hauge M, Harvald B. Heredity in gout and hyperuricemia. *Acta Med Scand* 1955; **152**: 247–257.

84. Lawrence JS. *Rheumatism in populations*. London: Heinemann Medical Books, 1977: 352–85.

85. Jensen J, Blankenhorn DH, Sturgeon P, Chin HP, Ware AG. Serum lipids and serum uric acid in human twins. *J Lipid Res* 1965; **6**: 193–205.

86. Boyle JA, Greig WR, Jasani MK, Duncan A, Diver M, Buchanan WW. Relative roles of genetic and environmental factors in the control of serum uric acid levels in normouricaemic subjects. *Ann Rheum Dis* 1967; **26**: 234–238.

87. Talbott JH, Lillienfeld A. Longevity in gout. *Geriatrics* 1959; **14**: 409–420.

88. Darlington LG, Slack J, Scott JT. Vascular mortality in patients with gout and in their families. *Ann Rheum Dis* 1983; **42**: 270–273.

89. Gelber AC, Klag MJ, Mead LA, *et al*. Gout and risk for subsequent coronary heart disease. The Meharry-Hopkins Study. *Arch Intern Med* 1997; **157**: 1436–1440.

90. Bengtsson C, Lapidus L, Stendahl C, Waldenstrom J. Hyperuricaemia and risk of cardiovascular disease and overall death. A 12 -year follow-up of participants in the population study of women in Gothenburg, Sweden. *Acta Med Scand* 1988; **224**: 549–555.

91. Levine W, Dyer AR, Shekelle RB, Schoenberger JA, Stamler J. Serum uric acid and 11.5-year mortality of middle-aged women: findings of the Chicago Heart Association Detection Project in Industry. *J Clin Epidemiol* 1989; **42**: 257–267.

92. Freedman DS, Williamson DF, Gunter EW, Byers T. Relation of serum uric acid to mortality and ischemic heart disease. The NHANES I Epidemiologic Follow-up Study. *Am J Epidemiol* 1995; **141**: 637–644.

93. Culleton BF, Larson MG, Kannel WB, Levy D. Serum uric acid and risk for cardiovascular disease and death: The Framingham heart study. *Ann Intern Med* 1999; **131**: 7–13.

94. Liese AD, Hense HW, Lowel H, Doring A, Tietze M, Keil U. Association of serum uric acid with all-cause and cardiovascular disease mortality and incident myocardial infarction in the MONICA Augsburg cohort. World Health Organization Monitoring Trends and Determinants in Cardiovascular Diseases. *Epidemiology* 1999; **10**: 391–397.

95. Fang J, Alderman MH. Serum uric acid and cardiovascular mortality. The NHANES I epidemiologic follow-up study, 1971–1992. National Health and Nutrition Examination Survey. JAMA 2000; **283**: 2404–2410.

96. Franse LV, Pahor M, Di Bari M, *et al.* Serum uric acid, diuretic treatment and risk of cardiovascular events in the Systolic Hypertension in the Elderly Program (SHEP). *J Hypertension* 2000; **18**: 1149–1154.

97. Myers AR, Epstein FH, Dodge HJ, *et al.* The relationship of serum uric acid to risk factors in coronary heart disease. *Am J Med* 1968; **45**: 520–528.

98. Klein R, Klein BE, Cornoni JC, Maready J, Cassel JC, Tyroler HA. Serum uric acid. Its relationship to coronary heart disease risk factors and cardiovascular disease, Evans County, Georgia. *Arch Intern Med* 1973; **132**: 401–410.

99. Beard JT. Serum uric acid and coronary heart disease. *Am Heart J* 1983; **106**: 397–400.

100. Brand FN, McGee DL, Kannel WB, Stokes J, Castelli WP. Hyperuricemia as a risk factor of coronary heart disease: the Framingham Study. *Am J Epidemiol* 1985; **121**: 11–18.

101. Cigolini M, Targher G, Tonoli M, Manara F, Muggeo M, De Sandre G. Hyperuricaemia: relationships to body fat distribution and other components of the insulin resistance syndrome in 38-year-old healthy men and women. *Int J Obes* 1995; **19**: 92–96.

102. Clausen JO, Borch JK, Ibsen H, Pedersen O. Analysis of the relationship between fasting serum uric acid and the insulin sensitivity index in a population-based sample of 380 young healthy Caucasians. *Eur J Endocrinol* 1998; **138**: 63–69.

103. Rathmann W, Funkhouser E, Dyer AR, Roseman JM. Relations of hyperuricemia with the various components of the insulin resistance syndrome in young black and white adults: The CARDIA study. *Ann Epidemiol* 1998; **8**: 250–261.

104. Schmidt MI, Watson RL, Duncan BB, *et al.* Clustering of dyslipidemia, hyperuricemia, diabetes, and hypertension and its association with fasting insulin and central and overall obesity in a general population. *Metab Clin Exp* 1996; **45**: 699–706.

105. Tzonchev VT, Shubarov K, Ilinov P. Prevalence of gout and hyperuricaemia in Bulgaria. In: Bennett PH, Wood PHN, eds. *Population studies of the rheumatic diseases: proceedings of the third international symposium, New York, June 5th—10th, 1966.* Amsterdam: Excerpta Medica Foundation, 1968: 363–364.

106. Schaffalitsky De Muckadell OB, Gyntelberg F. Occurrence of gout in Copenhagen males aged 40–59. *Int J Epidemiol* 1976; **5**: 153–158.

107. Gardner MJ, Power C, Barker DJ, Padday R. The prevalence of gout in 3 English towns. *Int J Epidemiol* 1982; **11**: 71–75.

108. Steven MM. Prevalence of chronic arthritis in four geographical areas of the Scottish Highlands. *Ann Rheum Dis* 1992; **51**: 186–194.

109. Mikkelsen WM. The possible association of hyperuricemia and/or gout with diabetes mellitus. *Arthritis Rheum* 1965; **8**: 853–864.

110. O'Sullivan JB. Gout in a New England town: a prevalence study in Sudbury, Massachusetts. *Ann Rheum Dis* 1972; **31**: 166–169.

111. Lennane GAQ, Rose BS, Isdale IC. Gout in the Maori. *Ann Rheum Dis* 1960; **19**: 120–125.

112. Burch TA, O'Brien WM, Need R, Kurland LT. Hyperuricaemia and gout in the Mariana Islands. *Ann Rheum Dis* 1966; **25**: 114–116.

113. Shichikawa K. The prevalence of gout in Japan. In: Bennett PH, Wood PHN, eds. *Population studies of the rheumatic diseases: proceedings of the third international symposium, New York, June 5th—10th, 1966.* Amsterdam: Excerpta Medica Foundation, 1968: 354–357.

114. Rose BS, Prior IAM, Davidson F. Gout and hyperuricaemia in New Zealand and Polynesia. In: Bennett PH, Wood PHN, eds. *Population studies of the rheumatic diseases: proceedings of the third international symposium, New York, June 5th—10th, 1966.* Amsterdam: Excerpta Medica Foundation, 1968: 344–353.

115. Kato H, Duff IF, Russell WJ, *et al.* Rheumatoid arthritis and gout in Hiroshima and Nagasaki, Japan: a prevalence and incidence study. *J Chronic Dis* 1971; **23**: 659–679.

116. Jeremy R, Towson J, Kato H, *et al.* Serum urate levels and gout in Australian males. *Med J Aust* 1971; **1**: 1116–1118.

117. Brauer GW, Prior IA. A prospective study of gout in New Zealand Maoris. *Ann Rheum Dis* 1978; **37**: 466–472.

118. Zimmet PZ, Whitehouse S, Jackson L, Thoma K. High prevalence of hyperuricaemia and gout in an urbanised Micronesian population. *Br Med J* 1978; **1**: 1237–1239.

119. Akizuki S. A population study of hyperuricaemia and gout in Japan: analysis of sex, age and occupational differences in thirty-four thousand people living in Nagano Prefecture. *Ryumachi* 1982; **22**: 201–208.

120. Beighton P, Soskolne CL, Solomon L, Sweet B. Serum uric acid levels in a Nama (Hottentot) community in South West Africa. *S Afr J Sci* 1974; **70**: 281–283.

121. Beighton P, Solomon L, Soskolne CL, Sweet B. Serum uric acid concentrations in a rural Tswana community in Southern Africa. *Ann Rheum Dis* 1973; **32**: 346–350.

122. Beighton P, Daynes G, Soskolne CL. Serum uric acid concentrations in a Xhosa community in the Transkei of Southern Africa. *Ann Rheum Dis* 1976; **35**: 77–80.

123. Muller AS. *Population studies on the prevalence of rheumatic disease in Liberia and Nigeria.* University of Leiden, 1970.

124. Sturge RA, Scott JT, Kennedy AC, Hart DP, Buchanan WW. Serum uric acid in England and Scotland. *Ann Rheum Dis* 1977; **36**: 420–427.

125. Mertz DP, Loewer H. [First indications of decrease in the incidence of hyperuricemia in North Germany]. *Versicherungsmedizin* 1992; **44**: 211–214.

126. Cobb S. Hyperuricemia in executives. In: Kellgren JH, Jeffrey MR, Ball J, eds. *The epidemiology of chronic rheumatism.* Oxford: Blackwell, 1963: 182–188.

127. Acheson RM, O'Brien WM. Some factors associated with serum uric acid in the New Haven survey of joint disease. In: Bennett PH, Wood PHN, eds. *Population studies of the rheumatic diseases: proceedings of the third international symposium, New York, June 5th–10th, 1966.* Amsterdam: Excerpta Medica Foundation, 1968: 365–370.

128. Munan L, Kelly A, Petitclerc C. Population serum urate levels and their correlates. The Sherbrooke regional study. *Am J Epidemiol* 1976; **103**: 369–382.

129. Healey LA, Caner JEZ, Bassett DR, Decker JL. Serum uric acid and obesity in Hawaiians. *JAMA* 1966; **196**: 364–365.

130. Talbott JH. Serum urate in relatives of gouty patients. *J Clin Invest* 1940; **19**: 645–648.

131. Shun JC, Ying CK, Tsu NW, Fown TC, Cinkotal FF, Chung JC. High prevalence of gout and related risk factors in Taiwan's aborigines. *J Rheumatol* 1997; **24**: 1364–1369.

14 Calcium pyrophosphate dihydrate (CPPD) deposition disease

Alan J. Silman

Definition and criteria

This review covers a number of linked pathological, radiological, and clinical entities, and it is this linkage of conceptually distinct entities that creates confusion in determining epidemiology (Fig. 14.1). The pathological entity is deposition of calcium salt crystals in articular, including meniscal, cartilage. The crystals are predominantly of the calcium phosphate family [1], mainly calcium pyrophosphate dihydrate (CPPD), though other calcium salts are found, including hydroxyapatite [2].

The term basic calcium phosphate (BCP) associated syndrome is now the preferred term to describe the deposition of hydroxyapatite as well as octacalcium phosphate and tricalcium phosphate in the articular and periarticular tissues [3]. This review will focus on the more frequent CPPD deposition disorders. CPPD crystal deposition can be one cause of the radiological observation of chondrocalcinosis, that is the radiological appearance of calcified deposits in specific cartilaginous sites such as the meniscal cartilages of the knee, the wrist, pelvis, and other peripheral joints. Clinically, most of the calcified deposits are silent but the syndrome of pseudogout[1] is well recognized—an acute mono or oligoarthritis, resembling gout but where the synovial fluid contains CPPD crystals

rather than urate ones. Uric acid arthropathy probably coexists with CPPD arthropathy more often than expected by chance [4]. Both crystal types may be found in up to 2 per cent of synovial fluids, further clouding case definition [5]. The diagnosis of pseudogout is normally based indirectly on finding crystals in the synovial fluid which, under polarized light, are either weakly or negatively birefringent compared to the positive birefringence of urate crystals. During attacks there is an increase in the number and size of crystals and a shift to the monoclinic rather than triclinic morphology [6]. In addition to the clinical presentation of pseudogout, there are a number of other clinical patterns of presentation. These include: (i) a polyarticular osteoarthritis, though the exact relationship between CPPD and osteoarthritis is unclear [7]; (ii) a widespread inflammatory polyarthritis mimicking rheumatoid arthritis (including, in 10 per cent, a positive reaction for rheumatoid factor); and (iii) a more localized arthritis which may be restricted to non-peripheral joint sites including the temporomandibular joints and the cervical spine, [8–10] and, rarely, a neuropathic picture resembling a Charcot joint [4]. The term CPPD is used as a broad term covering all these entities.

Criteria

In the presence of such diversity, epidemiological study is complex. McCarty tried to produce a coherent criteria set which have been used by many investigators (Table 14.1). The criteria are deceptively simple and have difficulties in practice. Firstly, radiological diffraction is probably too specialized a technique for

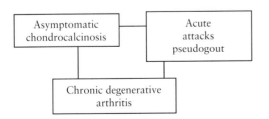

Fig. 14.1 Epidemiological dilemma for crystal deposition disease.

[1] Pseudogout is used by some authors to refer to CPPD deposition irrespective of its clinical sequelae.

Table 14.1   Criteria for crystal deposition disease

A Identification of calcium phosphate crystals by X-ray
   diffraction from joint aspiration or biopsy
B Identification of absent or weakly birefringent crystals
   from joint aspirate
C Radiological evidence of polyarticular chondrocalcinosis

Definite disease = A or B and C
Source: [1]

widespread use. Secondly, even with newer techniques there is only a sensitivity of 67 per cent to detect CPPD crystals [11]. Thirdly, there is considerable debate about the accuracy of conventional radiology in detecting calcification. Thus, the type of film used, for example Kodak type M as compared to AA, can make a substantial difference to the sensitivity [12]. Fourthly, the prevalence of individuals with calcification is dependent on the number of sites X-rayed. It is, however, a useful feature of CPPD that it is relatively rare not to have meniscal involvement in the face of calcification at other sites [13]. Finally, in population prevalence surveys, including those for genetic and family studies, recalled episodes of pseudogout are difficult to verify.

Chondrocalcinosis and osteoarthritis

There is considerable overlap between these two disorders. Firstly, as stated above, the clinical expression in many patients from unselected series with radiological calcification is frequently one of osteoarthritis [7,14]. Specifically, widespread osteoarthritic change is the end result of chondrocalcinosis [15]. The alternative hypothesis is that crystal deposition occurs as a result of previous joint damage including osteoarthritis which then sets up a vicious cycle causing further joint damage [7]. In a cross-sectional analysis of the Framingham survey data there was an increased risk of around two to three for osteoarthritis in the presence of chondrocalcinosis, after age adjustment, though the latter was not associated with an increased prevalence of symptoms. More importantly, the overlap between the two disorders was small: only 4 per cent of radiographic osteoarthritis could be attributed to chondrocalcinosis and only 6 per cent of symptomatic osteoarthritis could be similarly attributed [16]. In an Italian study of primary care referrals for hand and knee X-rays comparing 26 individuals with chondrocalcinosis and 104 unaffected individuals, there was an age and gender adjusted odds ratio for knee osteo-

arthritis of 4.3 (95 per cent CI 1.6–11.3) but a variable effect on hand osteoarthritis [17]. The nature of the selection of subjects for this study makes it impossible to extrapolate the results to the population. By contrast, in a recent report of a 10-year follow-up of those initially free of knee osteoarthritis at baseline, there was no increased risk of incident knee osteoarthritis in those 8 per cent who had baseline radiographic evidence of chondrocalcinosis [18].

Occurrence

Incidence-based studies on episodes of pseudogout are either not available or insufficiently soundly based to be of value. Thus, much of the data relies on point prevalence surveys using X-rays. In addition, there have been a number of post-mortem surveys of cartilage, either by histology or radiology, which can be used as a surrogate for lifetime, or cumulative, incidence.

Radiological prevalence surveys of chondrocalcinosis

There have been a considerable number of these (Table 14.2). They vary considerably in the population studied, their age distribution, the joints X-rayed, and the results obtained. Many studies have assumed, given that much calcification is likely to be asymptomatic, that screening either an in- or outpatient population, being treated for an apparently unrelated disorder, is an acceptable substitute for taking a population sample. This is, of course, an uncorroborated assumption and the point of being asymptomatic is irrelevant. There may very well be an association between the conditions leading to medical care and the radiological occurrence of calcification. The small study by Ellman and Levin [21] is frequently cited as an example of a carefully conducted survey using a sensitive method of investigation in a 'healthy' elderly population. Their reported prevalence rate of 26 per cent for meniscal involvement is relatively high compared to other reports. There is obviously an age effect on prevalence (Table 14.3) and differences in crude rates may be explained by differences in the age structure of the population studied.

Frequently, however, an age-specific breakdown is not given and the numbers studied are too small for reliable estimates within age groups. However, when

Table 14.2 Prevalence of radiological calcification in population surveys

Reference	No. studied	Source	Age	Sites examined	Prevalence (%)
Wolke et al 1935[a]	12,268	'Routine' knee X-rays	All	Knee	0.4
[19]	455	Elderly institution	Mean 80	Knee	7.0
Zinn *et al.* 1969[b]	131	N/S	65+	Knee	4.6
Mariakakis 1969[c]	1834	N/S	35+	Knee	0.6
[20]	360	Elderly institution	60–94	Knee	6.1
[21]	58	Elderly institution	70–94	Knee	26
				Knee/pelvis/wrists	28
[22]	100	N/S	50+	Wrists	2
			70+		5
[23]	108	Geriatric ward	80+	Knee	23
[24]	62	Elderly institution	80+	Knee	29
[25]	100	Population survey	75+	Knee	26
[13]	272	N/S	50+	Knee	13.9
[26]	100	Acute geriatric ward	60 – 95	Knee/hand	11
[27]	104	Trauma patients	20–79	Knee	3.4
[28]	200	Elderly population	65+	Knee	10.5
[14]	100	Acute geriatric admissions	Mean 78	Knee	21
				Knee/wrists/hands/pelvis	34
[29]	127	Hospital inpatients	55+	Knee	14.2
				Knee/wrists/pelvis	15.8
[30]	81	Population survey	70, 75, 79	Knee	11.5
[16]	1402	Population survey	63–93	Knee	8.1
[31]	261	Primary care attenders	60+	Knee, hand	10

[a] Quoted by [32].
[b] Quoted by [33].
[c] Personal communication quoted by [34].

Table 14.3 Effect of age on radiological chondrocalcinosis

Reference	Age	Prevalence (%)
[20]	60–69	1.6
	70–79	6.8
	80–89	9.1
	90+	13.6
[30]	70	7.5
	75	10
	79	16
[16]	63–64	3.6
	65–69	3.2
	70–74	7.3
	75–79	9.8
	80–84	16.5
	85+	27.1
[31]	60–69	7
	80+	43

attempts have been made to reconcile differences in prevalence by adjusting for age [35] substantial differences persist. It would seem reasonable to assume from the more robust and recent studies that the crude radiographic prevalence in a population aged over 65 is at least 10 per cent, with the age-specific rates being substantially less at age 65 than they are at age 80, when a prevalence of 20 per cent would be more likely. The highest recorded prevalence, in those over 80, of 43 per cent [31] was based on a small sample size and restricted to those referred for X-ray. It seems that chondrocalcinosis at ages below 65 is rare apart from its occurrence at a very young age in some of the multi-case families reported (see below) as a result of a presumed specific mutation.

The process of calcium deposition is, however, a dynamic one and can decrease in time and thus tending to reduce the prevalence with increasing age. This is, in part, due both to actual crystal shedding but also to a loss of cartilage with age. The latter, if substantial, would result in a lack of available material to calcify and hence prevalence at age 80 cannot be taken as cumulative lifetime occurrence.

Post-mortem surveys

Post-mortem surveys (Table 14.4) have again yielded different results but a large proportion of the diversity might be methodological in origin [2]. The identification of tiny areas of calcification by X-ray of post

Table 14.4   Prevalence of cartilage calcification at post-mortem in knee menisci

Reference	No. studied	Age	Sites examined	Prevalence %
[36]	100	All ages	Histological calcification	25 (of menisci)
Bennett *et al.* 1942[a]	63	All ages	Crystals identified	4
[2]	215	All ages	Radiological calcification	35
[37][a]	320	40–90	CPPD crystals identified	6.3
[38]	100	All ages	Radiological calcification	8
[35]	108	Elderly mean 72	Radiological calcification	18.5
[39]	130	All ages	Radiological calcification	20.7
		60+		26

[a] Quoted by [33].

mortem menisci, by a sensitive investigator, can yield very high prevalence rates [2]. By contrast, the histological demonstration of CPPD crystals is more difficult to achieve and hence rates from this approach yield prevalence estimates of 4–6 per cent. The question here is one of specificity: radiological to determine calcification of excised post-mortem cartilage, although by definition is chondrocalcinosis, may have only a weak relationship to the disease process of interest.

Gender influences

Differences in the prevalence between males and females need to take into account that in an elderly population there is an excess of women; thus demonstration of a sex difference requires a comparison of age-adjusted rates. Bergstrom *et al.* [30], in their population-based study, found a female excess at all ages, which interestingly increased from 1.5:1 at age 70 to 4:1 at age 79. This female excess (Table 14.5) is sup-

ported by the results from other studies including the one from Ellman and Levin [21], referred to above, when no male sufferer was found in 32 males examined compared to a rate of 32 per cent in females. There might be a site effect. Thus in a post-mortem study there was an almost two-fold female excess in chondrocalcinosis when the involvement was restricted to knee meniscus, whereas there was an equal sex occurrence when other sites were considered [35]. Sex hormones and pregnancy influences have not been widely investigated, though rarely pregnancy may predispose to an acute attack [40].

Geographical and ethnic influences

Data have not been collected in a sufficiently standardized way between populations to permit informed comment on the relative occurrence of disease in different populations. The disease has been described in relative similar frequencies in the North American, Western, Eastern, and European populations previously cited (Table 14.2). The condition is also well recognized in Japan [41] but there are limited data from other non-Caucasian populations. Clinical case series from populations of African origin, in the United States, suggest a relative occurrence similar to that expected from the general population [42,43].

Clusters of cases have been described in some population groups; the most typical example is the Chiloe islanders off the coast of Chile [44]. Interestingly, investigation of those affected suggests that it is genetic factors that are likely to be important, as some of the affected individuals had migrated from the islands while others had been raised substantially outside the islands. Further studies of families in Spain suggest that the origin of this Chilean cluster lies in the migration of

Table 14.5   Sex ratio and radiological chondrocalcinosis

Reference	Age	Male : Female (prevalence rate ratio)
[21]	70–94	No male cases 32% in females
[29]	55+	1 : 6
[30]	70	1 : 1.5
	75	1 : 2.9
	79	1 : 4.0
[16]	65–69	1 : 1.6
	70–74	1 : 1.4
	75–79	1 : 1.6
	80–84	1 : 1
	85+	1 : 1
[31]	60+	1 : 2.3

susceptible individuals from Spain some years previously [45]. Between regions in Spain there are no obvious differences in occurrence [31].

Time trends

There are no data on time trends in this disorder. One investigation showed no seasonal influence on the incidence of acute attacks in contrast to the pattern in 'true' gout [46].

Genetics

Introduction

It is the genetic aspects of the aetiology of this condition that provide the most interest epidemiologically. Much of the work has come from studies of populations of Spanish and Italian origin living in both Europe, and North and South America. It is useful to consider the genetics of this disorder under a number of different headings, although clearly these are intra-related. Firstly, there is the frequency of familial aggregation. Secondly, there are the studies of large, multimember, multigeneration families. Thirdly, there is a specific investigation of presumed susceptibility alleles that, in relation to CPPD, have involved investigation of both genes within the HLA region as well as other candidate genes associated with bone metabolism and cartilage. Finally, there is considerable interest in the role of specific metabolic and endocrine disorders which may be associated with CPPD, some of which will have their own genetic basis.

Frequency of familial aggregation

There have been a number of studies, particularly from Spain (Table 14.6), to determine the proportion of probands with the disease that have an affected first-degree relative. The results in the four studies shown do show considerable variability, with the most recent study of 44 pedigrees suggesting that 21 have at least one affected relative. Furthermore, in a further 10 of these pedigrees, there were features in first-degree relatives of other suggestive features of disease such as possible history of pseudogout or X-ray evidence of arthritis in the MCP joints [49,50]. The ascertainment of disease in first-degree relatives to some extent depends on the intensity of the investigation and also whether any selection factors are involved in determin-

Table 14.6 Frequency of multimember families in patient series

Reference	Country	Number probands	N (%) affected relative
[47]	Spain	46	5 (11)
[45]	Spain	32	9 (28)
[48]	Spain	35	9 (26)
[49]	Spain	44	21 (48)

ing which relatives are agreeable to have radiographic examination, for example. Nevertheless, the studies do seem to be fairly persuasive in suggesting that CPPD is fairly frequently, at least in Spanish populations, associated with a familial history. There does not appear to be any obvious difference between the clinical phenotype in individuals who appear to be sporadic compared to those with a family history.

Investigation of multimember multicase families

Multimember, multigenerational families with CPPD have been identified from many parts of the world and the literature has been outstandingly reviewed by Reginato *et al.* [50]. They noted that very few families had been described in pedigrees of African or Asian origin. A summary of the families published in the literature, from Europe, the Americas, and the Middle East and Far East (Table 14.7), reveals that for most families the disease was thought to have an autosomal dominant transmission. In a number of the families, there is incomplete penetrance but almost certainly this is due to too short a follow-up in the younger members. As an example, follow-up of the Chiloe Islanders revealed a substantial number developing disease over a 26-year follow-up period, many of whom had developed a severe disabling arthritis [50].

There are some interesting features in these families. In some of them, the disease appears to be severe with an early age at onset, for example [54,72], but in other pedigrees, for example [48], the disease was mild. There does not appear to be any female excess in these families, the disease segregating equally in males and females [63,73].

Some of these families seem to have a very specific phenotype disease, probably unrelated to 'typical' CPPD. Thus, in one Argentinean pedigree [70], the disease seemed to segregate with a Marfan's type hypermobility. In studies of a Gurani Indian

Table 14.7 Families reported with familial aggregation

Reference	Country	Group	Mode of transmission
A Europe			
[15]	Slovakia		Not stated
[51]	France		AD
[52]	Netherlands		AD
[53]	Germany		AD
[54]	Sweden		AD
[47]	Spain		Not stated
[45]	Spain		Not stated
[48]	Spain		AR
[55]	Spain	Catalonia	Not stated
[56]	Switzerland		AD
[57]	Italy		AD
[58]	United Kingdom		AD
[59]	Italy		AD
B America			
[60]	US	European	Not stated
[61]	US	European	Not stated
[62]	US	Northern European	AD
[63]	US	Mexican	AD
[64]	US	Ashkenazi-Jewish	Not stated
[65]	US	Italian	AR
[66]	Canada	French	AD
[67]	Chile	Chiloe Islanders	AD
[50]	Chile	Mapuche Indians	AD
[68]	Argentina	Italian	AD
[69]	Argentina	Italian	AD
[50]	Argentina	Guarani Indians	AD
[70]	Argentina		AD
C Other			
[41]	Japan		AD
[71]	Tunisia		AD
[72]	Israel	Ashkenazi Jews	AD

AD = Autosomal dominant.
AR = Autosomal recessive.
Source: [50].

population from Argentina [50], the disease was associated with an ankylosing type of arthritis. In the English family reported [58], the disease was associated with fits and particularly with childhood onset. These observations suggest that specific mutations may be associated with the occurrence of the particular disease phenotypes in these pedigrees.

Influence of HLA genes

CPPD disease is not thought to have any immune basis to its pathogenesis and therefore it seems unlikely that there would be any association between disease risk and genes within the HLA region. Despite this, there have been a large number of studies, particularly in

relation to segregation within multicase families, examining the role of HLA. Unfortunately, the results are conflicting but this might be consistent with genetic heterogeneity rather than some studies having the correct, and others the incorrect, result. In the first series of families to be identified, from Slovakia [74], a relationship was observed between the disease and the HLA class I haplotype A2 B35. In a small series of unrelated patients there is also the suggestion of an increase in A2 B18 [74], but the numbers were too small (n = 13) for robust estimates. In one Tunisian family [75], all seven affected subjects carried the A1 B12 DR3 haplotype with a maximum Lod score (MLS) of 2.7, just failing to reach statistical significance. However, a number of other large studies have not shown any segregation of multicase families with HLA [48,49,51,66,76].

Non-HLA susceptibility gene loci

As discussed below, there is considered to be a strong metabolic element, at least in some cases, to the occurrence of this disorder. One mark of the genetic defect is to determine the segregation of disease with abnormalities in biochemical markers of bone turnover. Thus, it is interesting to know that in two pedigrees there was evidence of segregation with an increase in the intracellular concentration of inorganic phosphate [62,77]. This, however, is not a universal finding [58]. Others have suggested a linkage with abnormalities in nucleotide triphosphate pyrophosphohydrolase (NTPPPHase) [58] although others [62] have not shown such a link. The recent advances in molecular genetics have enabled both detailed genotype screening within multicase families to search for possible susceptibility loci as well as identifying the potential role of possible candidate genes.

Reginato *et al.* [50] summarized a list of potential genetic targets for investigation covering a large number of different candidate molecules (Table 14.8). In the Chilian families studied [78], it was suggested that there was a linkage to a mutation in the type II procollagen gene (COL2A1) with a substitution of arginine to cysteine in one allele of exon 11. However, linkage with this mutation has not been found consistently in such families [67]. In a large family from the United States, with early-onset CPPD associated

Table 14.8   Potential candidate genes

Molecule Type	Candidates
Enzymes	Pyrophosphatase
	Alkaline phosphatase
	5′ nucleotidase
	NTPPPHase
Collagens	Type II
	Type IX
	Type X
	Type XI
Proteoglycans	Aggrecan
	Biglycan
	Decoran
Cellular proteins	Fibronectin
	Integrins
	TGFB
Growth Factors	Morphogenic bone protein

Source: [50].

Table 14.9   Metabolic and endocrine disorders associated with CPPD

Hypothyroidism
Diabetes mellitis
Primary hyperparathyroidism
Haemochromatase
Hypomagnesaemia (Bartter's syndrome)
Hypophosphatasia
Hypophosphoraemic rickets
Familial hypercalcaemia/hypocalciuria syndrome

Source: [50].

with severe degenerative disease, linkage was observed with a marker in 8q with a Lod score of four [79]. Similarly, in a study of a large three-generation family with early-onset disease, associated with seizures, linkage was observed to a locus in 5p15 with a Lod score of 4.6 [80]. It seems increasingly likely with the availability of molecular typing methods and the associated rapid technology that more of the multicase families mentioned above will be investigated and specific mutations or polymorphisms demonstrated to explain their occurrence. The relevance of such alleles for sporadic disease remains to be considered.

Non-genetic host factors

Metabolic and endocrine disorders

A number of metabolic and endocrine disorders have been associated with CPPD (see Table 14.9). The pathogenic question is whether the metabolic abnormality associated with these disorders increases the likelihood of crystal deposition.

Diabetes mellitus

Although it has been suggested that CPPD is associated with diabetes mellitus (observed in 70 per cent of patients in one series [43]) in a study comparing 184 subjects with diabetes with the matched controls referred for radiographs of knees and hands, there was no evidence of increased occurrence of chondrocalcinosis [81].

Hypothyroidism

It has long been suggested that hypothyroidism is associated with the occurrence of CPPD [82] and in a more recent study 17 per cent of patients with hypo-thyroidism had CPPD compared with age and sex-matched controls based on X-rays of the hands, knees, and pelvis [83]. However, others have found no such association [84,85]. In the latter study, based on the Framingham cohort, there was no relationship between TSH level either measured 6 years prior to X-rays or at the time of X-ray, with the occurrence of chondro-calcinosis in the knees. If anything, there was evidence of a reversed association with those with the highest TSH level having the lowest risk of chondrocalcinosis and *vice versa*, although in neither instances would these risks be particularly significant.

Hypomagnesaemia

Hypomagnesaemia is thought to be of relevance in the pathogenesis of CPPD as extracellular inorganic pyro-phosphate is complexed with magnesium, which is processed to orthophosphate by pyrophosphatase [86]. A number of case reports have suggested an association between hypomagnesaemia and CPPD [87–89]. Hypo-magnesaemia is often considered part of Bartter's syn-drome and in one study of 43 members of a family with the syndrome [90] all seven subjects with a low magnesium level had chondrocalcinosis. More import-antly, the provision of magnesium supplements led to an amelioration of the joint symptoms. Others have questioned whether Bartter's syndrome *per se* is associ-ated with low magnesium levels. Such a phenomenon is not always observed with Bartter's syndrome [91] and others have argued that the association of a hypo-magnesia with this syndrome could be termed Gitelman's variant and it is only that condition which is associated with CPPD.

Hypercalcaemia and hyperparathyroidism

A high risk of chondrocalcinosis from hyperparathy-roidism has been established in a number of surveys, although the occurrence varies from 18 per cent [92] to 24 per cent [93] to 40 per cent [94]. Studies of patients after a parathyroidectomy have suggested that there is an increased risk of associated chondrocalcinosis occurring at a young age [26]. Interestingly, those who are older and have a high alkaline phosphatase pre-operatively have an increased risk. In one study, 30 per cent of hyperparathyroid patients had chondro-calcinosis compared to 4 per cent of controls [27]. It appears that it is the surgical operation of para-thyroidectomy which is associated with an immediate

risk, due to the sudden drop in synovial fluid calcium. Such cases continue to be reported [95].

Haemochromatosis

As increased iron concentration inhibits alkaline phosphatase [86]. It has been suggested that there may be a link between these two disorders, based on case reports [86]. The distinct radiographic features of the arthropathy have been well described [96].

Summary of metabolic disorders

It does appear that with a number of these disorders there is an increased risk, although undoubtedly most cases of CPPD occur in the absence of any endocrine or metabolic abnormality that has been determined. For example in one series of 105 cases only two had hyper-parathyroidism, suggesting the vast majority of cases occur in euparathyroid individuals [82]. Similarly, hypomagnesaemia and haemochromatosis are also exceptionally rare as causes of CPPD.

Other host factors

The presence of local joint disease is thought to be par-ticularly important in the onset of chondrocalcinosis. For example in a series of 105 patients with CPPD, eight had had knee surgery many years prior to the onset of symptoms and in three patients the CPPD had been confined to the operated knee [7]. The most common surgical procedure on the knee, particularly in young adults, is meniscectomy and in one study the occurrence of chondrocalcinosis was compared in the operated and non-operated side in 100 post-meniscectomy patients, the surgery having occurred 25 years earlier. CPPD was five times more likely in the operated than the non-operated knee as well as the occurrence of osteoarthritis (90 per cent versus 54 per cent) [97]. It was argued that the trauma of the initial cartilage damage, in combination with the operation, were pathogenically responsible both for the crystal deposition and the subsequent degenerative disease. A similar high frequency of long-term development of chondrocalcinosis was seen at a mean of 33 years follow-up after surgery for osteochondritis dessicans [98]. Chondrocalcinosis may indeed occur within a very short time following anterior cruciate ligament repair as illustrated in one recent case [99]. There has been some suggestion that patients who have hyper-mobile joints present an increased risk [100] and

12 per cent of patients with CPPD in one series either had past or current evidence of joint laxity [7]. This is interesting given the possible association with Marfan's syndrome discussed above.

Infection

Infection in the joint is also associated with an increased risk of CPPD, as illustrated in one case report [101] following occurrence of septic arthritis and in another case where infection with *Actinobacillus* had occurred [102]. Others have also shown the co-existence with infection [103].

Drug therapy

Corticosteroid therapy is a frequent finding in uncontrolled hospital series [7]. Although in many of these patients the steroids had been given for suppression of presumed joint inflammation, used for the treatment of these disorders. Recent reports have suggested that the use of granulocyte colony stimulating factor, occasionally used for treatment of some cancers, may be associated with precipitation of acute arthritis after a short interval, perhaps related to an increased phagocytosis of crystals. Another suggestion is that drugs that cause rapid lowering of serum calcium, for example IV pamidromate, may also be associated with presentation of the disease [104].

References

1. McCarty DJ, Kohn NN, Faires JS. The significance of calcium phosphate crystals in the synovial fluid of arthritic patients: The pseudogout syndrome. *Ann Intern Med* 1962; 56: 711–737.
2. McCarty DJ, Hogan JM, Gatter RA, Grossman M. Studies on pathological calcifications in human cartilage. *J Bone Joint Surg Br* 1966; 48: 309–325.
3. Halverson PB, McCarty DJ. Basic calcium phosphate (apatite, octacalcium phosphate, tricalcium phosphate) crystal deposition diseases; calcinosis. In: Koopman WJ, editor. *Arthritis and allied conditions.* Baltimore: Lippincott, Williams and Wilkins, 1996: 2127–2145.
4. McCarty DJ. Diagnostic mimicry in arthritis—patterns of joint involvement associated with calcium pyrophosphate dihydrate crystal deposits. *Bull Rheum Dis* 1975; 25: 804–809.
5. Jaccard YB, Gerster JC, Calame L. Mixed monosodium urate and calcium pyrophosphate crystal-induced arthropathy. A review of seventeen cases. *Rev Rhum Engl Ed* 1996; 63: 331–335.

6. Swan A, Heywood B, Chapman B, Seward H, Dieppe P. Evidence for a casual relationship between the structure, size, and load of calcium pyrophosphate dihydrate crystals, and attacks of pseudogout. *Ann Rheum Dis* 1995; 54: 825–830.
7. Dieppe PA, Alexander GJM, Jones HE, Doherty M, Scott DGI. Pyrophosphate arthropathy: a clinical and radiological study of 105 cases. *Ann Rheum Dis* 1982; 41: 371–376.
8. Ishida T, Dorfman HD, Bullough PG. Tophaceous pseudogout (tumoral calcium pyrophosphate dihydrate crystal deposition disease). *Hum Pathol* 1995; 26: 587–593.
9. Fye KH, Weinstein PR, Donald F. Compressive cervical myelopathy due to calcium pyrophosphate dihydrate deposition disease: report of a case and review of the literature. *Arch Intern Med* 1999; 159: 189–193.
10. Constantin A, Bouteiller G. Acute neck pain and fever as the first manifestation of chondrocalcinosis with calcification of the transverse ligament of the atlas. Five case-reports with a literature review. *Rev Rhum Engl Ed* 1998; 65: 583–585.
11. McGill NW, York HF. Reproducibility of synovial fluid examination for crystals. *Aust N Z J Med* 1991; 21: 710–713.
12. Genant HK. Roentgenographic aspects of calcium pyrophosphate dihydrate crystal deposition disease (pseudogout). *Arthritis Rheum* 1976; 19: 307–328.
13. Leonard A, Solnica J, Cauvin M, Houdent G, Mallet E, Brunelle PH. La Chondrocalcinose: Etude de sa frequence radiologique et de ses rapports avec L'arthrose etude de taux de la parathormone (1)r1150. *Rev Rhum Mal Osteoartic* 1977; 44: 559–564.
14. Wilkins E, Dieppe P, Maddison P, Evison G. Osteoarthritis and articular chondrocalcinosis in the elderly. *Ann Rheum Dis* 1983; 42: 280–284.
15. Zitnan D, Sitaj S. Natural course of articular chondrocalcinosis. *Arthritis Rheum* 1976; 19: 363–390.
16. Felson DT, Anderson JJ, Naimark A, Kannel W, Meenan RF. The prevalence of chondrocalcinosis in the elderly and its association with knee osteoarthritis: the Framingham study. *J Rheumatol* 1989; 16: 1241–1245.
17. Sanmarti R, Kanterewicz E, Pladevall M, Panella D, Tarradellas JB, Gomez JM. Analysis of the association between chondrocalcinosis and osteoarthritis: A community based study. *Ann Rheum Dis* 1996; 55: 30–33.
18. Felson DT, Zhang Y, Hannan MT *et al.* Risk factors for incident radiographic knee osteoarthritis in the elderly: the Framingham Study. *Arthritis Rheum* 1997; 40: 728–733.
19. Bocher J, Mankin HJ, Berk RN, Rodnan GP. Prevalence of calcified meniscal cartilage in elderly persons. *N Engl J Med* 1965; 272: 1093–1097.
20. Cabanel G, Phelip X, Gras JP, Verdier JM. Frequence des calcifications meniscales et leur signification pathologique. *Rhumatologie* 1970; 22: 255–262.
21. Ellman MH, Levin B. Chondrocalcinosis in elderly persons. *Arthritis Rheum* 1975; 18: 43–47.
22. Trentham DE, Masi AT, Hamm RL. Roentgenographic prevalence of chondrocalcinosis. *Arthritis Rheum* 1975; 18: 627–628.

23. Memin Y, Monville C, Ryckewaert A. Chrondo-calcinosis over eighty. *Arthritis Rheum* 1975; **18**: 43.

24. Delauche MC, Stehle B, Cassou B, Verret JM, Kahn MF. Frequence de la chondrocalcinose radiologique apres 80 ans. *Rev Rhum Ed Fr* 1977; **44**: 555–557.

25. Emeriau JP, Bordec EC, Chapoulart H *et al*. Chondrocalcinose articulaire asymptomatique chez le sujet age. *Bordeaux Med* 1977; **10**: 825.

26. Pritchard MH, Jessop JD. Chondrocalcinosis in primary hyperparathyroidism. *Ann Rheum Dis* 1977; **36**: 146–151.

27. Rynes RI, Merzig EG. Calcium pyrophosphate crystal deposition disease and hyperparathyroidism: a controlled, prospective study. *J Rheumatol* 1978; **5**: 460–468.

28. Megard M, Vignon E, Arlot M, Pont P, Moos S, Betuel H. Etude de la chondrocalcinose articulaire dans une population de 200 viellards. *Lyon Medical* 1981; **245**: 365–370.

29. Gordon TP, Smith M, Ebert B, McCredie M, Brooks PM. Articular chondrocalcinosis in a hospital population: an Australian experience. *Aust N Z J Med* 1984; **14**: 655–659.

30. Bergstrom G, Bjelle A, Sorensen LB, Sundh V, Svanborg A. Prevalence of rheumatoid arthritis, osteoarthritis, chondrocalcinosis and gouty arthritis at age 79. *J Rheumatol* 1986; **13**: 527–534.

31. Sanmarti R, Panella D, Brancos MA, Canela J, Collado A, Brugues J. Prevalence of articular chondrocalcinosis in elderly subjects in a rural area of Catalonia. *Ann Rheum Dis* 1993; **52**: 418–422.

32. Weaver JB. Calcification and ossification of the menisci. *J Bone Joint Surg Br* 1942; **24**: 873–882.

33. McCarty DJ. Calcium pyrophosphate dihydrate crystal deposition disease—1975. *Arthritis Rheum* 1976; **19**: 275–285.

34. Atkins CJ, McIvor J, Smith PM, Hamilton E, Williams R. Chondrocalcinosis and arthropathy: studies in haemochromatosis and in idiopathic chondrocalcinosis. *QJM* 1970; **39**: 71–82.

35. Mitrovic D, Stankovic A, Morin J *et al*. Frequence anatomique de la menisco-chondrocalcinose du genou. *Rev Rhum Mal Osteoartic* 1982; **49**: 495–499.

36. Tobler T. Makroskopische und histologische befunde am kniegelenksmeniskus in verschiedenen lebensaltern. *Schweiz Med Wochenschr* 1929; **10**: 1359–1366.

37. Lagier R, Baud CA. Pathological calcifications of the locomotor system. Status of articular chrondocalcinosis. In: Milhaud G, Owen M, Blackwood H, editors. *Reports and communications of the IV European symposis of calcified tissues. Bordeaux 1967*. Paris: Sedes, 1968.

38. Fondimare A, Talon JP, Deshayes P. Etude anatomopathologique de la chondrocalcinose articulaire A propos de 11 observations. *Presse Med* 1971; **79**: 707–710.

39. Mitrovic DR, Stankovic A, Iriarte-Borda O *et al*. The prevalence of chondrocalcinosis in the human knee joint. An autopsy survey. *J Rheumatol* 1988; **15**: 633–641.

40. Regan M, Clarke AK, Doherty M. Pseudogout provoked by pregnancy. *Br J Rheumatol* 1993; **32**: 245–247.

41. Sakaguchi M, Ishikawa K, Mizuta HS, Kitagawa T. Familial pseudogout oil destructive arthropathy. *Arch Intern Med* 1982; **123**: 636–644.

42. Moskowitz RW, Garcia F. Chondrocalcinosis articularis (pseudogout syndrome). *Arch Intern Med* 1973; **132**: 87–91.

43. Skinner M, Cohen AS. Calcium pyrophosphate dihydrate crystal deposition disease. *Arch Intern Med* 1969; **123**: 636–644.

44. Reginato AJ, Hollander JL, Martinez V *et al*. Familial chondrocalcinosis in the Chiloe Islands, Chile. *Ann Rheum Dis* 1975; **34**: 260–268.

45. Fernandez-Dapica MP, Gomez-Reino JJ. Familial chondrocalcinosis in the Spanish population. *J Rheumatol* 1986; **13**: 631–633.

46. Schlesinger N, Gowin KM, Baker DG, Beutler AM, Hoffman BI, Schumacher HRJr. Acute gouty arthritis is seasonal. *J Rheumatol* 1998; **25**: 342–344.

47. Rodriguez-Valverde V, Tinture T, Zuniga M, Pena J, Gonzalez A. Familial chondrocalcinosis. Prevalence in northern Spain and clinical features in five pedigrees. *Arthritis Rheum* 1980; **23**: 471–478.

48. Balsa A, Martin-Mola E, Gonzalez T, Cruz A, Ojeda S, Gijon Banos J. Familial articular chondrocalcinosis in Spain. *Ann Rheum Dis* 1990; **49**: 531–535.

49. Fernandez-Dapica MP, Reginato AJ. Familial and sporadic calcium pyrophosphate deposition disease (CPPDD) in Spain: a unified hypothesis about an Iberian mutation. *Arthritis Rheum* 1992; **35**: S119.

50. Reginato AJ, Reginato AM, Fernandez-Dapica MP, Ramachandrula A. Familial calcium pyrophosphate crystal deposition disease or calcium pyrophosphate gout. *Rev Rhum Ed Fr* 1995; **62**: 397–412.

51. Gaucher A, Faure G, Netter P *et al*. Hereditary diffuse articular chondrocalcinosis. *Scand J Rheumatol* 1977; **6**: 217–221.

52. van der Korst JK, Geerards J. Articular chondrocalcinosis in a Dutch pedigree. *Arthritis Rheum* 1976; **19**: 405–409.

53. Aschoff H, Bohm P, Schoen E, Schurholz K. Hereditare chondrocalcinosis articularis. Untersuchung einer familie. *Humangenetik* 1966; **3**: 98–103.

54. Bjelle A, Edvinsson U, Hagstam A. Pyrophosphate arthropathy in two Swedish families. *Arthritis Rheum* 1982; **25**: 66–74.

55. Sanmarti R, Panella D, Brancos MA, Anglada A. Condrocalcinosis articular hereditaria en la comarca de Osona (Barcelona): presentacion de tres familias. *Med Clin Barc* 1989; **92**: 780–783.

56. Gerster JC, Schmied PA. Hereditary chondrocalcinosis in a Swiss family. *Schweiz Med Wochenschr* 1987; **117**: 402–405.

57. Adamo V, Grassi W, Cervini C. Chrondocalcinosi familiare. *Reumatismo* 1986; **36**: 262–267.

58. Doherty M, Hamilton E, Henderson J, Misra H, Dixey J. Familial chondrocalcinosis due to calcium pyrophosphate dihydrate crystals deposition in English families. *Br J Rheumatol* 1991; **30**: 10–15.

59. Fantechi V, Lazzeri S, Baldoni D, Maranghi P. Condrocalcinosi o malattia da deposizione di cristalli di pirofosfato diidrato di calcio (CPPD). Descrizione di un caso con familiarita. *Radiol Med Torino* 1993; **85**: 850–853.

60. Moskowitz RW, Katz D. Chondrocalcinosis (pseudogout syndrome). A family study. *JAMA* 1964; **188**: 867–871.

61. Mathews JL, Samuelson CO, Manis S. Familial brachydactyly and chondrocalcinosis—report of a patient, pedigree and review of the literature. *J Rheumatol* 1983; **10**: 819–822.

62. Ryan LM, Wortmann RL, Karas B, Lynch MP, McCarty DJ. Pyrophosphohydrolase activity and inorganic pyrophosphate content of cultured human skin fibroblasts. Elevated levels in some patients with calcium pyrophosphate dihydrate deposition disease. *J Clin Invest* 1986; **77**: 1689–1693.

63. Richardson BC, Chafetz NI, Ferrell LD, Zulman JI, Genant HK. Hereditary chondrocalcinosis in a Mexican-American family. *Arthritis Rheum* 1983; **26**: 1387–1396.

64. Brem JB. Vertebral ankylosis in a patient with hereditary chondrocalcinosis: A chance association? *Arthritis Rheum* 1982; **25**: 1257–1263.

65. Reginato AJ, Zmijewski CM, Dalinka MK. Calcium pyrophosphate dihydrate deposition disease (CPDD) in an Italo-north American. *Arthritis Rheum* 1982; **25**: S76.

66. Gaudreau A, Camerlain M, Pibarot M, Beauregard G, Lebrun A, Petitclerc C. Familial articular chondrocalcinosis in Quebec. *Arthritis Rheum* 1981; **24**: 611–615.

67. Reginato AJ, Knowlton RG, Jimenez SA, Weaver E, Venegas Passano GM, Prockop DJ. Calcium pyrophosphate deposition disease in the Chiloe Islanders. Follow-up and restriction length polymorphism studies in the procollagen II and in the liver-bone alkaline phosphatase gene. *Arthritis Rheum* 1990; **33** (Suppl. 9): S54.

68. Caeiro F, Babini A, Marchegiani R, Alvarelos A. Familial calcium pyrophosphate deposition disease (CPPDD) and marfanoid features in a kindred of Northern Italian-Argentinean ancestry. *Arthritis Rheum* 1994; **37**: S413.

69. Pons-Estel B, Sacnum M, Gentiletti S, Battagliotti C. Familial chronic shoulder destructive arthropathy (ChSDA), calcium pyrophosphate and apatite deposition. *Arthritis Rheum* 1994; **37**: S414.

70. Babini CF, Marchegiani R, Alvarelos A. Familial calcium pyrophosphate deposition disease (CPPDD) and marfanoid features in a kindred of Northern Italian-Argentinean ancestry. *Arthritis Rheum* 1994; **37**: 1512.

71. Hamza M, Meddeb N, Bardin T. Hereditary chondrocalcinosis in a Tunisian family. *Clin Exp Rheumatol* 1992; **10**: 43–49.

72. Eshel G, Gulik A, Halperin N *et al.* Hereditary chondrocalcinosis in an Ashkenazi Jewish family. *Ann Rheum Dis* 1990; **49**: 528–530.

73. Riestra JL, Sanchez A, Rodriguez-Valverde V, Alonso JL, de la Hera M, Merino J. Radiographic features of hereditary articular chondrocalcinosis. A comparative study with the sporadic type. *Clin Exp Rheumatol* 1988; **6**: 369–372.

74. Nyulassy S, Stefanovic J, Sitaj S, Zitnan D. HLA system in articular chondrocalcinosis. *Arthritis Rheum* 1976; **19**: 391–393.

75. Hamza M, Ayed K, Bardi R *et al.* HLA-antigens in a Tunisian familial chondrocalcinosis. *Dis Markers* 1990; **8**: 109–112.

76. Nunez-Roldan A. Familial chondrocalcinosis and HLA system. *Arthritis Rheum* 1981; **24**: 1590–1591.

77. Lust G, Faure G, Netter P, Gaucher A, Seegmiller JE. Evidence of a generalized metabolic defect in patients with hereditary chondrocalcinosis. Increased inorganic pyrophosphate in cultured fibroblasts and lymphoblasts. *Arthritis Rheum* 1981; **24**: 1517–1521.

78. Basualdo J, Munoz S, Reginato AJ, Williams CJ, Prockop DJ. Familial precocious osteoarthritis (POA) spondyloepiphyseal dysphagia (SED) and calcium pyrophosphate deposition disease (CPPD) linked to a point mutation in type II procollagen gene (COL2A1). *Arthritis Rheum* 1993; **37**: 149.

79. Baldwin CT, Farrer LA, Adair R, Dharmavaram R, Jimenez S, Anderson L. Linkage of early onset osteoarthritis and chondrocalcinosis to human chromosome 8Q. *Am J Hum Genet* 1995; **56**: 692–697.

80. Doherty M, Hughes A, McGibbon D, Woodward E. Localization of a gene for familial chondrocalcinosisin a UK kindred to chromosome 5P. *Arthritis Rheum* 1995; **38**: 42.

81. Silveri F, Adamo V, Corsi M *et al.* Chondrocalcinosis and diabetes mellitus. The clinico-statistical data. *Recenti Prog Med* 1994; **85**: 91–95.

82. Alexander GM, Dieppe PA, Doherty M, Scott GI. Pyrophosphate arthropathy: a study of metabolic associations and laboratory data. *Ann Rheum Dis* 1982; **41**: 377–381.

83. Deslandre C, Menkes CJ, Guinot M, Luton JP. Does hypothyroidism increase the prevalence of chondrocalcinosis? *Br J Rheumatol* 1993; **32**: 197–198.

84. Visinoni RA, Ferraz MB, Furlanetto RP, Fernandes AR, Oliveira HC, Atra E. Hypothyroidism and chondrocalcinosis: new evidence for lack of association between the 2 pathologies. *J Rheumatol* 1993; **20**: 1991–1992.

85. Chaisson CE, McAlindon TE, Felson DT, Naimark A, Wilson PW, Sawin CT. Lack of association between thyroid status and chondrocalcinosis or osteoarthritis: the Framingham Osteoarthritis Study. *J Rheumatol* 1996; **23**: 711–715.

86. Wright GD, Doherty M. Calcium pyrophosphate crystal deposition is not always 'wear and tear' or aging. *Ann Rheum Dis* 1997; **56**: 586–588.

87. Runeberg L, Collan Y, Jokinen EJ, Lahdevirta J, Aro A. Hypomagnesemia due to renal disease of unknown etiology. *Am J Med* 1975; **59**: 873–881.

88. Ellman MH, Brown NL, Porat AP. Laboratory investigations in pseudogout patients and controls. *J Rheumatol* 1980; **7**: 77–81.

89. Milazzo SC, Ahern MJ, Cleland LG, Henderson RF. Calcium pyrophosphate dihydrate deposition disease and familial hypomagnesemia. *J Rheumatol* 1981; **8**: 767–771.

90. Smilde TJ, Haverman JF, Schipper P, Hermus A. Familial hypokalemia/hypomagnesemia and chondrocalcinosis. *J Rheumatol* 1994; **21**: 1515–1519.

91. Fam AG. Calcium pyrophosphate crystal deposition disease and other crystal deposition diseases. *Curr Opin Rheumatol* 1995; 7: 364–368.

92. Dodds EJ, Steinbach HL. Primary hyperparathyroidism and articular calcification. *Am J Roent Radium There and Nuc Med* 1968; **104**: 884–892.

93. Rickewaert A, Solnica J, Lanham C, de Seze S. Articular manifestations of hyperparathyroidism. *Presse Med* 1966; **74**: 2599–2603.

94. Glass JS, Grahame R. Chondrocalcinosis after parathyroidectomy. *Ann Rheum Dis* 1976; **35**: 521–525.

95. Gantes-Mora MA, Rodriquez-Lorano B, Trujillo-Martin E, Bustabad-Reyes S, Gonzalez-Garcia T. Post parathyroidectomy pseudogout in primary hyperparathyroidism. *An Med Internat* 1998; **15**: 376–378.

96. Jager HJ, Mehring UM, Gotz GF *et al.* Radiological features of the visceral and skeletal involvement of hemochromatosis. *Eur Radiol* 1997; 7: 1199–1206.

97. Doherty M, Watt I, Dieppe PA. Localised chondrocalcinosis in post-meniscectomy knees. *Lancet* 1982; 1: 1207–1210.

98. Linden B, Nilsson BE. Chondrocalcinosis following osteochondritis dissecans in the femur condyles. *Clin Orthop* 1977; **130**: 223–227.

99. Minezaki T, Tomatsu T, Hanada K. Calcium pyrophosphate dihydrate crystal deposition disease after anterior cruciate ligament reconstruction. *Arthroscopy* 1998; **14**: 634–636.

100. Bird HA, Tribe CR, Bacon PA. Joint hypermobility leading to osteoarthritis and chondrocalcinosis. *Ann Rheum Dis* 1978; **37**: 203–211.

101. Ilahi OA, Swarna U, Hamill RJ, Young EJ, Tullos HS. Concomitant crystal and septic arthritis. *Orthopedics* 1996; **19**: 613–617.

102. Cuende E, de Pablos M, Gomez M, Burgaleta S, Michaus L, Vesga JC. Coexistence of pseudogout and arthritis due to Actinobacillus actinomycetemcomitans. *Clin Infect Dis* 1996; **23**: 657–658.

103. Razzaq A, Kokko K, Agudelo CA. Case report: coexistence of acute calcific periarthritis and infection. *Am J Med Sci* 1996; **312**: 140–141.

104. Malnick SD, Ariel Ronen S, Evron E, Sthoeger ZM. Acute pseudogout as a complication of pamidronate. *Ann Pharmacother* 1997; **31**: 499–500.

Introduction

Historically, the term 'osteoporosis' first entered medical parlance in France and Germany in the nineteenth century, where it was coined as a descriptive term emphasizing the porosity of the histological appearances of aged human bone. Predating this was Sir Astley Cooper's treatise on hip fracture published more than 150 years ago, which suggested that types of fracture might result from an age-related reduction in bone mass or quality [1]. He gave the original description of the classical epidemiological hallmarks of these fractures: incidence rates which increase with age; rates which are higher among women than men; and fractures which are associated with moderate trauma at sites containing large amounts of trabecular bone. These features are typified by fractures of the proximal femur, distal radius, and vertebrae: the three 'traditional' sites, but fractures at other sites, such as the pelvis, proximal humerus, and proximal tibia, also show similar patterns. Osteoporosis is of major public health significance because of its association with fracture. These fractures are the serious, costly, and important outcome of the condition, leading to severe mortality and morbidity and a considerable burden on society.

Definition of osteoporosis

The currently accepted definition of osteoporosis is: 'A systemic skeletal disorder characterized by low bone mass and micro-architectural deterioration of bone tissue, with a consequent increase in bone fragility and susceptibility to fracture risk' [2].

Critically, this definition encompasses the clinically significant aspect of osteoporosis, namely fracture, but also the relationship between fracture and low bone mass. This chapter will review the epidemiological aspects of osteoporosis, commencing with the public health significance in terms of mortality, morbidity,

and financial costs. It will then review the epidemiology of fractures, concentrating on those sites where the majority of age-related fractures occur. The chapter will then provide an overview of the determinants of fracture, aiming to emphasize the important role of bone mass. The relationship between bone mass and fracture will be clarified. Currently, the best method of assessing bone mass is by non-invasive densitometric techniques, therefore the pros and cons of the available techniques will be briefly described. Finally, the risk factors for osteoporosis will be discussed in terms of genetic factors, non-genetic host factors, environmental factors, and falls. Many of the studies of risk factors have examined the relationship of one or more factors with bone mass as a surrogate for fracture risk. Therefore, the risk factor sections will summarize the current epidemiological evidence both for effects on fracture risk and bone mass.

Occurrence: health burden

Mortality

Mortality patterns have been studied for the three most frequent osteoporotic fractures (Fig. 15.1) [3]. Survival rates 5 years after hip and vertebral fractures were found, in Rochester, Minnesota, to be around 80 per cent of those expected for men and women of similar age without fractures [3]. Mortality after Colles' fracture is not thought to deviate from the expected rate.

Hip fracture

Hip fracture mortality is higher for men than for women, increases with age [3], and is greater for those with coexisting illness and poor prefracture functional status [4]. There are about 31 000 excess deaths within 6 months of the approximately 300 000 hip fractures

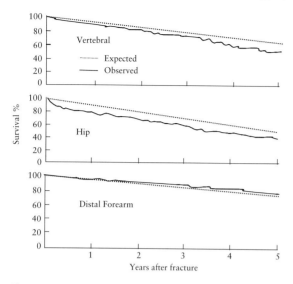

Fig. 15.1 Survival rates after the diagnosis of hip, vertebral, or distal forearm fracture among residents of Rochester, Minnesota. Both the observed survival and that expected using the 1980 death rates of residents of the West North Central United States are shown. Reproduced with permission of Oxford University Press from [3].

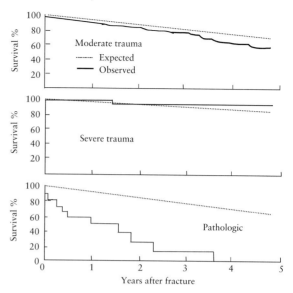

Fig. 15.2 Survival rates after the diagnosis of vertebral fracture among residents of Rochester, Minnesota. Fracture resulted from mild to moderate trauma, severe trauma, or a pathologic bone lesion. Reproduced with permission of Oxford University Press from [3].

that occur annually in the United States. About 8 per cent of men and 3 per cent of women over 50 years of age die while hospitalized for their fracture. One year after hip fracture, mortality is 36 per cent for men and 21 per cent for women and is much higher in older men. One French study reported that 21 per cent of hip fracture patients studied died within 3 months of their fracture, and mortality was twice as high in men as women [5]. Two years after hip fracture, mortality rates become comparable with people of the same age without hip fractures, although higher rates persist longer among elderly patients and among men. The interaction of acute injury or surgery with co-morbid conditions may contribute substantially to the excess mortality early after hip fracture. Both high levels of comorbidity and the presence of mental confusion during hospitalization are associated with an increased risk of dying after a hip fracture [5–7].

Vertebral fracture

Excess mortality after vertebral fracture appears to increase progressively after diagnosis of the fracture. This has been observed in studies based on clinically diagnosed vertebral deformities [3], and in those using radiological morphometric approaches to classify vertebral deformity [8]. Impaired survival is more pronounced for vertebral fractures that follow mild or moderate, rather than severe, trauma (Fig. 15.2) [3]. Five-year survival appears to be worse for men (72 per cent) than for women (84 per cent). Among patients with vertebral fractures secondary to mild or moderate trauma, only a small proportion (8 per cent) can be attributed to osteoporosis. The pattern of divergence between observed and expected survival suggests that the fractures are less the cause of death than an indicator of the presence of comorbid pathology and that it is the comorbidity that is responsible for the observed increased risk of death. There are an estimated 263 000 vertebral fractures annually in white US citizens followed within 6 months by about 11 000 excess deaths [3]. Furthermore, there is evidence of a relationship between mortality and low spinal bone mass in the absence of fracture: in a cohort of white women greater than 65 years of age, there was a 20 per cent increase in mortality for each standard deviation reduction in bone mineral density [9]. Further investigation is warranted of the complex relationships between bone mineral density (BMD), fracture, and excess deaths.

Morbidity

In the United States, about 7 per cent of survivors of all types of fragility fractures have some degree of permanent disability, and 8 per cent require long-term nursing home care. Overall, a 50-year old US white woman has a 13 per cent chance of experiencing fracture-related functional decline after any fracture [10]. However, the greatest fracture-attributable morbidity arises from hip fracture.

Hip fracture

Inability to walk after a hip fracture makes this a particularly disabling event with a pronounced effect on quality of life. Hip fractures invariably require hospitalization. The degree of functional recovery after a hip fracture is age-dependent. In the US, the proportion of hip fracture patients who were discharged from hospital to nursing homes was 14 per cent for those aged 50–55 years, but 55 per cent of those aged > 90 years and the length of stay was also related to age [11]. One year after hip fracture, 40 per cent of patients are still unable to walk independently, 60 per cent require assistance in at least one essential activity of daily living (e.g. dressing, bathing), and 80 per cent are unable to perform at least one instrumental activity of daily living (e.g. driving, shopping). Prefracture status is a strong predictor of outcome. In the US, for example, about 25 per cent of formerly independent people become at least partially dependent, 50 per cent of those who were dependent prefracture are admitted to nursing homes, and those who were in nursing homes predictably remain there. Similarly, in France, 20 per cent of those who had been independent prefracture required some form of assisted living afterwards [5].

Vertebral fracture

The clinical impact of a single vertebral fracture may be minimal, but the effects of multiple fractures are cumulative, leading to acute and chronic back pain, limitation of physical activity, progressive kyphosis, and loss of height. These, in turn, lead to a loss of functional capacities and an inability to take part in recreational activities, which leads to social isolation, depression, and low self-esteem. Pain and fear of additional fractures cause decreased physical activity, exacerbating further the underlying osteoporosis and leading to an increased risk of further fractures [12–14].

Distal forearm fracture

Distal forearm fractures are not associated with increased mortality, but they do cause significant morbidity. One study showed that only 50 per cent of patients report good functional recovery 1 year post fracture, and 1 per cent become dependent [15]. The poor recovery results from long-term complications such as reflex sympathetic dystrophy, neuropathies, and post-traumatic arthritis.

Occurrence: epidemiology of fractures

This section will review the epidemiology of fractures generally, and then focus on the specific characteristics of those age-related fractures that occur most frequently and consequently pose the most pressing public health problem.

Data from the US suggest that overall, around 40 per cent of all white women and 13 per cent of white men aged 50 years will experience at least one clinically apparent fragility fracture in their lifetimes (Table 15.1) [16]. However, taking into account sites other than the hip, spine, and distal forearm, the lifetime risk among women aged 50 years might be as high as 70 per cent. Estimates for the British population are around 20 per cent lower [4].

Epidemiology of all fractures

Recent data from the UK suggest that there is an overall fracture incidence of 21.1/1000 per year (23.5/1000 in men and 18.8/1000 in women) [17]. Fracture incidence in the community is bimodal, with peaks in youth and in the very elderly [18–21] (Fig. 15.3). In young people, fractures of the long bones predominate, usually after substantial trauma, more frequently in males than females. None of these

Table 15.1 Estimated lifetime risk of fracture in 50-year-old white men and women. Modified from [16].

Fracture site	Lifetime risk	
	Men (%)	Women (%)
Hip fracture	6.0	17.5
Clinically diagnosed vertebral fracture	5.0	15.6
Distal forearm fracture	2.5	16.0
Any of the above	13.1	39.7

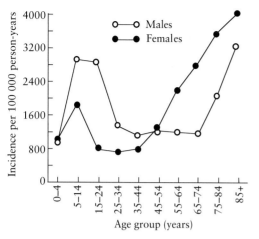

Fig. 15.3 Average annual age- and sex- specific incidence of all limb fractures among residents of Rochester, Minnesota. Reproduced with permission of Lippincott Williams and Wilkins from Melton LJ, in Riggs, Melton LJ (eds) *Osteoporosis: etiology, diagnosis and management* 1988 [29].

fractures seem to be related to osteoporosis. As the forces involved are substantial the question of bone strength rarely arises. Over the age of 35 years, overall fracture incidence in women climbs steeply, so that rates become twice those in men [22]. Hip and distal forearm fractures are the main contributors to this later peak, which also includes proximal humeral, pelvic, and proximal tibial fractures. It is within this latter group that osteoporosis makes a substantial impact. There are, however, differences in the patterns of these fractures by age and sex suggesting the influence of different aetiological factors, as will be detailed in the following site-specific sections.

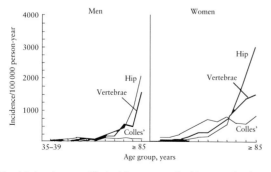

Fig. 15.4 Age-specific incidence rates for hip, vertebral, and distal forearm fractures in men and women. Data derived from the population of Rochester, Minnesota. Reprinted from Cooper C, Melton LJ, Epidemiology of osteoporosis. *Trends in Endocrinology and Metabolism*, 3, 224–29. Copyright (1992), with permission from Elsevier Science [27].

Epidemiology of hip fracture

Worldwide, there were an estimated 1.66 million hip fractures in 1990 [23], about 1 197 000 in women and 463 000 in men. Typically, hip fractures occur through the neck of the femur (cervical or intracapsular) or in the region between the greater and lesser trochanters (intertrochanteric or extracapsular). The incidence of cervical and trochanteric fractures is approximately equal, although some studies suggest a slight excess of trochanteric fractures (ratio of 1:1.03 in Swiss women; ratio of 1:1.12 in Swiss men [24]; ratio of 1:1.13 in Sweden [25]; ratio 1:1 in Spain [26].

Age

In most populations, hip fracture incidence rates increase exponentially with age after 60 years, so that overall about 98 per cent of all hip fractures occur among people aged 35 years and above (Fig. 15.4) [27].

Gender

In Western populations, above 50 years of age, there is a female-to-male incidence ratio of approximately 2:1 [28–30]. However, around 80 per cent of all hip fractures occur in women, partly because there are more elderly women. These gender differences are not seen in all ethnic groups: the female-to-male ratio for hip fracture in Chinese is 1:1.

Geographical

Examination of hospital records of age- and sex-standardized discharge rates after hip fracture in the UK [31] and in the US [32] reveal considerable geographical variation in both populations. In the UK, the variation was not explained by differences in water fluoride content or by dietary consumption of calcium (assessed from a national food survey). In the US, there is a north–south gradient of fracture risk with a cluster of high incidence in the southeast. An association was detected between hip fracture incidence and southerly latitude, socio-economic deprivation, proportion of agricultural land, reduced sunlight exposure, and soft, fluoridated water supply. Differences in body weight, smoking, and alcohol consumption do not reveal parallel geographic trends [33]. In Europe, hip fracture rates vary more than seven-fold from one country to another [34]. However, variation in activity levels, obesity, cig-

Table 15.2 Age-adjusted incidence rates per 100 000 person-years for hip fractures in women of different populations; modified from [35]

Reference	Population	Rate/100 000	
		Women	Men
[35]	Norway (1983–4)	1290	550
	Stockholm (1972–81)	620	290
	California whites (1983–4)	560	210
	Rochester, Minn (1965–74)	510	170
	Hong Kong (1965–7)	150	100
	Hong Kong (1985)	350	180
	Singapore (1955–62)	80	100
	California Asians (1983–4)	340	100
	California Blacks (1983–4)	220	140
	California Hispanics (1983–4)	200	90
	Beijing, China (1990–2)	90	100
[36]	Canada (1993–4)	480	190
[37]	Kuwait (1992–5)	295	200
[38]	Japan (1986–8)	115	41
	Japan (1992–4)	145	60

Incidence rates age-standardized to US population

arette smoking, alcohol consumption, or migration status have not provided explanations of these wide geographical variations.

Ethnicity

Internationally, comparisons of rates of hip fracture reveal a consistent trend in which ethnic group plays a major part. Wherever these have been examined, rates of hip fracture are higher among Caucasians than among populations of African origin (Table 15.2), although there are differences within populations of a given gender or race. Within African populations, both in South Africa and in North America, rates in men and women are similar [39–41]. Urbanization in certain parts of Africa has led to an increase in hip fracture incidence, but even recently derived urban African rates for hip fracture are considerably lower than those found in western Caucasians [42]. The highest recorded rates of hip fracture, after age-adjustment, come from Sweden and the northern US (Fig. 15.5) [43]. Rates in southern Europe and Israel are substantially lower [29]. In Asian populations, rates overall are intermediate between those found in Caucasians and Africans. The reasons for these ethnic patterns are uncertain.

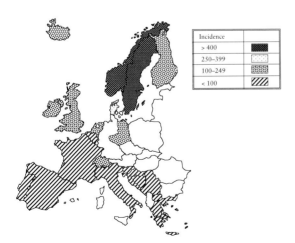

Incidence	
> 400	
250–399	
100–249	
< 100	

Fig. 15.5 Incidence of hip fracture in Europe (women, crude rate /100 000 of the population aged 50 years or over). Reproduced with permission of Martin Dunitz Publishers from [43].

Seasonality

Hip fractures show marked seasonality in their incidence, tending to occur more frequently in the winter in temperate countries [32]. However, the majority of the hip fractures occur indoors and not as a result of slipping on icy pavements.

Time trends

Analyses of age-adjusted hip fracture incidence rates in the US, Scandinavia, and the UK suggest an approxi-

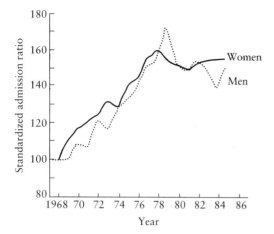

Fig. 15.6   Secular trends in hip fracture incidence in England and Wales, UK. (Ratio of observed to expected numbers of patients aged over 45 admitted to hospital with hip fracture in England and Wales, 1968–85. Data obtained from Hospital Inpatient Enquiry and standardized for age on basis of age-specific rates in 1968). Reproduced from *BMJ* 1990; **300**: 1178–1184, with permission from the BMJ Publishing Group [52].

mate doubling between 1955 and 1985 [44–48]. Similar rates of increase have been observed in men and women. This time trend was first documented in the population of Rochester, Minnesota, where rates increased steeply between 1930 and 1960 [45]. Age-adjusted rates thereafter appear to have stabilized, or possibly declined, in the northern region of the United States [49], in parts of Sweden [50,51], and in Great Britain (Fig. 15.6) [48,52]. These secular trends are currently unexplained although there are three main hypotheses. Firstly, they might reflect the influence of one or more risk factors for osteoporosis or falls, which is increasing. Of all the candidate risk factors, physical activity would appear to be the only one that follows similar trends of variance. A second possible explanation is that the elderly population is becoming increasingly frail. It is recognized that the prevalence of disability rises with age and is greater in women than men at any given age. Many of the causes of frailty are independently associated with an increased predisposition to osteoporosis, or falling. The third possible explanation is that this represents a cohort phenomenon. Hip fracture is influenced by bone mineralization of the skeleton in the first 20 years of life as well as by rates of bone loss and risk of falling later in life. Therefore, a cohort effect could occur as a result of either an adverse influence on bone mineralization or falling risk acting at an earlier time, manifesting sub-

sequently as rising incidence in successive generations of the elderly [53–55].

Epidemiology of vertebral fractures

Vertebral fractures have been synonymous with the diagnosis of osteoporosis since its earliest description as a metabolic bone disease [56]. However, our understanding of the epidemiology of vertebral fractures has been scant for two reasons. Firstly, a significant proportion of vertebral fractures are asymptomatic, so that a proportion do not reach clinical attention. Secondly, there has been difficulty achieving consensus as to the definition of vertebral deformities from lateral thoracolumbar radiographs [57]. Three broad categories of vertebral fracture have been described: compression (or crush) fractures, in which there is loss of both anterior and posterior vertebral height, wedge (or partial) fractures, in which anterior height tends to be lost, and biconcave (balloon) fractures, where loss of central bony tissue leads to a concavity of both vertebral endplates (Fig. 15.7, Table 15.3 and Table 15.4) [58,59]. Morphometric and semiquantitative visual techniques have now been evolved for use in large epidemiological surveys and use of these techniques in Europe has improved our understanding of the epidemiology of prevalent and incident deformities [60].

One early estimate of the age-adjusted incidence of vertebral fracture came from the US, where a figure of 18 per 1000 person years was obtained [61]. It had long been clear that a proportion of vertebral fractures

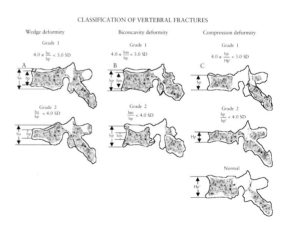

Fig. 15.7   Classification of vertebral fractures by type and grade. Reproduced from *J Bone Miner Res* 1991; 6: 207–215 [58] with permission of the American Society for Bone and Mineral Research.

Table 15.3 Classification of vertebral deformities: prevalent

Type of deformation	Abnormal ratio (s)	Assignment of deformity
None	None	Normal
Posterior alone	P/P	Normal
Middle alone	M/P	Biconcave
Anterior and posterior	A/P, P/P	Crush
Anterior, middle, and posterior	A/P, M/P, P/P	Crush
Anterior alone	A/P	Wedge
Anterior and middle	A/P, M/P	Wedge
Middle and posterior	M/P, P/P	Wedge

A, anterior; M, middle; P, posterior
From: [58]

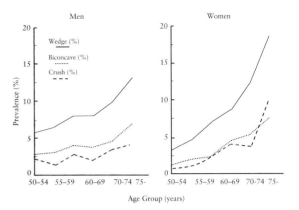

Fig. 15.8 Prevalence of vertebral deformity by type and sex. Reproduced with permission of the International Osteoporosis Foundation and National Osteoporosis Foundation USA from [13].

do not reach clinical attention, but the size of this fraction was unknown. However, the corresponding age-adjusted incidence of clinically ascertained vertebral fractures was 5.3 per 1000 person years [62], suggesting that only one-third of vertebral fractures reach clinical attention.

Age and gender

In the European Vertebral Osteoporosis Study (EVOS), 15 570 men and women aged 50–79 years were enrolled from population registers in 36 countries [63]. The overall prevalence of vertebral deformities in both men and women was found to be 12 per cent. Prevalence was seen to increase in both sexes with age, but the curve was steeper in women (Fig. 15.8) [13]. Thus, the frequency of deformities in men aged 50–54 years was around 10 per cent, rising to 18 per cent at age 75–79 years. The prevalence among women aged 50–54 years was only 5 per cent, but this rose to over 24 per cent at age 75–79 years. These findings were similar to those in a Hiroshima study, which detected

only moderately lower frequencies of vertebral deformities among Japanese men than women [64].

Geographical

The European Vertebral Osteoporosis Study found three-fold variations in the prevalence of vertebral deformities between countries, with the highest rates in Scandinavian countries. This between-centre range of prevalence was seen in both men (range 7.5–19.8 per cent) and women (range 6.2–20.7 per cent). The geographical variation was not as great as that seen in rates of hip fractures across Europe. Some of the variation across Europe could be explained by differences in physical activity levels and body mass index.

Time trends

Studies of secular trends in vertebral fractures have been hampered by the lack of consensus definition of prevalent and incident vertebral deformities. There

Table 15.4 Classification of vertebral deformities: incident; modified from [59]

Threshold	Relative height reduction (%)	Absolute height reduction (mm)	Relative (%) and absolute (mm) height reduction	Absolute height ratio reduction
1	≥ 15	≥ 3	≥ 15 + 3	≥ 0.12
2	≥ 17.5	≥ 4	≥ 17.5 + 3	≥ 0.14
3	≥ 20	≥ 5	≥ 20 + 4	≥ 0.16
4	≥ 25	≥ 6	≥ 25 + 4	≥ 0.18

All criteria applied to follow-up radiographs in comparison with corresponding baseline films.
Absolute height ratio reduction: h_a/h_p, h_m/h_p, h_p/h_{p+1} or h_p/h_{p-1}.

is some evidence to suggest that the prevalence of vertebral fractures is increasing [23].

Aetiology

The risk of vertebral deformity among men is significantly elevated in those with high levels of physical activity [65], suggesting the aetiological importance of trauma. In contrast, women with higher levels of customary physical activity have a reduced risk of deformity. Risk is elevated among women in the highest quintile of menarche (OR 1.5; 95% CI 1.2–1.9) and reduced among those with later menopause (OR 0.8; 95% CI 0.6–1.0) and those who have used the oral contraceptive pill (OR 0.8; 95% CI 0.6–1.0) [66]. Other factors that seem to be of importance include maternal history of hip fracture and low body mass index [60].

Epidemiology of distal forearm fracture

Most of these fractures are of the Colles' type, with displacement of the distal radial segment. They display a different pattern of incidence to that of hip and vertebral fractures [67–70].

Age

Several epidemiological studies in Caucasian women suggested that the incidence of distal forearm fractures in women increased linearly from approximately age 40 years to about the mid sixties, at which point there seemed to be a plateau [22,67,69]. Recently, however, some studies in the UK [68] and in Scandinavia [71,72] found that the age-adjusted incidence of forearm fractures increases progressively after the postmenopausal period. These data appear to suggest that there has been a change in the pattern of incidence with age, at least in Europe, although this currently remains unexplained. In men, incidence rates of distal forearm fracture are much lower, and more constant until later life (>75 years).

Gender

The majority of distal forearm fractures occur in women (age-adjusted female to male ratio of 4 to 1) and around one-half occur among women aged 65 years and over. At age greater than 35 years, the age-adjusted incidence rates in the UK are 36.8/10 000

person years in women and 9.0/10 000 person years among men.

Seasonality

As with hip fractures, distal forearm fractures show seasonality, so that there is a winter peak in incidence [73]. However, the current evidence suggests that wrist fractures are more clearly related to falls outdoors during periods of icy weather [74,75].

Time trends

The secular trends in age-adjusted incidence rates of distal forearm fractures have been studied in several different populations. Data from Rochester, Minnesota over the 50-year period 1945–94 show an overall doubling in incidence rates of distal forearm fractures among men but only a modest 7 per cent increase in the incidence rates among women [29]. Further examination of these data shows that most of the increases among men were explained by fractures after severe levels of trauma. Data recorded over a similar time period in Malmö, Sweden show a dramatic increase in the incidence rates of forearm fractures among women between the 1950s and the 1980s, but a subsequent reduction in the incidence by 1991–2 [76]. Among the men in Sweden, the incidence rates continued to rise throughout the 40-year period of study. Data from Japan (1986–1995) [38] suggest an increasing age-adjusted incidence in both genders.

Aetiology

Distal forearm fractures are slightly more common on the left than the right, possibly reflecting lower bone mass in the non-dominant arm. Distal forearm fractures almost always follow a fall on the outstretched arm and fall-related factors may be important, since there is evidence that individuals who are left handed may have an increased risk of distal forearm fracture [77].

Epidemiology of other age-related fractures

The incidence rates of proximal humeral, pelvic, and proximal tibial fractures also rise steeply with age, and are greater in women than men. Proximal humeral fractures typically (around 75 per cent) occur following a fall from standing height or less, but severe trauma

Table 15.5 Clustering of fractures

Reference	Baseline fracture	Fracture rates at follow-up	Number	Relative risk (95% CI)
[80]	1 prevalent crush deformity (n = 13)	New vertebral deformity	NS	5.3 (1.9–15.2)
	1 prevalent wedge deformity (n = 15)	New vertebral deformity	NS	4.1 (2.1–8.1)
	> 2 crush or wedge deformities (n = 12)	New vertebral deformity	NS	11.8 (5.1–26.8)
[81]	Clinical vertebral deformity (n = 621)	Hip fracture	58	1.7 (1.3–2.2)
		Forearm fracture	48	1.4 (1.0–1.8)
		Proximal humerus	71	4.5 (3.5–5.7)
		Any limb fracture	293	1.5 (1.3–1.8)
[82]	Distal forearm fracture (n = 1288)	Hip fracture (women)	72	1.4 (1.1–1.8)
		Hip fracture (men)	6	2.7 (0.98–5.8)
		Vertebral deformity (women)	217	5.2 (4.5–5.9)
		Vertebral deformity (men)	22	10.7 (6.7–16.3)
[83]	Clinical vertebral deformity (n = 820)	Hip fracture	75	2.3 (1.8–2.9)
		New vertebral deformity	282	12.6 (11–14)
		Distal forearm	24	1.6 (1.01–2.4)

NS = not stated.

might occur in a greater proportion of proximal tibial and pelvic fractures [29,78]. Furthermore, there is some direct evidence that these fractures are associated with low BMD [79].

Clustering of fractures in individuals

There is evidence from several epidemiological studies that patients with different types of fragility fractures are at increased risk of developing further osteoporotic fractures, both at the same site and at other sites (Table 15.5). The earliest evidence came from a study of patients with prevalent radiological vertebral deformities, who were found to have a seven to ten-fold increase in the risk of subsequent vertebral deformities [80]. This is a comparable level of increased risk to that seen for individuals who have sustained one hip fracture to then sustain a second hip fracture. Vertebral deformities were then shown to predispose to subsequent limb fractures [81]. The increased risk was apparent in men and women and was more marked in those people who had sustained vertebral deformities after mild or moderate, rather than severe, trauma. Cuddihy *et al.* demonstrated that if people with a distal forearm fracture are followed up, the risk of a subsequent hip or vertebral fracture is increased [82]. In women, the relationship between distal forearm fracture and subsequent hip fracture was found to be an age-related phenomenon, such that those aged over 70 years at the time of their distal forearm fracture had a 1.6-fold increase in their risk of hip fracture, but

those who were aged less than 70 years had no increased risk.

These data emphasize the importance of a previous fracture in the prediction of a subsequent fracture. Although the risk of a future hip fracture among those with vertebral fractures is not as high as the risk of subsequent vertebral deformities, the predictive capacity is sufficient to justify the cost-effective use of a prevalent vertebral deformity in any therapeutic algorithm that aims to prevent hip fractures. However, the correspondence between different fractures is sufficiently disparate to suggest that there is not a uniform aetiological model for fractures at all sites. As the next section will discuss, fractures at any one site are influenced by both the patterns of involutional bone loss and the patterns of external trauma experienced and the influences on both of these are heterogeneous at different skeletal sites.

Determinants of fracture risk

Ultimately, the probability of fracture in any bone will depend upon the force applied to the bone and its strength [84]. All bones will fracture if sufficient trauma is applied to them, though the level of trauma required to fracture pathologically weak bone may be low. The variable shape, composition, and load-bearing properties of bones in the skeleton require that aetiological models for fracture are site-specific. Thus, for example, external trauma through a fall may play a

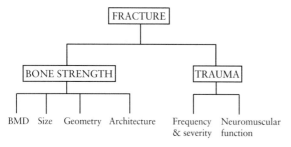

Fig. 15.9　Determinants of fracture risk.

greater role in causing distal forearm fractures than vertebral fractures.

Although pathological processes may sometimes weaken a bone to such an extent that it fractures following forces from gravity and muscle contraction, the majority of age-related fractures are associated with an injury. This most frequently takes the form of a fall from standing height or less. However, only 1 in every 100 falls of this type in elderly people culminates in a fracture, and the potential energy generated by such falls far exceeds the breaking strength of most bones in the body [85]. These observations highlight the importance of a variety of energy-absorbing mechanisms that

operate to prevent bony injury [86]. These mechanisms include the padding effect of adipose and other soft tissues, as well as neuromuscular reflexes, which absorb the forces generated during a fall (Fig. 15.9). Clearly, qualitative aspects of bone structure, such as geometry, architecture and size influence bone strength. Properties such as internal trabecular connectivity, repair of bone tissue microdamage, and impairment of mineralization all contribute to the mechanical strength of bone and thereby to the potential for fracture in the event of a specified level of trauma [87]. However, bone mineral density accounts for 75–90 per cent of the variance in bone strength [88]. Moreover, of all these factors, it is only bone mass quantified as bone mineral density, which can currently be measured with precision and accuracy. Consequently, it is this measurement that forms the basis for the diagnosis of osteoporosis.

Bone mineral density and fracture

The distribution of BMD in a population is approximately normal at any age, and in each sex. Many prospective and cross-sectional epidemiological studies

Table 15.6　Correlation between bone mineral density and fracture at different skeletal sites; modified from [95]

Reference	Size of cohort	Mean age	Site of BMD measurement	Type of fracture (No. of women with fracture)	Relative risk
[89]	386	57	Proximal radius	Forearm (17)	4.4 (2.2–8.7)
				All non-spine (89)	2.6 (2.0–3.4)
[90]	1098	63	Distal radius	Vertebral (61)	2.0 (1.5–2.6)
			Proximal radius	Vertebral (61)	2.0 (1.5–2.7)
			Calcaneus	Vertebral (61)	2.4 (1.8–3.2)
			Lumbar spine	Vertebral (61)	2.2 (1.7–3.0)
			Spine	All non-spine (15)	2.0 (1.2–3.0)
[91]	1076	63	Proximal radius	Hip (43)	2.5 (1.3–4.8)
				Vertebral (70)	1.9 (1.05–3.5)
				Fragility (154)	1.9 (1.05–3.5)
			Distal radius	Hip (43)	2.1 (1.06–4.1)
				Vertebral (70)	2.4 (1.1–5.2)
				Fragility (154)	2.6 (1.6–4.1)
[92]	1080	69	Femoral neck	All (192)	2.4 (1.9–3.0)
[93]	8134	73	Middle radius	Hip (65)	1.5 (1.2–1.9)
			Distal radius	Hip (65)	1.6 (1.2–2.1)
			Calcaneus	Hip (65)	2.0 (1.5–2.7)
			Proximal femur	Hip (65)	2.7 (2.0–3.6)
			Lumbar spine	Hip (65)	1.6 (1.2–2.2)
[94]	304	60	Lumbar spine	Vertebral (37)	1.9 (1.3–3.0)
			Lumbar spine	Proximal femur (<15)	1.9 (0.9–3.7)
			Lumbar spine	All (93)	1.4 (1.1–1.8)
			Femoral neck	Vertebral (37)	1.5 (1.1–2.7)
			Femoral neck	Proximal femur (<15)	2.3 (1.2–4.5)
			Femoral neck	All (93)	1.2 (1.0–1.8)

Table 15.7 Relative risk of fracture (with 95% CI in parentheses) for each standard deviation decrease in BMD; data derived from a meta-analysis of prospective studies; modified from [95]

Site of measurement	Wrist fracture	Hip fracture	Vertebral fracture	All fractures
Distal radius	1.7 (1.4–2.0)	1.8 (1.4–2.2)	1.7 (1.4–2.1)	1.4 (1.3–1.6)
Hip	1.4 (1.4–1.6)	2.6 (2.0–3.5)	1.8 (1.1–2.7)	1.6 (1.4–1.8)
Lumbar spine	1.5 (1.3–1.8)	1.6 (1.2–2.2)	2.3 (1.9–2.8)	1.5 (1.4–1.7)

have shown that there is an inverse and continuous relationship between bone mass and fracture risk, such that a reduction in BMD is associated with an increasing risk of fracture (Table 15.6). Marshall *et al.* [95] performed a meta-analysis of the prospective studies (Table 15.7). From Table 15.7, it can be deduced that the risk of hip fracture increases 2.6-fold for each standard deviation decrease in hip BMD. Thus, a woman at the age of the menopause whose hip BMD is one standard deviation below average will have a greater than 30 per cent remaining lifetime risk of hip fracture (Fig. 15.10) [96].

Thus, the relationship between BMD and osteoporosis can be compared to that between blood pressure and stroke. Elevated blood pressure is an important risk factor for stroke, but strokes occur in the absence of elevated blood pressure. Similarly, fractures occur in the absence of osteoporosis but the risk of fracture is considerably increased in the presence of low bone mass. Therefore, as with blood pressure, appropriate cut-off values can be defined so as to direct appropriate intervention towards 'at risk' individuals. Accordingly, a World Health Organization study group was convened in 1994 with the objective of incorporat-

Table 15.8 Diagnostic categories for osteoporosis based on WHO criteria

Category	Definition by bone density
Normal	A value for BMD that is not more than 1 s.d. below the young adult mean value
Osteopenia	A value for BMD that lies between 1 and 2.5 s.d. below the young adult mean value
Osteoporosis	A value for BMD that is more than 2.5 s.d. below the young adult mean value
Severe osteoporosis (established)	A value for BMD more than 2.5 s.d. below the young adult mean value in the presence of one or more fragility fractures

Source: [97]

ing both bone mass and fracture into a simple, stratified definition of osteoporosis [97]. Four categories were recommended (Table 15.8 and Fig. 15.11) [97,98].

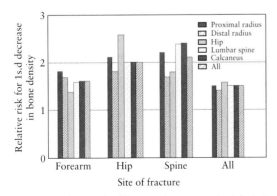

Fig. 15.10 Relative risk of fracture for one standard deviation decrease in bone density below the age-adjusted mean (data from [95]). The results are given for various fracture sites as well as various sites of bone density measurements. Reproduced with permission of Martin Dunitz Pulishers from [96].

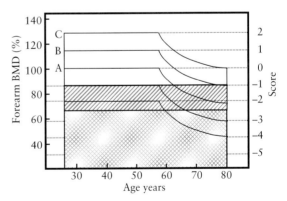

Fig. 15.11 Bone mineral content at the distal forearm in women expressed as a percentage of young healthy adults. The solid lines denote the mean values with age (category A) ± 2 s.d. (categories B and C). The hatched area denotes women with osteopenia and the cross-hatched area women with osteoporosis. From Kanis JA, Melton LJ, Christiansen C, Johnston CC, Khaltaev N. The diagnosis of osteoporosis. *J Bone Miner Res* 1994; **9**: 1137–1141 [98] reproduced with the permission of the American Society of Bone and Mineral Research.

Bone density measurement is the best currently available method of predicting future fracture. Alternatives, such as historical risk factors, biochemical markers of bone turnover, measurements of bone geometry, and quantitative ultrasound, are likely to serve as adjuncts to bone densitometry for fracture prediction. However, evidence to support their use lags a long way behind that for BMD measurement, and explicit clinical algorithms for their utilization and interpretation have not been developed. In contrast, the WHO definition has been incorporated into clear guidelines for the management of osteoporosis and the cost-effectiveness of this approach has been established [99].

Limitations of bone densitometry

The correlation between BMD measured at different skeletal sites is not sufficient to permit accurate determination at one site from measurements at another [100]. However, BMD measurements are capable of predicting fractures at distant skeletal sites sufficiently well to have clinical utility [101]. The future risk of fracture at any one site is optimally predicted by a measurement at the same site [95] (Table 15.7).

Although a useful theoretical concept for clinical diagnosis in individuals, there is no convincing evidence of a threshold in the BMD–fracture relationship. In fact, the relationship between BMD and the risk of fracture is continuous, and there is significant overlap between normal and fracture-prone populations. For example, among cases of vertebral fracture, a lumbar spine BMD that is two standard deviations below the young adult mean value has a specificity and sensitivity

for fracture of only around 60 per cent [102]. Furthermore, a woman aged 50 years with a radial BMD that is equal to the young adult mean has a 15 per cent lifetime risk of hip fracture, compared with a 25 per cent lifetime risk for a 50-year old woman with a radial BMD that is 2.5 standard deviations below the young adult mean [103]. Therefore, BMD will not reliably predict all those individuals who will sustain a fracture from all those who will not, reflecting the multifactorial pathogenesis of osteoporotic fractures. It may be, of course, that within certain narrowly defined ranges of external trauma, the breaking strength of various bones can be fairly precisely represented by a given value for their BMD. However, this deficiency in bone mineral measurement militates against the use of bone screening programmes in the general population, since a 'safe' threshold cannot be defined. Rather, bone densitometry should be used for individual clinical decision-making in circumstances where knowledge of the test result influences a therapeutic decision [104].

Non-invasive assessment of bone density

The earliest non-invasive techniques for assessing bone mineral density involved plain radiography, most notably of the hand, lumbar spine, and proximal femur [105]. However, radiographic techniques were not sufficiently accurate or reproducible to lend themselves to sequential studies in individuals. These techniques have been superseded by: (a) absorptiometric methods: single and dual photon absorptiometry (SPA/DPA), single and dual energy X-ray absorptiometry (SXA/DXA); (b) quantitative computed tomography (QCT); (c) ultrasound (Table 15.9).

Table 15.9 Methods for the non-invasive assessment of skeletal status

Technique	Site	Trabecular Bone (%)	Precision error *in vivo* (%)	Accuracy error *in vivo* (%)	Scan time (mins)	Effective dose (μSv)
DXA[a]	Forearm—distal	5	1–2	2–5	10	<1
	Forearm—ultradistal	40	1–2	2–5	10	<1
	Heel	95	1–2	2–5	10	<1
	Lumbar spine	50	1–3	5–8	10	1
	Lumbar—lateral	90	3	5–10	20	5
	Femur—proximal	40	1–2	5–8	10	1
	Total body	20	1	1–2	20	3
QCT	Spine—single-energy	100	2–4	5–10	15	60
	Spine—dual-energy	100	4–5	3–6	20	90

[a] DXA has largely superseded DPA, SPA and SXA

Absorptiometric methods

In single-energy absorptiometry, bone mineral is measured using an isotope source at peripheral sites, such as the heel or wrist. It is useful both at sites where cortical bone predominates (such as the radial midshaft) and at sites where a mixture of cortical and trabecular bone is found (such as the distal radius or calcaneus). Single-energy X-ray absorptiometry (SXA) is based on the same principles as SPA, but utilizes an X-ray beam, making it more precise and avoiding the use of isotopes.

Dual-energy absorptiometry involves photons in dual-energy photon absorptiometry (DPA), or X-rays in DXA, to measure bone mineral at sites such as the spine or hip. DPA is capable of scanning thicker body parts and can be corrected for soft tissue dimensions but, although reasonably accurate, this technique is subject to poor reproducibility. DXA produces a higher beam intensity, and therefore a faster scan with better spatial resolution, so that it has considerably better reproducibility and is more convenient, particularly for sequential estimates of axial bone loss [106]. This technique has rapidly become the norm for measurement of the spine and hip and has also been adapted for measurements at the forearm. In all the absorptiometric techniques, the primary measurement value is the amount of bone mineral present in the region scanned. The size of the bone clearly contributes to this parameter, and various size corrections are used to approximate true mineral density. As none of the methods currently assesses the thickness of bone scanned, these size corrections relate total mineral content to the width of the bone (grams of hydroxyapatite per cm) or to its area (grams per cm^2). The derived measurements obtained by these methods—bone mineral content (BMC), bone mineral density (BMD), and bone mineral apparent density (BMAD)—have all been found to be associated with fracture, especially in women.

Quantitative computed tomography

Quantitative computed tomography (QCT) assesses true volumetric bone mineral density [107] rather than an area-corrected result. An area of purely trabecular bone can be measured at the skeletal periphery or at the spine. This technique cannot currently be used at the proximal femur, but the introduction of new spiral CT scanners may change this. Widespread use of this method, however, is limited by its cost, high radiation dose, and scanning time.

Ultrasound

Quantitative ultrasonography (QUS) is a more recent innovation in the assessment of osteoporosis. This technique, applied in the form of speed of sound (SOS) and broadband ultrasound attenuation (BUA) measurements, evolved from methods used in industrial materials testing. The major advantages are that these techniques do not use radiation, are inexpensive, and relatively portable. It is clear that ultrasound measures do not provide a direct estimate of bone mineral density and they may assess structural properties of bone. To date, evidence supports the use of QUS by water-based calcaneal systems for the assessment of fracture risk in elderly, institutionalized women. The predictive ability of other systems is not yet known and the role of QUS in monitoring the progression of disease, or response to treatment, is uncertain. Further research is needed to define the role of QUS in the diagnostic assessment and monitoring of osteoporosis [108].

Changes in bone mineral with ageing

Peak bone mass

The outline of the skeleton is apparent early in fetal development and the long bones attain their future shape and proportions by about 26 weeks of gestation [109]. From conception to epiphyseal closure, there is a progressive increase in cortical and trabecular bone which is accelerated during the prepubertal growth spurt (Fig. 15.12) [110–113]. This growth phase produces about 90 per cent of the peak bone mass attained during adult life. The pubertal acceleration of bone gain commences earlier in girls than boys, but by age 20 the difference in vertebral BMD between men and

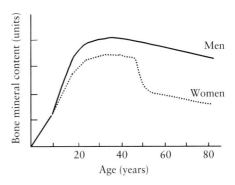

Fig. 15.12 Changes in bone mineral with age in men and women. Reproduced with permission of the Institute of Physics and Engineering in Medicine from [120].

women is slight [114,115]. The precise physiological mechanism of the accelerated bone growth of adolescence is unknown; the spurt in mineral growth parallels the spurt in height, but appears to last longer. In boys, it coincides with a steep rise in serum testosterone concentration, but this is accompanied by a myriad of other endocrinological changes [116]. Following the adolescent growth spurt, BMD undergoes a consolidative phase during which it continues to increase for a 5–15 year period [117,118]. This phase may be critical in determining the overall peak density achieved, as it occurs during a period of significant lifestyle changes [119].

Loss of bone mineral mass

Skeletal growth and consolidation are followed by a transient period of stability until about the age of 35 years, after which bone loss commences (Fig. 15.12) [120]. This bone loss is universal [121] in all races and in both sexes but includes an accelerated phase in the immediate postmenopausal years in women. The differential rates of loss of cortical and trabecular bone and the varying patterns of loss at different skeletal sites have not been precisely defined. However, there have now been a few published longitudinal studies of bone loss rates at the hip and lumbar spine [122–124]. From these studies in Caucasian ambulatory females in the postmenopause, estimates of loss range from 0.35 per cent to 0.96 per cent loss/year at the femoral neck, 0.32 per cent to 0.95 per cent at the total hip region, 0.3 per cent to 0.75 per cent at the trochanteric region, and 0.36 per cent to 1.14 per cent at the intertrochanteric region. Fewer data are available for men, but a mean annual loss rate of 0.82 per cent at the femoral neck [124] was reported in an Australian cohort aged around 70 years. Over a lifetime, BMD of the femoral neck declines an estimated 58 per cent in women and 39 per cent in men, while BMD of the intertrochanteric region of the proximal femur falls about 53 per cent and 35 per cent in women and men respectively [84]. Estimates of lumbar spine loss rates among women range from 0.39 per cent/year to gains of 0.94 per cent/year; longitudinal studies of men show gains of around 0.5 per cent/year; these 'gains' are artefactual due to osteophytosis [125]. Bone loss is continuous throughout later life, with rates of bone loss increasing at the hip region from 0.32 per cent/year at age 67–69 years to 1.64 per cent/year from age 85 years onwards [123].

Falls and fracture

Occurrence

The likelihood of falling rises with age and is greater in women than men: a survey in Oxford, England reported that about 1 in 3 women aged 80–84 years had fallen in the previous year, and this rose to nearly half of women aged 85 years and over [126]. There is some evidence from a study in a white population that the incidence of fall-induced injuries is increasing at a rate beyond that which would be expected if it were due to demographic changes [127].

Risk factors for falls

Medication

Falling is more likely in those taking psychotropic medications, with the strongest evidence for an effect of antidepressants [128] and benzodiazepines [129]. Some observational studies have suggested that some cardiovascular drugs, particularly those with a hypotensive effect, and non-steroidal anti-inflammatory drugs may be implicated as causes of falling in the elderly, but the evidence is less clear. A possible protective effect of thiazide diuretics against hip fracture after a fall has been investigated, but the evidence for this is currently contradictory [130,131].

Physical activity

There is evidence that physical activity can improve gait, balance, co-ordination, proprioception, reaction time, and muscle strength, even in the very old and frail population [127]. Despite this, the evidence that these improvements lead to a beneficial reduction in the risk of falling, or of injurious, fracture-inducing falling in particular, has remained questionable [132].

Falls as a cause of hip fracture

Only about 1 per cent of falls lead to a hip fracture, and studies suggest that this is because the amount of trauma delivered to the proximal femur depends upon the orientation of the fall [133]. The vast majority of hip fracture patients fall sideways, leading to direct impact on the greater trochanter, and fail to break their fall with an outstretched arm [134]. A recent case–control study in men found that the most important predictor of a hip fracture following a fall was the orientation of the fall. The factors which were found to protect against a hip fracture occurring were: higher levels of physical activity in the previous year, greater body mass index and a history of fracture at aged 45 years or over [135].

Risk factors for osteoporosis

This section of the chapter will present an overview of the risk factors for susceptibility to osteoporosis. As discussed previously, the relationship between bone mineral and fracture is closely intertwined and many of the studies which will be reviewed in this section have examined the relationship between a putative risk factor and bone mass, using this as a surrogate for fracture risk. Where fracture data are available, these will be highlighted accordingly.

Genetic factors

Evidence from several sources suggests a genetic influence on bone density and fracture.

Family studies

In an extensive series of studies performed in adults and children, Garn [136] found that the metacarpal dimensions of siblings were more highly correlated than were those of parents with their children. Australian studies [137,138] then showed familial clustering of low spinal BMD among relatives of osteoporotic parents and daughters of osteoporotic mothers (Table 15.10). More recently, it has been shown that a

family history of an osteoporotic fracture predicts low bone mass in men and women [139] and that a family history of fracture is an independent predictor of fracture at that site with relative risks of 1.5–3.0 [140]. This relationship appears strongest for a maternal history of hip fracture.

Twin studies

Twin studies allow a more detailed study of genetic influences, by comparing monozygotic and dizygotic twins (Table 15.11). As the table shows, these studies consistently demonstrate that monozygotic twin pairs have a greater concordance for axial and appendicular BMD than dizygotic twin pairs, with corresponding estimates of heritability suggesting that 70 to 85 per cent of the variance in BMD might be genetic. Anatomical sites with a high trabecular bone content appear to have a greater genetic influence than those sites composed predominantly of cortical bone. Those studies undertaken in postmenopausal twins show that BMD after the menopause also has a genetic component, but that this effect is not as strong as that premenopausally. Twin studies have also provided some evidence that bone turnover and bone loss may have genetic influences [147,148].

Genetic markers

As might be expected from the heterogeneous pathogenesis of osteoporosis, there is no single genetic marker denoting an inherited susceptibility to the condition. To date, the genes that regulate bone mass are incompletely defined. There are many potential candi-

Table 15.10 Studies of familial clustering of osteoporosis

Reference	Outcome	Relationship	Cases (95% CI)	Controls (95% CI)	Significance
[137]	L. spine BMD	Male relatives of osteoporotics	91 (75,107)	129 (108,150)	p<0.001
		Female relatives of osteoporotics	96 (79, 113)	126 (107, 145)	p<0.001
[138]	L. spine BMC	Daughters of osteoporotic mothers	34.3 (33.3,35.3)	37.0 (36.1,37.9)	p=0.03
	F. neck BMC	Daughters of osteoporotic mothers	2.31 (2.26,2.36)	2.44 (2.39,2.49)	NS
[139]	L. spine BMD	Sons of osteoporotic mothers	1.041(0.02)	1.044 (0.017)	NS
	Total hip BMD	Sons of osteoporotic mothers	0.905 (0.015)	0.937 (0.012)	p<0.05
	L. spine BMD	Sons of osteoporotic fathers	1.011 (0.03)	1.074 (0.010)	p<0.05
	Total hip BMD	Sons of osteoporotic fathers	0.913 (0.022)	0.930 (0.008)	NS
	L. spine BMD	Daughters of osteoporotic mothers	0.859 (0.013)	0.878 (0.012)	NS
	Total hip BMD	Daughters of osteoporotic mothers	0.764 (0.009)	0.773 (0.008)	p=0.02
	L. spine BMD	Daughters of osteoporotic fathers	0.842 (0.020)	0.896 (0.007)	p<0.05
	F. neck BMD	Daughters of osteoporotic fathers	0.756 (0.014)	0.781 (0.005)	p<0.10

NS = Not statistically significant

Table 15.11   Twin studies of the genetic effects and heritability of bone mineral

Reference	Outcome	rMZ twins	rDZ twins	Heritability
[141]	Radial mid-shaft bone mass:			
	Juvenile	0.962	0.966	0.75
	Adult	0.698	0.451	0.49
[142]	Lumbar spine BMD: postmenopausal	0.68	0.29	0.78
	Femoral neck BMD: postmenopausal	0.61	0.19	0.84
	Distal forearm BMD: postmenopausal	0.63	0.32	0.61
[143]	Lumbar spine BMD: elderly women	0.74	0.33	0.73
	Femoral neck BMD: elderly women	0.74	0.52	0.66
[144]	Lumbar spine BMD: premenopausal	0.92	0.36	0.92
	Femoral neck BMD: premenopausal	0.77	0.56	0.46
	Lumbar spine BMD: all ages	0.92	0.36	0.92
	Femoral neck BMD: all ages	0.73	0.33	0.73
[145]	Lumbar spine BMD: all ages	0.85	0.33	1.05
	Femoral neck BMD: all ages	0.81	0.37	0.88
[146]	Distal radial BMC: <25 years	0.925	0.899	0.47
	Distal radial BMC: >25 years	1.129	1.020	0.75
	Lumbar spine BMC: <25 years	39.3	35.1	0.88
	Lumbar spine BMC: >25 years	41.6	37.2	−0.57

rMZ: Within-twin pair correlation for monozygotic twins.
rDZ: Within-twin pair correlation for dizygotic twins.

date genes for the regulation of bone mass, including those that code for cytokines, growth factors, matrix components, and the receptors for gonadotrophin and calcitropic hormones. Current data suggest that several genes are involved, each with relatively modest effects individually, rather than one or two genes with major effects. The exact number of genes involved and their relative effects remain unclear [149]. Familial clustering occurs frequently, but this may reflect both genetic factors and shared environmental influences which, in combination, determine the risk of fracture. Hence, there is considerable potential for beneficial environmental modulation of peak bone density.

The vitamin D receptor gene

The first studies of the vitamin D receptor (VDR) gene polymorphisms [150] found an association between these polymorphisms and circulating levels of osteocalcin. They have subsequently been studied in relation to bone mass in both twin and population studies, some of which have demonstrated a positive effect of VDR genotypes on bone mass, but others of which revealed no association, or an inverse association (Table 15.12). It may be that these variable results can be explained through modification of the effect of VDR genotype by dietary intakes of calcium and vitamin D [162].

However, even taking this into account, the effects of the VDR genotype on bone mass appear to be weak and there is currently little evidence linking VDR status to osteoporotic fracture.

The collagen I α1 gene

Initial information about the genes encoding type I collagen emerged from studies of osteogenesis imperfecta. The main fibrillar collagen in bone (Type I) is a heteropolymer of three chains, which are coded for by different genes on different chromosomes. Mutations in these genes cause osteogenesis imperfecta, a heterogeneous disorder with an incidence of approximately 1 in 20 000 births, which exists in several forms [163]. These range from a mild variant associated with vertebral osteoporosis in women through to a lethal perinatal disease with a functionally useless skeleton. Mutations of the collagen Iα1 (COLIA1) genotype appeared very likely candidates for the genetic regulation of bone mass because of these phenotypic manifestations. However, mutations of the coding regions of collagen have not been identified in the majority of osteoporotic patients [164]. More recently, a G/T polymorphism in the promoter region was found to be associated with low BMD and fracture [165]. A large population-based study in the Netherlands confirmed the association [166]. The data support the hypothesis

Table 15.12 Vitamin D receptor polymorphisms and bone mineral density; modified from [161]

Reference	Population	Age	Number		% difference in BMD	p value
Premenopausal						
[151]	US white twins	35.3	126	Hip	−2.3	0.58
				Spine	1.7	0.55
				Radius	0.0	1.0
[152]	US black	30.4	72	Hip	−13.4	0.03
				Spine	−5.8	0.30
	US white	29.5	83	Hip	−5.2	0.24
				Spine	−3.5	0.30
[153]	US white	39.8	46	Hip	−9.9	0.07
				Spine	5.9	0.21
[154]	France	40.4	189	Hip	−1.2	0.65
				Spine	0.0	1.0
[155]	US white	36.9	32	Spine	−17.3	0.02
[156]	US white	46.9	470	Hip	2.2	0.18
				Spine	2.5	0.07
[157]	Japan	30.1	488	Hip	−3.9	0.05
				Spine	−5.9	0.002
Postmenopausal						
[158]	Sweden	69.8	76	Hip	6.3	0.40
				Spine	−3.0	0.70
[151]	US white	52.0	124	Hip	−0.1	0.98
				Spine	3.0	0.55
				Radius	−7.2	0.07
[159]	UK twins	58.7	190	Hip	−6.8	0.01
				Spine	−7.5	0.03
				Radius	−3.6	0.21
[153]	US white	62.0	81	Hip	−1.6	0.78
				Spine	−2.2	0.72
[160]	France	58.4	268	Hip	0.0	1.0
				Spine	2.3	0.45
				Radius	0.0	1.0

that COLIA1 is a determinant of bone mass, possibly through an effect on collagen synthesis.

Other genes

Several other candidate genes have been investigated, including those for the oestrogen receptor, interleukin-6, and transforming growth factor beta. However, none of these genotypes currently appear to be associated with marked increases in the risk of osteoporotic fracture [167].

Non-genetic host factors

The four non-genetic host factors associated with osteoporosis are body build, reproductive variables, diseases and drugs predisposing to bone loss, and intrauterine programming.

Body build

Skeletal development until the prepubertal growth spurt is closely related to changes in height and weight. Body mass index in later years remains associated with BMD in both the axial and appendicular skeleton [119,168–170], and thin body build has been demonstrated to be a risk factor for fragility fractures (Table 15.13). Although the protective effect of obesity against fracture is greater in women, thin body build acts as a risk factor even in men [174]. Prospective data have recently become available demonstrating that rates of bone loss in postmenopausal women [180,181] and in men and women in the age group 60–75 years [122] are related to body mass index (BMI) at baseline and to the rate of change in BMI over time. Generally, lower baseline BMI and a greater rate of loss of adiposity over the follow-up period are associated with greater rates of bone loss, especially at the

Table 15.13 Studies of the relationship between anthropometric variables and osteoporotic fractures

Reference	Outcome	Variable	Cases	Controls	p value
[171]	Hip and distal forearm fractures	Height (in)	63.4 (61.2,65.6)	63.5 (60.8,66.2)	NS
		Weight (lb)	129 (97.6,160.4)	148 (121.8,174.2)	p<0.001
		BMI	12.6 (11.7,13.5)	12.1 (11.3,12.9)	p<0.001
[172]	Vertebral deformity	Height (m)	1.61(1.6,1.62)	1.54 (1.53,1.55)	p<0.001
		Weight (kg)	65.6 (64,67.2)	60.6 (58.9,62.3)	p<0.05
[173]	Hip fractures	Height (cm)	156.4 (148.8, 164)	155.8 (148.1,163.5)	0.004
		Weight (kg)	58.2 (46.2,70.2)	61.0 (49.2,72.8)	0.0001
		BMI (kg/m²)	23.6 (18.9,28.3)	25.1 (20.4,29.8)	0.0001
[174]	Vertebral deformity	Height (cm)	153.3 (152.4,154.2)	160.4 (157.7,161.1)	p<0.001
		Weight (kg)	55.7 (54.4, 57)	60.3 (59.3,61.3)	p<0.001

Reference	Outcome	Anthropometric variable	Relative risk	95% CI
[173]	Hip fractures	BMI <25	1.0	–
		BMI >25	0.51	0.44–0.58
[175]	Vertebral deformity	Height: shortest quintile (men)	1.0	–
		Height: tallest quintile (men)	0.85	0.68–1.08
		Height: shortest quintile (women)	1.0	–
		Height: tallest quintile (women)	0.74	0.58–0.93
		Weight: lightest quintile (men)	1.0	–
		Weight: heaviest quintile (men)	0.75	0.60–0.94
		Weight: lightest quintile (women)	1.0	–
		Weight: heaviest quintile (women)	0.67	0.53–0.83
		BMI: lowest quintile (men)	1.0	–
		BMI: highest quintile (men)	0.80	0.64–0.99
		BMI: lowest quintile (women)	1.0	–
		BMI: highest quintile (women)	0.74	0.59–0.92
[176]	Hip fractures	Height: lowest tertile	1.0	–
		Height: highest tertile	2.76	NS
		Quetelet's index: lowest tertile	1.0	–
		Quetelet's index: highest tertile	0.61	NS
[177]	Hip fracture	Height at age 25 (per 6 cm)	1.2	1.1–1.4
		Increase in weight since age 25 (per 20%)	0.6	0.5–0.7
[178]	Hip and distal forearm fractures	Ponderal index: thin and average	1.0	–
		Ponderal index: obese	0.5	(0.4–0.7)
[179]	Hip fracture	Weight gain 1.3–5.5 kg in 11 years (women)	1.0	–
		Loss of >3 kg weight in 11 years (women)	2.26	1.4–3.7
		Gain of >5.6 kg weight in 11 years (women)	2.33	1.38–3.95
		Weight gain 1.3–5.5 kg in 11 years (men)	1.0	–
		Loss of >3 kg weight in 11 years (men)	2.12	1.01–4.44
		Increase in weight >5.6 kg in 11 years (men)	1.67	0.73–3.81

NS = Not stated
95% confidence intervals given in parentheses

proximal femur. At all sites, bone loss rate is generally more closely associated with change in BMI than baseline BMI (Fig. 15.13) [122].

The importance of other aspects of body build is unclear. Case–control studies have generally reported that hip and distal forearm fracture cases are taller than controls [173] but those patients with vertebral fractures are shorter [172] (Table 15.13). Osteoporotic subjects also have a higher prevalence of edentulous-

ness (a marker of mandibular bone loss) [182] and lower skinfold thickness [183].

Reproductive variables

Since Albright's classical description of the clinical presentation of osteoporosis, it has been recognized that loss of ovarian function is accompanied by accelerated bone loss. The most dramatic manifestation of this

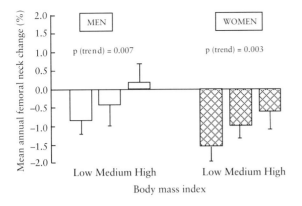

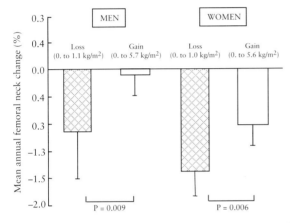

Fig. 15.13 Determinants of bone loss in elderly men and women. Reproduced with permission of the International Osteoporosis Foundation and National Osteoporosis Foundation USA from [122].

phenomenon is found in women who have undergone bilateral oophorectomy before age 45 years. These women have an increased risk of hip fracture, as well as markedly reduced cortical and trabecular bone density [184–186]. The changes in bone density accompanying a natural menopause are less striking. While most cross-sectional studies demonstrate acceleration in cortical bone loss during the first postmenopausal decade, a trabecular acceleration has been more difficult to demonstrate [19], and one prospective study suggests substantial trabecular bone loss prior to the menopause in women [112]. In a similar fashion, it is uncertain whether an early menopause is a risk factor for osteoporotic fracture. One study [176] has reported a doubling in risk of hip fracture in women undergoing natural menopause before the age of 59 years, as compared with those who were older than 60, but others

have found no difference between the menopausal age of hip fracture cases and controls [187] (Table 15.14).

Less attention has been paid to the role of other reproductive factors in the aetiology of osteoporosis (Table 15.14). There may be protective effects of both high parity and lactation, but the data are inconsistent. Use of the oral contraceptive pill has been associated with greater bone density in some, but not all, studies [188] but does not appear to protect against fracture [189]. Number of fertile years (time from age at menarche to age at menopause) has been found to be associated with a reduced risk of hip fracture [173]. More recently, the effects of reproductive variables were studied as part of the European Vertebral Osteoporosis Study [66]. After adjusting for age, BMI and smoking, those in the highest quintile of age at menarche (>16 years) had an increased risk of vertebral deformity. Furthermore, late menopause, use of hormone replacement therapy or use of the oral contraceptive pill were found to be protective. No apparent effect was demonstrated of parity or breast feeding on the risk of deformity. These findings suggest that oestrogen status, as defined by several different reproductive variables, is an important determinant of osteoporosis in women.

Diseases and drugs

Osteoporosis is a feature of many diseases (Table 15.15). The designation 'secondary' osteoporosis has traditionally been used when medical conditions are present which might have been responsible for bone loss [19]. In many cases, documentation of the association between a chronic disease and osteoporosis is patchy, due to poor or inappropriate methodology. Consequently, the numerical significance of some clinical associations remains uncertain. The evidence is most persuasive for a relationship between osteoporosis and thyrotoxicosis, Cushing's disease, partial gastrectomy, stroke, and male hypogonadism. In a second group of conditions, for example rheumatoid arthritis, osteoporosis appears to be a sequel of lifestyle changes such as immobility.

Among medications, the strongest evidence exists to support an association with chronic glucocorticoid therapy [190] and anticonvulsants. Thiazide diuretics are protective against bone loss [191].

Programming during early life

'Programming' is the term used for persisting changes in structure and function caused by environmental stimuli during critical periods of early development

Table 15.14 Studies of the relationship between reproductive variables and risk of osteoporotic fractures

Reference	Outcome	Reproductive variable	Relative risk	95% CI
[176]	Hip fracture	HRT use: Never	1.0	–
		HRT use: <5 years	0.97	NS
		HRT use: >5 years	0.42	p=0.03
		Postoophorectomy HRT use: Never	1.65	NS
		Postoophorectomy HRT use: <5 years	0.70	NS
		Postoophorectomy HRT use: >5 years	0.14	p=0.01
[187]	Hip or wrist fracture	HRT use: Never	1.0	–
		HRT use: >15 years	0.6	0.4–1.0
		Parity: 0	1.0	–
		Parity: 5–8	1.2	0.7–2.22
		Lactation: 0 months	1.0	–
		Lactation: 1–12 months	1.2	0.73–1.95
[33]	Hip fracture	Menarche: age >12 years	1.38	1.13–1.7
		Breast-feeding	0.94	0.78–1.12
		Parity	1.06	0.91–1.23
		Menopause: age > 45 years	0.81	0.68–0.96
[66]	Vertebral deformity	Menarche: age lowest quintile (<12 years)	1.0	–
		Menarche: age highest quintile (>16 years)	1.48	1.16–1.88
		OCP use: Never	1.0	–
		OCP use: Ever	0.76	0.58–0.99
		Menopause: age lowest quintile	1.0	–
		Menopause: age highest quintile (>52.5 years)	0.78	0.6–1.00
		HRT use: Never	1.0	–
		HRT use: <1 year	0.98	0.74–1.30
		HRT use: >1 year	0.86	0.65–1.13

Table 15.15 Causes of secondary osteoporosis

Early oophorectomy (women)
Hypogonadism (men)
Hyperthyroidism
Partial gastrectomy and malabsorption syndromes
Stroke
Use of corticosteroids
Use of anticonvulsants

[192]. One of the best examples of this phenomenon is the life-long effect of early exposure to sex hormones on sexual physiology. A female rat injected with testosterone propionate on the fifth day after birth develops normally until puberty, but fails to ovulate or show normal patterns of female sexual behaviour thereafter [193]. Pituitary and ovarian function are normal, but the release of gonadotrophin by the hypothalamus has been irreversibly altered from the cyclical female pattern of release to the tonic male pattern. If the same injection is given at 20 days of age, there is no effect. Thus, there appears to be a critical time period at which the animal's sexual physiology is sensitive and can be permanently altered. Other animal studies have

shown that restriction of maternal nutrient intake at critical periods of pregnancy leads to effects on the birth size of the offspring [194].

The most likely candidate mechanism for programming of osteoporosis is through alteration of endocrine set points during critical periods of early development, with the most likely pathways being the growth hormone/insulin-like growth factor-1 (IGF-1) axis, the hypothalamic/pituitary/adrenal (HPA) axis, or the parathyroid/vitamin D axis. In elderly men and women, statistically significant relationships are seen between various parameters of the growth hormone/IGF-1 axis and femoral neck bone density and, furthermore, the concentration of median growth hormone correlates very strongly with weight in infancy [195]. It has been shown that the umbilical cord concentrations of cortisol in infants born small for gestational age are higher than those of normal infants. Furthermore, mean fasting plasma cortisol in elderly men is statistically significantly inversely associated with birthweight [196]. Finally, in a study of 37 elderly men, basal levels of cortisol over a 24-h period were found to be negatively associated with hip BMD but positively correlated with bone loss rate measured at the same site over 4 years [197]. These findings point to the potential clinical importance of programming of the endocrine axes.

Evidence of programming of osteoporotic risk is demonstrated in a study of 144 neonates, born to mothers who had been characterized at 18 and 28 weeks of gestation for their anthropometry, physical activity, and nutrition. Neonatal BMC is found to be strongly, positively associated with birthweight, birth length, and placental weight. Maternal smoking and maternal energy intake at 18 weeks gestation are negative predictors of neonatal BMC at the whole body and spine [198]. This would seem to suggest that maternal nutrition and body build are able to modify foetal nutrient supply and subsequent bone accretion. From other epidemiological studies, a group of 153 women born in Bath who were followed up to the age of 21 years [199] were found to have statistically significant associations between weight at 1 year and bone mineral content (BMC) at age 21 years; the relationships were independent of BMI, diet, and lifestyle. Similar findings were demonstrated in Swedish boys and girls aged 15 years [200], and the relationships were found to persist in men and women aged between 63 and 73 years [201].

Environmental factors

This section groups together some of the individual risk factors for osteoporosis and age-related fracture. The specific profile of risk factors differs for fractures at different sites, largely as a result of varying pathogenetic contributions from osteoporosis and the risk of falls. Four broad risk factor categories are included here: cigarette smoking, alcohol consumption, physical inactivity, and nutrition.

Cigarette smoking

As long ago as 1976, lower cortical bone mass was demonstrated in women who were cigarette smokers [168,202]. There have since been many published trials showing that men and women who smoke have a higher rate of hip and vertebral fractures than non-smokers (Table 15.16). A recent meta-analysis of 29 published studies of 2156 smokers and 9705 non-smokers found that premenopausal smokers have similar BMD to non-smokers, but that postmenopausal rates of bone loss were greater in current smokers than non-smokers [220]. This analysis also showed that risk of hip fracture was similar in smokers and in non-

Table 15.16 Studies of the relationship between cigarette smoking and the risk of hip fracture in female subjects

Study	Mean age	Relative risk	95% CI
Cohort studies			
[203]	53	0.97	0.83–1.14
[204]	56	1.16	0.83–1.62
[205]	75	1.10	0.46–2.64
[207]	75	1.19	0.84–1.69
[177]	78	2.10	1.40–3.30
[208]	78	1.74	1.19–2.54
[209]	82	1.83	1.31–2.57
[210]	88	5.60	1.80–17.70
Case–control studies			
[211]	62	1.60	1.00–2.30
[178]	64	1.34	0.93–1.91
[185] [212]	66	1.29	0.79–2.11
[213]	68	1.87	1.27–2.75
[214]	74	1.73	0.90–3.32
[215]	75	1.30	0.70–2.60
[176]	75	1.25	0.71–2.18
[216]	75	1.48	1.05–2.07
[217]	76	1.30	1.00–1.70
[218]	78	1.70	1.20–2.30
[219]	82	2.20	1.10–4.60

Data from [206].

smokers at age 50 years, but greater among smokers thereafter, by an estimated 17 per cent at age 60, 41 per cent at 70, 71 per cent at 80 and 108 per cent at 90 years. One hypothesis is that the effect of smoking may be indirect, mediated through earlier age at menopause or low BMI [221,222]. Some studies have suggested that smoking is only important in women receiving hormone replacement therapy [207,223]. However, the results of the meta-analysis suggest that the lifetime risk of fracture in postmenopausal women who smoke is increased by around 50 per cent. It therefore currently appears that cigarette smoking is an important, potentially modifiable, risk factor for osteoporosis and fracture.

Alcohol consumption

Alcohol consumption is another lifestyle variable that has been implicated in the causation of age-related fractures [224,225]. Hutchinson *et al.* reported that a history of alcoholism substantially increased hip fracture risk [171] and Paganini-Hill *et al.* found a doubling of risk in women with alcohol consumption greater than eight measures weekly [176]. Alcoholic men have been shown to have lower bone mass and a greater rate of bone loss than non-alcoholics. Mechanisms for the association between excess alcohol and osteoporosis include a direct toxic effect of alcohol on the osteoblast, reduced BMI, increased frequency of trauma, associations with smoking, poor nutrition, reduced activity, and chronic liver disease.

The influence of more moderate levels of alcohol consumption on bone mass are less clear, with some studies even showing protective effects [226,227]. In the European Vertebral Osteoporosis Study there was no detectable association between the frequency of alcohol intake and vertebral deformity in men or women [228]. After stratifying for age, women over 65 years who consumed alcohol frequently (five days/week) had a lower risk of vertebral deformity than those who consumed alcohol less than once each week. There was a weaker effect in the same direction for men aged over 65 years. It is not clear from these data at what level of alcohol intake the benefits are maximized.

Physical activity

Inactivity has been linked with hip fracture in several epidemiological surveys (Table 15.17), possibly as a result of changes in bone density, the risk of falling, or both. Furthermore, rates of hip fracture rose dramatically in Hong Kong in the period between 1966 and 1985 at a time during which substantial declines occurred in the level of customary physical activity [217].

The suggestion that mechanical factors influence bone mass is not new: Wólff [231] stated that any bone becomes adapted to the functional forces acting upon it. The need for a rigid skeleton, the specific requirements for its architecture, and the necessity for a particular level of bone density are all related exclusively to the role of bone as a load-bearing organ, rather than as a mineral reservoir. It is thus reasonable to expect that the features of the skeletal environment primarily responsible for determining its mass should be mechanical rather than hormonal [232].

The role of physical activity in preventing osteoporosis is a difficult issue to study [182,233,234]. There are few controlled trials in the literature, and in many instances the exercise regimens adopted stress a particular skeletal site while measurements are taken at another. Nevertheless, there appears to be a consensus that increased functional loading is associated with increased bone density. Three of four controlled trials have found a beneficial effect of 30–60 min exercise

Table 15.17 Studies of the relationship between customary physical activity and the risk of hip fracture; modified from [230]

Reference	Activity level	Relative risk of hip fracture	95% CI
[209]	Outdoor sports		
	low	1.0	–
	medium	0.5	–
	high	0.3	–
[218]	Productive activity		
	<2 hours/week	2.1	1.4–3.2
	3–4 hours/week	1.1	0.7–1.6
	>5 hours/week	1.0	–
[217]	Walking with a load		
	< once/day	2.3	1.2–4.7
	> once/day	1.0	–
[229]	Standing <2 hours/day	7.1	2.9–17.0
	Standing >4 hours/day	1.0	–
	Walking – none	3.4	1.7–6.8
	Walking >1 hour/day	1.0	–
[219]	No work	1.0	–
	>3 hours/day	0.5	0.3–1.0
[216]	Past inactivity	1.0	–
	Past very active	0.54	0.33–0.88
[179]	Climbing stairs – none	3.43	1.58–7.42
	Climbing stairs >9 times/day	1.0	–
[177]	Walking <4 hours/day	1.0	–
	Walking >4 hours/day	1.7	1.2–2.4

three to five days a week on bone density or total body calcium.

Studies *in vitro* suggest that strain magnitude, rate, and distribution are independent determinants of the osteogenic potential of a strain regime. The normal skeleton appears to adapt rapidly to the stimuli associated with physiological loading, thus repetitions of habitual activities are unlikely to confer additional benefits. In fact, short periods of loading in non-physiological directions appear to be most osteogenic.

Physical activity is something we do throughout life and at all hours when awake, making it very difficult to classify by type, intensity, frequency, duration, or complexity. A recent meta-analysis of physical activity and its relationship with hip fracture reviewed 18 studies [230]. All suggested a protective effect of physical activity against hip fracture, with a strong and consistent association across several geographical locations, and including activity from childhood through to old age (Table 15.17).

Nutrition

Dietary intake of calcium and vitamin D
Almost 99 per cent of the 1.2 kg calcium in the human body is in the bones and teeth, where its primary role is structural. The remainder is in tissues and body fluid where it is essential for cellular structure and function. Approximately 400 mg of calcium enter the skeleton daily through growth. As calcium absorption is inefficient, and substantial urinary loss occurs, calcium nutrition could become a critical factor in skeletal development.

Evidence from balance studies is supportive of a role for calcium deficiency in the aetiology of osteoporosis. The majority of such studies have measured balance response to manipulated calcium intake [235,236]. Estimated mean requirements from such studies range from 200 to 1700 mg/day. However, many of them, particularly those at the lower end of the scale for calcium requirement, were performed in young healthy individuals, and are of uncertain relevance in the elderly.

Very few balance studies have been performed in individuals on their self-selected home calcium intakes. Heaney *et al.* [237] in 233 balances obtained on 150 oestrogen replete perimenopausal women observed a mean requirement of 990 mg/day, and in 41 balances from oestrogen deprived women of the same general age, a mean requirement of 1504 mg/day. When the relationship between calcium intake and calcium balance was examined under conditions of oestrogen presence and oestrogen deficiency, a linear relationship was found in both groups, but a shift was found in the regression line suggesting an increased calcium requirement for zero balance in oestrogen deficiency.

Calcium intake and skeletal development
Evidence does exist that calcium nutrition is important to skeletal development in humans [238]. It has long been recognized that milk supplements given to school children increase their gain in height when compared with controls given the same caloric intake. This has been documented in Japan, where, prior to 1950, calcium intake was very low at about 200 mg/day. After 1960, the Japanese authorities began fortifying school bread with calcium and issuing free milk to school children. Twenty years later, 12-year old Japanese boys averaged about 4 inches taller in height. In the Yugoslavian study already outlined, bone density was greater in the high calcium district by the age of 30 years, suggesting that any nutritional advantage was achieved early in life. More recently, positive associations have been documented between milk consumption in childhood and bone density in adult life [239]. A trial of calcium supplementation in American twins of school age also reported a 22 per cent greater gain in radial BMD among twins treated with a gram of calcium carbonate daily over 3 years, when compared with twins given a placebo [240]. This finding has been replicated in pubertal girls using pharmacological [241] and dietary (milk) supplementation [242].

Calcium intake and osteoporosis
Two basic approaches have been used to study the relationship between calcium requirements and bone health in the elderly: epidemiological methods and balance studies [243]. Epidemiological studies have sought the effects of self-selected differences in calcium intake on bone density, rate of bone loss, osteoporotic fracture incidence, or, conversely, differences in calcium intake between osteoporotics and age-matched controls.

Several early studies failed to detect a relationship between current calcium intake and current bone density. Garn [136], in several studies in North and Central America, found no appreciable effect of calcium intake on bone density in persons across a broad age range. Similarly, Smith and Frame [244] found no significant relationship between current intake and femoral cortical thickness, metacarpal cortical thickness, or vertebral density in women with calcium intakes ranging from 150 to 2100 mg/dl. Hurxthal and Vost [245] found a weak positive correlation of lumbar vertebral density with lifetime calcium intake calculated by diet history in 404 subjects and the results of the 10-State Nutrition Survey also showed a weak but significant positive correlation of calcium intake with metacarpal cortical area.

By contrast, Matkovic *et al.* [246] found clear differences in bone mass and fracture rates in two Yugoslav communities distinguished primarily by an approximately two-fold difference in calcium intake. In both rural districts, nutritional data on intakes of protein, calories, fat, calcium, and phosphorus were obtained by diet histories in 200 subjects. Bone density was measured by metacarpal morphometry, and incidence rates for femoral and forearm fractures were recorded over a 6-year period. Bone density was found to be higher at all ages in men and women in the high calcium district. Apparent rate of loss with age was the same in both districts for men and women, and the principal reason for the density difference appeared to be the fact that persons in the high calcium district started with a higher peak bone density than did persons in the low calcium district.

It is noteworthy that the majority of such studies have used radiogrammetric methods of measuring bone mass. Metacarpal morphometry takes no account of intracortical porosity, or of trabecular bone, and correlates less well than radial photon absorptiometry with either ash weight at the examined site, or total body calcium. The results of studies which have use photon absorptiometric techniques to study the relationship between customary calcium intake and current bone density have also been equivocal [247,248].

With regard to the relationship between calcium intake and rate of bone loss, Garn's studies of over 5000 subjects in seven countries showed a similar rate of cortical bone loss in all groups despite wide variation in calcium intake. Other data also fail to support an association between current calcium consumption and spinal trabecular bone loss [249,250]. By contrast, several recent randomized controlled trials have found that bone loss was retarded by calcium supplementation in postmenopausal women, especially those who already have low bone density [251–253].

Geographic studies of calcium intake and the incidence of osteoporotic fracture also appear inconsistent. Despite some evidence for a relationship between intake and fracture risk within populations, international rates suggest higher fracture incidence in

countries where calcium consumption is high [254]. Such comparisons are complicated, however, by ascertainment bias, ethnic diversity, and cultural differences.

Calcium intake and fracture

The final piece of epidemiological evidence comes from studies comparing the calcium intakes of subjects with fractures and controls without fracture. Several studies have addressed the issue as to whether reduced calcium intake is a risk factor for hip fracture (Table 15.18). A recent meta-analysis [264] reviewed 23 of these, which were found to give inconsistent results. The overall effect of increasing dietary calcium intake by 300 mg/day (a glass of milk daily) was an 8 per cent reduction in hip fracture risk; increasing by 1000 mg/day was associated with a 24 per cent reduction in risk. It is noteworthy that those studies where a positive effect of calcium was apparent had low intakes in the control groups. It may be that there is a threshold level below which calcium consumption becomes critical. In large trials of calcium and vitamin D among elderly French nursing-home residents, significant reductions in fracture incidence have been reported [251,265] suggesting that such interventions in individuals with particularly low calcium or vitamin D intake might be beneficial. Unfortunately, the only large randomized controlled trial to examine the effect of vitamin D supplementation alone in the prevention of hip fracture did not confirm a benefit [266]. The extent to which vitamin D supplementation should be recommended in the institutionalized elderly (a highly cost-effective intervention) [267] is therefore, controversial.

In conclusion, the relation between calcium intake and bone density remains controversial. The evidence from metabolic studies fully supports a high calcium requirement in the elderly and randomized controlled trials confirm that calcium reduces bone loss in osteoporotic patients. This must be contrasted with the epidemiological data suggesting only a weak correlation between calcium intake and fracture risk in the non-institutionalized or healthy elderly, and limited trial evidence for the effectiveness of either calcium or vitamin D in the primary prevention of hip fracture.

Water fluoride concentration

Fluoride has potent effects on bone cell function, bone structure and bone strength; theoretically, these effects could serve to increase or decrease fracture risk. They are mediated by the incorporation of fluoride ions into bone crystals to form fluoroapatite (a more brittle bone tissue), and by inducing an increase in the activity of

Table 15.18 Studies of the relationship between dietary calcium intake and the risk of fracture; modified from [264]

Reference	Calcium intake (mg/day)	Relative risk of fractures	95% CI
Hip fracture			
[255]	992 mg	Higher calcium intake in cases	
[218]	Highest fifth	1.0	–
	Lowest fifth	0.8	0.5–1.4
[205]	Lower two thirds	1.0	–
	Highest third	0.6	0.4–0.9
[217]	Highest fifth	1.0	–
	Lowest fifth	0.5	0.3–0.8
[210]	Highest fifth	1.0	–
	Lowest third	1.4	0.3–10.0
[256]	1023 mg	Higher calcium intake in cases	
[209]	Highest third	1.0	–
	Lowest third	1.1	0.9–1.4
[214]	Highest third	1.0	–
	Lowest third	1.9	0.8–4.7
[257]	Highest fifth	1.0	–
	Lowest fifth	1.2	0.6–2.6
[216]	Highest third	1.0	
	Lowest third	0.8	0.4–1.4
[258]	Highest quartile	1.0	–
	Lowest quartile	0.7	0.5–5.4
[177]	713 mg	1.0	–
	450 mg	0.9	0.8–1.1
[173]	Highest quartile	1.0	–
	Lowest quartile	0.8	0.7–0.9
[179]	697 mg	1.0	0.8–1.3
[213]	Highest quartile	1.0	–
	Lowest quartile	1.5	0.9–2.8
[259]	Highest quintile	1.0	–
	Lowest quintile	1.2	0.8–2.0
[260]	Highest quartile	1.0	–
	Lowest quartile	0.7	0.4–1.1
Forearm fractures			
[261]	713 mg	1.0	0.8–1.3
[214]	Highest third	1.0	
	Lowest third	0.2	0.1–0.8
Proximal humerus fractures			
[261]	713 mg	0.9	0.7–1.4
Vertebral fractures			
[262]	Highest quartile	1.0	–
	Lowest quartile	0.5	0.3–0.9
All fractures			
[263]	Highest	1.0	–
	Lowest	0.3	0.1–0.7

osteoblasts (potentially increasing bone strength). Most fluoride ingested by humans is derived from drinking water, tea, and small fish. Fluoridation of water to around 1 ppm has been widely proposed to prevent dental caries, but concerns have arisen as to whether fluoridation to this level might increase fracture risk.

Animal studies suggest that low-level fluoride intake (0–3 ppm) has little effect on bone strength [268]. Randomized controlled trials using high doses of fluoride in patients with osteoporosis have shown that, despite substantial increases in trabecular bone density, there is no concomitant reduction in vertebral

Table 15.19 Ecological studies investigating the association between water fluoridation and hip fracture; modified from [271]

Reference	Location	Sample size	Duration	Association	
				Direction	Significance
[272]	Sweden	109	Not stated	–ve	NS
[273]	US	93	3 years	–	NS
[274]	US	96 314	5 years	–	NS
[275]	Finland	395	12 years	–ve	p<0.001
[276]	Finland	61	Not stated	–	NS
[32]	US	514 985	4 years	+ve	p<0.009
[277]	UK	20 393	5 years	+ve	p<0.001
[278]	US	4999	7 years	+ve	RR 1.27 (1.00–1.46)
[279]	US	218 951	4 years	+ve	RR 1.08(1.06–1.10)
[280]	Canada	4915	7 years	–	NS
[281]	France	3777	Not stated	+ve	p<0.04

NS = Not statistically significant

fracture [269,270]. Furthermore, the increases in bone density found in the axial skeleton may be occurring at the expense of appendicular sites. Consequently, high-dose sodium fluoride (>80 mg daily) is no longer recommended for the treatment of osteoporosis.

The majority of the evidence that water fluoridation may have an adverse influence on hip fracture risk is based on geographical epidemiological studies comparing regions with different levels of fluoride in the drinking water [271]. Table 15.19 shows these studies; they are clearly inconsistent. If anything, they reveal a weak positive association between water fluoride concentration and hip fracture risk. Data based on individuals are more scarce. However, a recent large, case–control study from the North of England suggested no association between lifelong water fluoride and hip fracture risk [282]. It is becoming more widely accepted, therefore, that concerns over hip fracture risk should not serve as a limitation to public health programmes aiming to promote water fluoridation to levels around 1 ppm.

Conclusion

This review has shown that osteoporosis is a major public health problem because of its association with fracture. It is now possible to predict future risk of fracture by measuring bone mineral density with non-invasive techniques. The relationship between BMD and fracture is comparable to that between blood pressure and stroke so that fracture risk can be assessed from a definition of osteoporosis using bone mass and

past history of fracture. Since some of the risk factors for peak bone mass, involutional bone loss, and fracture are now characterized, coupled with innovative agents which are capable of retarding bone loss, it is becoming possible to generate preventive strategies, both for the entire population and those at the highest risk.

References

1. Cooper AP. *A treatise on dislocations and fractures of the joints.* London: John Churchill, 1842.
2. Consensus Development Conference. Diagnosis, prophylaxis, and treatment of osteoporosis. *Am J Med* 1993; **94**: 646–650.
3. Cooper C, Atkinson EJ, Jacobsen SJ, O'Fallon WM, Melton LJ. Population-based study of survival after osteoporotic fractures. *Am J Epidemiol* 1993; **137**: 1001–1005.
4. Cooper C. The crippling consequences of fractures and their impact on quality of life. *Am J Med* 1997; **103**: 12S–17S.
5. Baudoin C, Fardellone P, Bean K, Ostertag-Ezembe A, Hervy F. Clinical outcomes and mortality after hip fracture: a 2-year follow-up study. *Bone* 1996; **18**: 149S–157S.
6. Magaziner J, Simonsick EM, Kashner TM, Hebel JR, Kenzora JE. Survival experience of aged hip fracture patients. *Am J Public Health* 1989; **79**: 274–278.
7. Poor G, Atkinson EJ, O'Fallon WM, Melton LJ, III. Predictors of hip fractures in elderly men. *J Bone Miner Res* 1995; **10**: 1900–1907.
8. Ismail AA, O'Neill TW, Cooper C *et al.* Mortality associated with vertebral deformity in men and women: results from the European Prospective Osteoporosis Study (EPOS). *Osteoporos Int* 1998; **8**: 291–297.

9. Browner WS, Seeley DG, Vogt TM, Cummings SR. Non-trauma mortality in elderly women with low bone mineral density. Study of Osteoporotic Fractures Research Group. *Lancet* 1991; **338**: 355–358.

10. Chrischilles EA, Butler CD, Davis CS, Wallace RB. A model of lifetime osteoporosis impact. *Arch Intern Med* 1991; **151**: 2026–2032.

11. Washington Office of Technology Assessment, US. *Hip fracture outcomes in people aged 50 and over: mortality, service use, expenditures and long-term functional impairment.* Washington DC: 1993.

12. Gold DT. The clinical impact of vertebral fractures: quality of life in women with osteoporosis. *Bone* 1996; **18**: 185S–189S.

13. Ismail AA, Cooper C, Felsenberg D *et al.* Number and type of vertebral deformities: epidemiological characteristics and relation to back pain and height loss. European Vertebral Osteoporosis Study Group. *Osteoporos Int* 1999; **9**: 206–213.

14. Tromp AM, Smit JH, Deeg DJ, Bouter LM, Lips P. Predictors for falls and fractures in the Longitudinal Aging Study Amsterdam. *J Bone Miner Res* 1998; **13**: 1932–1939.

15. Kaukonen JP, Karaharju EO, Porras M, Luthje P, Jakobsson A. Functional recovery after fractures of the distal forearm. Analysis of radiographic and other factors affecting the outcome. *Ann Chir Gynaecol* 1988; **77**: 27–31.

16. Melton LJ, Chrischilles EA, Cooper C, Lane AW, Riggs BL. How many women have osteoporosis. *J Bone Miner Res* 1992; 7: 1005–1010.

17. Johansen A, Evans RJ, Stone MD, Richmond PW, Lo SV, Woodhouse KW. Fracture incidence in England and Wales: a study based on the population of Cardiff. *Injury* 1997; **28**: 655–660.

18. Garraway WM, Stauffer RN, Kurland LT, O'Fallon WM. Limb fractures in a defined population. I. Frequency and distribution. *Mayo Clin Proc* 1979; **54**: 701–707.

19. Riggs BL, Melton LJ. Involutional osteoporosis. *N Engl J Med* 1986; **314**: 1676–1686.

20. Garraway WM, Stauffer RN, Kurland LT, O'Fallon WM. Limb fractures in a defined population. II. Orthopedic treatment and utilization of health care. *Mayo Clin Proc* 1979; **54**: 708–713.

21. Anonymous. Fracture patterns revisited. *Lancet* 1990; **336**: 1290–1291.

22. Donaldson LJ, Cook A, Thomson RG. Incidence of fractures in a geographically defined population. *J Epidemiol Community Health* 1990; **44**: 241–245.

23. Cooper C, Atkinson EJ, Kotowicz M, O'Fallon WM, Melton LJ. Secular trends in the incidence of postmenopausal vertebral fractures. *Calcif Tissue Int* 1992; **51**: 100–104.

24. Nydegger V, Rizzoli R, Rapin CH, Vasey H, Bonjour JP. Epidemiology of fractures of the proximal femur in Geneva: incidence, clinical and social aspects. *Osteoporos Int* 1991; **2**: 42–47.

25. Rogmark C, Sernbo I, Johnell O, Nilsson JA. Incidence of hip fractures in Malmo, Sweden, 1992–1995. A trend-break. *Acta Orthop Scand* 1999; **70**: 19–22.

26. Arboleya LR, Castro MA, Bartolome E, Gervas L, Vega R. Epidemiology of the osteoporotic fracture of the hip in the province of Palencia. *Rev Clin Esp* 1997; **197**: 611–617.

27. Cooper C, Melton LJ. Epidemiology of osteoporosis. *Trends Endocrinol Metab* 1992; **3**: 224–229.

28. Alffram PA. An epidemiological study of cervical and trochanteric fractures of the femur in an urban population. Analysis of 1664 cases with special reference to aetiologic factors. *Acta Orthop Scand* 1964; **65** (Suppl.): 1–109.

29. Melton LJ. Epidemiology of fractures. In: Riggs BL, Melton LJ, editors. *Osteoporosis: etiology, diagnosis and management.* New York: Raven Press, 1988: 133–154.

30. Stewart IM. Fractures of neck of femur: incidence and implications. *BMJ* 1955; **1**: 698–701.

31. Cooper C, Wickham C, Lacey RF, Barker DJ. Water fluoride concentration and fracture of the proximal femur. *J Epidemiol Community Health* 1990; **44**: 17–19.

32. Jacobsen SJ, Goldberg J, Miles TP, Brody JA, Stiers W, Rimm AA. Seasonal variation in the incidence of hip fracture among white persons aged 65 years and older in the United States, 1984–1987. *Am J Epidemiol* 1991; **133**: 996–1004.

33. Melton LJ, Bryant SC, Wahner HW *et al.* Influence of breastfeeding and other reproductive factors on bone mass later in life. *Osteoporos Int* 1993; **3**: 76–83.

34. Johnell O, Gullberg B, Allander E, Kanis JA. The apparent incidence of hip fracture in Europe: a study of national register sources. MEDOS Study Group. *Osteoporos Int* 1992; **2**: 298–302.

35. Lau EM. The epidemiology of hip fracture in Asia: an update. *Osteoporos Int* 1996; **3** (Suppl.): S19–23.

36. Papadimitropoulos EA, Coyte PC, Josse RG, Greenwood CE. Current and projected rates of hip fracture in Canada. *Can Med Assoc J* 1997; **157**: 1357–1363.

37. Memon A, Pospula WM, Tantawy AY, AbdulGhafar S, Suresh A, AlRowaih A. Incidence of hip fracture in Kuwait. *Int J Epidemiol* 1998; **27**: 860–865.

38. Hagino H, Yamamoto K, Ohsiro H, Nakamura T, Kishimoto H, Nose T. Changing incidence of hip, distal radius and proximal humerus fractures in Tottori prefecture, Japan. *Bone* 1999; **24**: 265–270.

39. Farmer ME, White LR, Brody JA, Bailey KR. Race and sex differences in hip fracture incidence. *Am J Public Health* 1984; **74**: 1374–1380.

40. Solomon L. Osteoporosis and the fracture of the femoral neck in the South African Bantu. *J Bone Jt Surg* 1969; **50B**: 2–13.

41. Bollet AJ, Engh G, Parson W. Epidemiology of osteoporosis: sex and race incidence of hip fractures. *Arch Intern Med* 1965; **116**: 191–194.

42. Adebajo AO, Cooper C, Evans JG. Fractures of the hip and distal forearm in West Africa and the United Kingdom. *Age Ageing* 1991; **20**: 435–438.

43. Arden N, Cooper C. Present and future of osteoporosis: epidemiology. In: Meunier P, editor. *Osteoporosis: diagnosis and management.* London: Martin Dunitz, 1998: 1–16.

44. Boyce WJ, Vessey MP. Rising incidence of fracture of the proximal femur. *Lancet* 1985; **1**: 150–151.

45. Melton LJ, Ilstrup DM, Riggs BL, Beckenbaugh RD. Fifty-year trend in hip fracture incidence. *Clin Orthop* 1982; **50**: 144–149.

46. Melton LJ, O'Fallon WM, Riggs BL. Secular trends in the incidence of hip fractures. *Calcif Tissue Int* 1987; **41**: 57–64.

47. Obrant KJ, Bengner U, Johnell O, Nilsson BE, Sernbo I. Increasing age-adjusted risk of fragility fractures: a sign of increasing osteoporosis in successive generations? *Calcif Tissue Int* 1989; **44**: 157–167.

48. Spector TD, Cooper C, Lewis AF. Trends in admissions for hip fracture in England and Wales, 1968–85. *BMJ* 1990; **300**: 1173–1174.

49. Melton LJ, III, Atkinson EJ, Madhok R. Downturn in hip fracture incidence. *Public Health Rep* 1996; **111**: 146–150.

50. Naessen T, Parker R, Persson I, Zack M, Adami HO. Time trends in incidence rates of first hip fracture in the Uppsala Health Care Region, Sweden, 1965–1983. *Am J Epidemiol* 1989; **130**: 289–299.

51. Rehnberg L, Nungu S, Olerud C. The incidence of femoral neck fractures in women is decreasing. *Acta Orthop Scand* 1992; **63** (Suppl. 248): 92–93.

52. Spector TD, Cooper C, Lewis AF. Recent changes in hip fracture incidence in England and Wales 1968–85. *BMJ* 1990; **300**: 1178–1184.

53. Evans JG, Seagroatt V, Goldacre MJ. Secular trends in proximal femoral fracture, Oxford record linkage study area and England 1968–86. *J Epidemiol Community Health* 1997; **51**: 424–429.

54. Martyn CN, Cooper C. Prediction of burden of hip fracture. *Lancet* 1999; **353**: 769–770.

55. Reid IR, Chin K, Evans MC, Jones JG. Relation between increase in length of hip axis in older women between 1950s and 1990s and increase in age specific rates of hip fracture. *BMJ* 1994; **309**: 508–509.

56. Albright F, Smith PH, Richardson AM. Postmenopausal osteoporosis—its clinical features. *JAMA* 1941; **116**: 2465–2474.

57. Cooper C, O'Neill T, Silman A. The epidemiology of vertebral fractures. European Vertebral Osteoporosis Study Group. *Bone* 1993; **14** (Suppl. 1): S89–S97.

58. Eastell R, Cedel SL, Wahner HW, Riggs BL, Melton LJ. Classification of vertebral fractures. *J Bone Miner Res* 1991; **6**: 207–215.

59. Wu CY, Li J, Jergas M, Genant HK. Diagnosing incident vertebral fractures: a comparison between quantitative morphometry and a standardised visual (semiquantitative) approach. In: Genant HK, Jergas M, van Kuijk C, editors. *Vertebral fracture in osteoporosis.* California: Radiology Research and Education Foundation, 1995: 281–291.

60. Cooper C. Epidemiology of osteoporosis. *Osteoporos Int* 1999; **9** (Suppl. 2): S2–S8.

61. Melton LJ, Lane AW, Cooper C, Eastell R, O'Fallon WM, Riggs BL. Prevalence and incidence of vertebral deformities. *Osteoporos Int* 1993; **3**: 113–119.

62. Cooper C, Atkinson EJ, O'Fallon WM, Melton LJ. Incidence of clinically diagnosed vertebral fractures: a population-based study in Rochester, Minnesota, 1985–1989. *J Bone Miner Res* 1992; **7**: 221–227.

63. O'Neill TW, Felsenberg D, Varlow J, Cooper C, Kanis JA, Silman AJ. The prevalence of vertebral deformity in European men and women: the European Vertebral Osteoporosis Study. *J Bone Miner Res* 1996; **11**: 1010–1018.

64. Fujiwara S, Mizuno S, Ochi Y *et al.* The incidence of thoracic vertebral fractures in a Japanese population, Hiroshima and Nagasaki, 1958–86. *J Clin Epidemiol* 1991; **44**: 1007–1014.

65. Silman AJ, O'Neill TW, Cooper C, Kanis JA, Felsenberg D. Influence of physical activity on vertebral deformity in men and women: results from the European vertebral Osteoporosis Study. *J Bone Miner Res* 1997; **12**: 813–819.

66. O'Neill TW, Silman AJ, Naves-Diaz M, Cooper C, Kanis J, Felsenberg D. Influence of hormonal and reproductive factors on the risk of vertebral deformity in European women. European Vertebral Osteoporosis Study Group. *Osteoporos Int* 1997; **7**: 72–78.

67. Miller SW, Evans JG. Fractures of the distal forearm in Newcastle: an epidemiological study. *Age Ageing* 1985; **14**: 155–158.

68. O'Neill TW, Cooper C, Finn JD *et al.* Incidence of distal forearm fracture in British men and women. In press, 2000.

69. Owen RA, Melton LJ, Johnson KA, Ilstrup DM, Riggs BL. Incidence of Colles' fracture in a North American community. *Am J Public Health* 1982; **72**: 605–607.

70. Solgaard S, Petersen VS. Epidemiology of distal radius fractures. *Acta Orthop Scand* 1985; **56**: 391–393.

71. Bengner U, Johnell O. Increasing incidence of forearm fractures. A comparison of epidemiological patterns 25 years apart. *Acta Orthop Scand* 1985; **56**: 158–160.

72. Mallmin H, Ljunghall S, Naessen T. Colles' fracture associated with reduced bone mineral content. *Acta Orthop Scand* 1992; **63**: 552–554.

73. Ralis ZA. Epidemic of fractures during period of snow and ice. *Br Med J Clin Res Ed* 1981; **282**: 603–605.

74. Cooper C. Osteoporosis—an epidemiological perspective: a review. *J R Soc Med* 1989; **82**: 753–757.

75. Jacobsen SJ, Sargent DJ, Atkinson EJ, O'Fallon WM, Melton LJ. Contribution of weather to the seasonality of distal forearm fractures: a population-based study in Rochester, Minnesota. *Osteoporos Int* 1999; **9**: 254–259.

76. Jonsson B, Bengner U, Redlund-Johnell I, Johnell O. Forearm fractures in Malmo, Sweden—changes in the incidence occurring during the 1950s, 1980s and 1990s. *Acta Orthop Scand* 1999; **70**: 129–132.

77. Hemenway D, Azrael DR, Rimm EB, Feskanich D, Willett WC. Risk factors for wrist fracture: effect of age, cigarettes, alcohol, body height, relative weight, and handedness on the risk of distal forearm fractures in men. *Am J Epidemiol* 1994; **140**: 361–367.

78. Rose SH, Melton LJ, Morrey BF, Ilstrup DM, Riggs BL. Epidemiologic features of humeral fractures. *Clin Orthop* 1982; **168**: 24–30.

79. Seeley DG, Browner WS, Nevitt MC, Genant HK, Scott JC, Cummings SR. Which fractures are associated with low appendicular bone mass in elderly women? The

Study of Osteoporotic Fractures Research Group. *Ann Intern Med* 1991; **115**: 837–842.

80. Ross PD, Davis JW, Epstein RS, Wasnich RD. Pre-existing fractures and bone mass predict vertebral fracture incidence in women. *Ann Intern Med* 1991; **114**: 919–923.

81. Cooper C, Kotowicz M, Atkinson EJ, O'Fallon WM, Riggs BL, Melton LJ. Risk of limb fractures among men and women with vertebral fractures. In: Papapoulos SE, Lips P, Pols HAP, Johnston CC, Delmas PD, editors. *Osteoporosis '96.* Amsterdam: Elsevier Science, 1996: 101–104.

82. Cuddihy MT, Gabriel SE, Crowson CS, O'Fallon WM, Melton LJ, III. Forearm fractures as predictors of subsequent osteoporotic fractures. *Osteoporos Int* 1999; **9**: 469–475.

83. Melton LJ, Atkinson EJ, Cooper C, O'Fallon WM, Riggs BL. Vertebral fractures predict subsequent fractures. *Osteoporos Int* 1999; **10**: 214–221.

84. Cooper C, Melton LJ. Magnitude and impact of osteoporosis and fractures. In: Marcus R, Feldman D, Kelsey J, editors. *Osteoporosis.* San Diego: Academic Press, 1996: 419–434.

85. Melton LJ, Riggs BL. Risk factors for injury after a fall. *Clin Geriatr Med* 1985; **1**: 525–539.

86. Cooper C, Barker DJ, Morris J, Briggs RS. Osteoporosis, falls, and age in fracture of the proximal femur. *Br Med J Clin Res Ed* 1987; **295**: 13–15.

87. Heaney RP. Qualitative factors in osteoporotic fracture: the state of the question. In: Christiansen C, editor. *Osteoporosis 1987, I. Proceedings of the international symposium on osteoporosis, Denmark.* Copenhagen: Osteoporosis ApS, 1987: 281–287.

88. Lauritzen JB. Hip fractures: incidence, risk factors, energy absorption, and prevention. *Bone* 1996; **18**: 65S–75S.

89. Hui SL, Slemenda CW, Johnston CCJr. Baseline measurement of bone mass predicts fracture in white women. *Ann Intern Med* 1989; **111**: 355–361.

90. Wasnich RD, Ross PD, Davis JW, Vogel JM. A comparison of single and multi-site BMC measurements for assessment of spine fracture probability. *J Nucl Med* 1989; **30**: 1166–1171.

91. Gardsell P, Johnell O, Nilsson BE, Gullberg B. Predicting various fragility fractures in women by forearm bone densitometry: a follow-up study. *Calcif Tissue Int* 1993; **52**: 348–353.

92. Nguyen T, Sambrook P, Kelly P *et al.* Prediction of osteoporotic fractures by postural instability and bone density. *BMJ* 1993; **307**: 1111–1115.

93. Cummings SR, Black DM, Nevitt MC *et al.* Bone density at various sites for prediction of hip fractures. The Study of Osteoporotic Fractures Research Group. *Lancet* 1993; **341**: 72–75.

94. Melton LJ, Atkinson EJ, O'Fallon WM, Wahner HW, Riggs BL. Long-term fracture prediction by bone mineral assessed at different skeletal sites. *J Bone Miner Res* 1993; **8**: 1227–1233.

95. Marshall D, Johnell O, Wedel H. Meta-analysis of how well measures of bone mineral density predict occurrence of osteoporotic fractures. *BMJ* 1996; **312**: 1254–1259.

96. Jergas M, Genant HK. Contributions of bone mass measurements by densitometry in the definition and diagnosis of osteoporosis. In: Meunier P, editor. *Osteoporosis: diagnosis and management.* London: Martin Dunitz; 1998. p. 37–57.

97. World Health Organisation. *Assessment of fracture risk and its application to screening for postmenopausal osteoporosis.* Geneva: WHO, 1994.

98. Kanis JA, Melton LJ, Christiansen C, Johnston CC, Khaltaev N. The diagnosis of osteoporosis. *J Bone Miner Res* 1994; **9**: 1137–1141.

99. Kanis JA, Delmas P, Burckhardt P, Cooper C, Torgerson D. Guidelines for diagnosis and management of osteoporosis: EFFO report. *Osteoporos Int* 1997; **7**: 390–406.

100. Seldin DW, Esser PD, Alderson PO. Comparison of bone density measurements from different skeletal sites. *J Nucl Med* 1988; **29**: 168–173.

101. Black DM, Cummings SR, Genant HK, Nevitt MC, Palermo L, Browner W. Axial and appendicular bone density predict fractures in older women. *J Bone Miner Res* 1992; **7**: 633–638.

102. Overgaard K, Hansen MA, Riis BJ, Christiansen C. Discriminatory ability of bone mass measurements (SPA and DXA) for fractures in elderly postmenopausal women. *Calcif Tissue Int* 1992; **50**: 30–35.

103. Suman V, Atkinson EJ, O'Fallon WM, Black DM, Melton LJ. A nomogram for predicting lifetime risk from radius bone mineral density and age. *Bone* 1993; **14**: 834–846.

104. Compston JE, Cooper C, Kanis JA. Bone densitometry in clinical practice. *BMJ* 1995; **310**: 1507–1510.

105. Barnett E, Nordin BEC. The radiological diagnosis of osteoporosis. *Clin Radiol* 1960; **11**: 166–174.

106. Wahner HW, Dunn WL, Brown ML, Morin RL, Riggs BL. Comparison of dual-energy x-ray absorptiometry and dual photon absorptiometry for bone mineral measurements of the lumbar spine. *Mayo Clin Proc* 1988; **63**: 1075–1084.

107. Genant HK, Block JE, Steiger P, Glueer CC, Ettinger B, Harris ST. Appropriate use of bone densitometry. *Radiology* 1989; **170**: 817–822.

108. Gluer CC. Quantitative ultrasound techniques for the assessment of osteoporosis: expert agreement on current status. The International Quantitative Ultrasound Consensus Group. *J Bone Miner Res* 1997; **12**: 1280–1288.

109. Cooper C. Bone mass throughout life: bone growth and involution. In: Francis R, editor. *Osteoporosis: pathogenesis and management.* London: Kluwer, 1990: 1–26.

110. Landin L, Nilsson BE. Forearm bone mineral content in children. Normative data. *Acta Paediatr Scand* 1981; **70**: 919–923.

111. Mazess RB, Cameron JR. Growth of bone in school children: comparison of radiographic morphometry and photon absorptiometry. *Growth* 1972; **36**: 77–92.

112. Riggs BL, Wahner HW, Melton LJ, Richelson LS, Judd HL, Offord KP. Rates of bone loss in the appendicular and axial skeletons of women. Evidence of substantial vertebral bone loss before menopause. *J Clin Invest* 1986; **77**: 1487–1491.

113. Specker BL, Brazerol W, Tsang RC, Levin R, Searcy J, Steichen J. Bone mineral content in children 1 to 6 years of age. Detectable sex differences after 4 years of age. *Am J Dis Child* 1987; **141**: 343–344.

114. Kelly PJ, Eisman JA, Sambrook PN. Interaction of genetic and environmental influences on peak bone density. *Osteoporos Int* 1990; **1**: 56–60.

115. Kelly PJ, Twomey L, Sambrook PN, Eisman JA. Sex differences in peak adult bone mineral density. *J Bone Miner Res* 1990; **5**: 1169–1175.

116. Krabbe S, Christiansen C, Rodbro P, Transbol I. Effect of puberty on rates of bone growth and mineralisation: with observations in male delayed puberty. *Arch Dis Child* 1979; **54**: 950–953.

117. Kleerekoper M, Tolia K, Parfitt AM. Nutritional, endocrine, and demographic aspects of osteoporosis. *Orthop Clin North Am* 1981; **12**: 547–558.

118. Recker RR, Davies KM, Hinders SM, Heaney RP, Stegman MR, Kimmel DB. Bone gain in young adult women. *JAMA* 1992; **268**: 2403–2408.

119. Slemenda C, Johnston CC, Hui SL. Patterns of bone loss and physiologic growing. In. *Proceedings of the third international symposium on osteoporosis.* Copenhagen: Osteoporosis ApS, 1990: 99.

120. Cooper C. Epidemiological aspects of osteoporosis and age-related fractures. In: Ring EFJ, Evans WD, Dixon AS, editors. *Osteoporosis and bone mineral measurement.* York: IPSM Publications, 1989.

121. Garn SM, Rohmann CG, Wagner B. Bone loss as a general phenomenon in man. *Fed Proc* 1967; **26**: 1729–1736.

122. Dennison E, Eastell R, Fall CHD, Kellingray S, Wood PJ, Cooper C. Determinants of bone loss in elderly men and women: A prospective population-based study. *Osteoporos Int* 1999; **10**: 384–391.

123. Ensrud KE, Palermo L, Black DM *et al.* Hip and calcaneal bone loss increase with advancing age: longitudinal results from the study of osteoporotic fractures. *J Bone Miner Res* 1995; **10**: 1778–1787.

124. Jones G, Nguyen T, Sambrook P, Kelly PJ, Eisman JA. Progressive loss of bone in the femoral neck in elderly people: longitudinal findings from the Dubbo osteoporosis epidemiology study. *BMJ* 1994; **309**: 691–695.

125. Slemenda CW, Christian JC, Reed T, Reister TK, Williams CJ, Johnston CCJr. Long-term bone loss in men: effects of genetic and environmental factors. *Ann Intern Med* 1992; **117**: 286–291.

126. Winner SJ, Morgan CA, Evans JG. Perimenopausal risk of falling and incidence of distal forearm fracture. *BMJ* 1989; **298**: 1486–1488.

127. Kannus P, Parkkari J, Koskinen S, Niemi S, Palvanen M, Jarvinen M. Fall-induced injuries and deaths among older adults. *JAMA* 1999; **281**: 1895–1899.

128. Liu B, Anderson G, Mittmann N, To T, Axcell T, Shear N. Use of selective serotonin-reuptake inhibitors or tricyclic antidepressants and risk of hip fractures in elderly people. *Lancet* 1998; **351**: 1303–1307.

129. Cumming RG. Epidemiology of medication-related falls and fractures in the elderly. *Drugs Aging* 1998; **12**: 43–53.

130. Feskanich D, Willett WC, Stampfer MJ, Colditz GA. A prospective study of thiazide use and fractures in women. *Osteoporos Int* 1997; **7**: 79–84.

131. Weiland SK, Ruckmann A, Keil U, Lewis M, Dennler HJ, Welzel D. Thiazide diuretics and the risk of hip fracture among 70–79 year old women treated for hypertension. *Eur J Public Health* 1997; **7**: 335–340.

132. Gillespie LD, Gillespie WJ, Cumming R, Lamb SE, Rowe BH. Interventions to reduce the incidence of falling in the elderly. *The Cochrane Library, Cochrane Collaboration; Issue 4.* Oxford: Update Software, 1997.

133. Gibson MJ. The prevention of falls in later life. *Dan Med Bull* 1987; **34** (Suppl. 4): 1–24.

134. Parkkari J, Kannus P, Palvanen M *et al.* Majority of hip fractures occur as a result of a fall and impact on the greater trochanter of the femur: a prospective controlled hip fracture study with 206 consecutive patients. *Calcif Tissue Int* 1999; **65**: 183–187.

135. Schwartz AV, Kelsey JL, Sidney S, Grisso JA. Characteristics of falls and risk of hip fracture in elderly men. *Osteoporos Int* 1998; **8**: 240–246.

136. Garn SM. The earlier gain and later loss of cortical bone. Springfield: CC Thomas, 1970.

137. Evans RA, Marel GM, Lancaster EK, Kos S, Evans M, Wong SY. Bone mass is low in relatives of osteoporotic patients. *Ann Intern Med* 1988; **109**: 870–873.

138. Seeman E, Hopper JL, Bach LA *et al.* Reduced bone mass in daughters of women with osteoporosis. *N Engl J Med* 1989; **320**: 554–558.

139. Soroko SB, Barrett-Connor E, Edelstein SL, Kritz-Silverstein D. Family history of osteoporosis and bone mineral density at the axial skeleton: the Rancho Bernardo Study. *J Bone Miner Res* 1994; **9**: 761–769.

140. Fox KM, Cummings SR, Threets K. Family history and risk of osteoporotic fracture. *J Bone Miner Res* 1994; **9** (Suppl. 1): S153.

141. Smith DM, Nance WE, Kang KW, Christian JC, Johnston CCJr. Genetic factors in determining bone mass. *J Clin Invest* 1973; **52**: 2800–2808.

142. Arden NK, Baker J, Hogg C, Baan K, Spector TD. The heritability of bone mineral density, ultrasound of the calcaneus and hip axis length: a study of postmenopausal twins. *J Bone Miner Res* 1996; **11**: 530–534.

143. Flicker L, Hopper JL, Rodgers L, Kaymakci B, Green RM, Wark JD. Bone density determinants in elderly women: a twin study. *J Bone Miner Res* 1995; **10**: 1607–1613.

144. Pocock NA, Eisman JA, Hopper JL, Yeates MG, Sambrook PN, Eberl S. Genetic determinants of bone mass in adults. A twin study. *J Clin Invest* 1987; **80**: 706–710.

145. Slemenda CW, Christian JC, Williams CJ, Norton JA, Johnston CCJr. Genetic determinants of bone mass in adult women: a reevaluation of the twin model and the potential importance of gene interaction on heritability estimates. *J Bone Miner Res* 1991; **6**: 561–567.

146. Dequeker J, Nijs J, Verstraeten A, Geusens P, Gevers G. Genetic determinants of bone mineral content at the spine and radius: a twin study. *Bone* 1987; **8**: 207–209.

147. Kelly PJ, Hopper JL, Macaskill GT, Pocock NA, Sambrook PN, Eisman JA. Genetic factors in bone turnover. *J Clin Endocrinol Metab* 1991; **72**: 808–813.

148. Kelly PJ, Nguyen T, Hopper J, Pocock N, Sambrook P, Eisman J. Changes in axial bone density with age: a twin study. *J Bone Miner Res* 1993; **8**: 11–17.

149. Gueguen R, Jouanny P, Guillemin F, Kuntz C, Pourel J, Siest G. Segregation analysis and variance components analysis of bone mineral density in healthy families. *J Bone Miner Res* 1995; **10**: 2017–2022.

150. Morrison NA, Yeoman R, Kelly PJ, Eisman JA. Contribution of trans-acting factor alleles to normal physiological variability: vitamin D receptor gene polymorphism and circulating osteocalcin. *Proc Natl Acad Sci U S A* 1992; **89**: 6665–6669.

151. Hustmeyer FG, Peacock M, Hui S, Johnston CC, Christian J. Bone mineral density in relation to polymorphism at the vitamin D receptor gene locus. *J Clin Invest* 1994; **94**: 2130–2134.

152. Fleet JC, Harris SS, Wood RJ, Dawson-Hughes B. The BsmI vitamin D receptor restriction fragment polymorphism (BB) predicts low bone density in premenopausal black and white women. *J Bone Miner Res* 1995; **10**: 985–990.

153. Riggs BL, Ngyuen TV, Melton LJ *et al.* The contribution of the vitamin D receptor gene alleles to the determination of bone mineral density in normal and osteoporotic women. *J Bone Miner Res* 1995; **10**: 991–996.

154. Garnerno P, Borel O, Sornay-Rendu E, Delmas PD. Vitamin D receptor polymorphisms do not predict bone turnover and bone mass in healthy premenopausal women. *J Bone Miner Res* 1995; **10**: 1283–1288.

155. Barger-Lux MJ, Heaney RP, Hayes J, DeLuca HF, Johnson ML, Gong G. Vitamin D receptor polymorphism, bone mass, body size and vitamin D receptor density. *Calcif Tissue Int* 1995; **57**: 161–162.

156. Salamone LM, Ferrel R, Black DM *et al.* The association between vitamin D receptor gene polymorphisms and bone mineral density at the spine, hip, and whole body in premenopausal women. *Osteoporos Int* 1996; **6**: 187–188.

157. Tokita A, Matsumoto H, Morrison NA *et al.* Vitamin D receptor alleles, bone mineral density and turnover in premenopausal Japanese women. *J Bone Miner Res* 1996; **11**: 1003–1009.

158. Melhus H, Kindmark A, Amér S, Wilén B, Lindh E, Ljunghall S. Vitamin D receptor genotypes in osteoporosis. *Lancet* 1994; **344**: 949–950.

159. Spector TD, Keen RW, Arden NK *et al.* Influence of vitamin D receptor genotype on bone mineral density in postmenopausal women: a twin study in Britain. *BMJ* 1995; **310**: 1357–1360.

160. Garnerno P, Borel O, Sornay-Rendu E, Arlot ME, Delmas P. Vitamin D receptor polymorphisms are not related to bone turnover, rate of bone loss, and bone mass in postmenopausal women: the OFELY study. *J Bone Miner Res* 1996; **11**: 827–834.

161. Cooper GS, Umbach DM. Are vitamin D receptor polymorphisms associated with bone mineral density? A meta-analysis. *J Bone Miner Res* 1996; **11**: 1841–1849.

162. Eisman JA. Vitamin D receptor gene alleles and osteoporosis: an affirmative view. *J Bone Miner Res* 1995; **10**: 1289–1293.

163. Smith R. Osteoporosis: lessons from rare causes. In: Smith R, editor. *Osteoporosis*. London: Royal College of Physicians of London, 1990.

164. Spotila LD, Colige A, Sereda L *et al.* Mutation analysis of coding sequences for type I procollagen in individuals with low bone density. *J Bone Miner Res* 1994; **9**: 923–932.

165. Grant SF, Reid DM, Blake G, Herd R, Fogelman I, Ralston SH. Reduced bone density and osteoporosis associated with a polymorphic Sp1 binding site in the collagen type I alpha 1 gene. *Nat Genet* 1996; **14**: 203–205.

166. Uitterlinden AG, Burger H, Huang Q *et al.* Relation of alleles of the collagen type Ialpha1 gene to bone density and the risk of osteoporotic fractures in postmenopausal women. *N Engl J Med* 1998; **338**: 1016–1021.

167. Ralston SH. Do genetic markers aid in risk assessment? *Osteoporos Int* 1998; **8**: S37–S42.

168. Daniell HW. Osteoporosis of the slender smoker. Vertebral compression fractures and loss of metacarpal cortex in relation to postmenopausal cigarette smoking and lack of obesity. *Arch Intern Med* 1976; **136**: 298–304.

169. Saville PD, Nilsson BE. Height and weight in symptomatic postmenopausal osteoporosis. *Clin Orthop* 1966; **45**: 49–54.

170. Slemenda CW, Hui SL, Longcope C, Wellman H, Johnston CCJr. Predictors of bone mass in perimenopausal women. A prospective study of clinical data using photon absorptiometry. *Ann Intern Med* 1990; **112**: 96–101.

171. Hutchinson TA, Polansky SM, Feinstein AR. Postmenopausal oestrogens protect against fractures of hip and distal radius. A case-control study. *Lancet* 1979; **2**: 705–709.

172. Aloia JF, Cohn SH, Vaswani A, Yeh JK, Yuen K, Ellis K. Risk factors for postmenopausal osteoporosis. *Am J Med* 1985; **78**: 95–100.

173. Johnell O, Gullberg B, Kanis JA *et al.* Risk factors for hip fracture in European women: the MEDOS Study. Mediterranean Osteoporosis Study. *J Bone Miner Res* 1995; **10**: 1802–1815.

174. Seeman E, Melton LJ, O'Fallon WM, Riggs BL. Risk factors for spinal osteoporosis in men. *Am J Med* 1983; **75**: 977–983.

175. Johnell O, O'Neill T, Felsenberg D, Kanis J, Cooper C, Silman AJ. Anthropometric measurements and vertebral deformities. European Vertebral Osteoporosis Study (EVOS) Group. *Am J Epidemiol* 1997; **146**: 287–293.

176. Paganini-Hill A, Ross RK, Gerkins VR, Henderson BE, Arthur M, Mack TM. Menopausal estrogen therapy and hip fractures. *Ann Intern Med* 1981; **95**: 28–31.

177. Cummings SR, Nevitt MC, Browner WS *et al.* Risk factors for hip fracture in white women. Study of Osteoporotic Fractures Research Group. *N Engl J Med* 1995; **332**: 767–773.

178. Williams AR, Weiss NS, Ure CL, Ballard J, Daling JR. Effect of weight, smoking, and estrogen use on the risk

of hip and forearm fractures in postmenopausal women. *Obstet Gynecol* 1982; **60**: 695–699.

179. Meyer HE, Henriksen C, Falch JA, Pedersen JI, Tverdal A. Risk factors for hip fracture in a high incidence area: a case-control study from Oslo, Norway. *Osteoporos Int* 1995; **5**: 239–246.

180. Reid IR, Ames RW, Evans MC, Sharpe SJ, Gamble GD. Determinants of the rate of bone loss in normal postmenopausal women. *J Clin Endocrinol Metab* 1994; **79**: 950–954.

181. Tremollieres FA, Pouilles JM, Ribot C. Vertebral postmenopausal bone loss is reduced in overweight women: a longitudinal study in 155 early postmenopausal women. *J Clin Endocrinol Metab* 1993; **77**: 683–686.

182. Cummings SR, Kelsey JL, Nevitt MC, O'Dowd KJ. Epidemiology of osteoporosis and osteoporotic fractures. *Epidemiol Rev* 1985; **7**: 178–208.

183. Wootton R, Bryson E, Elsasser U *et al.* Risk factors for fractured neck of femur in the elderly. *Age Ageing* 1982; **11**: 160–168.

184. Cann CE, Genant HK, Ettinger B, Gordan GS. Spinal mineral loss in oophorectomized women. Determination by quantitative computed tomography. *JAMA* 1980; **244**: 2056–2059.

185. Kreiger N, Kelsey JL, Holford TR, O'Connor T. An epidemiologic study of hip fracture in postmenopausal women. *Am J Epidemiol* 1982; **116**: 141–148.

186. Lindsay R, Hart DM, Forrest C, Baird C. Prevention of spinal osteoporosis in oophorectomised women. *Lancet* 1980; **2**: 1151–1154.

187. Alderman BW, Weiss NS, Daling JR, Ure CL, Ballard JH. Reproductive history and postmenopausal risk of hip and forearm fracture. *Am J Epidemiol* 1986; **124**: 262–267.

188. Lloyd T, Buchanan JR, Ursino GR, Myers C, Woodward G, Halbert DR. Long-term oral contraceptive use does not affect trabecular bone density. *Am J Obstet Gynecol* 1989; **160**: 402–404.

189. Cooper C, Hannaford P, Croft P, Kay CR. Oral contraceptive pill use and fractures in women: a prospective study. *Bone* 1993; **14**: 41–45.

190. Eastell R, Reid DM, Compston J *et al.* A UK Consensus Group on management of glucocorticoid-induced osteoporosis: an update. *J Intern Med* 1998; **244**: 271–292.

191. Cauley JA, Cummings SR, Seeley DG *et al.* Effects of thiazide diuretic therapy on bone mass, fractures, and falls. The Study of Osteoporotic Fractures Research Group. *Ann Intern Med* 1993; **118**: 666–673.

192. Barker DJP. Programming the baby. In: Barker DJP, editor. *Mothers, babies and disease in later life*. London: BMJ publishing group, 1994: 14–36.

193. Barraclough CA. Production of anovulatory, sterile rats by single injections of testosterone propionate. *Endocrinology* 1961; **68**: 62–67.

194. Widdowson EM, McCance RA. The effect of finite periods of undernutrition at different ages on the composition and subsequent development of the rat. *Proc R Soc Lond (Biol)* 1963; **158**: 329–342.

195. Fall C, Hindmarsh P, Dennison E, Kellingray S, Barker D, Cooper C. Programming of growth hormone secretion and bone mineral density in elderly men: a hypothesis. *J Clin Endocrinol Metab* 1998; **83**: 135–139.

196. Phillips DIW, Barker DJP, Fall CHD *et al.* Elevated plasma cortisol concentrations: A link between low birth weight and the insulin resistance syndrome? *J Clin Endocrinol Metab* 1998; **83**: 757–760.

197. Dennison E, Hindmarsh P, Fall C *et al.* Profiles of endogenous circulating cortisol and bone mineral density in healthy elderly men. *J Clin Endocrinol Metab* 1999; **84**: 3058–3063.

198. Godfrey K, Breier B, Cooper C. Constraints of the materno-placental supply of nutrients: causes and consequences. In: O'Brien PMS, Wheeler T, Barker DJP, editors. *Fetal programming: influences on development and disease in later life*. London: RCOG Press, 1999.

199. Cooper C, Cawley M, Bhalla A *et al.* Childhood growth, physical activity, and peak bone mass in women. *J Bone Miner Res* 1995; **10**: 940–947.

200. Duppe H, Cooper C, Gardsell P, Johnell O. The relationship between childhood growth, bone mass, and muscle strength in male and female adolescents. *Calcif Tissue Int* 1997; **60**: 405–409.

201. Cooper C, Fall C, Egger P, Hobbs R, Eastell R, Barker D. Growth in infancy and bone mass in later life. *Ann Rheum Dis* 1997; **56**: 17–21.

202. Lindsay R. The influence of cigarette smoking on bone mass and bone loss. In: DeLuca HF, Frost HM, Jee WSS, Johnston CC, Parfitt AM, editors. *Osteoporosis: recent advances in pathogenesis and treatment* . Baltimore: University Park Press, 1981: 481.

203. Hemenway D, Colditz GA, Willett WC, Stampfer MJ, Speizer FE. Fractures and lifestyle: effect of cigarette smoking, alcohol intake, and relative weight on the risk of hip and forearm fractures in middle-aged women. *Am J Public Health* 1988; **78**: 1554–1558.

204. Meyer HE, Tverdal A, Falch JA. Risk factors for hip fracture in middle-aged Norwegian women and men. *Am J Epidemiol* 1993; **137**: 1203–1211.

205. Holbrook TL, Barrett-Connor E, Wingard DL. Dietary calcium and risk of hip fracture: 14-year prospective population study. *Lancet* 1988; **2**: 1046–1049.

206. Law MR. Personal communication.

207. Kiel DP, Baron JA, Anderson JJ, Hannan MT, Felson DT. Smoking eliminates the protective effect of oral estrogens on the risk for hip fracture among women. *Ann Intern Med* 1992; **116**: 716–721.

208. Forsen L, Bjorndal A, Bjartveit K *et al.* Interaction between current smoking, leanness, and physical inactivity in the prediction of hip fracture. *J Bone Miner Res* 1994; **9**: 1671–1678.

209. Paganini-Hill A, Chao A, Ross RK, Henderson BE. Exercise and other factors in the prevention of hip fracture: the Leisure World study. *Epidemiology* 1991; **2**: 16–25.

210. Wickham CAC, Walsh K, Cooper C *et al.* Dietary calcium, physical-activity, and risk of hip fracture—a prospective-study. *BMJ* 1989; **299**: 889–892.

211. La Vecchia C, Negri E, Levi F, Baron JA. Cigarette smoking, body mass and other risk factors for fractures of the hip in women. *Int J Epidemiol* 1991; **20**: 671–677.

212. Kreiger N, Hilditch S. Cigarette smoking and estrogen-dependent diseases. *Am J Epidemiol* 1986; **123**: 200.

213. Michaelsson K, Holmberg L, Mallmin H *et al.* Diet and hip fracture risk: a case-control study. Study Group of the Multiple Risk Survey on Swedish Women for Eating Assessment. *Int J Epidemiol* 1995; **24**: 771–782.

214. Kreiger N, Gross A, Hunter G. Dietary factors and fracture in postmenopausal women: a case-control study. *Int J Epidemiol* 1992; **21**: 953–958.

215. Grisso JA, Kelsey JL, Strom BL *et al.* Risk factors for hip fracture in black women. *N Engl J Med* 1994; **330**: 1555–1559.

216. Jaglal SB, Kreiger N, Darlington G. Past and recent physical activity and risk of hip fracture. *Am J Epidemiol* 1993; **138**: 107–118.

217. Lau E, Donnan S, Barker DJ, Cooper C. Physical activity and calcium intake in fracture of the proximal femur in Hong Kong. *BMJ* 1988; **297**: 1441–1443.

218. Cooper C, Barker DJ, Wickham C. Physical activity, muscle strength, and calcium intake in fracture of the proximal femur in Britain. *BMJ* 1988; **297**: 1443–1446.

219. Cumming RG, Klineberg RJ. Case-control study of risk factors for hip fractures in the elderly. *Am J Epidemiol* 1994; **139**: 493–503.

220. Law MR, Hackshaw AK. A meta-analysis of cigarette smoking, bone mineral density and risk of hip fracture: recognition of a major effect. *BMJ* 1997; **315**: 841–846.

221. Jensen GF. Osteoporosis of the slender smoker revisited by epidemiologic approach. *Eur J Clin Invest* 1986; **16**: 239–242.

222. McDermott MT, Witte MC. Bone mineral content in smokers. *South Med J* 1988; **81**: 477–480.

223. Jensen J, Christiansen C, Rodbro P. Cigarette smoking, serum estrogens, and bone loss during hormone-replacement therapy early after menopause. *N Engl J Med* 1985; **313**: 973–975.

224. Bikle DD, Genant HK, Cann C, *et al.* Bone disease in alcohol abuse. *Ann Intern Med* 1986; **103**: 42–48.

225. Spencer H, Rubio N, Rubio E, Indreika M, Seitam A. Chronic alcoholism. Frequently overlooked cause of osteoporosis in men. *Am J Med* 1986; **80**: 393–397.

226. Felson DT, Kiel DP, Anderson JJ, Kannel WB. Alcohol consumption and hip fractures: the Framingham Study. *Am J Epidemiol* 1988; **128**: 1102–1110.

227. Holbrook TL, Barrett-Connor E. A prospective study of alcohol consumption and bone mineral density. *BMJ* 1993; **306**: 1506–1509.

228. Naves-Diaz M, O'Neill TW, Silman AJ. The influence of alcohol consumption on the risk of vertebral deformity. European Vertebral Osteoporosis Study Group. *Osteoporos Int* 1997; **7**: 65–71.

229. Coupland C, Wood D, Cooper C. Physical inactivity is an independent risk factor for hip fracture in the elderly. *J Epidemiol Community Health* 1993; **47**: 441–443.

230. Joakimsen RM, Magnus JH, Fonnebo V. Physical activity and predisposition for hip fractures: a review. *Osteoporos Int* 1997; **7**: 503–513.

231. Wólff J. Das gesetz der transformation der knochen. Hirschwald, Berlin, 1892. Cited in: Aloia J. Exercise and skeletal health. *J Am Geriatr Soc* 1981; **29**: 104–107.

232. Cooper C, Eastell R. Bone gain and loss in premenopausal women. *BMJ* 1993; **306**: 1357–1358.

233. Chow R, Harrison JE, Notarius C. Effect of two randomised exercise programmes on bone mass of healthy postmenopausal women. *Br Med J Clin Res Ed* 1987; **295**: 1441–1444.

234. Smith EL, Raab DM. Osteoporosis and physical activity. *Acta Med Scand Suppl* 1986; **711**: 149–156.

235. Kanis JA, Passmore R. Calcium supplementation of the diet—II. *BMJ* 1989; **298**: 205–208.

236. Kanis JA, Passmore R. Calcium supplementation of the diet—I. *BMJ* 1989; **298**: 137–140.

237. Heaney RP, Recker RR, Saville PD. Menopausal changes in calcium balance performance. *J Lab Clin Med* 1978; **92**: 953–963.

238. Kanders B, Dempster DW, Lindsay R. Interaction of calcium nutrition and physical activity on bone mass in young women. *J Bone Miner Res* 1988; **3**: 145–149.

239. Sandler RB, Slemenda CW, LaPorte RE *et al.* Postmenopausal bone density and milk consumption in childhood and adolescence. *Am J Clin Nutr* 1985; **42**: 270–274.

240. Johnston CCJr, Miller JZ, Slemenda CW *et al.* Calcium supplementation and increases in bone mineral density in children. *N Engl J Med* 1992; **327**: 82–87.

241. Bonjour JP, Carrie AL, Ferrari S *et al.* Calcium-enriched foods and bone mass growth in prepubertal girls: a randomized, double-blind, placebo-controlled trial. *J Clin Invest* 1997; **99**: 1287–1294.

242. Cadogan J, Eastell R, Jones N, Barker ME. Milk intake and bone mineral acquisition in adolescent girls: randomised, controlled intervention trial. *BMJ* 1997; **315**: 1255–1260.

243. Heaney RP, Gallagher JC, Johnston CC, Neer R, Parfitt AM, Whedon GD. Calcium nutrition and bone health in the elderly. *Am J Clin Nutr* 1982; **36**: 986–1013.

244. Smith RW, Frame B. Concurrent axial and appendicular osteoporosis: its relation to calcium consumption. *N Engl J Med* 1965; **273**: 72–78.

245. Hurxthal LM, Vose GP. The relationship of dietary calcium intake to radiographic bone density in normal and osteoporotic persons. *Calcif Tissue Res* 1969; **4**: 245–256.

246. Matkovic V, Kostial K, Simonovic I, Buzina R, Brodarec A, Nordin BE. Bone status and fracture rates in two regions of Yugoslavia. *Am J Clin Nutr* 1979; **32**: 540–549.

247. Anderson JJB, Tylavsky FA. Diet and osteopenia in elderly Caucasian women. In: Christiansen C, *et al.*, editors. *Osteoporosis I. Proceedings of the Copenhagen international symposium on osteoporosis.* Copenhagen: Glostrup Hospital, 1984: 299–304.

248. Lavel-Jeantet AM, Paul G, Bergot C, Lamarque JL, Ghiania MN. Correlation between vertebral bone density measurements and nutritional status. In: Christiansen C, editor. *Osteoporosis I. Proceedings of the Copenhagen international symposium on osteoporosis.* Copenhagen: Glostrup Hospital, 1984: 305–310.

249. Riggs BL, Wahner HW, Melton LJ, Richelson LS, Judd HL, O'Fallon WM. Dietary calcium intake and rates of bone loss in women. *J Clin Invest* 1987; **80**: 979–982.

250. Stevenson JC, Whitehead MI, Padwick M *et al.* Dietary intake of calcium and postmenopausal bone loss. *BMJ* 1988; **297**: 15–17.

251. Dawson-Hughes B, Harris SS, Krall EA, Dallal GE. Effect of calcium and vitamin D supplementation on bone density in men and women 65 years of age or older. *N Engl J Med* 1997; **337**: 670–676.

252. Reid IR, Ames RW, Evans MC, Gamble GD, Sharpe SJ. Effect of calcium supplementation on bone loss in postmenopausal women. *N Engl J Med* 1993; **328**: 460–464.

253. Royal College of Physicians of London. *Osteoporosis clinical guidelines for prevention and treatment.* London: Royal College of Physicians of London, 1999.

254. Hegsted DM. Calcium and osteoporosis. *J Nutr* 1986; **116**: 2316–2319.

255. Wootton R, Brereton PJ, Clark MB *et al.* Fractured neck of femur in the elderly: an attempt to identify patients at risk. *Clin Sci* 1979; **57**: 93–101.

256. Wheadon.M., Goulding A, Barbezat GO, Campbell AJ. Lactose malabsorption and calcium intake as risk factors for osteoporosis in elderly New Zealand women. *NZ Med J* 1991; **104**: 417–419.

257. Nieves JW, Grisso JA, Kelsey JL. A case-control study of hip fracture: evaluation of selected dietary variables and teenage physical activity. *Osteoporos Int* 1992; **2**: 122–127.

258. Looker AC, Harris TB, Madans JH, Sempos CT. Dietary calcium and hip fracture risk: the NHANES I epidemiologic follow-up study. *Osteoporos Int* 1995; **3**: 177–184.

259. Tavani A, Negri E, La Vecchia C. Calcium, dairy products, and the risk of hip fracture in women in northern Italy. *Epidemiology* 1995; **6**: 554–557.

260. Meyer HE, Pedersen JI, Loken EB, Tverdal A. Dietary factors and the incidence of hip fractures among middle-aged Norwegians. *Am J Epidemiol* 1997; **145**: 117–123.

261. Kelsey JL, Browner WS, Seeley DG, Nevitt MC, Cummings SR. Risk factors for fractures of the distal forearm and proximal humerus. The Study of Osteoporotic Fractures Research Group. *Am J Epidemiol* 1992; **135**: 477–489.

262. Chan HH, Lau EM, Woo J, Lin F, Sham A, Leung PC. Dietary calcium intake, physical activity and the risk of vertebral fracture in Chinese. *Osteoporos Int* 1996; **6**: 228–232.

263. Chi I, Pun KK. Dietary calcium intake and other risk factors: study of the fractured patients in Hong Kong. *J Nutr Elder* 1991; **10**: 73–87.

264. Cumming RG, Nevitt MC. Calcium for prevention of osteoporotic fractures in postmenopausal women. *J Bone Miner Res* 1997; **12**: 1321–1329.

265. Chapuy MC, Arlot ME, Duboeuf F *et al.* Vitamin D3 and calcium to prevent hip fractures in the elderly women. *N Engl J Med* 1992; **327**: 1637–1642.

266. Lips P, Graafmans WC, Ooms ME, Bezemer PD, Bouter LM. Vitamin D supplementation and fracture incidence in elderly persons. A randomized, placebo-controlled clinical trial. *Ann Intern Med* 1996; **124**: 400–406.

267. Torgerson DJ, Kanis JA. Cost-effectiveness of preventing hip fractures in the elderly population using vitamin D and calcium. *QJM* 1995; **88**: 135–139.

268. Turner CH, Akhter MP, Heaney RP. The effects of fluoridated water on bone strength. *J Orthop Res* 1992; **10**: 581–587.

269. Kleerekoper M, Peterson E, Phillips E, Nelson D, Tilley B, Parfitt AM. Continuous sodium fluoride therapy does not reduce vertebral fracture rate in postmenopausal osteoporosis. *J Bone Miner Res* 1989; **4** (Suppl. 1): 1035.

270. Riggs BL, Hodgson SF, O'Fallon WM *et al.* Effect of fluoride treatment on the fracture rate in postmenopausal women with osteoporosis. *N Engl J Med* 1990; **322**: 802–809.

271. Hillier S, Inskip H, Coggon D, Cooper C. Water fluoridation and osteoporotic fracture. *Community Dent Health* 1996; **13** (Suppl. 2): 63–68.

272. Alffram PA, Hernborg J, Nilsson BE. The influence of a high fluoride content in the drinking water on the bone mineral mass in man. *Acta Orthop Scand* 1969; **40**: 137–142.

273. Korns RF. Relationship of water fluoridation to bone density in two N.Y. towns. *Public Health Rep* 1969; **84**: 815–825.

274. Madans J, Kleinman JC, Cornoni-Huntley J. The relationship between hip fracture and water fluoridation: an analysis of national data. *Am J Public Health* 1983; **73**: 296–298.

275. Simonen O, Laitinen O. Does fluoridation of drinking-water prevent bone fragility and osteoporosis? *Lancet* 1985; **2**: 432–434.

276. Arnala I, Alhava EM, Kivivuori R, Kauranen P. Hip fracture incidence not affected by fluoridation. Osteofluorosis studied in Finland. *Acta Orthop Scand* 1986; **57**: 344–348.

277. Cooper C, Wickham CA, Barker DJ, Jacobsen SJ. Water fluoridation and hip fracture. *JAMA* 1991; **266**: 513–514.

278. Danielson C, Lyon JL, Egger M, Goodenough GK. Hip fractures and fluoridation in Utah's elderly population. *JAMA* 1992; **268**: 746–748.

279. Jacobsen SJ, Goldberg J, Cooper C, Lockwood SA. The association between water fluoridation and hip fracture among white women and men aged 65 years and older. A national ecologic study. *Ann Epidemiol* 1992; **2**: 617–626.

280. Suarez-Almazor ME, Flowerdew G, Saunders LD, Soskolne CL, Russell AS. The fluoridation of drinking water and hip fracture hospitalization rates in two Canadian communities. *Am J Public Health* 1993; **83**: 689–693.

281. Jacqmin-Gadda H, Commenges D, Dartigues JF. Fluorine concentration in drinking water and fractures in the elderly. *JAMA* 1995; **273**: 775–776.

282. Hillier S, Kellingray S, Coggon D *et al.* Water fluoridation and fracture of the proximal femur. *J Bone Miner Res* 1997; **12**: 44–44.

16 | Paget's disease

Terence W. O'Neill

It begins in middle age or later, is very slow in progress, may continue for many years without influence on the general health, and may give no other trouble than those which are due to the changes of shape, size, and direction of the diseased bones.

Sir James Paget, 1877

Introduction

Paget's disease of bone is a focal disorder characterized by rapid bone remodelling and the formation of structurally abnormal bone. The first detailed description of the disease was made by Sir James Paget in 1876 in a presentation to the Royal Medical and Chirurgical Society of London, [1], though cases of the disease had been reported previously by others [1,2]. Paget [1] suggested that the disease be called 'osteitis deformans', however, although the term remains in use, it is now more widely known as Paget's disease of bone.

Paget's disease may affect any bone, though the lumbosacral spine, skull, pelvis, and femur are the most frequently affected sites, see Table 16.1 [3]. The majority of individuals with the disease are asymptomatic. Pain and skeletal deformity are the most common pre-

senting symptoms [4]. Affected bones are structurally abnormal, and there is an increased risk of fracture, particularly of the long bones. Other complications of the disease include deafness, various neurological syndromes, and degenerative joint disease. A small proportion of individuals develop malignant bone tumours.

Diagnostic criteria

The majority of individuals with Paget's disease are asymptomatic and the disease is recognized clinically usually only in an advanced stage. Clinical assessment is therefore an unreliable indicator of disease status. Standardized criteria for diagnosis of Paget's disease have been developed based on qualitative radiographic features of the disease [5–9], see Table 16.2.

Although subjective, the reproducibility of these criteria has been reported as excellent in several studies [8,10–12]. As a test of their validity, bone biopsy specimens were taken at necropsy from the iliac blades of 21 subjects in whom post-mortem pelvic radiographs had shown evidence of Paget's disease according to the criteria [13]. In 19 of the 21 specimens the biopsy showed histological signs of the disease. It is possible that patchy distribution of the pathological changes of Paget's disease within the pelvis may explain the lack of concordance in the other two cases.

Table 16.1 Anatomic distribution of Paget's disease[a]; reproduced with permission from Collins D. H. *Lancet* 1956; 2: 51–57 © by the Lancet Ltd [3]

Skeletal site	Prevalence %
Lumbosacral spine	76
Skull	65
Pelvis	43
Femur	35
Tibia	30
Clavicle	11
Sternum	7
Fibula	4

[a] Analysis of 46 post-mortem specimens.

Table 16.2 Radiographic criteria for diagnosis of Paget's disease; reprinted from Cooper C., Dennison E., Schafheutle K., Kellingray S., Guyer P., Barker D. *Bone* 1999; 24: 3S-5S with permission from Elsevier Science [6]

Increase in bone density/areas of decreased radiolucency
Increase in bone size
Bone deformity
Cortical thickening
Enhanced trabecular pattern

One limitation of the criteria, however, is that in cases with early disease, radiographs may appear normal.

Lawrence [14] developed a standard atlas of pelvis and lumbar spine radiographs for grading Paget's disease according to severity. The reproducibility of assessment of the gradings was reported to be good.

Occurrence

Early estimates of disease occurrence were derived from hospital statistics. However, because a large proportion of cases are asymptomatic, these considerably underestimated the true frequency of the disease. Most of our knowledge about the population occurrence of the disease is based on prevalence data obtained either from post-mortem studies or limited radiological skeletal surveys. Other investigators have used screening (with serum alkaline phosphatase) to target radiological investigations (Table 16.3). Each of these approaches, discussed in the following section, are subject, however, to different biases which may over or underestimate the true population prevalence of the disease.

Post-mortem studies

Two large post-mortem series have been reported. Schmorl [15] working in Dresden (Germany) studied 4614 post-mortem specimens of men and women, aged 40 years and over, for evidence of various skeletal disorders; 138 (3 per cent) were found to have Paget's disease. Similar results were obtained by Collins [3] who reported that among 650 post-mortem specimens aged 40 years and over, from Leeds and Sheffield (UK), 24 (3.7 per cent) had evidence of the disease. Subjects undergoing autopsy are not, however, representative of the underlying population—inclusion of those with symptoms or skeletal abnormalities may have resulted in an over-estimation of disease frequency.

Radiological surveys

Paget's disease may affect any bone, however, for practical and ethical reasons it is not possible to X-ray every bone and estimates of the radiological prevalence of the disease are based on assessment of a relatively limited number of skeletal sites. There are few data from community surveys. In the largest of these, a series of 3936 pelvic radiographs taken during the course of the first National Health and Nutrition Examination Survey (NHANES-1) were reviewed for evidence of the disease. The overall prevalence of Paget's disease was 1.2 per cent in men and 1.0 per cent in women aged 45–74 years [16]. In a smaller UK survey (comprising radiographs of the pelvis, lumbar spine, and knees), Lawrence [14] reported a prevalence, among those aged 45 years and over, of 2.7 per cent in men and 1.1 per cent in women. Limited skeletal surveys will underestimate the true frequency of the

Table 16.3 Prevalence (%) of Paget's disease by methodologic approach

Reference	Year	Age (years)	N	Prevalence (%)		
				Male	Female	Both
Autopsy series						
[15]	1932	40+	4614	3.5	2.5	3.0
[3]	1956	40+	650	3.5	4.0	3.7
Radiological surveys						
i) Population						
[14]	1977	45+	1412	2.7	1.1	1.8
[16]	2000	45–74	2854	1.2	1.0	1.1
ii) Hospital[a]						
[17]	1957	45+	9775	3.5	1.9	2.9
[10]	1980	55+	29 054	6.2	3.9	5.0
[8]	1999	55+	9828	2.5	1.6	2.0
Screening with alkaline phosphatase						
[18]	1955	60+	162	8.6	2.2	4.9
[19]	1990	40+	670			6.4
[20]	1997	40+	378			5.7

[a] See also Tables 16.5–16.7

disease (because only a portion of the skeleton is assessed), and may in part explain the lower observed frequency compared with the more extensive post-mortem studies.

Population radiological surveys are costly and involve exposing large numbers of 'normal' individuals to potentially harmful radiation. A more widely used approach to characterize disease frequency—which avoids the need to undertake screening surveys—is to review series of radiographs that have already been taken for clinical purposes. This approach is usable because the majority of individuals with the disease are asymptomatic, and the radiographs will have been taken for purposes unrelated to the disease.

Pygott [17] studied a series of radiographic reports of the lumbar spine and pelvis from a London hospital taken over a 6-year period. The prevalence of Paget's disease, among those aged 45 years and over, was 3.5 per cent in men and 1.9 per cent in women. Case ascertainment in the study, however, relied on contemporary radiological opinion and it is possible that cases with mild disease may have been overlooked.

Barker [10] obtained series of stored films from radiology departments in different UK hospitals. Radiographs were included for assessment if they showed the complete pelvis, sacrum, both femoral heads, and all lumbar vertebrae (the films included IVPs, barium studies, abdominal X-rays, and those taken specifically to show the skeleton). These sites were chosen as it was estimated that 95 per cent of individuals with Paget's have involvement of one of these sites [5], thereby reducing underascertainment. All of the radiographs were subsequently assessed for evidence of Paget's disease using standard diagnostic criteria [5]. Using this approach Barker [10] reported that in 31 UK towns, among those aged 55 years and over, the prevalence of disease was 6.2 per cent in men, and 3.9 per cent in women.

The main methodological limitation with this approach is that while the majority of individuals with Paget's disease are indeed asymptomatic, those with Paget's may be more likely (because of symptoms of the disease) to have had radiological investigations performed. Such selection bias would tend to result in an overestimation of the true frequency of the disease. There was some evidence for this in relation to radiographs which had been taken for skeletal purposes (which comprised about 20 per cent of all radiographs)—the prevalence of Paget's being higher than in radiographs taken for non-skeletal purposes (6.3 versus 4.6 per cent) [10]. Additionally, the estimate that

95 per cent of individuals with Paget's have involvement of the lumbar spine, sacrum, pelvis, or femoral heads has been questioned, others suggesting that the proportion of Paget's cases with involvement of these sites is lower [4,21,22].

Screening

Serum alkaline phosphatase (AP) is a marker of bone formation and is increased in individuals with active Paget's disease. It is not, however, specific for the disease and may be elevated in other skeletal (and liver) diseases. Several investigators have characterized disease prevalence using a two-stage screening strategy—initial assessment of AP followed by radiological/clinical assessment in those found to have elevated levels.

Hobson and Pemberton [18], in a small survey of 162 elderly men and women living in Sheffield (UK), found 11 with elevated levels of AP of whom eight were subsequently confirmed as having Paget's disease—a prevalence of 4.9 per cent though, because of the small number of cases, the confidence intervals around this estimate are relatively wide. In a population survey in Sierra de la Cabrera (Spain), among 670 men and women aged 40 years and over who were screened, 133 were found to have elevated AP levels of whom 40 were subsequently confirmed as having Paget's, resulting in an age-adjusted prevalence of 6.4 per cent (one case with a normal AP level was also detected) [19]. Using a similar approach Miron-Canelo [20] reported a prevalence of 5.7 per cent, among men and women aged 40 years and over in Salamanca (Spain).

One of the limitations of using AP as a screening tool is that individuals with early or limited disease—in whom AP can be within the normal range—may be missed, resulting in an underestimate of disease frequency.

Influence of age and sex

The prevalence of Paget's disease increases with age in both men and in women (Table 16.4). As far as is known, the disease does not spontaneously remit and the progressive increase in prevalence with age reflects an accumulation of cases in old age. The disease is uncommon under the age of 40 years. Cases of Paget's disease in children and young adults have been reported, however, some of these may be due to diseases that are similar to Paget's, such as congenital

Table 16.4   Prevalence (%) of Paget's disease by age and sex

Post-mortem series[a]			Radiology survey[b]		
Age (years)	Men	Women	Age (years)	Men	Women
40–49	1.2	0.8			
50–59	2.8	2.5	45–54	0.4	0.5
60–69	3.6	3.1	55–64	2.9	1.4
70–79	3.9	1.7	65–74	7.4	3.6
80–89	7.8	4.2	75–84	7.0	2.9
90+	11.1	10.0	85+	8.6	11.4

[a]Source: [15]
[b]Source: [17]

hyperphosphatasia [23,24] or familial expansile osteolysis [25].

Most population surveys suggest that Paget's is more common in men—estimates of the male to female ratio range from 1.4 to 1.9 [8,10,15,17]. There is some evidence, however, that among those with clinically diagnosed disease, the male excess is less marked [4].

Influence of race and geography

The frequency of Paget's disease varies widely in the different regions and populations of the world. Data are available from several sources; however, the best evidence derives from a series of surveys of stored clinical radiographs, which were undertaken using the standard methods of sampling and diagnosis described by Barker *et al.* [10]. The main findings from these hospital-based radiographic surveys are presented in Tables 16.5–16.7 and are discussed below, together with data from other sources.

United Kingdom

Barker *et al.* [10] found evidence of marked variation in occurrence of Paget's disease within the UK, ranging from 2.3 per cent (both sexes) in Aberdeen to 8.3 per cent in Lancaster, see Table 16.5. The highest frequency was observed in Lancashire—a county in the North-west of England with rates over 6 per cent occurring in a cluster of six towns in the area.

Selection bias is unlikely to explain the findings. Standardization to allow for the different proportions of radiographs performed for musculoskeletal reasons at individual centres had little effect on the ranking of towns according to prevalence, and if anything the 'Lancashire focus' became more marked. In a repeat UK survey 20 years later, using similar methodology,

Table 16.5   Prevalence (%) of Paget's disease among men and women aged 55 years and over in 31 towns in the United Kingdom; reproduced by permission of BMJ Publishing Group from Barker D.J., Chamberlain A.T., Guyer P.B., Gardner M.J. *BMJ* 1980; 280: 1105–1107[10]

Town	No. of patients	Prevalence (%)		
		Men[a]	Women[a]	Both[b]
Aberdeen	899	2.0	2.6	2.3
Bath	998	5.3	4.7	5.0
Birkenhead	994	4.4	3.2	3.8
Blackburn	595	8.8	3.8	6.3
Blackpool	949	6.5	4.1	5.3
Bolton	602	7.7	6.4	7.1
Bradford	1000	7.9	3.6	5.8
Burnley	979	8.2	4.9	6.5
Cardiff	999	6.6	3.3	4.9
Carlisle	1482	3.9	1.5	2.7
Chester	970	5.6	2.9	4.2
Glasgow	938	6.3	4.6	5.4
Hull	1000	7.6	3.1	5.3
Ipswich	997	6.5	3.8	5.1
Lancaster	626	6.5	10.0	8.3
Leicester	1021	7.8	3.1	5.5
Macclesfield	890	5.3	4.4	4.8
Middlesborough	734	5.9	3.9	4.9
Newcastle	1002	3.9	2.6	3.2
Oldham	917	5.4	3.2	4.3
Plymouth	959	6.8	2.7	4.7
Portsmouth	999	5.4	3.9	4.6
Preston	1000	8.6	6.3	7.5
Reading	989	7.3	2.7	5.0
Rochdale	1104	4.0	3.1	3.5
Southampton	1000	6.6	3.6	5.1
Stoke	1000	4.7	4.2	4.5
Warrington	809	4.5	3.9	4.2
Whitehaven	1002	7.1	3.4	5.2
Wigan	600	8.1	5.4	6.8
York	1000	5.8	2.5	4.2
All	29 054	6.2	3.9	5.0

[a] Age standardized
[b] Age and sex standardized

Table 16.6 Prevalence (%) of Paget's disease among men and women aged 55 years and over in European populations

Reference	Country/centre	No. of patients	Men[a]	Women[a]	Both[b]
[26]	Ireland				
	Dublin	938	1.8	1.6	1.7
	Galway	714	0.6	0.7	0.7
[11]	France				
	Bordeaux	946	3.9	1.5	2.7
	Rennes	934	3.7	1.0	2.4
	Nancy	939	2.7	1.2	2.0
	Spain				
	Valencia	749	0.7	1.9	1.3
	La Coruna	1017	1.0	0.9	0.9
	Germany				
	Essen	972	1.4	1.2	1.3
	Denmark				
	Copenhagen	1006	1.4	0.8	1.1
	Italy				
	Milan	1061	1.6	0.4	1.0
	Palermo	509	0.3	0.7	0.5
	Austria				
	Innsbruck	1041	0.7	0.6	0.7
	Holland				
	Drachten	716	1.3	0.0	0.6
	Greece				
	Athens	901	0.6	0.3	0.5
	Sweden				
	Malmo	1027	0.2	0.6	0.4

[a] Age standardized
[b] Age and sex standardized

Table 16.7 Prevalence (%) of Paget's disease among men and women aged 55 years and over in non-European populations

Reference	Country/centre	No. of patients	Men[a]	Women[a]	Both[b]
	Australia				
[27]	Perth	2145	5.1	3.1	4.1
	New Zealand				
[12]	Dunedin	1000	5.4	3.4	4.4
	South Africa				
[28]	Johannesburg				
	Whites	1003	2.6	2.2	2.4
	Blacks	1355	1.2	1.3	1.3
	US				
[29]	New York				
	Whites	1082	5.2	2.5	3.9
	Blacks	950	3.3	2.0	2.6
	Atlanta				
	Whites	1563	0.9	0.8	0.9
	Blacks	1111	1.9	0.6	1.2
	Israel				
[30]	Jerusalem				
	Jews	1013	1.3	0.6	1.0
	Arabs	370	0.0	0.0	0.0

[a] Age standardized
[b] Age and sex standardized
(except Australia where figures represent crude rates)

the overall frequency of the disease was less than in the earlier survey though the degree of geographic variation was similar and the disease remained most frequent in Lancashire (see below) [8].

Europe (non UK)

The frequency of Paget's disease is lower in the rest of Europe than the UK, though, as in the UK, there is evidence of variation in occurrence both within and between individual countries, see Table 16.6, [11]. Among European countries the disease appears to be most common in France, with rates in some towns approaching those in the UK. Perhaps surprisingly, despite the close geographic proximity to the UK, the disease appears to be infrequent in Ireland [26]. The disease is uncommon in Scandinavia and in southern Europe, though single centre studies, undertaken using differing methodology (initial screening using alkaline phosphatase with subsequent radiographic confirmation) suggest there are pockets with relatively high frequency in some areas of Spain including the Sierra de la Cabrera (Madrid) and Salamanca [19,20].

The findings, in relation to geographic heterogeneity, are supported by the results of a large postal questionnaire survey of radiologists across Europe, who were asked about the frequency with which they observed Paget's disease [11]. Outside the UK, the disease was most frequent in France and less common in Scandinavia and southern Europe.

North America, Australia, and New Zealand

Outside the UK, the countries with the highest frequency of Paget's disease are New Zealand and Australia [12,27], see Table 16.7, though within these countries the disease is very rare among the native aboriginal and Maori populations [31,32]. Within the US, as elsewhere, there is evidence of geographic variation in occurrence—in a comparative study the disease was more frequent among residents of New York than Atlanta [29]. The prevalence of the disease was similar in blacks and whites in these two cities, see Table 16.7. Among native Americans the disease appears to be rare [14].

Africa

In the past Paget's disease has been considered to be rare in native Africans [33,34]. In a radiological survey undertaken in Johannesburg (South Africa), however, Guyer *et al.* [28] reported a prevalence of 1.3 per cent among native Africans, see Table 16.7. Among white south Africans the prevalence of disease was 2.4 per cent. Elsewhere in the African subcontinent, though, there remain few reports of the disease [35–38].

Asia, Middle East, South America

Based on the available case reports and case series, Paget's disease appears rare in India, China, and Japan [39–45]. There are no population data, though in Japan a review of over 6900 radionucleotide scans suggested a frequency of 0.22 per cent [46].

In Israel, in a survey of stored hospital radiographs, the frequency of the disease among Jews was 1 per cent, see Table 16.7 [30]. In contrast, no evidence of the disease was found in a series of 370 Arabs. There are no population data from South America, though clinical series suggest heterogeneity in disease occurrence, being more frequent in and around Buenos Aries (Argentina) than other areas studied, including Chile and Venezuela [47].

Migrant studies

Studies of migrant groups are of help in determining the contribution of genetic and environmental factors to disease susceptibility. There has been substantial migration from Britain, an area of high frequency of the disease, to Australia, an area of lower frequency. Gardner *et al.* [27] looked at birth status (UK or Australian) among individuals who had been included in a hospital-based survey of Paget's disease in Perth, western Australia. The frequency of the disease was lower among those who had been born in the UK and then emigrated than those who continued to reside in the UK [5,27] (Table 16.8). The decline in prevalence

Table 16.8 Prevalence (%) of Paget's disease among men and women aged 55 years and over by place of birth and residence; reproduced by permission of BMJ Publishing Group from Gardner M.J., Guyer PB, Barker D.J. *BMJ* 1978; 1: 1655–1657[27]

Place of birth	Residence	Prevalence (%)		
		Men[a]	Women[a]	Both[b]
UK	UK	7.0	3.8	5.4
UK	Australia	5.7	2.3	4.0
Australia	Australia	3.5	2.8	3.2

[a] Age standardized
[b] Age and sex standardized

that follows migration from the United Kingdom suggests that environmental factors are important in pathogenesis.

The rates among the migrants did not, however, fall to the levels among Australian natives, suggesting, either that the migrants carried with them environmental risk factors which persisted, or that the disease had in fact developed (as either latent or sub-clinical disease) while they had been living in the UK. In a small study among the British migrants, there did not appear to be any difference in the age at migration between those with and without Paget's disease [13].

Secular trends

Paleopathologic evidence suggests that Paget's disease may have affected mankind since the Neolithic period [48]. However, the most convincing evidence of the antiquity of the disease is the finding of a virtually intact skeleton with classic features, excavated from an Anglo-Saxon burial ground in Durham (UK), dating to approximately AD 950 [49].

Despite its antiquity, there is circumstantial evidence that the epidemiology of Paget's disease may have changed during the last century, with a decline in frequency and severity of the disease. The evidence for this derives from several sources including population surveys, mortality statistics and clinical series. These are reviewed below.

Population surveys

In the UK, two cross-sectional prevalence surveys of stored radiographs, separated by a 20-year time period, were undertaken in men and women aged 55 years and over in 10 towns [8,10]. In the earlier survey, the age and sex adjusted prevalence of Paget's disease was 5 per cent, see Table 16.9. In the later survey, using similar methods (and indeed the same study radiologist) the prevalence was 2 per cent. The decrease in frequency was observed in both men and women and in all 10 towns studied.

Mortality

Paget's disease
Paget's disease is rarely fatal, and mortality statistics are an unreliable indicator of disease incidence, however, they provide some insight into the secular pattern of disease occurrence. In the UK there has

Table 16.9 Prevalence (%) of Paget's disease in men and women aged 55 years and over in 10 UK towns: 1974 and 1994

Centre	Prevalence (%)[a]		Ratio 1974/1994
	1974[b]	1994[c]	
Bath	5.0	2.2	2.3
Cardiff	4.9	1.5	3.3
Carlisle	2.7	1.2	2.3
Lancaster	8.3	3.7	2.2
Newcastle	3.2	3.1	1.0
Portsmouth	4.6	2.1	2.2
Preston	7.5	2.4	3.1
Southampton	5.1	2.7	1.9
Warrington	4.2	3.1	1.4
Wigan	6.8	3.5	1.9
All	5.0	2.0	2.5

[a] Age and sex standardized
[b] Source: [10]
[c] Source: [8]

been a gradual decline in mortality due to Paget's disease between 1951 and 1970 (Fig. 16.1) [50]. When analysed by birth cohort, death rates were highest among those born in the 1880s, and have declined progressively since then, (Fig. 16.2). A similar pattern of decline in mortality due to Paget's has been observed in the US [51].

Primary bone tumours
Paget's disease is associated with an increase in the risk of osteosarcoma [52]. The rise in mortality from primary bone tumours in middle age and later life is largely due to osteosarcoma linked with Paget's

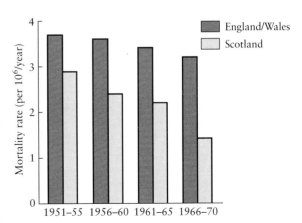

Fig. 16.1 Annual mortality rate (per 10[6]) from Paget's disease among men and women: England/Wales and Scotland, 1951–1970. Data from [50].

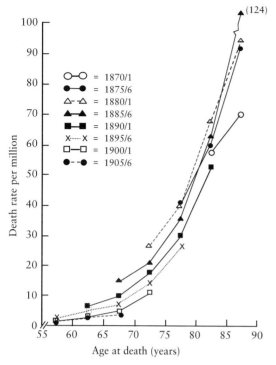

Fig. 16.2 Cohort mortality from Paget's disease in England and Wales in 5-year periods, 1951–1975, ages 55 years and over. Reproduced by permission of Oxford University Press from [51].

disease. Mortality statistics from both the UK and US suggest a gradual decline in deaths due to primary bone tumours between 1951 and 1975 [51]. When analysed by birth cohort, deaths from primary bone tumours have declined progressively since 1870. Some caution is required in interpreting this data—not all primary bone tumours are associated with Paget's disease and a proportion of primary tumours are actually secondary bone tumours which have been misclassified as primary. Nevertheless, the data are consistent with the Paget's mortality data indicating that there has been a recent decrease in the frequency of the disease.

Clinical series

Cundy *et al.* [53] reviewed records of 1041 patients referred to a Paget's clinic in New Zealand between 1973 and 1993. Over this time period there was a reduction in the number of patients referred to the clinic with severe disease as determined by the alkaline phosphatase level at presentation. In addition, the average age of newly referred patients increased. The

observations suggest the severity of the disease has declined in recent years.

Cyclic trends

In an analysis of 386 patients belonging to a UK patients' association, who were born between 1888 and 1924, there was evidence of a fluctuating distribution of years of birth with a periodicity of around 3 years. The periodicity was not, however, present over all years and did not attain conventional levels of statistical significance [54]. Nevertheless the finding is of interest—evidence of cyclic variation in disease occurrence would tend to support an infectious aetiology for the disease.

Genetic factors

Familial clustering

Data from studies of clinically diagnosed cases indicate that 1–14 per cent of affected individuals report a positive family history of Paget's disease [4,54–58]. Sofaer *et al.* [54], in a survey of members of a UK patient organization, found a 10-fold increase in the risk of disease among parents and siblings of index cases compared with spouse controls. Using a similar method, Siris *et al.* [58] reported a seven-fold increase in risk. One of the methodological limitations in assessing familial risk in Paget's disease is that the disease is often sub-clinical and affected relatives may be unaware they have it —the effect of this might be to tend to underestimate the strength of any familial risk. In a more comprehensive survey of relatives of affected cases, using a combination of alkaline phosphatase, and radionucleotide scans, Morales-Piga *et al.* [59] reported that of 35 index cases, 40 per cent had at least one first-degree relative with the disease.

Familial aggregation may be explained on the basis of genetic factors, a shared environment, or an interaction between them. Data from multicase families point to an autosomal dominant pattern of inheritance; however, such families are relatively uncommon [60].

Immunogenetics

Data from multicase families with up to three generations affected suggest probable linkage with the histocompatibility (HLA) loci on chromosome 6 [61,62]. More recent data, however, do not support evidence of linkage [63].

Studies looking at associations with specific HLA antigens have yielded conflicting results. Early studies revealed no evidence of an association between Paget's disease and either HLA-A or B antigens [64,65], though a later report suggested an association with A9 and B15 [4].

Singer *et al.* [66] studied 53 patients and a group of controls and found a significant risk associated with DQw1 (86.2 vs. 49.6 per cent) and DR2 (45.3 vs. 25.1 per cent) while DR3 (9.4 vs. 22.1 per cent) and DR7 (11.3 vs. 23.9 per cent) appeared protective. Gordon *et al.* [67] in a study of 81 cases and 29 controls, however, found no association with DR2, DR3, or DR7. DPw4 was more frequent among Paget's patients (82.7 vs. 62.1 per cent), while DPw6 was less frequent (2.5 vs. 13.7 per cent).

In an Israeli study, comprising 31 cases and 106 controls, there was a significant increase in the antigen frequency of HLA-A2, Bw52, and DR2 in Paget's patients compared with controls [68]. In a study of Ashkenazi Jews comprising 40 cases and 199 controls, Singer *et al.* [69] reported that DRβ1*1104 was associated with a 7.5-fold increase in risk of the disease.

Chromosome 18q

Familial expansile osteolysis (FEO) is a rare bone dysplasia which is inherited as an autosomal dominant trait [25]. There are similarities both clinically and histologically with Paget's disease though the disease differs in that it affects individuals at an earlier age and involves predominantly the appendicular skeleton. Based on a large kindred in Northern Ireland, the gene for the disease was found to show tight linkage with several polymorphic markers on chromosome 18q [70].

Cody *et al.* [71] looked at linkage of Paget's disease to chromosome 18q in a large multicase family. Analysis yielded a two point Lod score of 3.4 with the genetic marker D18S42—a marker tightly linked to the FEO locus, suggesting that within the family, the gene(s) for Paget's and FEO were either closely linked or the same locus. Similar linkage was observed in a large French pedigree [72]. Haslam *et al.* [60] looked in eight multicase families and found linkage with the susceptibility region in 18q in five families. Data from the other three families did not, however, support evidence of linkage at the site, suggesting the presence of additional loci. Further evidence for genetic heterogeneity in disease susceptibility has come from a larger study of 41 families, in which evidence of linkage with the susceptibility region in 18q, although present in some families, was uncommon [73].

Several genes have been mapped to the susceptibility region in 18q including Bcl-2—a suppressor of apoptosis [74]. Recently it has been shown that mutations in TNFRSF11A, the gene encoding receptor activator of nuclear factor-κ B (RANK), cause FEO [75].

Environmental factors

The major interest in relation to the study of the environmental determinants of Paget's disease has been the role of infectious agents. Evidence has been derived from a combination of direct and indirect sources and is reviewed below together with data concerning other environmental exposures.

Paramyxovirus infection

In 1974, using electron microscopy, Rebel reported evidence of inclusion bodies in Pagetic osteoclasts, a finding that has been confirmed by others [76–78]. Morphologically these inclusion bodies resembled inclusions observed in cells infected with paramyxoviruses, and suggested a possible role for these viruses in the pathogenesis of Paget's disease.

Paramyxoviruses are single stranded RNA viruses, found in a variety of human and animal diseases, including measles, parainfluenza, respiratory syncytial virus (RSV), and canine distemper virus (CDV) [79]. Despite intensive investigation, however, the role of paramyxovirus infection in the pathogenesis of Paget's disease remains uncertain.

The cellular inclusions are not specific for the disease and are found in other bone diseases including pycnodystosis [80], osteopetrosis [81], and primary oxalosis [82]. Serological studies show no difference in level of antibodies to common paramyxovirus infections among those with and those without Paget's disease, though this does not exclude a possible aetiological role for paramyxovirus infection [83–86].

Immunohistochemical studies have shown variously the presence of antigens of several paramyxoviruses in Pagetic bone including measles [87–89], RSV [90] or both [88] as well as simian virus 5 and parainfluenza [87]. *In situ* hybridization studies have shown evidence of measles [91] and CDV RNA [92,93] in Pagetic bone. Using reverse transcription polymerase chain reaction (RT-PCR), CDV or measles virus have been detected by different groups [94,95], and CDV also in 15/15 samples using *in situ* RT-PCR [96]. The RT-PCR findings have not, however, been replicated in other laboratories [97,98].

At present therefore, while there is evidence suggestive of viral involvement, there is currently insufficient evidence to implicate paramyxoviruses as causal agents in the pathogenesis of Paget's disease.

Pet ownership

Because of the putative viral aetiology, evidence of previous exposure to viral illnesses has been sought by several investigators. The main results are shown in Table 16.10. O'Driscoll and colleagues hypothesized that animals and, more particularly, domestic pets might be the source of infection [99]. They compared past exposure to pets among 50 Paget's patients and 50 age and sex-matched control subjects with diabetes mellitus. A history of previous dog ownership was significantly more common in the patients than controls (odds ratios [OR] at different ages varied between 4 and 8). There was no association with previous exposure to domestic cats or birds. Similar findings were observed in an extended study by the same group and using a different (general practice) control group [107]. The link with dog ownership suggested that if there

was a viral aetiology, then canine distemper virus may have been the responsible agent.

Other investigators who have studied the association between Paget's disease and domestic pets have found conflicting results. Several observational studies reported no link with previous dog ownership [100,102,104,108]. Others, however, provide some supportive evidence. Holdaway *et al.* [103] studied 112 Paget's patients and a similar number of community controls. Overall, there was no association with previous dog or cat ownership, however, in sub-group analyses, among those less than 60 years, dog ownership (OR = 3.8; 95% CI 1.4, 13.0) was associated with an increased risk of the disease.

Morales-Piga *et al.* [101] studied 41 Paget's patients and 629 controls, both recruited during the course of a community survey, and found a small, though non-significant, association with contact with domestic pets (OR = 2.5; 95% CI 0.9, 7.3), though individual pet types were not distinguished. Lopez-Abente *et al.* [106] studied 149 patients and 150 rheumatology outpatient controls in two areas of Spain—Madrid and La Rioja. Overall there was no association with previous contact with dogs, though in sub-group analyses, among those who lived in La Rioja there was an increased risk of the disease associated with previous contact with dogs (OR = 3.7; 95% CI 1.1, 11.8). There was an increased

Table 16.10   Studies of the relationship between pet ownership and the risk of Paget's disease

Reference	Cases	Controls	Exposure	OR[a] (95% CI[b])
[99]	50	50	Dog	4–8[c,d]
			Cat	1
			Budgerigar	2.3
[100]	36	72	Dog	0.8 (0.4,1.8)
	26	47	Dog	1.4 (0.6,3.6)
[101]	41	629	Pets	2.5 (0.9,7.3)
[102]	433	433	Dog	0.9–1.6[c]
			Cat	0.8–1.3[c]
[103]	112	112	Dog	1.7 (0.9,3.2)
			Cat	1.0 (0.6,1.8)
			Bird	0.7 (0.3,1.2)
[104]	247	281	Dog	1.0 (0.7,1.4)
			Cat	0.6 (0.4,0.9)
[105]	150	185	Dog (vaccinated)	1.1 (0.7,1.8)
			Dog (unvaccinated)	2.8 (1.7,4.5)
			Cat	2.2 (1.0,5.0)
			Bird	2.3 (1.0,5.3)
[106]	149	150	Dog	1.8 (1.0,3.4)
			Cat	2.2 (1.3,3.9)

[a] Odds ratio
[b] 95% confidence interval
[c] Range of ORs at different ages
[d] p <0.05

risk associated with previous contact with cats (OR = 2.2).

Other factors such as the type of dog or its vaccination status (to canine distemper virus) may be important. Khan *et al.* [105] studied 150 cases and 185 hospital based controls, and found that overall, past dog ownership did not increase the risk of Paget's disease. Ownership of a mongrel dog (OR = 1.7; 95% CI 1.1, 2.7) and an unvaccinated dog (OR = 2.8; 95% CI 1.7, 4.5) both increased the risk, though after taking into account vaccination status, the species of dog did not appear to matter. Ownership of a dog with a history of canine distemper virus infection was not associated with Paget's, however, the numbers with distemper were few and the illness may have not been recognized by some owners. In the same study, after excluding those who had owned a dog, ownership of cats (OR = 2.2) and birds (OR = 2.3) also increased the risk of Paget's.

Although these data are somewhat conflicting, they are consistent with an association between Paget's disease and exposure to domestic pets. The evidence appears stronger for previous dog ownership, and particularly unvaccinated dogs, than for other pets.

Childhood illness

Renier *et al.* [104] reported a significant association between Paget's disease and a history of measles in childhood (OR=2.5; 95% CI 1.5, 4.0), however, the finding was not confirmed in two other observational studies [102,107]. Other childhood infectious diseases which have been studied including varicella, mumps, polio, and rubella do not appear to be associated with the disease [104,109].

Diet

Results from two Spanish studies suggest that consumption of certain animal foods may confer an increased risk of Paget's disease. Morales-Piga *et al.* [101] reported that consumption of lamb and/or goat meat without adequate sanitary (veterinary) inspection was associated with an increased risk of Paget's disease (OR=2.2; 95% CI 1.1, 4.5). Lopez-Abente *et al.* [106] reported that consumption of meat traceable to sick livestock (OR=2.7; 95% CI 1.0, 7.4) and frequent consumption during youth of brains (OR=1.8; 95% CI 1.1, 3.0) and other animal viscera were associated with an increased risk of Paget's. In an American study,

milk consumption during childhood was lower among Paget's patients than a group of controls [102].

Other

Siris *et al.* [102] reported no difference in childhood environment (rural, urban, suburban) or socio-economic status between Paget's patients and a group of controls. To date, no association has been observed between Paget's disease and occupations linked with animals including vets [110], farmers, hunters, or taxidermists [101,106].

References

1. Paget J. On a form of chronic inflammation of bones. *Med Chir Trans* 1877; **60**: 37–63.
2. Wilks S. Osteitis deformans. *Lancet* 1909; **2**: 1627.
3. Collins DH. Paget's disease of bone. Incidence and subclinical forms. *Lancet* 1956; **2**: 51–57.
4. Kanis JA. *Pathophysiology and treatment of Paget's disease*. London: Martin Dunitz, 1998.
5. Barker DJ, Clough PW, Guyer PB, Gardner MJ. Paget's disease of bone in 14 British towns. *BMJ* 1977; **1**: 1181–1183.
6. Cooper C, Dennison E, Schafheutle K, Kellingray S, Guyer P, Barker D. Epidemiology of Paget's disease of bone. *Bone* 1999; **24**: 3S–5S.
7. Shanks SC, Kerley P. *A textbook of X-ray diagnosis*. London: Lewis, 1971.
8. Cooper C, Schafheutle K, Dennison E, Kellingray S, Guyer P, Barker D. The epidemiology of Paget's disease in Britain: is the prevalence decreasing? *J Bone Miner Res* 1999; **14**: 192–197.
9. Murray RO, Jacobson HG. *The radiology of skeletal disorders*. London: Churchill Livingstone, 1972.
10. Barker DJ, Chamberlain AT, Guyer PB, Gardner MJ. Paget's disease of bone: the Lancashire focus. *BMJ* 1980; **280**: 1105–1107.
11. Detheridge FM, Guyer PB, Barker DJ. European distribution of Paget's disease of bone. *BMJ* 1982; **285**: 1005–1008.
12. Reasbeck JC, Goulding A, Campbell DR, Beale LR, Stewart RD. Radiological prevalence of Paget's disease in Dunedin, New Zealand. *BMJ* 1983; **286**: 1937.
13. Barker DJ. The epidemiology of Paget's disease of bone. *Br Med Bull* 1984; **40**: 396–400.
14. Lawrence JS. *Rheumatism in populations*. London: Heinemann, 1977.
15. Schmorl G. Uber osteitis deformans Paget. *Virchows Arch Pathol Anat Physiol* 1932; **283**: 694–751.
16. Altman RD, Bloch DA, Hochberg MC, Murphy WA. Prevalence of pelvic Paget's disease of bone in the United States. *J Bone Miner Res* 2000; **15**: 461–465.
17. Pygott F. Paget's disease of the bone. The radiological incidence. *Lancet* 1957; **1**: 1170–1171.

18. Hobson W, Pemberton J. *The health of the elderly at home*. London: Butterworths, 1955.

19. Morales-Piga A, Lopez-Abente G, Vadillo AG, Ibanez AE, Lanza MG. Features of Paget's disease of bone in a new high-prevalence focus. *Med Clin (Barc)* 1990; **95**: 169–174.

20. Miron-Canelo JA, Del Pino-Montes J, Vicente-Arroyo M, Saenz-Gonzalez MC. Epidemiological study of Paget's disease of bone in a zone of the province of Salamanca (Spain). The Paget's disease of the bone study group of Salamanca. *Eur J Epidemiol* 1997; **13**: 801–805.

21. Guyer PB, Clough PW. Paget's diseases of bone: some observations on the relation of the skeletal distribution to pathogenesis. *Clin Radiol* 1978; **29**: 421–426.

22. Merrick MV, Merrick JM. Observations on the natural history of Paget's disease. *Clin Radiol* 1985; **36**: 169–174.

23. Eyring EJ, Eisenberg E. Congenital hyperphosphatasia. A clinical, pathological, and biochemical study of two cases. *J Bone Joint Surg Am* 1968; **50**: 1099–1117.

24. Golob DS, McAlister WH, Mills BG *et al*. Juvenile Paget disease: life-long features of a mildly affected young woman. *J Bone Miner Res* 1996; **11**: 132–142.

25. Osterberg PH, Wallace RG, Adams DA *et al*. Familial expansile osteolysis. A new dysplasia. *J Bone Joint Surg Br* 1988; **70**: 255–260.

26. Detheridge FM, Barker DJ, Guyer PB. Paget's disease of bone in Ireland. *BMJ* 1983; **287**: 1345–1346.

27. Gardner MJ, Guyer PB, Barker DJ. Radiological prevalence of Paget's disease of bone in British migrants to Australia. *BMJ* 1978; **1**: 1655–1657.

28. Guyer PB, Chamberlain AT. Paget's disease of bone in South Africa. *Clin Radiol* 1988; **39**: 51–52.

29. Guyer PB, Chamberlain AT. Paget's disease of bone in two American cities. *BMJ* 1980; **280**: 985.

30. Bloom RA, Libson E, Blank P, Nubani N. Prevalence of Paget's disease of bone in hospital patients in Jerusalem: an epidemiologic study. *Isr J Med Sci* 1985; **21**: 954–956.

31. Barry HC. Paget's disease of bone in an aboriginal. *Med J Aust* 1968; **1**: 955.

32. Barry HC. *Paget's disease of the bone*. Edinburgh and London: E and S Livingstone, 1969.

33. Robertson MM, Thomas AF. Osteitis deformans in the South African negro. A report of 3 cases. *S Afr Med J* 1978; **53**: 183–185.

34. van Meerdervoort HFP, Richter GG. Paget's disease of bone in South African Blacks. *S Afr Med J* 1976; **50**: 1897–1899.

35. Bohrer SP. Osteitis deformans in Nigerians. *Afr J Med Sci* 1970; **1**: 109–113.

36. Collomb H, Dumas M, Peytral G, Jabiol M, Petit M. Paget's disease of bone in the Senegal (4 cases of which one was complicated by Pott's disease). *Bull Soc Med Afr Noire Lang Fr* 1967; **12**: 125–130.

37. Dahniya MH. Paget's disease of bone in Africans. *Br J Radiol* 1987; **60**: 113–116.

38. Dodge OG. Bone tumours in Uganda Africans. *Br J Cancer* 1964; **18**: 627–633.

39. Barry HC. Orthopaedic surgery in modern China. *J Bone Joint Surg Br* 1957; **39B**: 800–802.

40. Bhardwaj OP. Monostotic Paget's disease of the bone. *J Indian Med Assoc* 1964; **43**: 341–342.

41. Chakrabarty RP, Bhardwaj OP. Paget's disease of the bone. *J Indian Med Assoc* 1963; **41**: 126–127.

42. Ehara S. Paget's disease of bone in Japan. *Am J Roentgenol* 1998; **170**: 1110.

43. Hsu LF, Rajasoorya C. A case series of Paget's disease of bone: diagnosing a rather uncommon condition in Singapore. *Ann Acad Med Singapore* 1998; **27**: 289–293.

44. Kumar K. Paget's disease of bone. *J Indian Med Assoc* 1986; **84**: 316–318.

45. Yip KM, Lee YL, Kumta SM, Lin J. The second case of Paget's disease (osteitis deformans) in a Chinese lady. *Singapore Med J* 1996; **37**: 665–667.

46. Ishikawa Y, Tsukuma H, Miller RW. Low rates of Paget's disease of bone and osteosarcoma in elderly Japanese. *Lancet* 1996; **347**: 1559.

47. Mautalen C, Pumarino H, Blanco MC, Gonzalez D, Ghiringhelli G, Fromm G. Paget's disease: the South American experience. *Semin Arthritis Rheum* 1994; **23**: 226–227.

48. Pales L. Maldie de Paget prehistorique. *Anthropologie* 1929; **39**: 263–270.

49. Wells C, Woodhouse N. Paget's disease in an Anglo-Saxon. *Med Hist* 1975; **19**: 396–400.

50. Barker DJ, Gardner MJ. Distribution of Paget's disease in England, Wales and Scotland and a possible relationship with vitamin D deficiency in childhood. *Br J Prev Soc Med* 1974; **28**: 226–232.

51. Gardner MJ, Barker DJ. Mortality from malignant tumours of bone and Paget's disease in the United States and in England and Wales. *Int J Epidemiol* 1978; **7**: 121–130.

52. Price CHG. The incidence of oestrogenic sarcoma in Southwest England and its relationship to Paget's disease of the bone. *J Bone Joint Surg Br* 1962; **44B**: 366–376.

53. Cundy T, McAnulty K, Wattie D, Gamble G, Rutland M, Ibbertson HK. Evidence for secular change in Paget's disease. *Bone* 1997; **20**: 69–71.

54. Sofaer JA, Holloway SM, Emery AE. A family study of Paget's disease of bone. *J Epidemiol Community Health* 1983; **37**: 226–231.

55. Dickson DD, Camp JD, Ghormley RK. Osteitis deformans: Paget's disease of the bone. *Radiology* 1945; **44**: 449–470.

56. Galbraith HJ, Evans EC, Lacey J. Paget's disease of bone—a clinical and genetic study. *Postgrad Med J* 1977; **53**: 33–39.

57. Rosenkrantz JA, Wolf J, Kaicher JJ. Paget's disease (osteitis deformans). Review of 111 cases. *Arch Intern Med* 1952; **90**: 610–633.

58. Siris ES, Ottman R, Flaster E, Kelsey JL. Familial aggregation of Paget's disease of bone. *J Bone Miner Res* 1991; **6**: 495–499.

59. Morales-Piga A, Rey-Rey JS, Corres-Gonzalez J, Garcia-Sagredo JM, Lopez-Abente G. Frequency and characteristics of familial aggregation of Paget's disease of the bone. *J Bone Miner Res* 1995; **10**: 663–670.

60. Haslam SI, Hul WV, Morales-Piga A *et al*. Paget's disease of bone: evidence for a susceptibility locus on

chromosome 18q and for genetic heterogeneity. *J Bone Miner Res* 1998; **13**: 911–917.

61. Fotino M, Haymovits A, Falk CT. Evidence for linkage between HLA and Paget's disease. *Transplant Proc* 1977; **9**: 1867–1868.

62. Tilyard MW, Gardner RJ, Milligan L, Cleary TA, Stewart RD. A probable linkage between familial Paget's disease and the HLA loci. *Aust N Z J Med* 1982; **12**: 498–500.

63. Moore SB, Hoffman DL. Absence of HLA linkage in a family with osteitis deformans (Paget's disease of bone). *Tissue Antigens* 1988; **31**: 69–70.

64. Cullen P, Russell RG, Walton RJ, Whiteley J. Frequencies of HLA-A and HLA-B histocompatibility antigens in Paget's disease of bone. *Tissue Antigens* 1976; **7**: 55–56.

65. Roux H, Mercier P, Maestracci D, Eisinger J, Recordier AM. HLA and Paget's disease. *Rev Rhum Mal Osteoartic* 1975; **42**: 661–662.

66. Singer FR, Mills BG, Park MS, Takemura S, Terasaki PI. Increased HLA-DQW1 antigen pattern in Paget's disease of the bone. *Clin Res* 1985; **33**: 574A.

67. Gordon MT, Cartwright EJ, Mercer S, Anderson DC, Sharpe PT. HLA polymorphisms in Paget's disease of bone. *Semin Arthritis Rheum* 1994; **23**: 229.

68. Foldes J, Shamir S, Scherman L, Menczel J, Brautbar C. Histocompatibility antigens and Paget's disease of the bone. *Calcif Tissue Int* 1987; **41**: 59.

69. Singer FR, Siris ES, Knieriem A, Gjertson D, Terasaki PI. The HLA DR beta1*1104 gene frequency is increased in Ashkenazi Jews with Paget's disease of bone. *J Bone Miner Res* 1996; **11**: M752–M752.

70. Hughes AE, Shearman AM, Weber JL *et al.* Genetic linkage of familial expansile osteolysis to chromosome 18q. *Hum Mol Genet* 1994; **3**: 359–361.

71. Cody JD, Singer FR, Roodman GD *et al.* Genetic linkage of Paget disease of the bone to chromosome 18q. *Am J Hum Genet* 1997; **61**: 1117–1122.

72. Lucotte G. Genetic linkage of Paget's disease to chromosome 18q in a French pedigree. *Bone* 1999; **24**: 31S.

73. Hocking LJ, Slee F, van Hul W *et al.* A multicentre study of chromosome 18q linkage in familial Paget's disease. *Bone* 1999; **24**: 31S.

74. Reed JC. Double identity for proteins of the Bcl-2 family. *Nature* 1997; **387**: 773–776.

75. Hughes AE, Ralston SH, Marken J *et al.* Mutations in TNFRSF11A, affecting the signal peptide of RANK, cause familial expansile osteolysis. *Nat Genet* 2000; **24**: 45–48.

76. Gherardi G, Lo-Cascio V, Bonucci E. Fine structure of nuclei and cytoplasm of osteoclasts in Paget's disease of bone. *Histopathology* 1980; **4**: 63–74.

77. Mills BG, Singer FR. Nuclear inclusions in Paget's disease of bone. *Science* 1976; **194**: 201–202.

78. Rebel A, Malkani K, Basle M. Nuclear anomalies in osteoclasts in Paget's bone disease. *Nouv Presse Med* 1974; **3**: 1299–1301.

79. Mee AP. Paramyxoviruses and their possible role in Paget's disease. In: Sharpe PT, editor. *The molecular biology of Paget's disease*. Texas: Springer, 1996: 59–99.

80. Beneton MN, Harris S, Kanis JA. Paramyxovirus-like inclusions in two cases of Pycnodysostosis. *Bone* 1987; **8**: 211–217.

81. Mills BG, Yabe H, Singer FR. Osteoclasts in human osteopetrosis contain viral-nucleocapsid-like nuclear inclusions. *J Bone Miner Res* 1988; **3**: 101–106.

82. Bianco P, Silvestrini G, Ballanti P, Bonucci E. Paramyxovirus-like nuclear inclusions identical to those of Paget's disease of bone detected in giant cells of primary oxalosis. *Virchows Arch A Pathol Anat Histopathol* 1992; **421**: 427–433.

83. Gordon MT, Bell SC, Mee AP, Mercer S, Carter SD, Sharpe PT. Prevalence of canine distemper antibodies in the Pagetic population. *J Med Virol* 1993; **40**: 313–317.

84. Hamill RJ, Baughn RE, Mallette LE, Musher DM, Wilson DB. Serological evidence against role for canine distemper virus in pathogenesis of Paget's disease of bone. *Lancet* 1986; **2**: 1399.

85. Morgan-Capner P, Robinson P, Clewley G, Darby A, Pettingale K. Measles antibody in Paget's disease. *Lancet* 1981; **1**: 733.

86. Winfield J, Sutherland S. Measles antibody in Paget's disease. *Lancet* 1981; **1**: 891.

87. Basle MF, Russell WC, Goswami KK *et al.* Para-myxovirus antigens in osteoclasts from Paget's bone tissue detected by monoclonal antibodies. *J Gen Virol* 1985; **66**: 2103–2110.

88. Mills BG, Singer FR, Weiner LP, Suffin SC, Stabile E, Holst P. Evidence for both respiratory syncytial virus and measles virus antigens in the osteoclasts of patients with Paget's disease of bone. *Clin Orthop* 1984; **183**: 303–311.

89. Rebel A, Basle M, Pouplard A, Kouyoumdjian S, Filmon R, Lepatezour A. Viral antigens in osteo-clasts from Paget's disease of bone. *Lancet* 1980; **2**: 344–346.

90. Mills BG, Singer FR, Weiner LP, Holst PA. Immuno-histological demonstration of respiratory syncytial virus antigens in Paget disease of bone. *Proc Natl Acad Sci U S A* 1981; **78**: 1209–1213.

91. Basle MF, Fournier JG, Rozenblatt S, Rebel A, Bouteille M. Measles virus RNA detected in Paget's disease bone tissue by in situ hybridization. *J Gen Virol* 1986; **67**: 907–913.

92. Cartwright EJ, Gordon MT, Freemont AJ, Anderson DC, Sharpe PT. Paramyxoviruses and Paget's disease. *J Med Virol* 1993; **40**: 133–141.

93. Gordon MT, Anderson DC, Sharpe PT. Canine dis-temper virus localised in bone cells of patients with Paget's disease. *Bone* 1991; **12**: 195–201.

94. Gordon MT, Mee AP, Anderson DC, Sharpe PT. Canine distemper virus transcripts sequenced from Pagetic bone. *Bone Miner* 1992; **19**: 159–174.

95. Reddy SV, Singer FR, Roodman GD. Bone marrow mononuclear cells from patients with Paget's disease contain measles virus nucleocapsid messenger ribo-nucleic acid that has mutations in a specific region of the sequence. *J Clin Endocrinol Metab* 1995; **80**: 2108–2111.

96. Mee AP, Dixon JA, Hoyland JA, Davies M, Selby PL, Mawer EB. Detection of canine distemper virus in 100% of Paget's disease samples by in situ-reverse

transcriptase-polymerase chain reaction. *Bone* 1998; **23**: 171–175.

97. Birch MA, Taylor W, Fraser WD, Ralston SH, Hart CA, Gallagher JA. Absence of paramyxovirus RNA in cultures of Pagetic bone cells and in Pagetic bone. *J Bone Miner Res* 1994; **9**: 11–16.

98. Ralston SH, Digiovine FS, Gallacher SJ, Boyle IT, Duff GW. Failure to detect paramyxovirus sequences in Paget's disease of bone using the polymerase chain reaction. *J Bone Miner Res* 1991; **6**: 1243–1248.

99. O'Driscoll JB, Anderson DC. Past pets and Paget's disease. *Lancet* 1985; **2**: 919–921.

100. Barker DJ, Detheridge FM. Dogs and Paget's disease. *Lancet* 1985; **2**: 1245.

101. Morales-Piga A, Lopez-Abente G, Ibanez AE, Vadillo AG, Lanza MG, Jodra VM. Risk factors for Paget's disease: a new hypothesis. *Int J Epidemiol* 1988; **17**: 198–201.

102. Siris ES, Kelsey JL, Flaster E, Parker S. Paget's disease of bone and previous pet ownership in the United States: dogs exonerated. *Int J Epidemiol* 1990; **19**: 455–458.

103. Holdaway IM, Ibbertson HK, Wattie D, Scragg R, Graham P. Previous pet ownership and Paget's disease. *Bone Miner* 1990; **8**: 53–58.

104. Renier JC, Fanello S, Bos C, Audran M. An etiologic study of Paget's disease. *Rev Rhum Engl Ed* 1996; **63**: 606–611.

105. Khan SA, Brennan P, Newman J, Gray RE, McCloskey EV, Kanis JA. Paget's disease of bone and unvaccinated dogs. *Bone* 1996; **19**: 47–50.

106. Lopez-Abente G, Morales-Piga A, Ibanez EA, Rey-Rey JS, Corres-Gonzalez J. Cattle, pets, and Paget's disease of bone. *Epidemiology* 1997; **8**: 247–251.

107. O'Driscoll JB, Buckler HM, Jeacock J, Anderson DC. Dogs, distemper and osteitis deformans: a further epidemiological study. *Bone Miner* 1990; **11**: 209–216.

108. Stamp TC, Mackney PH, Kelsey CR. Innocent pets and Paget's disease? *Lancet* 1986; **2**: 917.

109. Siris ES. Epidemiological aspects of Paget's disease: family history and relationship to other medical conditions. *Semin Arthritis Rheum* 1994; **23**: 222–225.

110. Holt PE. Dogs and Paget's disease. *Lancet* 1985; **2**: 1245.

PART IV

Regional and widespread pain disorders

| *Back pain*

Heiner Raspe

Introduction

There is a vast literature on the epidemiology of back pain but this chapter restricts itself to back pain in the general population. It concentrates mainly on investigations that have included both sexes, a broad range of age groups, all types of work (including housework), and work status including schooling, unemployment, and retirement. Thus studies of back pain in patient groups (for example [1]) as well as 'back pain in workers' (for example [2–7]) are virtually excluded. The subject of back pain in specific occupational groups is so extensive as to be outside the scope of this book. The review will, however, also cover many areas relevant to those who are mainly interested in the epidemiology of occupational back pain.

Since the first edition of this volume research in some areas has increased, including studies of the course and prognosis of back pain in populations, though a still neglected field is that of health economics. Valid data are scarce and, if available (as for the UK [8]) highly specific for the country and social system studied and thus hardly generalizable. They give the impression that back pain is one of the most costly conditions for which an economic analysis has been carried out in the UK [9]. For detailed discussion of these areas the readers may turn to other sources [10–23]. An historical perspective on low back pain and sciatica is also described elsewhere [24].

Assessing back pain in populations

Back pain is a symptom and an assessment of its occurrence necessitates a detailed understanding of the measurement of its dimensions. The following section summarizes basic descriptors of back pain for epidemiological studies. These are listed in Table 17.1. The use

Table 17.1 Selected dimensions of back pain (sufferers) for population studies

Characteristic	Dimensions of variability
Back pain	Ever/within last 12 months and/or currently
Time	Age at first attack
	Mode of onset, course pattern
	Days of pain and number of episodes in specified period
	Duration of current/last episode
Topography	Location and size of area in the back
	Radiation (e.g. to one/both legs, sciatica)
Intensity	Actual/ average/ highest intensity
Concomitant complaints	Other (musculoskeletal) pains
	Other bodily sensations
Psychological distress	Depression, anxiety
	Dysfunctional cognitions/ beliefs
Pain behaviour	Medical consultations, self treatment
	Physical (in)activity
	Inappropriate symptoms and signs
Disability, handicap	Limited activities of daily living
	Work disability, work loss
General health	Subjective health status
	Health related quality of life
	Concurrent morbidity, signs
	Somatic: red flags
	Psychiatric
	Actual and previous health care
	Types and density of contacts with professionals
	Types and density of diagnostic and therapeutic interventions

of existing instruments is nearly always to be preferred to developing new ones. Recently, clinically relevant outcome measures for low back pain research have been proposed [19,25–26] and may be especially relevant in the context of health services research [see 16,27]. This type of research may additionally profit from a new type of scientific literature, evidence-based clinical guidelines (e.g. [28,29]), mainly by providing a normative background for evaluative studies.

Back pain

The first issue to address is whether the study is on past and/or current back pain. An elegant way to combine the two interests is to enquire initially on back pain 'ever', then 'during the last 12 months' and finally 'today'. The *a priori* restriction to certain forms of back pain (as e.g. occurring 'on most days for at least 2 weeks [27], leading 'to a consultation with a doctor...' [30], or 'lasting for one day or longer' [31]), that is the use of implicit grading schemes, should be avoided. Questions are to be kept as simple as possible (e.g. 'do you have back pain today?'). Since the concept of 'the back' differs between and within populations the use of 'region of interest drawings' seems to be helpful [32] (Fig. 17.1).

Temporal characteristics

Back pain in populations usually has a very long overall history. Its lifetime prevalence approached (in a German study) 90% in the youngest age group (25 to 29 years) [33] (Fig. 17.2). Back pain is thus a common problem by the second and third decade of life [34]. Hence the recall of age and mode of first onset is likely to become less reliable with advancing age [35,36]. Many have pointed to the often fluctuating course of back pain with remissions and exacerbations (see

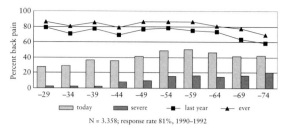

N = 3.358; response rate 81%, 1990–1992

Fig. 17.2 Present and past back pain in Luebeck (Germany) in 10 age groups (1990—1992).

below). The previous course of present pain seems to be among the best predictors of outcome of current pain. Chronic back pain sufferers seem to keep their track. Though clinicians usually distinguish between different course pattern, for example recurrent, fluctuating, continuous, or progressive [37], such a taxonomy has not systematically been developed for cross-sectional or longitudinal back pain studies. The reliability and validity of respective questions are yet to be clarified. The same seems true for questions concerning the number of 'pain days' and/or episodes over a specified period of time. Thus, also not rigorously tested, questions on the duration and course of a current episode seem to have the highest (face) validity.

Definition of chronicity

The previous duration of back pain present at survey is often used to distinguish 'acute' from 'chronic' forms (chronic if present for more than 3 or 6 months [37]). A major problem remains of the divergent definitions of the term 'chronic'. To identify 'chronic' back pain for the analysis of the First National Health and Nutrition Examination Survey [38] pain 'on most days for at least 1 month in the 12 months preceding the interview' was required. According to the Quebec Task Force [39], back pain should be considered chronic if absence from work exceeds more than 7 weeks. Besides these time-related definitions, Bonica [40] has referred to time of 'normal healing', whereas others have identified chronic pain with 'psychologic–physiologic disability' (see [41]) or dysfunctional pain [42,43]. Category 10 of The Quebec Task Force defines a 'chronic pain syndrome' where 'pain, with its consequences, has become the patient's main preoccupation, limiting his/her daily activities'. None of these approaches is totally satisfactory. Definitions with a simple time cut off seem epidemiologically preferable since they are not burdened with uncertain descriptions

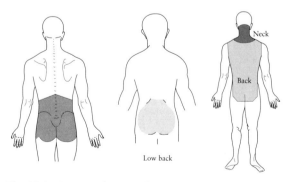

Fig. 17.1 Region of interest drawings and pain mannequins in back pain research. Reproduced from Raspe HH, Kohlmann T. *J Epidemiol Community Health* 1994; **48**: 531–537, by permission of the BMJ Publishing Group [32].

or hypotheses. The author recommends Waddell's definition (acute: less than 6 weeks; subacute 6–12 weeks, chronic more than 3 months duration of a current episode [19] but proposes to complement it with a more sophisticated system of staging (see below). It has, however, to be decided what 'duration' actually means: for example has 'continuous' back pain to be present at least once a week or daily, once a day or for at least 2 h, do days with menstrual periods or a feverish illness count [44]?

Topography

A precise recording of the location and size of painful areas in the back (e.g. sacral versus lumbar versus thoracic back pain) may require 'pain drawing' techniques as recently used in the UK [45]. Drawings show a high reliability both within subjects and between observers [46,47]. Spontaneous pain drawings provide more than topographic information. They can be used to identify non-organic pain, symmetric involvement, radiation or widespread pain pattern, for example according to the fibromyalgia definition of the ACR [48] (see Chapter 19). The method was used on 160 back pain sufferers from the Malmö Longitudinal Population Study of Musculoskeletal Symptoms [47]. Of those 28 per cent with back pain, 5 per cent had an unequivocal—and a further 5 per cent a possible—non-organic drawing. By contrast, 7 per cent displayed a possible, and the remaining 83 per cent a clear, organic pattern.

The spatial distribution of pain, for example whether and how it radiates to the legs can also be assessed by questionnaire or interview techniques (for example [25,49–52]). The concurrent validity of these approaches, however, deserves further study.

Pain intensity

A numeric rating scale (NRS) is a simple, concrete, and robust method to measure the intensity aspect of pain experience in clinical [53,54] as well as epidemiological studies. Usually such a scale ranges from 0 = 'no pain' to 10 = 'intolerable pain'. It seems preferable to the more abstract visual analogue scale (VAS) [55]. In clinic patients, for example, a considerable proportion had needed help in using a VAS [54,55].

In the Puget Sound Study [56] a questionnaire was sent to a stratified random sample of 1500 enrolees of the Health Group Cooperative of Puget Sound in the greater area of Seattle/Washington (US) aged 18–75, of

which 1016 were returned. The questionnaire included questions on pain problems at each of five sites (back, head, abdomen, face, chest) in the prior 6 months, but asked only for pains that had lasted a whole day or more or had occurred several times in a year. A further question covered the average pain intensity on a 1–10 point scale. The mean for back pain reached 4.7 (SD 1.9) with 15 per cent recording intensities of 7 and more. Several German surveys produced mean intensities of actual back pain mostly between 4 and 5 (Berger-Schmidt *et al.* 1996). In the European Vertebral Osteoporosis Study (EVOS) there were no differences between actual pain intensities of those with back pain amongst 2255 British and 3980 German respondents aged 50 to 79 (5.3 versus 5.4) [57].

The values are, in general, lower than those of patients with active rheumatoid arthritis (mean usually between 5.5 and 6 points), but the prevalence of intensive or intolerable back pain is still substantial. Taylor and Curran [58] have used an identical NRS to assess overall 'severity' of back pain in the respondents to the Nuprin Pain Report, a population-based telephone interview study of a stratified systematic random sample of 1254 Americans aged 18 or over. In all, 37 per cent of those with six or more back pain days within the last 12 months gave values of 7 to 10.

Concomitant complaints

Many back pain surveys have concentrated exclusively on backaches and have neglected that back pain (as one type of pain) is most often part of more complex pain and complaint syndromes as shown early by Valkenburg and Haanen [50]. It may well be that back pain, though present, is actually not the most prominent problem.

Forty-seven per cent of the subjects with pain from the Puget Sound Study recorded simultaneous pains in two or more (of a total of five listed) sites [59]. And the degree of their psychological distress (anxiety, depression, somatization) as measured with a symptom checklist and of impaired subjective health status correlated highly positively with the number of pain complaints.

A similar result was obtained in a postal pain survey in one Swedish county (N = 1009, aged 18–84) [60]. Six out of ten among those 44 per cent with recent and 'obvious pain' of at least 1 month's duration reported pain from more than one site. Table 17.2 gives more evidence from other population-based studies. The Nuprin Pain Report [58] included other pain types and

Table 17.2 Prevalence of back pain in two population pain surveys

Reference	Year	Country	N	Prevalence (%) of back pain	
				All subjects	Pain restricted to back
[58]	1985	US	1254	34[a]	10
[61]	1990	FRG	3426	31[b]	19

[a] Figure is for percentage with >5 days in past year. Figure for at least 1 day is 56%.
[b] Pain on day of survey.

sites such as headache, muscle pain, stomach pain, pre-menstrual, and menstrual pain) whereas a German postal study [61] (N = 4037; response rate 85 per cent) asked additionally for neck and joint pain and swelling and morning stiffness around joints. A later study demonstrated that subjects with current back pain scored significantly higher on a (German) symptom checklist compared to those actually free of it [62]. A close relationship between the number of physical (including back pain) and psychological symptoms has also been reported from an international study at 15 primary care centres [63].

It is still an important task for the future to model statistically the complex response pattern, since it is not clear whether these responses reflect clinical syndromes with distinct biological backgrounds or rather response characteristics dependent on personal 'traits' or cultural patterns [64–66]. In summary, the combined empirical evidence argues strongly against the artificial separation of pain in the back from pain in other sites and other bodily and psychic complaints. Back pain is virtually always more than pain in the back.

Psychological distress

One way to estimate the extent of emotional involvement in (back) pain surveys is to measure the affective quality of pain. This can be accomplished by adjective lists as in the original or short-form of the McGill Pain Questionnaire [67]. Also psychological tests such as the revised version of the Symptom Check List (SCL 90) [68,69], Beck's Depression Inventory [70], Centre for Epidemiologic Studies Depression Scale (CES-D scale) [71], or State-Trait Anxiety Inventory [72] seem suitable, even if disturbances can by no means solely be attributed to pain experience. So far, they have seldom been used in back pain epidemiology [38,59,73–74]. Additionally, data on the psychiatric co-morbidity (major depression, panic disorder, agrophobia; based on DSM-IIIR) of back pain sufferers in a general population has been published [75].

A new class of instruments and variables aims at assessing 'dysfunctional' beliefs and cognitions. Prominent examples are 'catastrophizing cognitions' [76], a paradigmatic item being 'I am a hopeless case', and a set of beliefs around what Waddell and Main have called 'fear of pain' [77]. This can be assessed by the 'Fear Avoidance Beliefs Questionnaire' [78] which includes such items as 'Physical activity makes my pain worse'. Such beliefs are strong predictors of future pain and disability [79].

Other and more indirect ways to assess psychological distress are the use of pain drawings ([47,80] see above) or the assessment of 'non-organic/inappropriate' signs and symptoms [81,82]. Finally, a large number of concomitant bodily complaints has been interpreted as indicative for constructs such as psychological distress, disturbance, or overlay.

The different methods and instruments obviously do not refer to one and the same underlying dimension. Their concurrent validity is still to be tested.

Pain behaviour

Pain behaviour is a very broad concept. It refers to verbal, paraverbal, and non-verbal expressions (for example [83]) to involuntary (for example 'non-organic physical signs') [81] as well as intentional utterances; it covers complex social activities as pain talks, medical consultations, drug use, and work absenteeism, and some behavioural psychologists would also include, as 'covert behaviour', the pain-related self-statements and cognitions referred to above [76,84].

Disabilities and handicaps

Disabilities and handicaps [85,86] are relevant and frequent consequences of back pain experiences. Disabilities are usually assessed as perceived limitations in every day activities 'considered normal for a human being' such as moving around, lifting and carrying objects, washing oneself, housekeeping, having sexual relations, etc. In accordance with the basic concept of WHO's International Classification of Impairments, Disabilities, and Handicaps [85,86] disability appears to act as the link between the somatic and the psychosocial status of individuals with painful chronic disorders.

The measurement of disability has a long tradition in rheumatology and orthopaedics reaching back to the third decade of the last century [87]. Currently, activity limitations can easily, reliably, and validly be assessed by paper and pencil tests, so called ADL or IADL questionnaires ((I)ADL = (instrumental) activities of daily living). Personal interviews and functional (obstacle) tests (e.g. [88]) are more objective but also more expensive in terms of equipment, time, and personnel.

Since the first edition of this book, more back-specific questionnaires have been developed, tested and published (e.g. The Quebec Back Pain Disability Scale [89,90] or the Bournemouth Questionnaire [91]. Comparative overviews of these and earlier instruments have been undertaken [89–94].

Instruments constructed or modified earlier to assess back-related disability include the Oswestry Low Back Pain Disability Questionnaire [96], a visual item analogue scales [97], and the Roland and Morris questionnaire based on a selection of items from the Sickness Impact Profile [98]. Other instruments were developed for back pain spondyloarthro-pathies [99–100]. Kohlmann and Raspe [101] developed a 12-item ADL-list (Table 17.3) specifically for back pain sufferers. Each item is to be answered with 'yes, without difficulty' (= 2 points) or 'yes, but with some difficulty' (= 1 point) or 'either unable to do, or able only with help' (= 0 points). The actual sum is (in case of no missing values) divided by 24 and multiplied with 100 to get an estimate of the current functional capacity expressed as a percentage. The instrument has been used in several epidemiological studies.

Related to but not identical with disability measures are measures of handicap [85], now referred to as 'participation restriction'—following ICIDH-2, [86]. One central indicator of occupational handicap among subjects gainfully employed is medically certified work loss [8,102]. Its validity seems limited due to concurrent reasons for work disability and errors in medical coding. One global measure for both the working and non-working part of the population is the number of disability days over a specified period of time. Respective questions have become part of national health surveys, for example NHANES II [103]. Indicators of disabilities and handicaps give overlapping but not equivalent information [104].

General health, health-related quality of life

There is no syndrome-specific quality of life (QoL) instrument for back pain victims. This is surprising as such instruments have been developed for nearly every clinical condition. The Maine Lumbar Spain Study reported on the usefulness of the Short Form 36, a generic QoL instrument with eight dimensions and 36 items [105]. The first dimension relates to general health perceptions and includes a first item on general health status which is often used separately.

Assessment of associated disorders and physical disease

Since the early investigations of Lawrence in the late 1940s [106], Laine in the late 1950s [107], and Valkenburg in the late 1970s [50] only few epidemiological surveys of back pain have included medical interviews, clinical and laboratory tests, and/or imaging techniques. Their use (Table 17.4) increases the study costs considerably and needs both a careful justification and a very strict protocol.

Table 17.3 Items in the Hannover ADL-questionnaire to determine back-related disability

1. Can you reach up and get for example a book from a high shelf or cupboard?
2. Can you lift a full suitcase and carry it for 10 m?
3. Can you wash and dry yourself from head to toe?
4. Can you bend forward to pick up a small lightweight object from the floor?
5. Can you wash your hair over a wash basin?
6. Can you sit for 1 h on a hard chair?
7. Can you stand continuously for 30 min (for example in a queue)?
8. Can you raise yourself in bed from a lying position?
9. Can you put on and take off socks or similar garments?
10. Can you bend sideways from a seated position to pick up a small object on the floor just beside your chair?
11. Can you lift a box containing six litre bottles on to a table?
12. Can you run 100 m fast without stopping in order to catch a bus?

Table 17.4 Options for other data acquisition in back pain survey

- Demonstrate the presence of functional or structural deficits of the spine, i.e. quantify spinal impairment [108]
- objective assessment of disability/activity limitations by means of performance tests [88]
- measure the extent of hyperalgesia/allodynia, e.g. by a tender point score [48]
- identify underlying somatic or psychiatric disorders, e.g. via 'red flags' [28]
- search for somatic or behavioural risk factors such as vertebral deformities [109] or 'non-organic signs' [81]

Health care use

An increasing number of studies report on the epidemiology of health care in relation to back pain, be it care-seeking [110–117], medication use in primary care [118], self-care and medication [119], hospitalizations and operations [120,121], or use of diagnostic testing [122], including imaging [123]. At present there seems to be no national or international standard for how to best capture different types of health care, though the first methodological studies have appeared [124].

Classification of back pain (sufferers)

The next stage is to consider how these dimensions can be used to define homogeneous groups of cases for investigation. Classification refers to the assignment of cases ('elements') to predefined, nominal groups ('classes') within a broader taxonomy, based on ,for example, aetiological, prognostic, pragmatic, evaluative, or, most often, mixed concepts and interests.

Some classifications are generic, such as the International Classification of Diseases (ICD, now in its 10th revision), the American Rheumatism Association Nomenclature and Classification of Arthritis and Rheumatism [125], or the multiaxial Classification of Chronic Pain of the International Association of the Study of Pain (IASP; [37]). They are useful either to indicate disorders actually underlying back pain (which in this case is conceived as a symptom) or to describe back pain syndromes along different axes (IASP: region–system–pattern of occurrence–time since onset/intensity–aetiology).

When no underlying disorder can be detected, back pain has been variously described as 'of unknown or uncertain origin'(IASP), 'non-specific'(ICD 10), or

'idiopathic'(ARA classification), 'common' [126], or 'simple' [19]. The relative frequency of this 'temporary diagnosis' [37] partly depends on the intensity of the diagnostic procedure. For many reasons it will be limited in epidemiological studies where, for example, expensive imaging techniques are not practical. Thus 'non-specific back pain' will be the main diagnosis in an epidemiological setting.

Non-specific back pain must not be assumed a nosological entity. If back pain is unequivocally modulated by mechanical factors the adjective 'mechanical' is often used [19]. If an unusual pain behaviour prevails 'chronic (back) pain syndrome' [51], '(back) pain of psychological origin' [37], or 'dysfunctional pain' [127] have been applied. If it recurs after surgical intervention it may be classified as back pain 'after failed spinal surgery'. Labels as such are not merely descriptive but express pathophysiological or aetiological conjectures. They should be used in epidemiological studies only under strict control of clear objectives and operational definitions.

The well-known 'Classification of Activity-related Spinal Disorders' of the Quebec Task Force (Table 17.5) [39] distinguishes 11 classes based on various patient recall and clinical data as well as aetiological assumptions. Categories 1–4 can additionally be specified by suffixes that code for duration of symptoms from onset and actual working status. So far it has (to the author's knowledge) not been used in epidemiological studies.

Waddell *et al.* recently proposed a set of seven clinical tests to quantify back-pain-related physical impairment for clinical use [19,108] (e.g. impaired flexion

Table 17.5 Classification of activity-related spinal disorders [51]

1. Pain without radiation
2. Pain plus radiation to extremity, proximally
3. Pain plus radiation to extremity, distally
4. Pain plus radiation to upper/ lower limb, neurological signs
5. Presumptive compression of spinal nerve root on plain X-ray
6. Compression of spinal nerve root confirmed by specific imaging and / or other diagnostic techniques
7. Spinal stenosis
8. Postsurgical status, 1–6 months after intervention
9. Postsurgical status, >6 months after intervention
   9.1 Asymptomatic
   9.2 Symptomatic
10. Chronic pain syndrome
11. Other diagnoses

and extension, muscle weaknesses). Epidemiological studies to assess these are in progress. The tests' validity and usefulness in this context is still to be proven. In one study, few clinical signs (out of 34 tested) showed a satisfactory association with the severity of back pain reported [128].

Grading and staging of back pain in surveys

Grading

As suggested above, back pain exhibits a wide spectrum of severity from barely perceptible discomfort to nearly intolerable, disabling pain. Grading refers to assessing the severity of present back pain, be it acute or chronic. Different schemes use different elements. Partly following von Korff *et al.* [129], we proposed to combine only two variables, actual pain intensity and disability (Table 17.6), the former measured by a numeric rating scale (see above), the latter by a specific disability questionnaire (see above).

A more complex, retrospective system, using data of the Puget Sound Study, distinguished six grades:

Table 17.6 Grading severity of current back pain [130]

Grade 0 no back pain present
Grade 1 back pain with low pain intensity (<5) **and** low disability (functional capacity >70%)
Grade 2 back pain with high pain intensity (5+) **or** high disability (functional capacity ≤70%)
Grade 3 back pain with high pain intensity **and** low functional capacity

(i) no pain problem; (ii) non-recurrent pain; (iii) recurrent pain; (iv) severe and persistent pain with no disability days in the prior 6 months; (v) severe and persistent pain with one to six pain-related disability days; (vi) severe and persistent pain with seven and more disability days [127,129], which was modified into a 5-grade system using seven questions [131].

Occurrence prevalence

The prevalence of back pain will be considered under three headings based on data derived from: (i) populations surveys of chronic pains and complaints; (ii) national health surveys with specific reference to back pain; (iii) surveys of back pain in sub-national areas.

Table 17.7 The prevalence of back pain in four pain surveys

Reference	Country	Number responding	Age range	Back pain definition	Prevalence of back pain (%)
[132]	Canada	827	18–91	Often troubled with pain and any noteworthy pain within the last 2 weeks ('persistent pain')	3.4
				Any noteworthy pain within the last 2 weeks ('temporary pain')	0.8
[58]	US	1254	18 +	Back pain in the last 12 months	
				1 or more days	56
				6 or more days	34
				31 or more days	15
				101 or more days	9
[56]	US	1016	18–75	Back pain in the last 6 months	41
				One brief episode	4
				2+ episodes	25
				More than half the days	12
[60]	Sweden	827	18–84	Any pain or discomfort in any part of your body, upper back:	
				All	13.4
				>6 months duration	10.2
				Obvious pain of >6 months lower back	7.5
				All	31.3
				>6 months duration	20.3
				Obvious pain of >6 months	16.1

Back pain in population pain surveys

Older surveys

As at 1990, the results of four major population-based pain surveys have been published [56,58,60,132]. This type of study offers the unique opportunity to analyse back pain in the context of other pain and discomfort.

Table 17.7 describes point and/or period prevalence of back pain derived from the surveys. The column 'definitions' quotes the authors' operational definitions of back pain available in the text. It clarifies which part of the total back pain spectrum was to be covered. The survey characteristics are described rather extensively. This gives the reader an impression of the fundamental lack of homogeneity between studies.

Crook *et al.* [132] drew a random sample of 500 English-speaking households from a group family practice clinic in Burlington, Canada. They used telephone interviews. The mean age was 41 and 52 per cent were female. The overall prevalence of 'persistent pain' was 11 per cent, that of 'temporary pain' 5 per cent. More than 60 per cent of all 'persistent pain' sufferers had had pain for 3 or more years. 'Back pain' indicates pain in the 'back/lower back'. The prevalence estimates were based on only 35 cases with back pain as the only or most severe complaint.

The Nuprin Pain Report [58] drew a stratified systematic sample of, eventually, 1254 Americans 18 years of age or over, probably representative for the entire adult population in the continental US (50 per cent females). They reached their probands by telephone interviews with the main question being, 'on roughly how many days—if any—in the last 12 months have you had … (seven different types of) pain'. Headaches were found to be the most common type (73 per cent with one or more episodes in the last 12 months), followed by backaches (56 per cent) and dental pains (27 per cent).

The Puget Sound Study [56] used postal questionnaires that had been mailed to 1500 enrolees of a Group Health Cooperative. This sample was 58 per cent female with a high proportion of middle-aged, well-educated, and actively-employed subjects. Persons were asked to report only pain problems that had either lasted a whole day or had occurred several times in a year at least. Back pain was the most frequent pain type within the last 6 months (41 per cent), followed by headaches (26 per cent). The cumulative lifetime prevalence by age 70 was estimated to reach 85 per cent for back pains and between 34 per cent and 46 per cent for the other types. The mean duration of back

pain since initial onset was 11 years (median 8 years). Only 9 per cent of the 411 back pain sufferers had experienced a single brief episode in the last 6 months, 62 per cent had two or more episodes, and 29 per cent had pain on more than half of the days.

Brattberg *et al.* [60] sent a postal questionnaire to 1009 randomly selected individuals, aged 18–84 years in a (not further specified) Swedish county. The central question was: 'Do you have /have you had any pain or discomfort in any part of your body?' Sixty-six per cent reported 'recent troubles', including both 'upper' and 'lower back'. In all 76 per cent of the actual pains in the upper back and 65 per cent of that in the lower parts could be traced back for at least 6 months. The actual intensity and consequences of recent back pain of at least 1 month' duration reached 79–91 per cent levels that qualified for the authors' criteria for 'obvious pain'. The overall prevalence of obvious pain with a duration of 7 and more months was 40 per cent; it affected (insignificantly) women more often than men and showed a significant U-shaped age dependence with a prevalence maximum in the age group 45–64 years.

The results of the four early surveys are not easy to summarize. The differences concerning target populations, data acquisition techniques, and wording, as well as temporal dimensions of the central questions, are profound. They are most probably responsible for equally profound differences in the prevalence rates that range from about 4–56 per cent.

Despite all methodological and technical differences it can be stated that:

1. Back pain is the most (or second most) prevalent pain complaint.

2. The average sufferer has a long history, often in form of multiple episodes. Chronic, continuous back pain accounts for maximally one-quarter of the total prevalence.

3. Back pains that occur more than occasionally manifest themselves in a broad range of seriousness and interference with ordinary activities with 15–37 per cent severe cases.

4. Females are generally more often affected than men.

5. There is no unequivocal influence of age: two studies point to an increase of more severe back pains with advancing age whereas back pain in general tends to peak before or around the age of 60.

Recent surveys

Since 1990 more data and a review of 15 studies on 'chronic benign pain disorders' among adults [133] have been published, making the picture even more complex. Eight studies addressed chronic pain or pain complaints in defined communities in New Zealand [30], Germany [134], Sweden [135], Spain [136], Canada [137], and Great Britain [138,139]. Again implicit grading schemes, definitions of chronicity, number and type of pains included, and hence results, vary markedly. In general, however, the broad results are in agreement with the conclusions of the earlier studies.

Some have restricted their focus to muculoskeletal pains [140–142] including 'chronic widespread pain' [140–143]. These recent studies support results from an earlier survey of regional adult population in the southwest of Finland (participation rate 93 per cent) [144]. Low back pain is the most prevalent conditions (about 18 per cent for 1-year-period-prevalence of at least 'fairly frequent' pain), and three to four times more frequent than thoracic pain. Pain radiating down to one or both legs was reported from less than half of the low back cases. A survey from Manchester, UK found back pain ('for more than 1 week in the past month' [142] the most common symptom (adjusted overall prevalence 23 per cent) in adults. Only 34 per cent experienced pain in only one site, with the most common combinations were back and knee pain, neck and shoulder pain, and back and hip pain—possibly indicating both semantic uncertainties (where does 'the neck' end and 'the shoulder' begin?) and actual clustering of discrete symptoms (back–knee). Similar overlaps had been reported by others [50,58,61].

Back pain and chronic widespread pain

The occurrence of chronic, widespread musculoskeletal pain which includes, by definition, axial, especially back pain [48] is described in detail in Chapter 19. This symptom complex is reported by 10–17 per cent of adults in studies from six countries: the UK [145], US [146], Sweden [147], Norway [148], Germany [149], and Israel [150]. A more stringent ('Manchester') definition resulted in a lower prevalence of 4–5 per cent [151].

Finally, one study from Scandinavian countries [154] assessed the occurrence and severity of 10 symptoms within the previous 30 days. In all, 35 and 22 per cent of subjects, aged 16 years or more, reported pain in the

low back and upper back, respectively, with a preponderance in females and the elderly, but no clear differences between the four countries. Further, 14 per cent and nearly 9 per cent complained of 'substantial' low and upper back pain, respectively. A comparable study was conducted among adults (18–60 years) from East and West Germany [155]. The main question addressed 'suffering' from any of 24 complaints without reference to duration. Sacral or back pain was reported by 62 per cent including 16 per cent with pains of at least considerable intensity. Prevalences of most symptoms were slightly higher among East Germans.

In summary the studies allow for an extension of the above summary:

6. Back pain is—in the majority of cases—part of more complex complaint syndromes comprising rheumatic and non-rheumatic pains and other bodily symptoms, suggesting synchronous disturbances of the nociceptive, proprioceptive, and enteroceptive system.

7. The more amplified the pain and complaint pattern the higher is the prevalence of psychological distress (and dysfunctional pain behaviour).

National surveys of back pain prevalence

Back pain has also been included as a target condition in different national health surveys (Table 17.8). Again, the definitions used and the occurrence measure derived vary substantially. The questions are in some cases stricter than in the pain surveys, thus concentrating on more chronic and serious forms of (low) back pain.

The Mini Finland Health Survey [156] included a physical (but not radiological) examination, of 52 per cent of all respondents. A clinical diagnosis of non-sciatic low back pain was made in 12 per cent, and of sciatica in 5 per cent. Definite or probable lumbar disc syndromes accounted for about 25 per cent of all clinically detectable low back syndromes. Males were significantly more often affected by such syndromes and reached their peak prevalence one decade (aged 45–54) earlier than females (55–64). The results of the Swedish National Central Bureau of Statistics' studies are based on reported symptoms, illnesses, and diseases [157] that were coded according to ICD 8. Data on reliability or validity are not given. The temporal reference of the central question ('are you suffering from

Table 17.8   The prevalence of back pain in national health surveys

Reference	Year of survey	Country	Age range	Pain definition	Prevalence of back pain (%)	Influence of	
						Sex	Age
[162]	1971–75	US (HANES I)	25–74	Past as well as current pain in back lasting at least 1 month	17	N/R	N/R
[157]	1975–78	Sweden	16–74	713.1, 717.0, 725, 728 (ICD 8) as reason of suffering as long-term illness, accident sequel, handicap or debility	6	N/R	N/R
[2]	1978–79	Canada (Canada Health Survey)	25+	Among long-term health problems: serious back or spine problems presently	7	m > f	f increase m peak at 45–54
[27]	1976–80	US (NHANES II)	25+	Pain in the back on most days for at least 2 weeks ever	17[a]	m > f	
				Primarily lower back pain ever	14		
				Severe pain	5		
				Pain lasting >6 months	5		
				Lower back pain last year	10		
				point prevalence[b]	7		
[165]	1977–80	Finland (Mini Finland Health Survey)	30+	Lifetime occurrence of low back pain	75	N/R	N/R
[156]				Actual definite or probable low back pain syndrome[c]	17	m > f	
				Lumber disc syndrome[c]	5	m > f	f peak at 55–64 m peak at 45–54
				Other low back syndromes[c]	13	f > m	m + f peak at 55–64
[158]	1984–86	West Germany	24–69	Do you suffer from low back or back pain	78		
				Severely	23	f > m	f increase m peak at 55–64
				Have you ever had lumbago or sciatica	25	f > m	f increase m peak at 55–64
				Currently	5		
				Disk disorder	23	f > m	f increase m peak at 55–64
				Currently	19		
[166]	1986–87	Denmark	16+	Do you suffer from long-standing back disorder (>6 months)	12	f > m	m + f peak at 45–66
				Pain or complaints of the back and loins during the past 2 weeks	23	f > m	N/R

[a] Unweighted estimate.
[b] Not further explained.
[c] Medical diagnosis.
N/R not reported; m = male; f = female.

any long-term illness ...') is not totally clear. The resulting low prevalence rate seems all the more astonishing.

The categories used in an early German survey [158] 'lumbago', 'sciatica', and 'disc disorder' refer to self-diagnosed 'subjective' morbidity and are part of a symptom check list. The differences in point prevalence of 'lumbago, sciatica' (5 per cent) versus 'disc disorders' (19 per cent) are as remarkable as unexplainable. This illustrates problems of epidemiological studies where rheumatological questions are included as a more or less incidental appendix. More stringent questions were used in two subsequent surveys, one in East Germany [52], the other in the whole of Germany (1998/99) [159–160]. In the latter study, back pain within the past 7 days 'including today' was reported by 39 per cent of all females and 31 per cent of all males (aged 18–80). In higher age groups (females 50+, males 40+) back pain becomes the most prominent problem. Overall prevalences showed a maximum in the age group 50–59 years with 44 per cent and 39 per cent for females and males, respectively. Back pain was more frequently reported from East than West Germans, confirming earlier observations from more heterogeneous and less comparable studies [52]. Data from the UK [161] concentrating on 'any back pain which lasted for more than one day' in the last 12 months yielded a prevalence overall of 37 per cent. Prevalence rates again peaked among those aged 55 to 64.

There have been a number of national health surveys from North America which have included back pain [27,103,162–164]. In NHANES II the cumulative life-time prevalence was estimated to be 14 per cent, compared to 75 per cent in the Mini Finland Health Survey [165]. The difference seems very likely to be explained by differences in definition. The Danish Health and Morbidity Survey screened for 'any long-standing illness (back disorders), i.e. lasting more than 6 months' and' pain or complaints of the back and loins during the past 2 weeks' [166]. This study too did not observe the expected/increase of cumulative lifetime prevalence of back pain with age. Respondents from the age group 55–64 years showed the highest rate of about 19 per cent; whereas the prevalence among subjects aged 65+ was below 16 per cent, a figure that is even lower than the results for those aged 45–54. The curves for point prevalence and cumulative lifetime prevalence run strictly parallel but on different levels. This, at first glance, illogical outcome ('paradoxical' pattern [27]) is possibly due to a true cohort effect, or

selective mortality (though this is unlikely) [167], non-specific recall errors, or, a more attractive hypothesis, from changes in the perception or reporting of past back pain experiences in the context of other and perhaps more serious health and life challenges in the elderly.

Back pain in sub-national surveys

Table 17.9 summarizes point and Table 17.10 period prevalences derived from surveys in a number of local or regional populations between 1948 and 1991. A critical overview of methods of 26 Nordic studies [168] highlighted recommendations for future research.

The influence of gender varied across the studies tabulated: females seem to be more often affected than males, especially with more chronic and severe back pain, but this difference is not always significant.

Although in a Danish survey [169] there was the intuitively convincing age pattern of a (nearly) linear increase with age in female lifetime and one year prevalence—several other studies confirm the 'paradoxical' result with prevalence tending to peak before or around the age of 60. This trend was first described by Lawrence [170], confirmed in several studies and was especially marked in females of one recent German study (Fig. 17.2 for both sexes).

The data of this Luebeck survey revealed 12-months period prevalence and prevalence of back pain 'ever' to be highest among females aged 25–34, 88 per cent and 89 per cent respectively, and lowest among those aged of 65–74 (67 per cent and 71 per cent respectively). This clear trend results primarily from an inverse relationship between age and the frequency of non-severe, and often episodic, back pain, whereas the prevalence of continuous back pain (within the last 12 months) and current severe back pain (Grade 3) show a steady increase with advancing age. The paradoxical pattern is also seen in retrospective pain data from another German region [149], Switzerland (females), the Netherlands (both sexes) [50], Denmark (males), and Sweden (both sexes) [135].

In the past decade, at least seven studies have been published. Indeed, in a comment on a recent Danish study [171] a commentator asked 'how long should we continue to repeat epidemiological cross-sectional investigations without clear new ideas or improvement...?'. The question seems justified as all studies confirmed established prevalence rates, age, and sex patterns, and risk factors (such as social class, see

Table 17.9 Point prevalence rates of back pain in sub-national population surveys

Reference	Year of survey	Country	Number responding	Age range	Males	Back pain definition	Point prevalence %	Influence of Sex	Influence of Age
[170]	1948–58	UK	1522	35+	47	Present back–hip–sciatic pain	15	f > m	f increase m constant after 40
[202]	1963	Switzerland	773	15+	51	Pain, weakness or fatigue within the last 2 weeks in the low back in the dorsal back (between scapulae)	26	f > m	f peak at 45–54 m peak at 45–49
[50]	1975–78	Netherlands	6584	20+	45	Low back pain now	7	f > m	N/A
[169]	1977–78	Denmark	928	30/40/50/60	48	Pain or in other ways trouble with the lower part of your back today (excluding menstrual pains)	26 14	f > m f > m	f + m peak at 55 f bimodal m peak at 40
[49]	1978	Sweden	716	40–47	100	Current conditions of pain, ache, stiffness or fatigue localized to the lower back, recurrent or at least once a month Daily pain > time/ week Less frequent	31 6 13 13	N/A	N/A
[225]	1979–81	Sweden	1414	38–64	0	All conditions of pain, ache, stiffness, or fatigue localized to the lower back within last month Low back pain for > 5 years Daily pain Pain > 1 time/ week Less frequent Severe or disabling pain	35 22 10 17 7 10	N/A	increase
[253]	1983	Sweden	552	55	56	Back pain > 12 months Exclusively low back pain[a] Sciatica[a]	29 15 12 5	f > m	N/R
[61]	1984–87	West Germany	3426	25–74	46	Back pain today (Hannover)	31	f > m	f peak at 45–54 m peak at 55–64
[130]	1991–92	Germany	3109	25–74	42	Back pain today	39	f > m	f peak at 45–54 m peak at 55–64
[286]	1978–86	Finland	1040	65+	41	Low back pain	32	m > f	N/R

[a] Based on pain drawings.

Table 17.10 Period prevalence rate of back pain in sub-national population surveys

Reference	Year of survey	Country	Number responding	Males %	Back pain definition	Point prevalence	Influence of Sex	Influence of Age
[170]	1948–58	UK	1522	47	Past or present back–hip–sciatic pain	51	f > m	f + m peak at 54
					Single episode	15		
					Episodic	29		
					>3 months duration (chronic)	7		
[202]	1963	Switzerland	773	51	Past or present pain, weakness or fatigue in the lower back	54	f = m	f peak 50–54 m increase
					In the dorsal back (between scapulae)	12	f > m	f polymodal m peak 40–44
[221]	N/R	US	1135	44	Often bothered with pain in your back	18	f > m	for both sexes increases f peak at 45
[50]	1975–78	Netherlands	6584	47	Low back pain ever	55	f > m	m peak at 55
[169]	1977–78	Denmark	928	48	Pain or in other way troubled with the lower part of your back ever	62	m > f	f increase m peak at 40
					Last 12 months	50	m > f	
					1–7 days	12	f > m	f increase
					Daily pain	9	f > m	
					Following 12 months	45		m peak at 40
[49]	1978	Sweden	716	100	Previous and/or present low back pain[a] sciatica	61 25	N/A	N/A
[225]	1979	Sweden	1414	0	Overall lifetime incidence of low back pain[a]	66	N/A	peak 38–39
[130]	1991/92	Germany	3109	49	Back pain today and/or during the last 12 months	75	f = m	f decrease

m constant after 45
[a] For precise definitions see Table 17.9.
N/R = not reported; N/A not applicable.

below). However, more recent studies tend to be methodologically more robust with more concern with implications for public health.

Methodological improvements include studies of repeatability, consider non-response bias [45, 114–116, 172–173], the use of validated region-of-interest drawings [172], free pain drawings [45,173], and accepted grading schemes [172]. The most important gains are of clearer distinctions between acute and chronic and between trivial and severe back pain. Similarly, the demonstration of non-response bias, which by self selection of back pain sufferers into study most probably leads to an inflation of prevalence rates. However, the neglect of previous back pain experiences and failure to take account of the time-course remain a major deficit of virtually all cross-sectional studies. Estimates of 'incidence' of any and prevalence of 'acute' back pain seem unreliable in the absence of any structured enquiry of history.

Prevalence of back pain in defined age-groups

Children and adolescents

The increasing number of cross-sectional back pain studies among children and adolescents yield results very similar to that of adults.

In Australia life-time prevalence reached 33 per cent by 10 years and 46 per cent by 12 years. The point and 'last month' prevalence rate was about 4.5 per cent and 12 per cent respectively, with 6.4 per cent reported sciatica, and in 3.2 per cent back pain interfered with daily activities [174]. Similar rates were observed in a Swiss Canton [175] and in a nation-wide Finnish study [176]. In a Swedish town as many as 8 per cent of 8-year-old school children answered 'yes' to the question 'do you often have back pain?'; the frequency rose steadily to reach 39 per cent of male and 58 per cent of female adolescents aged 17 [177]. A similar pattern was observed in the Finnish study, however at a much lower overall occurrence (1 year prevalence rate). Increasing age and female sex are (nearly) unanimously associated with higher rates, especially of recurrent/ continuous back pain [176]. Children aged 10 to 14 may provide a useful model to study the epidemiology of chronicity.

As in adults, back troubles in school children (aged 11–12 and 15–16 years) often comprised more than just pain in the back. Thus in Iceland [178] combinations of back pain with headache and stomach

pain were frequently observed. Weekly pain was reported by 40 per cent overall. About 60 per cent of the cases suffered back pain: one-fifth had only back pain, 13 per cent suffered from pain in the back and stomach pain or headache, and 28 per cent experienced all three pains combined. The experience of back pain was significantly associated with psychological and interpersonal problems [177] a finding in agreement with data from others [175]. Psychosocial risk factors appear to be more relevant than biomedical such as anthropometric characteristics [179–180] and spinal mobility and muscle strength [179]. However, early disc degeneration as assessed by magnetic resonance imaging may be a relevant risk factor and predictor of concurrent and subsequent back pain [181].

The elderly

There are also a few studies on acute and chronic 'geriatric pain' [182–184]. One systematic review of 'low back pain in the elderly' summarized 12 relevant studies of subjects aged 65 and older [185] published between 1985 and 1995. The results are again sobering, mainly because of the lack of standardized terminology and methodology. Prevalence estimates vary widely between 10 per cent and 50 per cent, dependent on implicit grading and variable time frames. The main conclusion related to 'a need to improve reporting of epidemiologic data with respect to low back pain in the elderly'.

Two more recent studies give additional evidence that females report more (multiple and severe) pain than males and that the frequency of back and other musculoskeletal pains decreases more (in males) or less (in females) beyond the age of 80 [186]. This latter trend could not be confirmed in elders of the Framingham cohort [187].

Time trends

Across all studies considered, there are higher prevalences from more recent experiences. The results suggest a 'rising tide' of back pain (see for example from Finland [188]). Detailed data from two German studies, both of which used the same wording: 'Do you have back pain today?' reinforce the impression: whereas around 1985 a prevalence of 33 per cent was observed (among German adults aged 25–74 years in Hannover) in 1991 it reached 40 per cent in a comparable sample from Luebeck, another north German city.

A similar picture emerges for measures of period prevalence. A slight increase was reported among Swedish females (but not males) between 1975 and 1981 (from 6.1 per cent to 8.1 per cent) [189]. Most recently a comparison of two heterogeneous British surveys from 1987/8 and 1997/8 suggested an increase of overall 1 year prevalence of back pain from 36 per cent to 49 per cent; [190]; though this is not a universal occurrence [191]. However, the frequency of more severe forms of back pain did not change and even fell by 0.7 per cent. A steady increase of frequent back, neck, or shoulder pain has been reported among Finish adolescents on the basis of biannual nation-wide surveys [192].

Other direct comparisons of equally consistent sequential surveys in one country do not support the hypothesis of a steadily increasing frequency of back pain at the population level. A Finnish study utilizing data from the North Karelia Project could not find any important difference between age-adjusted, 1 month prevalence rates between 1972 and 1992 [193]. Independent studies from the same country corroborate these findings for the period 1978/9 to 1992 from a national survey [194–195] with even a decrease of back pain reported in subgroups such as farmers. A German study that compared back pain prevalence (derived from representative populations samples in West Germany by means of a symptom check list [155] observed nearly identical overall rates in 1975 and 1994 among subjects in the age range 18–60 years. More severe back pains were even less frequent in 1994 (14.6 per cent vs. 19 per cent in 1975).

These population-based data are in sharp contrast to the increasing frequencies of back-related health-care use, work disability, and disability pensions observed in different countries such as the UK [8,194] and Germany. However in contrast to such, the European experience of an important increase of occupational low back pain was not observed in the US, based on claims data between 1987 and 1995 [196]. In view of these discrepancies, the question merits further periodic health surveys of stable populations under uniform protocols before any firm conclusions can be drawn.

Geographical trends

Currently, only few studies permit a direct comparison of prevalence rates between different regions or countries.

A study in eight areas of Scotland and England did not observe any important geographical variation of underlying prevalence rates [197], despite a marked variability in consultation rates. Comparisons of East and West Germany between 1991 and 1994 revealed substantial differences with lower rates from the East states [52]; with, for example, a prevalence of 27 per cent in the East versus 39 and 41 per cent for two Western communities. In view of a shared genetic background and more unfavourable physical living conditions in the former East Germany, so far unspecified sociocultural differences should become the most prominent target of further studies. These findings have been extended by data from the European Vertebral Osteoporosis Study [109]. They confirmed the German East–West difference and found equally substantial differences between males and females (50–79 years of age) from six British versus four West and four East German regions (e.g. 22 per cent vs. 48 and 42 per cent for current back pain among females in the pooled UK vs. West and East German centres respectively) [57]. Differences have also been observed between two Belgian language groups [198], between Hong Kong and Britain [199], between Scandinavian countries [154], and comparing developed countries and 'the rest of the world' [200]. Central European countries consistently provide high, and countries from the (Far) East and developing countries surprisingly low rates. A higher prevalence of severe lumbar degenerative changes was observed in a British compared to a Japanese community [201].

Compared to Western industrialized countries, too little data exist for 'the rest of the world'. The few available studies suggest an, at first glance, surprisingly low prevalence of back pain in underdeveloped and developing countries. There are too few studies which allow for a direct comparison of back pain occurrence across different countries, regions, and sociocultural groups [201].

Since most of the data are not directly comparable, further studies under common protocols are urgently needed. The fascinating question is why some populations produce, perceive, or report more pain than others. Hence the research methodology should aim at distinguishing between differences in nociception, pain perception, and pain reporting and use equivalent grading and staging schemes.

Incidence

Annual incidence has been studied, retrospectively and/or prospectively, with or without considering previous back pain experiences. Estimates were derived from point or 1-month or 1-year prevalence data among those who claim they had never experienced any back pain before. Thus 'incidence rates' of 'some 11 per cent annually' were reported in the youngest age group in a Dutch study declining to 2 per cent in the highest [50]. A prospective incidence study from Denmark [169] was undertaken on those who at first examination reported never to have had back pain before. This revealed 58 within 351 such cases, resulting in an annual incidence rate of overall 17 per cent (males 17 per cent, females 16 per cent), with the youngest age group (30 years) carrying the highest risk (24 per cent). Including all subjects into the denominator results in an incidence rate of overall 6 per cent. In a Swedish study [49] 15/716 male probands developed current but had not had previous back troubles, equivalent to a (monthly) incidence rate of 2.1 per cent for males aged 40–47. Back pain for the 'first time' was reported by 3.6 per cent, 773 probands, in a German study in respect to the last 14 days [202]. This leads to an unrealistically high annual incidence rate of 93.6 per cent.

The author's own studies in Hannover [61] and Luebeck [130] found 0.9 per cent and 0.4 per cent with back pain 'today' but without any indication of former back pain experiences. The duration of this (most probably) very first back pain episode varied however between <1 week and >12 months, so that the temporal reference of these incidence rates is not totally clear. If the results are combined and assuming that they relate 'in the average' to a 3-months period then we end up with a retrospectively obtained annual incidence rate of about 2 per cent—definitely lower than that of other European studies discussed [203–204]. A prospective cohort study [205–206] report an episode incidence rate of about 35 per cent in one year including 3 per cent for 'new consulting episodes', that is episodes which lead to primary care consultations.

Given a vulnerable phase of at least 60 years, that is to suppose that a first occurrence of back pain has a low probability outside the age range 10–70, any reported annual incidence rate of more than 10 per cent would be highly implausible since cumulative lifetime incidence would have approached 100 per cent already after 50 years. It has in fact always been found below 90 per cent, compatible with an average annual incidence rate of less than 4 per cent.

When does back pain start? According to the older data from NHANES II [27], in 11 per cent before the age of 20 and in another 28 per cent in the range 20–29. The relative frequency decreases from decade to decade down to 5 per cent for subjects aged 60 years or more. Forty-eight per cent of the 40–47-year-old men [49] reported their back pain commenced before the age of 30. Given the high frequency of back pain in children and adolescents, these retrospective data are far from being plausible [34].

Occurrence of persistence

Back pain as an acute, short-lived problem is of much lesser interest than the persistence of back pain. A very favourable prognosis was observed in a study of French primary care patients seen within 72 h after manifestation of low back pain without distal radiation [207]: 90 per cent recovered completely, that is with no residual pain or disability within a fortnight. A similar outcome was observed among a less selective sample of Dutch primary care patients [208]. Indeed 95 per cent of a large and heterogeneous group of patients with acute low back pain regained—within 6 months—a functional status 'equivalent to that before the onset of pain' [209]. A recent analysis presented data from five studies of acute back pain cases with return to work rates in back pain patients between 80 and 95 per cent at week twelve [20,148].

However, the concept of back pain as a generally benign condition is hardly compatible with its high point and 1-year prevalence. Though any single episode of acute back pain may resolve within a short time, partial and incomplete recovery and frequent recurrences seem to characterize the long-term course of the majority of GP and even community cases.

A first impression of the recurrent nature of back pain comes from recalled data of so-called acute cases. Many of them report of earlier episodes [42,73,207, 210,211]. Hence it is not surprising that the mean disease duration of prevalent cases approaches or even exceeds 12 years [212].

The following review focuses mainly on studies from primary care, especially to those whose sampling frames and procedures approximate to that of population-based studies. Studies prior to 1994 have been reviewed elsewhere [213]. Table 17.11 concentrates on the more recent ones.

The results of most studies are consistent with Croft's statement [214] that 'low back pain should be viewed as a chronic problem with an untidy pattern of grumbling symptoms and periods of relative freedom from pain and disability interspersed with acute episodes, exacerbations, and recurrences'.

325

Table 17.11 Course and outcome of back pain in prospective cohort studies from primary care

Study (country)	Duration of index episode	Follow-up	Course pattern	% Complete recovery	Outcomes % Functional	% Return to work
Acute back pain						
[207] (F)	– 72 h	3 months		98		about 90
[216] (UK)	– 1 week	12 months	Intermittent 72%	21		
[214] (UK)	new consulting episode[a]	12 months	Repeat consultation 41%	25		
[210] (NL)	new consulting episode	7 years	Chronic persistent 28%			
[211] (DK)	– 14 days	12 months	Repeat sick leave 15%	54	92	98
[215] (UK)	new consulting episode[a]	12 months	Persistent disabling 34%		58	
Acute and chronic back pain						
[73] (US)	I: – 6 months[b] P: ?	12 months		I: 21 P: 12	I: 86 P: 80	
[217] (UK)[c]	– 3 weeks 48% >52 weeks 12%	12 months	repeat consultation about 66% relapse 76%	47		
[208] (NL)	23% 7 weeks	12 months	md number relapses 2	90		
Chronic back pain						
[287] (NL)	>3 months	12 months	persistent 57% intermittent 37%	6		
[42] (US)	no recovery 12 weeks after acute index episode	19 months	unremitting 61%	16		

[a] 'New consulting episode': no prior consultation within past 3 months
[b] I = incidental cases; P = prevalent cases
[c] osteopathic patients

Nevertheless, it must not be forgotten that even patients with chronic dysfunctional back pain at entry are not inevitably condemned to further pain and dysfunction. In one study [73], 170 patients (from a population of 1128) reported high pain, moderate or severe disability, and more than 90 pain days at baseline. After 1 year, 5 per cent were pain free, a third showed a 'good outcome', and more than 50 per cent at least some improvement. In a similar recent study [42], the corresponding figures were 16 per cent (recovery) and 33 per cent (good function).

The most relevant risk factors of an unfavourable course and outcome of back pain episodes are a longer history and/or higher severity/intrusiveness of the actual episode, clinical characteristics (such as radiating pain/sciatica), restriction in spinal movements, and, especially important, psychological variables such as depression, somatization, perceived health status, fear avoidance, dysfunctional coping strategies, and somatic perceptions [42,208,212,215–217].

Risk factors

The interpretation of data on risk factors is difficult given some of the issues relating to case definition, defining subtypes of back pain, and case ascertainment mentioned earlier [218–219]. Further, given the lack of possible mechanisms for some 'risk' factors it is difficult to distinguish between those that are causally related from those that are statistically associated. Finally, much of the data has been accumulated from cross-sectional studies whereas prospective investigations might better define the causal sequence.

Genetics

There are remarkably few data on the genetic influences on back pain occurrence per se, although there are more studies on genetic influences on specific causes of back pain (see below). Race (white versus black and/or other) as a risk factor has been included in four studies from the US: HANES I [162,220]; NHANES II [27,221–222]; always with a negative result. There is a brief report from Finland indicating data from a nation-wide twin study demonstrating that 'environmental factors explained more than 80 per cent of the aetiology of sciatica'. By contrast genetic influences are by far the most relevant risk factor of lumbar disc degeneration in identical twins compared

to the influences from physical work and life style characteristics [223–224].

Non-genetic host factors
Reproductive history

Of all women with previous pregnancies from the Gothenburg study [225–226], 24 per cent reported mostly transient low back pain while having been pregnant. Of those with low back pain ever 10 per cent experienced their first attack during pregnancy, suggesting an annual incidence rate not too different from other reports concerning non-pregnant periods. A positive correlation between the occurrence of low back pain and the number of live births recalled could only be observed in an older age group (50–64 years), whereas the number of abortions was predictive in this group as well as among women aged 38–49. An association between the frequency of liveborn children and back pain was also observed in the South Manchester Survey, not only among mothers but also in fathers [227]. In contrast to these, others could not observe any influence of the number of childbirths [228–229]. A high proportion of the younger women indicated pregnancy or delivery as a cause of their back pain [203]. Assuming that pregnancy and childbirth carry a considerable risk but occur exclusively in females, one would expect a significant difference, especially during womens' later reproductive years. Data however do not confirm this hypothesis: the greater differences between the two sexes being in the age groups 25–35 [61]. Recently, an association between use of oral contraceptives and medical consultations for back pain was observed [189].

Body height

Among population-based investigations that analysed the influence of body height are the Mini Finland Health Survey [230] [231], the Glostrup study [232], and the Malmö study [229]. All found virtually no influence of that biological trait. Earlier 'positive' studies, for example [156,233], may suffer from selection bias in concentrating (in this case) exclusively on hospitalized patients with an officially registered discharge diagnosis of 'herniated lumbar intervertebral disk.' However, a more recent British study did find an association of symptom prevalence and increasing height in both men and women with a relative risk of 1.5 [234].

Other anatomical and structural influences

One hypothesis is that structural abnormalities independent of any underlying disorder are associated with back pain. However, few epidemiological studies have included a clinical examination with or (more often) without radiography. The presence and grade of clinically diagnosed kyphosis, lordosis or scoliosis, vertebral canal size, and lumbar anterolisthesis (in contrast to posterolisthesis) do not correlate with current or predict future back pain [50,229,235–238] In the EPOZ study only a decreased lumbar lordosis gave an odds ratio of 2.4 (women) and 3.8 (men) for current low back pain. In the Glostrup study [232] only unequal leg length was positively correlated with low back trouble 'ever' in both sexes. Fifteen other anthropometric variables, for example weight, femur epicondylar width, and clinical tests, for example Schober's test, muscle strength, showed no consistent associations and were predictive for first or recurrent persistent back trouble only sporadically. Results from a German population-based survey again revealed only weak associations between graded back pain and the results of multiple static, dynamic, neurological tests and non-organic physical signs [128]. It seems therefore that traditional physical measurements do not add substantially to our pathogenetic understanding of common back troubles.

Influence of lumbar spine disease on low back pain

Disc degeneration

The other major hypothesis is that lumbar spine pathology is a major contributor to the occurrence of back pain. The prevalence of radiologically assessed lumbar disc degeneration was more than 50 per cent in both sexes in a large Dutch population survey (EPOZ) [50]. Similar proportions, 65 and 52 per cent for males and females respectively, were reported from a study of four population samples in the UK [170].

The degenerative changes in the lumbar spine increased progressively with age. A statistically significant association between grade 3–4 X-ray changes and back–hip–sciatic pain 'ever' was found in men but not in women. Additionally, only men with grade 2 changes had reported more pain that those graded 0–1. By contrast, there was no such correlation for 'pain now'. A more detailed analysis revealed that 42 per cent of the men and 47 per cent of the women without any radiographic changes had had back–hip–sciatic pain at some time, whereas 37 per cent of the men and 35 per cent of the women with grade 3–4 changes could not remember any such pain. In the EPOZ-study the odds ratios for the associations between (pseudo) spondylolisthesis, (grade 2+) disc degeneration or rigid lumbar segments and actual or former back pain or sciatica were always below or around 2 for males and females [235]. The risks increased in men (but not in women) for disabling pains to a maximum of 4.2. In a subgroup comprising 477 women aged 45–64, one-half with chronic back pain at initial examination, the other with no former or present pains, the relative risk of those 222 subjects with grade 2+ disc disorder for back pain was 1.4 [239,240]. Disk degeneration occurred however in 38 per cent of the asymptomatic women. Over a follow-up period of 9 years the overall prevalence of disc disorder rose from 47 per cent to 64 per cent. Deterioration was more common in those with pre-existing disk degeneration, but group membership exerted no influence. This suggests that idiopathic back pain is unlikely to be a result of early, that is radiologically not yet detectable, disc disorder. Otherwise one would expect an excess incidence of disc degeneration among those with back pain at initial examination.

Taken together, the results indicate the limited value of conventional X-ray analyses in truly population-based epidemiological studies. Closer correlation between pain reports and a variety of structural changes have been reported from some studies with more selected populations [241–243]. The use of more advanced imaging techniques such as magnetic resonance do not seem to lead to completely different conclusions [244].

Osteoporosis

A relationship between back pain and vertebral osteoporosis has been proposed [169,226] based on clinical observations of an acute osteoporotic fracture which has lead to incapacitating pain. Osteoporosis itself may have little relevance. Thus one epidemiological study could not find any correlation between bone mineral content as measured by single photon absorptiometry over the left distal radius and current back pain [229]. Another study found no differences between two cohorts of women with and without recently active chronic back pains in respect to vertebral deformities between D12 and L5 at the beginning and the end of a 9-year follow-up period [240]. A (third) population-based case–control study identified even (significantly) more back pain during the last 10 years among controls than among the cases with a recently encountered hip fracture, though the cases showed more often vertebral fractures (43 per cent versus 22 per cent among controls) [245]. The authors conclude that 'there seems to be an inverse relationship between long-standing or severe back pain and spinal osteoporosis'. In an analysis of a study of white women who were solicited by newspaper advertisement in the San Francisco Bay area, a significant but overall small effect of a spinal deformity score on indicators of back-related disability and pain, maximally accounting for 4–10 per cent of their variance, was found [246]. Pains from other sites, as well as subjective health status and subjective co-morbidity, appeared more important again pointing to the syndromatic character of musculoskeletal complaints. Only severe or incident spinal deformities are therefore significant predictors of severe back pain [247–248]. These conclusions are supported by the Study of Osteoporotic Fractures [249] and the European Vertebral Osteoprosis Study (EVOS) [109]. In the latter significant but modest associations between the presence of unequivocal (morphometrically identified) vertebral deformities (between D4 to L4) and both actual back pain and disability were found, more pronounced in females than in males. Recently a modifying effect of the location of deformities on pain occurrence was described [250].

A rheumatic disorder with no demonstrable importance for actual or former back pains is diffuse idiopathic skeletal/spinal hyperostosis (DISH), though this has been studied only in clinical cases and controls [251], and no population studies have been conducted.

Psychological factors

Indicators of poor mental and emotional health [2,144,221], subjective stress and multiple daily hassles [58], as well as multiple somatic symptoms and a poor subjective health status [252] generally proved to be associated with a higher prevalence (or incidence) of back troubles.

Using data from HANES I [38], cases with chronic rheumatic pain in the previous year (prevalence 14 per cent) were at a higher risk for depressive symptoms (OR 2.3) and this association persisted after controlling for race, sex, income, and education. The authors of the Puget Sound Study [56] interpret comparable results in an opposite direction; they describe two distress measures, that is a poor self–rated health status and high scores on a somatization scale, as significant

predictors of retrospectively assessed back pain, with OR around 2.0. This illustrates the Achilles' heel of cross-sectional research, that is the possibility to reverse the direction of 'causality'. Depression or any other measure of distress may be an antecedent as well as a consequence of pain experiences, or even both.

Work dissatisfaction

The correlation with low work satisfaction seems equally consistent, but its temporal relationship can better be demonstrated. Low job satisfaction predicted back pain assessed at least 12 years later [253] in a Swedish study. This finding was recently confirmed by data from the South Manchester Back Pain Study [254]. The data from the prospective part of the Glostrup study [252] are similar, whereas in the cross-sectional, but multivariately analysed, Swedish study [49] 'work dissatisfaction did not remain directly associated with low back pain'. However, the correlation of work monotony with low back pain persisted in an analysis of co-variance. Since this variable should be interpreted as a psychological indicator of work-related distress, one can assume that job strain may play a pathogenic role [255] which however seems to loose relevance after retirement [256].

Psychological factors: cause or effect

Mechanic and Angel [220] studied the well-known discrepancy between subjective pain reports and the results of a medical examination, which had both been included in HANES I. They developed, tested, and confirmed the hypothesis that elderly subjects are 'less likely than their younger counterparts to complain of back pain relative to objective measure' whereas depression should augment or amplify chronic pain perception/report. In this study, complaints of back discomfort have again been much more frequent than physical findings that 'explain' such complaints. Only 23 per cent of those with pain reports have had two or more physical findings ($r = +0.28$ for two composite variables 'bad back' with 'bad complaints'). Depression was positively but weakly ($r < + 0.20$) correlated with back-related signs and symptoms, whereas age showed a positive correlation with signs and a negative with symptoms ($r < 0.15$). Age, physical findings, and depression explain about 10 per cent of the variance of back complaints. Further data from a prospective study of volunteers with no history of serious low back pain indicated that psychological problems precede rather than follow severe low back [257] confirming earlier results from the South Manchester Back Pain Survey [74] and from the US [73]. In a recent review of cohort studies on psychological risk factors in back pain there was moderate evidence that such factors predicted subsequent acute and chronic back (and neck) pain [116]. There has also been a recent systematic review of occupational related psychological factors predicting future back pain [258].

The results of psychosocially focused studies show that it is promising to include such variables, but it is theoretically and statistically demanding to disentangle the complexity of the association and interactions. In this field especially, theory-guided modelling should precede data acquisition and analysis.

Environmental factors

Work conditions

The type of actual or former occupations or work conditions has often been included in risk factor studies. Disc degeneration (grade 2+) was more prevalent among coal miners and outdoor workers than among textile workers, business, and professional men, whereas all groups of female workers (including housewives) showed similar frequencies [170]. Clinically diagnosed disc disorder followed a similar trend in a study 50 years ago [259]. Thus in females no clear differences in prevalence rates emerged considering varying occupational groups, but among men a higher frequency of back-related disorders could be identified again in coal miners and outdoor workers.

The EPOZ study [50] found no consistent correlation between the symptom of back pain and physical demands of former or recent occupations in male and females, a conclusion also observed by others [144]. By contrast to these negative results, others [221–253] described significantly higher point or period prevalence rates among unskilled labourers, truck drivers, and other types of blue collar workers, who are usually under physically more strenuous work conditions. Frequent and heavy lifting [260] as well as whole body vibration [261] seem especially dangerous. By contrast, others found no evidence for the popular opinion that associates sitting-at-work with back pain [262].

Lifestyle factors

Data from NHANES II, [263] addressed the influences of smoking and different measures of obesity. A significant trend toward greater back pain prevalence was found with greater smoking and more pack-years in the past, especially in younger subjects, even after controlling for pulmonary signs and symptoms. In most subjects smoking seemed to have preceded the first back pain attack. Similar data were found in Europe [230,252]. Smoking was also an important predictor of disc degeneration in a Finnish MRI Study of 20 identical male twin pairs. Since then several further studies [34,264–267] and at least two reviews [268–269] have generally confirmed smoking as a risk factor of back (and other musculoskeletal) pain.

In the NHANES II study the body mass index showed a non-linear dose–response relationship with the highest prevalence of back pain among the most obese (BMI >29.0) [263]. Multivariate analyses demonstrated that these lifestyle related factors carry a risk that is independent of each other, common sociodemographic variables and additional risk factors. Though not further explained, 'usual daily activity seemed to be correlated too with an odds ratio of 1.50 for the categories 'very active' versus 'quite inactive', contrary to the common notion that a high level of physical fitness and/or activity is protective [255]). The risk of obesity was recently confirmed [268,270–271] and an authoritative review on this topic has recently been published.

Social factors

There are only few studies on the influence of social network characteristics. In one study [253,256], no association was found between the presence of back pain and the (unspecified) quality of social relationships with family, relatives, or friends. In a further study, only small and inconsistent influence of social network/support characteristics were found on chronic back (and neck) pain in retired persons [256].

A lower prevalence of back pain among (already or still) married subjects has been observed [221–222]. Based on a logistic model the latter study calculated a higher prevalence for those 50–64-year-old males and females who were no longer married, irrespective of their educational level. A low prevalence was to be expected in married subjects with greater than high-school education, regardless of age. Nevertheless, another study did not find any influence of marital status [27]. The results of HANES I [162] show even an inverse relationship with the highest prevalence of vertebrogenic pain syndromes among the married, as found by others [272]. By contrast, relatively more subjects living alone were among those with a first back pain attack during 1 year of follow-up [252]. It is presently impossible to draw a clear conclusion, though in view of the inconsistent results it seems unlikely that structural or functional attributes of the social network exert a relevant and (therapeutically utilizable) influence.

Additionally, the medical profession and other parts of the health-care system may be understood as part of the back pain patients' social network. Experimental as well as observational studies point to the possibility of chronic back pain as an (in part) iatrogenic disorder [273–277]. The term 'nomogenic disorder' [278] suggests an even wider context for the manifestation and/or presentation of back pain. A paradoxical effect of new social benefits on back-pain-related sick leave rates was reported among pregnant women in Sweden [279] supporting earlier suggestions [280]. One promising preventive strategy could thus imply a demedicalization of uncomplicated, non-specific back pain.

Education and income

Indicators of socio-economic status such as education and income are considered important determinants of back pain. The available studies are mainly 'positive' and demonstrate an inverse relationship between the frequency or severity of back complaints and the level of education and/or income. Thus disproportionally more subjects with lower social status were observed among incident cases in a Danish study [252], and in a Swedish study the educational status at age 36 was predictive for actual back pain at age 55 [253]. Interestingly, neither the social background of the family, nor the parents' educational attitudes, nor the education of the father of the (male) subjects differed between those with, compared to those without, current back pain. This suggests an early blocked social achievement, unlikely to be caused by back pain. A similar result has been found in a satellite project of the Finnish Healthy Child Study [281]. As a risk factor, lower levels of education seems early and nearly irreversibly established.

Comparable observations have been described from cross-sectional studies by several authors [2,27,58, 221–222]. The effect may depend on an interaction with depression [27]. In contrast to these results a positive correlation was reported between education and vertobrogenic pain, and others did not find any significant association [50,56]. In general though, more recent studies mostly confirm the inverse relationship between indicators of social status and the occurrence of back pain [193,282–285]. According to one study [283] the effect of school education does not seem to be mediated by occupational factors in adult life.

In summary, it seems likely that low education per se or as a marker of social status increases the risk of becoming a back pain sufferer and disabled. The, sometimes observed, parallel or even dominant influence of income level may point more to the social status hypothesis; but this does not help to clarify the pathogenic mechanisms by which education, income, or social status 'realise' their risk. Bringing together the earlier reported, but weak and frequently unconfirmed, associations of back pain with unfavourable work conditions, distress, obesity, smoking, and the (statistical) influences of low education, income, and social status, back pain can be hypothesized as a symptom of a social disadvantage syndrome and an indicator of psychosocial inequality.

Acknowledgements

I am indebted to Dr Thomas Kohlmann for statistical analyses and permission to publish results from common studies, to Dr Alan Silman for very helpful (epidemiological as well as linguistic) comments and suggestions, and to his staff for technical assistance.

References

1. Frymoyer W *et al.*: Epidemiologic studies of low-back pain. *Spine* 1980; 5: 419–423.
2. Bombardier C, Balwin JA, Crull L: The epidemiology of regional musculoskelatal disorders: Canada. In: Hadler NM, Gillings DB (eds). *Arthritis and society.* London: Butterworths, 1985: 104–118.
3. Andersson GBJ: Epidemiologic aspects on low-back pain in industry. *Spine* 1981; 6: 53–60.
4. Deyo RA (ed): *Back pain in workers.* Philadelphia: Hanley and Belfus, 1988.
5. Carey TS: Occupational back pain: Issues in prevention and treatment. In: Balint GP, Buchanan WW (eds). *Occupational rheumatic diseases.* London: Bailliere Tindall, 1989.
6. Fordyce WE (ed.): *Back pain in the workplace.* Seattle: IASP Press, 1995.
7. Bernard BP: *Musculoskeletal disorders and workplace factors. A critical review of epidemiological evidence of work-related musculoskeletal disordes of the nack, upper extremity, and low back.* National Institute for Occupational Safety and Health: Cincinnati, 1997.

8. Clinical Standards Advisory Group: *Epidemiologic review: The epidemiology and cost of back pain.* London: HMSO, 1994.

9. Maniadakis N, Gray A: The economic burden of back pain in the UK. *Pain* 2000; **84**: 95–103 .

10. Benn RT, Wood PHN: Pain in the back: An attempt to estimate the size of the problem. *Rheumatol Rehabil* 1975; **14**: 121–128.

11. Kelsey JL: *Epidemiology of musculoskeletal disorders.* Oxford University Press: New York, 1982.

12. Steinberg GG: Epidemiology of low back pain. In: Stanton-Hicks M, Boas R (eds): *Chronic low back pain.* New York: Raven Press, 1982: 1–13.

13. Nachemson AL: Advances in low-back pain. *Clinical Orthop Rel Res* 1985; **200**: 266–278.

14. Frymoyer JW, Cats-Baril WL: An overview of the incidences and costs of low back pain. *Orthop Clin N Am* 1991; **22**: 263–271.

15. Kelsey JL, Golden AL, Mundt DJ: Low back pain/prolapsed lumbar intervertebral disc. In: Hochberg MC (ed). *Epidemiology of rheumatic disease.* WB Saunders Company: Philadelphia, 1990: 699–716.

16. Deyo RA, Cherkin D, Conrad D et al.: Cost, controversy, crisis: low back pain and the health of the public. *Ann Rev Publ Health* 1991; **12**: 141–156.

17. Loeser JD, Volinn E: Epidemiology of low back pain. *Neurosurg Clin N Am* 1991; **2**: 713–718.

18. Videman T, Battié MC: A critical review of the epidemiology of idiopathic low back pain. In: Weinstein JN, Gordon StL (eds). *Low back pain: A scientific and clinical overview.* Rosemont, IL: American Academy of Orthopaedic Surgeons, 1996.

19. Waddell G: *The back pain revolution.* Edinburg, London: Churchill Livingstone, 1998: 119–134.

20. Andersson GBJ: Epidemiological features of chronic low back pain. *Lancet* 1999; **354**: 581–585.

21. Dionne CE: Low back pain. In: Crombie IK (ed.). *Epidemiology of pain.* Seattle: IASP Press, 1999.

22. Loney PL, Stratford PW: The prevalence of low back pain adults: A methodological review of the literature. *Physical Therapy* 1999; **79**: 384–396.

23. Nachemson AL, Waddell G, Norlundt AI: Epidemiology of neck and low back pain. In: Nachemson AL, Jonsson E (eds). *Neck and back pain.* Philadelphia: Lippincott Williams and Wilkins, 2000: 165–187.

24. Waddell G, Allan DB: Back pain through history. In: Waddell G. *The back pain revolution.* Edinburgh, London: Churchill Livingstone, 1998: 45–67.

25. Deyo R, Battie M, Beurskens AJHM et al.: Outcome measures for low back pain research. *Spine* 1998; **23**: 2003–2013.

26. Daltroy LH, Cats-Baril WL, Katz JN et al.: The North American Spine Society Lumbar Spine Outcome Assessment Instrument. *Spine* 1996; **21**: 741–749.

27. Deyo RA, Tsui-Wu YJ: Descriptive epidemiology of low back pain and its related medical care in the United States. *Spine* 1987; **12**: 264–268.

28. Bigos S, Bowyer O, Braen G et al.: *Acute low back problems in adults.* Clinical Practice Guideline, Quick Reference Guide Number 14. Rockville MD: U.S. Department of Health and Human Services, Public Health Service, Agency for Health Care Policy and Research, AHCPR Pub No. 95–0643, 1994.

29. Waddell G, Feder G, McIntosh A et al.: *Low back pain evidence review.* London: Royal College of General Practitioners, 1996.

30. James FR, Large RG, Bushnell JA, Wells JE: Epidemiology of pain in New Zealand. *Pain* 1991; **44**: 279–283.

31. Hillman M, Wright A, Rajaratnam G, Tennant A: Prevalence of low back pain in the community: implications for service provision in Bradford, UK. *J Epidemiol Community Health* 1996; **50**: 347–352.

32. Raspe HH, Kohlmann T: Disorders characterized by pain: A methodological review of population surveys. *J Epidemiol Community Health* 1994; **48**: 531–537.

33. Raspe HH, Kohlmann T: Die aktuelle Rückenschmerzepidemie (The present back pain epidemic). *Therapeutische Umschau* 1994; **51**: 367.

34. Leboeuf-Yde Ch, Ohm Kyvik K: At what age does low back pain become a common problem? *Spine* 1998; **23**: 228–234.

35. Biering-Soerensen F, Hilden J: Reproducibility of the history of low-back trouble. *Spine* 1984; **9**: 280–286.

36. Walsh K, Coggon D: Reproducibility of histories of low back pain obtained by self-administered questionnaire. *Spine* 1991; **16**: 1075–1077.

37. Merskey H, Bogduk N (eds): *Classification of chronic pain*, 2nd edn. Seattle: IASP Press, 1994.

38. Magni G et al.: Chronic musculoskeletal pain and depressive symptoms in the general population. An analysis of the 1st National Health and Nutrition Examination Survey data. *Pain* 1990; **43**: 299–307.

39. Spitzer WO, LeBlanc FE, Dupuis M et al.: Scientific approach to the assessment and management of activity-related spinal disorders. *Spine* 1987; **12** (Suppl. 1).

40. Bonica JJ: Definitions and taxonomy of pain. In: Bonica JJ (ed.): *The management of pain*, 2nd edn. Philadelphia, London: Lea and Febiger 1990: 18–27.

41. Addison RG. Chronic pain syndrome. *Am J Med* 1984; Supp. **10**: 54–58.

42. Carey TS, Mills Garrett J, Jackman AM: Beyond the good prognosis. *Spine* 2000; **25**: 115–120.

43. Kröner-Herwig B: *Rückenschmerz.* Göttingen: Hogrefe, 2000.

44. Korff M von: Studying the natural history of back pain. *Spine* 1994; **19**: 2041–2046.

45. Papageorgiou AC, Croft PR, Ferry S et al.: Estimating the prevalence of low back pain in the general population. *Spine* 1995; **20**: 1889–1894.

46. Waddell G et al.: Normality and reliability in the clinical assessment of backache. *Br Med J* 1982; **284**: 1519–1523.

47. Udén A, Aström M, Bergenudd H: Pain drawings in chronic back pain. *Spine* 1988; **13**: 389–392.

48. Wolfe F, Smythe HA, Yunus MB et al.: The American College of Rheumatology 1990. Criteria for the classification of fibromyalgia. Report of the Multicenter Criteria Committee. *Arthritis Rheum* 1990; **33**: 160–172.

49. Svensson HO, Andersson GBJ: Low back pain in forty to forty-seven year old men. I. Frequency of occurrence

and impact on medical services. *Scand J Rehab Med* 1982; **14**: 47–53.

50. Valkenburg HA, Haanen HCM: The epidemiology of low back pain. In: White AA III, Gordon SL (eds). *Symptoms on idiopathic low back pain*. Miami, Florida: Mosby Company, 1982: 9–22.

51. Quebec Task Force on Spinal Disorders: Scientific approach to the assessment and management of activity-related spinal disorders. *Spine* 1987; Suppl. **1**: 12.

52. Berger-Schmitt R, Kohlmann T, Raspe HH: Rückenschmerzen in Ost- und Westdeutschland. *Gesundheitswesen* 1996; **58**: 519–524.

53. Downie WW *et al.*: Studies with pain rating scales. *Ann Rheum Dis* 1978; **37**: 378–381.

54. Strong J, Ashton R, Chant D: Pain intensity measurement in chronic low back pain. *Clin J Pain* 1991; **7**: 209–218.

55. Callaghan LF, Brooks RH, Summey JA, Pincus TH: Quantitative pain assessment for routine care of rheumatoid arthritis patients using a pain scale based on activities of daily living and a visual analog pain scale. *Arthritis Rheum* 1987; **30**: 630–636.

56. Korff M von, Dworkin SF, Le Resche L, Kruger A: An epidemiologic comparison of pain complaints. *Pain* 1988; **32**: 173–183.

57. Raspe H, Matthis Ch, Croft P *et al.*: Back pain in the United Kingdom and Germany – Are British tougher? submitted.

58. Taylor H, Curran NM: *The nuprin pain report*. New York: Louis Harris and Associates, 1985.

59. Dworkin SF, Korff M von, LeResche L: Multiple pains and psychiatric disturbance. *Arch Gen Psychiat* 1990; **47**: 239–244.

60. Brattberg G, Thorslund M, Wikman A: The prevalence of pain in general population. The results of a postal survey in a county of Sweden. *Pain* 1989; **37**: 215–222.

61. Raspe H, Wasmus A, Greif G, Kohlmann T, Kindel P, Mahrenholtz M: Rückenschmerzen in Hannover. *Akt Rheumatol* 1990; **15**: 32–37.

62. Raspe HH, Kohlmann T: Rückenschmerzen—eine Epidemie unserer Tage? *Deutsches Ärzteblatt* 1993; **90**: 2920–2925.

63. Simon GE, Korff M von, Piccinelli M *et al.*: An international study of the relation between somatic symptoms and depression. *New Eng J Med* 1999; **341**: 1329–1335.

64. Drury TF: Problems of meaning and measurement in cross-sectional interview surveys of chronic pain in the adult population. In: Chapman CR, Loeser JD (eds). *Issues in pain measurement*. New York: Raven Press, 1989: 489–518.

65. McArthur DL, Cohen MJ, Schandler SL: A philosophy for measurement of pain. In: Chapman CR, Loeser JD (eds). *Issues in pain measurement*. New York: Raven Press, 1989: 37–49.

66. Rudy TE: Innovations in pain psychometrics. In: Chapman CR, Loeser JD (eds). *Issues in pain measurement*. New York: Raven Press, 1989: 51–61.

67. Melzack R: The short-form McGill Pain Questionnaire. *Pain* 1987; **30**: 191–197.

68. Derogatis LR *et al.*: The Hopkins Symptom Checklist (HSCL): a self report inventory. *Behav Sci* 1974; **19**: 1–15.

69. Bernstein IH, Jaremko ME, Hinkley BS: On the utility of the SCL-90-R with low-back pain patients. *Spine* 1994; **19**: 42–48.

70. Beck AT, Ward CH, Mendelson H, Mock J, Erbraugh J: An inventory for measuring depression. *Arch Gen Psychiatr* 1961; **4**: 53–63.

71. Radloff LS: The CES-D scale: a self-report depression scale for research in the general population. *Appl Psychol Measurement* 1977; **1**: 385–401.

72. Spielberg CD, Gorsuch RL, Lushene RE: *STAI—manual for state-trait anxiety inventory*. Palo Alto, CA: Consulting Psychologists Press, 1970.

73. Korff M von, Le Resche L, Dworkin SF: First onset of common pain symptoms: a prospective study of depression as a risk factor. *Pain* 1993; **55**: 251–258.

74. Croft PR, Papageorgiou AC, Ferry S *et al.*: Psychologic distress and low back pain. *Spine* 1996; **20**: 2731–2737.

75. Walker EA, Katon WJ, Jemelka RP *et al.*: Comorbidity of gastrointestinal complaints, depression and anxiety in the epidemiological catchment area (ECA) study. *Am J Med* 1992; **92**: 265–305.

76. Flor H, Turk DC: Chronic back pain and rheumatoid arthritis: Predicting pain and disability from cognitive variables. *J Behav Med* 1988; **11**: 251–265.

77. Waddell G, Main CH: Beliefs about back pain. In: Waddell G: *The back pain revolution*. Edinburg, London: Churchill Livingstone, 1998.

78. Waddell G, Newton M, Henderson I *et al.*: A fear-avoidance beliefs questionnaire (FABQ) and the role of fear-avoidance beliefs in chronic low back pain and disability. *Pain* 1993; **52**: 157–168.

79. Main CJ, Wood PLR, Hollis S *et al.*: The distress and risk assessment method. A simple patient classification to identify distress and evaluate the risk of poor outcome. *Spine* 1992; **17**: 42–52.

80. Ohnmeiss DD: Repeatability of pain drawings in a low back pain population. *Spine* 2000; **25**: 980–988.

81. Waddell G, McCulloch JA, Kummel ED, Venner RM: Nonorganic physical signs in low-back pain. *Spine* 1980; **5**: 117–125.

82. Waddell G, Bircher M, Finlaysson D, Main C : Symptoms and signs: physical disease or illness behaviour? *Br Med J* 1984; **289**: 739–741.

83. Keefe FJ, Wilkins RH, Cook WA: Direct observation of pain behavior in low back pain patients during physical examination. *Pain* 1984; **20**: 59–68.

84. Pilowsky I: Low back pain and illness behavior (inappropriate, maladaptive, or abnormal). *Spine* 1995; **20**: 1522–1524.

85. World Health Organization: *International classification of impairments, disabilities, and handicaps*. Geneva: World Health Organization, 1980.

86. World Health Organizsation: *ICIDH-2: International classification of functioning and disability. Beta-2-draft*. Geneva: WHO, 1999.

87. Steinbrocker O, Traeger CH, Batterman RC: Therapeutic criteria in rheumatoid arthritis. *J Am Med Ass* 1949; **140**: 659–661.

88. Flores L, Gatchel RJ, Polatin PB: Objectification of functional improvement after nonoperative care. *Spine* 1997; **22**: 1622–1633.

89. Kopec JA, Esdaile JM, Abrahamowicz M *et al.*: The Quebec pain disability scale. *Spine* 1995; **20**: 341–352.

90. Kopec JA, Esdaile JM, Abrahamowicz M *et al.*: The Quebec pain disability scale. Conceptualization and development. *J Clin Epidemiol* 1996; **49**: 151–161.

91. Bolton JE, Breen AC: The Bournemouth questionnaire: A short-form comprehensive outcome measure. I. Psychometric properties in back pain patients. *J Manipulative Physiol Ther* 1999; **22**: 503–510.

92. Millard RW, Jones RH: Construct validity of practical questionnaires for assessing disability of low-back pain. *Spine* 1991; **16**: 835–838.

93. Kopec JA, Esdaile JM: Functional disability scales for back pain. *Spine* 1995; **20**: 1943–1949.

94. Beurskens AJ, de Vet HC, Köke AJ *et al.*: Measuring the functional status of patients with low back pain. *Spine* 1995; **20**: 1017–1028.

95. Katz RT, Rondinelli RD: Impairment and disability rating in low back pain. *Occup Med* 1998; **13**: 213–230.

96. Fairbanks JCT, Davies J, Coupar J, O'Brien JP: The Oswestry low back pain disability questionnaire. *Physiotherapy* 1980; **66**: 271–273.

97. Million R, Hall W, Nilsen H *et al.*: Assessment of the progress of the back-pain patient. *Spine* 1982; **7**: 204–212.

98. Roland M, Morris R: A study of the natural history of back pain. Part I: Development of a reliable and sensitive measure of disability in low back pain. *Spine* 1983; **8**: 141–144.

99. Dougados M *et al.*: Evaluation of a functional index and an articular index in ankylosing spondylitis. *J Rheumatol* 1988; **15**: 302–307.

100. Daltroy LH *et al.*: A modification of the health assessment questionnaire for the spondyloarthropathies. *J Rheumatol* 1990; **17**: 946–950.

101. Kohlmann T, Raspe H: Der Funktionsfragebogen Hannover zur alltagsnahen Diagnostik der Funktionsbeeinträchtigung durch Rückenschmerzen (FFbH-R). *Rehabilitation* 1996; **35**: 1–7.

102. Watson PJ, Main CJ, Waddell G *et al.*: Medically certified work loss, recurrence and costs of wage comprehension for back pain: A follow-up study of the working population of Jersey. *Br J Rheumatol* 1998; **37**: 82–86.

103. Deyo RA, Tsui-Wu YJ: Functional disability due to back pain. *Arthritis Rheum* 1987; **30**: 1247–1253.

104. Dionne CE, Korff M von, Koepsell TD *et al.*: A comparison of pain, functional limitations, and work status indices as outcome measures in back pain research. *Spine* 1999; **24**: 2339–2345.

105. Patrick DL, Deyo RA, Atlas StJ *et al.*: Assessing health-related quality of life in patients with sciatica. *Spine* 1995; **20**: 1899–1909.

106. Lawrence JS: *Rheumatism in populations*. London: William Heinemann Medical Books, 1977.

107. Laine VAI: Rheumatic complaints in an urban population in Finland. *Acta Rheum Scand* 1962; **8**: 81–88.

108. Waddell G, Somerville D, Henderson I *et al.*: Objective clinical evaluation of physical impairment in chronic low back pain. *Spine* 1992; **17**: 617–628.

109. Matthis C, Weber U, O'Neill TW, Raspe H *et al.*: Health impact associated with vertebral deformities: results from the European Vertebral Osteoporosis Study (EVOS) *Osteoporosis Int* 1998; **8**: 364–372.

110. Hart LG, Deyo RA, Cherkin DC: Physician office visits for low back pain. *Spine* 1995; **20**: 11–19.

111. Shekelle PG, Markovich M, Louie R: An epidemiologic study of episodes of back pain care. *Spine* 1995; **20**: 1668–1673.

112. Szpalski M, Nordin M, Skovron ML *et al.*: Health care utilization for low back pain in Belgium. *Spine* 1995; **20**: 431–442.

113. Wright D, Barrow S, Fisher AD *et al.*: Influence of physical, psychological and behavioural factors on consultations for back pain. *Br J Rheumatol* 1995; **34**: 156–161.

114. Carey TS, Evans AT, Hadler NM, Liebermann G: Acute severe low back pain. A population-based study of prevalence and care-seeking. *Spine* 1996; **1**: 339–344.

115. Carey TS, Garrett JM, Jackman A, Hadler N, and the North Carolina Back Pain Project: Recurrence and care seeking after acute back pain. *Med Care* 1999; **37**: 157–164.

116. Linton StJ, Hellsing AL, Halldén K: A population-based study of spinal pain among 35–45-year-old individuals. *Spine* 1998; **23**: 1457–1463.

117. Waxman R, Tennant A, Helliwell P: Community survey of factors associated with consultation for low back pain. *Br Med J* 1998; **317**: 1564–1567.

118. Cherkin DC, Wheeler KJ, Barlow W *et al.*: Medication use for low back pain in primary care. *Spine* 1998; **23**: 607–614.

119. Andersson HI, Ejlertson G, Leden I, Scherstén B: Impact of chronic pain on health care seeking, self care, and medication. Results from a popultion-based Swedish study. *J Epidemiol Community Health* 1999; **53**: 503–509.

120. Taylor V, Anderson GM, McNeney B *et al.*: Hospitalizations for back and neck problems: A comparison between the province of Ontario and Washington State. *Health Service Research* 1998; **33**: 929–945.

121. Zitting P, Rantakallio P, Vanharanta H: Cumulative incidence of lumbar disc diseases leading to hospitalization up to the age of 28 years. *Spine* 1998; **23**: 2337–2343.

122. Cherkin DC, Deyo RA, Wheeler K *et al.*: Physician variation in diagnostic testing for low back pain. *Arthritis Rheum* 1994; **37**: 15–22.

123. Ren XS, Selim AJ, Fincke G *et al.*: Assessment of functional status, low back disability, and use of diagnostic imaging in patients with low back pain and radiating leg pain. *J Clin Epidemiol* 1999; **52**: 1063–1071.

124. Guzmàn J, Peloso P, Bombardier C: Capturing health care utilization after occupational low back pain: Development of an interviewer-administered questionnaire. *J Clin Epidemiol* 1999; **52**: 419–427.

125. Decker J and the Glossary Subcommittee of the ARA Committee on Rheumatology Practice: American Rheumatism Association nomenclature and classification of

arthritis and rheumatism. *Arthritis Rheum* 1983; **26**: 1029–1032.

126. Nordin M, VischerTL (eds): Common low back pain: Prevention of chronicity. *Baillière's Clinical Rheumatology* 1992; **6**, No. 3. London: Ballière Tindall.

127. Korff MR von, Dworkin SF: Problems in measuring pain by survey: The classification of chronic pain in field research. In: Chapman CR, Loeser JD (eds): *Issues in pain measurement*. New York: Raven Press, 1989: 519–534.

128. Michel A, Kohlmann T, Raspe H: The association between clinical findings on physical examination and self-reported severity in back pain. *Spine* 1997; **22**: 296–304.

129. Korff M von, Dworkin SF, Le Resche L: Graded chronic pain status: an epidemiology evaluation. *Pain* 1990; **40**: 279–291.

130. Kohlmann T, Deck R, Raspe H: Prävalenz und Schweregrade von Rückenschmerzen in der Lübecker Bevölkerung. *Akt Rheumatol* 1995; **20**: 99–104.

131. Korff M von, Ormel J, Keefe F, Dworkin SF: Grading the severity of chronic pain. *Pain* 1992; **50**: 133–149.

132. Crook J, Rideout E, Browne G: The prevalence of pain complaints in a general population. *Pain* 1984; **18**: 299–314.

133. Verhaak PMM, Kerssens JJ, Dekker K *et al.*: Prevalence of chronic benign pain disorder among adults: a review of the literature. *Pain* 1998; **77**: 231–239.

134. Kohlmann T: Schmerzen in der Lübecker Bevölkerung. *Der Schmerz* 1991; **5**: 208–213.

135. Andersson HI: The epidemiology of chronic pain in a Swedish rural area. *Qual Life Res* 1994; **3** (Suppl. 1): 19–26.

136. Bassols A, Bosch F, Campillo M *et al.*: An epidemiological comparison of pain complaints in the general population of Catalonia (Spain). *Pain* 1999; **83**: 9–16.

137. Birse TM, Lander J: Prevalence of chronic pain. *Can J Public Health* 1998; **89**: 129–131.

138. Bowsher D, Rigge M, Sopp L: Prevalence of chronic pain in the British population: a telephone survey of 1037 households. *Pain Clinic* 1991; **4**: 223–230.

139. Elliott AM, Smith BH, Penny KI *et al.*: The epidemiology of chronic pain in the community. *Lancet* 1999; **354**: 1248–1252.

140. Jäckel WH, Gerdes N, Cziske R, Jacobi E: Epidemiologie rheumatischer Beschwerden in der Bundesrepublik Deutschland. Daten zur Prävalenz und zur körperlichen und psychosozialen Beeinträchtigung. *Z Rheumatol* 1993; **52**: 281–288.

141. Raspe A, Matthis Ch, Domarus UV *et al.*: Aktuelle muskuloskelettale Beschwerden bei peri- und postmenopausalen Frauen: Ergebnisse einer multizentrischen bevölkerungsepidemiologischen Studie. *Soz Präventivmed* 1994; **39**: 379–386.

142. Urwin M, Symmons D, Allison T *et al.*: Estimating the burden of musculoskeletal disorders in the community: the comparative prevalence of symptoms at different anatomical sites, and the relation to social deprivation. *Ann Rheum Dis* 1998; **57**: 649–655.

143. Macfarlane GJ: Fibromyalgia and chronic widespread pain. In: Task force on Epidemiology of the International Association for the Study of Pain (eds): *Epidemiology of pain*. Seattle: IASP Press, 1999: 113–123.

144. Takala J, Sievers K, Klaukka T: Rheumatic symptoms in the middle-aged population in southwestern Finland. *Scand J Rheumatol* 1982; **47** (Suppl.): 15–29.

145. Croft P, Rigby AS, Boswell R *et al.*: The prevalence of chronic widespread pain in the general population. *J Rheumatol* 1993; **20**: 710–713 .

146. Wolfe F, Ross K, Anderson J *et al.*: The prevalence and characteristics of fibromyalgia in the general population. *Arthritis Rheum* 1995; **38**: 19–28.

147. Andersson HI, Ejlertsson G, Leden I *et al.*: Characteristics of subjects with chronic pain, in relation to local and widespread pain report. *Scand J Rheumatol* 1996; **25**: 146–154.

148. Hagen KB, Thune O: Work incapacity from low back pain in the general population. *Spine* 1998; **23**: 2091–2095.

149. Schochat T: *Epidemiology of the criteria of fibromyalgia in the female population*. Unveröffentlichte Dissertation, University of North Carolina, 1999.

150. Buskila D, Abramov G, Biton A, Neumann L: The prevalence of pain complaints in a general population in Israel and its implications for utilization of health services. *J Rheumatol* 2000; **27**: 1521–1525.

151. Hunt S, Silman AJ, Benjamin S *et al.*: The prevalence and associated features of chronic widespread pain in the community using the 'Manchester' definition of chronic widespread pain. *Rheumatology* 1999; **38**: 275–279.

152. Macfarlane GJ, Croft PR, Schollum J, Silman AJ: Widespread pain: Is an improved classification possible? *J Rheumatol* 1996; **23**: 1628–1632.

153. Macfarlane GJ, Morris S, Hunt I *et al.*: Chronic widespread pain in the community: The influence of psychological symptoms and mental disorder on healthcare seeking behavior. *J Rheumatol* 1999; **26**: 413–419.

154. Eriksen HR, Svendsrød R, Ursin G, Ursin H: Prevalence of subjective health complaints in the Nordic European countries in 1993. *Eur J of Public Health* 1998; **8**: 294–298.

155. Schumacher J, Brähler E: Prävalenz von Schmerzen in der deutschen Bevölkerung. *Schmerz* 1999; **6**: 375–384.

156. Helioevaara M, Knekt P, Aromaa A: Incidence and risk factors of herniated lumbar intervertebral disc of sciatica leading to hospitalization. *J Chron Dis* 1987; **40**: 251–258.

157. Bjelle A, Allander E, Lundquist B: Geographic distribution of rheumatic disorders and working conditions in Sweden. *Scand J Soc Med* 1981; **9**: 119–126.

158. Bormann C, Hoeltz J, Hoffmeister H *et al.*: *Subjective morbidity*. München: Medizin-Verlag, 1990.

159. Robert Koch Institut: Bundes-Gesundheitssurvey 1998. *Gesundheitswesen* 1999; **61** (Suppl. 2).

160. Bellach BM, Ellert U, Radoschewski M: Epidemiologie des Schmerzes – Ergebnisse des Bundesgesundheitssurveys 1998. *Bundesgesundheitsbl–Gesundheitsforsch—Gesundheitsschutz* 2000; **6**: 424–431.

161. Mason V *et al.*: *The prevalence of back pain in Great Britain*. London: Office of Population Censuses and Surveys Social Survey Divison, HMSO, 1994.

162. Cunningham LS, Kelsey JL: Epidemiology of musculoskeletal impairments and associated disability. *AJPH* 1984; **74**: 574–579.

163. Lawrence RC, Helmick ChG, Arnett FC *et al.*: Estimates of the prevalence of arthritis and selected musculoskeletal disorders in the United States. *Arthritis Rheum* 1998; **41**: 778–799.

164. Millar WJ: Chronic pain. *Statistics Canada, Health Reports* 1996; **7**: 47–53.

165. Sievers K *et al.*: Musculoskeletal disorders and disability in Finland. *Scand J Rheumatol* 1988; **67** (Suppl.): 86–89.

166. Bredkjaer SR: Musculoskeletal disease in Denmark. The Danish health and morbidity survey 1986–7. *Acta Ortop Scand* 1991; **62** (Suppl. 241): 10–12.

167. Helioevaara M, Mäkela M, Aromaa A *et al.*: Low back pain and subsequent cardiovascular mortality. *Spine* 1995; **20**: 2109–2111.

168. Leboeuf-Yde CH, Lauritsen JM: The prevalence of low back pain in the literature. *Spine* 1995; **20**: 2112–2118.

169. Biering-Soerensen F: Low back trouble in a general population of 30-, 40-, 50-, and 60-year-old men and women. *Dan Med Bull* 1982; **29**: 289–299.

170. Lawrence JS: Disc degeneration. Its frequency and relationship to symptoms. *Ann Rheum Dis* 1969; **28**: 121–137.

171. Leboeuf-Yde Ch, Klougart N, Lauritzen T: How common is low back pain in the Nordic population? *Spine* 1996; **21**: 1518–1526.

172. Cassidy JD, Carroll LJ, Côté P: The Saskatchewan health and back pain survey. *Spine* 1998; **23**: 1860–1867.

173. Reigo T, Timpka T, Tropp H: The epidemiology of back pain in vocational age groups. *Scand J Prim Health Care* 1999; **17**: 17–21.

174. Chan S, Ryan MD: Low back pain in school children in the fifth and sixth grade. *J Orthop Rheumatol* 1992; **5**: 43–47.

175. Balagué F, Skovron M-L, Nordin M *et al.*: Low back pain in schoolchildren. *Spine* 1995; **20**: 1265–1270.

176. Taimela S, Kujala UM, Salminen JJ *et al.*: The prevalence of low back pain among children and adolescents. *Spine* 1997; **22**: 1132–1136.

177. Brattberg G: The incidence of back pain and headache among Swedish school children. *Qual Life Res* 1994; **3**: 27–31.

178. Kristjansdottir G: Prevalence of pain combinations and overall pain: a study of headache, stomache pain and back pain among school children. *Scand J Soc Med* 1997; **25**: 58–63.

179. Salminen JJ, Maki P, Oksanen A, Pentti J: Spinal mobility and trunk muscle strength in 15-year-old schoolchildren with and without low back pain. *Spine* 1992; **17**: 405–411.

180. Nissinen M, Heliövaara M, Seitsamo J *et al.*: Anthropometric measurements and the incidence of low back pain in a cohort of pubertal children. *Spine* 1994; **19**: 1367–1370.

181. Salminen JJ, Erkintalo MO, Pentti J *et al.*: Recurrent low back pain and early disc degeneration in the young. *Spine* 1999; **24**: 1316–1321.

182. Harkins SW, Price DD, Bush FM, Small RE: Geriatric pain. In: Wall PD, Melzack R (eds): *Textbook of pain.* Edinburgh, London, Madrid: Churchill Livingstone, 1994: 769–784.

183. Gagliese L, Melzack R: Chronic pain in elderly people. *Pain* 1997; **70**: 3–14.

184. Fox PL, Raina P, Jadad AR: Prevalence and treatment of pain in older adults in nursing homes and other long-term care institutions: a systematic review. *Can Med Assoc J* 1999; **160**: 329–333.

185. Bressler HB, Keyes WJ, Rochon PA, Badley E: The prevalence of low back pain in the elderly. *Spine* 1999; **24**: 1813–1819.

186. Brattberg G, Parker MG, Thorslund M: The prevalence of pain among the oldest old in Sweden. *Pain* 1996; **67**: 29–34.

187. Edmond SL, Felson DT: Prevalence of back symptoms in elders. *J Rheumatol* 2000; **27**: 220–225.

188. Sievers K, Klaukka T: Back pain and arthrosis in Finland. How many patients by the year 2000? *Acta Orth Scand* 1991; **62** (Suppl. 24): 3–5.

189. Wreje U, Isacsson D, Åberg H: Oral contraceptives and back pain in women in a Swedish Community. *Int J Epidemiol* 1997; **26**: 71–74.

190. Palmer KT, Walsh K, Bendall H *et al.*: Back Pain in Britain: comparison of two prevalence surveys at an interval of 10 years. *Br Med J* 2000; **320**: 1577–1578.

191. Macfarlane GJ, McBeth J, Garrow A, Silman AJ: Life is as much a pain as it ever was. *Br Med J* 2000; **321**: 897.

192. Vikat A, Rimpelä M, Salminen JJ *et al.*: Neck or shoulder pain and low back pain in Finnish adolescents. *Scand J Public Health* 2000; **28**:164–173.

193. Heistaro S, Vartiainen E, Heliövaara M, Puska P: Trends of back pain in Eastern Finland, 1972–1992, in relation to socioeconomic status and behavioral risk factors. *Am J Emidemiol* 1998; **148**: 671–682.

194. Leino PI, Berg M-A, Puska P: Is back pain increasing? *Scand J Rheumatol* 1994; **23**: 269–276.

195. Manninen P, Riihimäki H, Heliövaara M: Has musculoskeletal pain become less prevalent? *Scand J Rheumatol* 1996; **25**: 37–41.

196. Murphy PL, Volinn E: Is occupational low back pain on the rise? *Spine* 199; **24**: 691–697.

197. Walsh K, Cruddas M, Coggon D: Low back pain in eight areas of Britain. *J Epidemiol Community Health* 1992; **46**: 227–230.

198. Skovron ML, Szpalski M, Nordin M *et al.*: Socio-cultural factors and back pain. A population-based study in Belgian adults. *Spine* 1994; **19**: 129–137.

199. Lau EMC, Egger P, Coggon D *et al.*: Low back pain in Hong Kong: Prevalence and characteristics compared with Britain. *J Epidemiol Community Health* 1995; **49**: 492–494.

200. Volinn E: The epidemiology of low back pain in the rest of the world. *Spine* 1997; **22**: 1747–1754.

201. Yoshimura N, Dennison E, Wilman C *et al.*: Epidemiology of chronic disc degeneration and osteoarthritis of the lumbar spine in Britain and Japan: A comparative study. *J Rheumatol* 2000; **27**: 429–433.

202. Wagenhäuser SJ: *Die Rheumamorbidität.* Bern: Huber, 1969.

203. Biering-Soerensen F: A prospective study of low back pain in a general population. I. Occurrence, recurrence and aetiology. *Scand J Rehab Med* 1983; **15**: 71–29.

204. Waxman R, Tennant A, Helliwell P: A prospective follow-up study of low back pain in the community. *Spine* 2000; **25**: 2085–2090.

205. Papageorgiou A, Croft P, Thomas E *et al.* (1996): Influence of previous pain experience on the episode incidence of low back pain: results from the South Manchester Back Pain Study. *Pain* 1996; **66**: 181–185.

206. Croft PR, Papageorgiou AC, Thomas E *et al.*: Short-term physical risk factors for new episodes of low back pain. *Spine* 1999; **24**: 1556–1561.

207. Coste J, Delecoeuillerie D, Cohen de Lara A, LeParc JM, Paolaggi JB: Clinical course and prognostic factors in acute low back pain: an inception cohort study in primary care patients. *Br Med J* 1994; **308**: 577–580.

208. Hoogen HJM van den, Koes BW, Devillé W, Eijk JTM van, Bouter LM: The prognosis of low back pain in general practice. *Spine* 1997; 22: 1515–1521.

209. Carey TS, Garrett J, Lachman A, McLaughlin C *et al.*: The outcomes and costs of care for acute low back pain among patients seen by primary care practitioners, chiropractors, and orthopedic surgeons. *New Eng J Med* 1995; **333**: 913–917.

210. Miedema HS, Chorus AMJ, Wevers CWJ, Linden, S van der: Chronicity of back problems during working life. *Spine* 1998; **23**: 2021–2029.

211. Schiottz-Christensen B, Nilesen GL, Kjaer Hansen V, Schoedt T *et al.*: Long-term prognosis of acute low back pain in patients seen in general practice: a 1-year prospective follow-up study. *Family Practice* 1999; **16**: 223–232.

212. Dionne CE, Koepsell TD, Korff M von, Deyo RA *et al.*: Predicting long-term functional limitations among back pain patients in primary care settings. *J Clin Epidemiol* 1997; **50**: 31–43.

213. Korff M von, Saunders K: The course of back pain in primary care. *Spine* 1996; **21**: 2833–2839.

214. Croft P, Macfarlane GJ, Papageorgiou A C, Thomas E., Silman AJ: Outcome of low back pain in general practice: a prospective study. *Br Med J* 1998; **316**: 1356–1359.

215. Thomas E, Silman AJ, Croft PR, Papageorgiou AC, Jayson MIV: Predicting who develops chronic low back pain in primary care: a prospective study. *Br Med J* 1999; **318**: 1662–1667.

216. Klenerman L, Slade PD, Stanley IM, Pennie B *et al.*: The prediction of chronicity in patients with an acute attack of low back pain in a general practice setting. *Spine* 1995; **20**: 478–484.

217. Burton AK, Tillotson KM, Main Ch J, Hollis S: Psychosocial predictors of outcome in acute and subchronic low back trouble. *Spine* 1995; **20**: 722–728.

218. Leboeuf-Yde Ch, Lauritsen JM, Lauritsen T: Why has the search for causes of low back pain largely been non-conclusive? *Spine* 1997; **22**: 877–81.

219. Ozguler A, Leclerc A, Landre MF *et al.*: Individual and occupational determinants of low back pain according to various definitions of low back pain. *J Epidemiol Community Health* 2000; **54**: 215–220.

220. Mechanic D, Angel RJ: Some factors associated with the report and evaluation of back pain. *J Health and Soc Behav* 1987; **28**: 131–139.

221. Nagi SZ, Riley LE, Newby LG: A social epidemiology of back pain in a general population. *J Chron Dis* 1973; **26**: 269–279.

222. Reisbord LS, Greenland S: Factors associated with self-reported back-pain prevalence: A population-based study, *J Chron Dis* 1985; **38**: 691 – 702.

223. Helioevaara M: Risk factors for low back pain and sciatica. *Ann Med* 1989; **21**: 257–264.

224. Battié MC, Videman T, Gibbons LA *et al.*: Determinants of lumbar disc degeneration. *Spine* 1995; **20**: 2601–2612.

225. Svensson HO *et al.*: A retrospective study of low back pain in 38- to 64-year-old women. *Spine* 1988; **13**: 548–552.

226. Svensson HO *et al.*: The relationship of low back pain to pregnancy and gynecologic factors. *Spine* 1990; **15**: 371–375.

227. Silman AJ, Ferry S, Papageorgiou A *et al.*: Number of children as a risk factor for low back pain in men and women. *Arth Rheum* 1995; **38**: 1232–1235.

228. Ostgaard HC, Andersson GBJ, Karlsson K: Prevalence of back pain in pregnancy. *Spine* 1991; **16**: 549–552.

229. Bergenudd H *et al.*: Bone mineral content, gender body posture, and build in relation to back pain in middle age. *Spine* 1989; **14**: 599–579.

230. Heliovaara M, Mäkelä M, Knekt P *et al.*: Determinants of sciatica and low back pain. *Spine* 1991; **16**: 608–614.

231. Heliovaara M: Risk factors for low back pain and sciatica. *Ann Med* 1989; **21**: 257–264.

232. Biering-Soerensen F: Physical measurement as risk indicators for low-back trouble over a one-year period. *Spine* 1984; **9**: 106–119.

233. Heliovaara M: Body height, obesity, and risk of herniated lumbar intervertebral disc. *Spine* 1987; **12**: 469–472.

234. Kuh DJL, Coggan D, Mann S *et al.*: Height, occupation and back pain in a national prospective study. *Br J Rheumatol* 1993; **32**: 911–916.

235. Horal J: The clinical appearance of low back disorders in the city of Gothenburg, Sweden. *Acta Orthop Scand* 1969; **118** (Suppl.): 7–109.

236. Dieck GS *et al.*: An epidemiologic study of the relationship between postural asymmetry in the teen years and subsequent back and neck pain. *Spine* 1985; **10**: 872–877.

237. Porter RW, Bewley B: A ten-year prospective study of vertebral canal size as a predictor of back pain. *Spine* 1994; **19**: 173–175.

238. Vogt MT, Rubin D, San Valentin R *et al.*: Lumbar olisthesis and lower back symptoms in elderly white women. *Spine* 1998; **23**: 2640–2647.

239. Symmons DPM *et al.*: A longitudinal study of back pain and radiological changes in the lumbar spines of middle aged women. I. Clinical findings. *Ann Rheum Dis* 1991; **50**: 158–161.

240. Symmons DPM, van Hemert AM, Vandenbroucke JP, Valkenburg HA: A longitudinal study of back pain and radiological changes in the lumbar spines of middle

aged women. II. Radiographic findings. *Ann Rheum Dis* 1991; **50**: 162–166.

241. Torgerson WR, Dotter WE: Comparative roentgenographic study of the asymptomatic lumar spine. *J Bone Joint Surg* 1976; **56-A**: 850–853.

242. Magora A, Schwartz A: Relation between low back pain and X-ray changes. *Scand J Rehab Med* 1980; **12**: 47–52.

243. Frymoyer JW *et al.*: Spine radiographics in patients with low-back pain. *J Bone Joint Surg* 1984; **66-A**: 1048–1055.

244. Nachemson AL, Vingård E: Assessment of patients with neck and back pain: A best evidence synthesis. In: Nachemson AL, Jonsson E (eds): *Neck and back pain*. Philadelphia: Lippincott Williams and Wilkins, 2000: 189–235.

245. Zetterberg C *et al.*: Osteoporosis and back pain in the elderly. A controlled epidemiologic and radiographic study. *Spine* 1990; **15**: 783–786.

246. Ettinger B *et al.*: An examination of the association between vertebral deformities, physical disabilities and psychosocial problems. *Maturitas* 1988; **10**: 283–296.

247. Ross PD, Davis JW, Epstein RS, Wasnich RD: Preexisting fractures and bone mass predict vertebral fracture incidence in women. *Ann Intern Med* 1991; **114**: 919–923.

248. Ross PD, Davis JW, Epstein RS *et al.*: Pain and disability associated with new vertebral fractures and other spinal conditions. *J Clin Epidemiol* 1994; **47**: 231–239.

249. Ettinger B, Black DM, Nevitt MC *et al.*: Contribution of vertebral deformities to chronic back pain and disability. *J Bone Min Res* 1992; **7**: 449–456.

250. Cockerill W, Ismail AA, Cooper C, Matthis C, Raspe H *et al.*: Does location of vertebral deformity within the spine influence back pain and disability? *Ann Rheum Dis* 2000; **59**: 368–371.

251. Schlapbach P *et al.*: Diffuse idiopathic skeletal hyperostosis (DISK) of the spine: A cause of back pain? A controlled study. *Br J Rheumatol* 1989; **28**: 299–303.

252. Biering-Soerensen F, Thomsen C: Medical, social and occupational history as risk indicators for low-back trouble in a general population. *Spine* 1986; **11**: 720–725.

253. Bergenudd H, Nilsson B: Back pain in middle age; occupational workload and psychologic factors: an epidemiologic survey. *Spine* 1988; **13**: 58–60.

254. Papageorgiou AC, Macfarlane GJ, Thomas E *et al.*: Psychosocial factors in the workplace – do they predict new episodes of low back pain? Evidence from the South Manchester Back Pain Study. *Spine* 1997; **22**: 1137–1142.

255. Barnekow-Bergkvist M, Hedberg GE, Janlert U, Jansson E: Determinants of self-reported neck-shoulder and low back symptoms in a general population. *Spine* 1998; **23**: 235–243.

256. Isacsson A, Hanson BS, Ranstam J *et al.*: Social network, social support and the prevalence of neck and low back pain after retirement. *Scand J Soc Med* 1995; **23**: 17–22.

257. Mannion AF, Dolan P, Adams MA: Psychological questionnaire: Do 'abnormal' scores precede or follow first-time low back pain? *Spine* 1996; **21**: 2603–2611.

258. Hoogendooorn WE, Poppel MN van, Bongers PM *et al.*: Systematic review of psychosocial factors at work and private life as risk factors for back pain. *Spine* 2000; **25**: 2114–2125.

259. Kellgren JH, Lawrence JS, Aitken-Swan J: Rheumatic complaints in an urban population. *Ann Rheum Dis* 1953; **12**: 5–15.

260. Svensson HO, Andersson GBJ: Low back pain in forty to forty-seven year old men: Work history and work environment factors. *Spine* 1983; **8**: 272–276.

261. Pope MH, Wilder DG, Magnussen ML: A review of studies on seated whole body vibration and low back pain. *Proc Inst Mech Eng* 1999; (**H**) **213**: 435–446.

262. Hartvigsen J, Leboeuf-Yde Ch, Lings S, Corder EH: Is sitting-while-at-work associated with low back pain? A systematic, critical literature review. *Scand J Public Health* 2000; **28**: 230–239.

263. Deyo RA, Bass JE: Lifestyle and low back pain. The influence of smoking and obesity. *Spine* 1989; **14**: 501–506.

264. Battié MC, Videman T, Gill K *et al.*: Smoking and lumbar intervertebral disc degeneration: An MRI Study of identical twins. *Spine* 1991; **16**: 1015–1021.

265. Boshuizen HC, Verbeek JHAM, Broersen JPJ, Weel ANNH: Do smokers get more back pain? *Spine* 1993; **18**: 35–40.

266. Brage S, Bjerkedal T: Musculoskeletal pain and smoking in Norway. *J Epidemiol Community Health* 1996; **50**: 166–169.

267. Ehrmann Feldman D, Rossignol M, Shrier I *et al.*: Smoking. A risk factor for development of low back pain in adolescents. *Spine* 1999; **24**: 2492–2496.

268. Leboeuf-Yde Ch, Ohm Kyvik K, Bruun NH: Low back pain and lifestyle. Part II – Obesity *Spine* 1999; **24**: 779–784.

269. Goldberg MS, Scott SC, Mayo NE: A review of the association between cigarette smoking and the development of nonspecific back pain and related outcomes. *Spine* 2000; **25**: 995–1014.

270. Lake JK, Power Ch, Cole TJ: Back pain and obesitiy in the 1958 British birth cohort: cause or effect? *J Clin Epidemiol* 2000; **53**: 245–250.

271. Leboeuf-Yde CH: Body weight and low back pain. *Spine* 2000; **25**: 226–237.

272. Kramer JS, Yelin ED, Epstein WV: Social and economic impacts of four musculoskeletal conditions. *Arthritis Rheum* 1983; **26**: 901–907.

273. Deyo RA, Diehl AK, Rosenthal M: How many days of bed rest for acute low back pain? *New Engl J Med* 1986; **315**: 1064–1070.

274. Indahl A, Velund L, Reikeraas O: Good prognosis for low back pain when left untampered. *Spine* 1995; **20**: 473–477.

275. Malmivaara A, Häkkinen U, Aro T *et al.*: The treatment of acute low back pain—bed rest, exercises, or ordinary activity? *New Engl J Med* 1995; **332**: 351–355.

276. Korff M von, LeResche L, Saunders K: *Medical care and risks of dysfunctional chronic pain*. Final Report, R01-HS07759. Spingfiled, VA: National Technical Information Service, 1997.

277. Waddell G, Feder G, Lewis M: Systematic reviews of bed rest and advice to stay active for acute low back pain. *Br J Gen Practice* 1997; **47**: 647–652.

278. Hayes B, Solyom CAE, Wing PC *et al*.: Use of psychometric measures and nonorganic signs testing in detecting nomogenic disorders in low back pain patients. *Spine* 1993; **18**: 1254–1262.

279. Sydsjö A, Sydsjö G, Wijma B: Increase in sick leave rates caused by back pain among pregnant Swedish women after amelioration of social benefits. *Spine* 1998; **23**: 1986–1990.

280. Hadler NM: The disabling backache. An international perspective. *Spine* 1995; **20**: 640–649.

281. Viikari-Juntura E, Vuori J, Silverstein BA *et al*.: Lifelong prospective study on the role of psychosocial factors in neck-shoulder and low-back pain. *Spine* 1991; **16**: 1056–1061.

282. Croft PR, Rigby AS: Socioeconomic influences on back problems in the community in Britain. *J Epidemiol Community Health* 1994; **48**: 166–170.

283. Latza U, Kohlmann T, Deck R, Raspe H: Influence of occupational factors on the relation between socioeconomic status and self-reported back pain in a population-based sample of German adults with back pain. *Spine* 2000; **25**: 1390–1397.

284. Badley EM, Ibanez D: Socioeconomic risk factors and musculoskeletal disability. *J Rheumatol* 1994; **21**: 515–522.

285. Dionne C, Koepsell TD, Korff M von *et al*.: Formal education and back-related disability. *Spine* 1995; **20**: 2721–2730.

286. Anttila SK. Diseases and symptoms as predictors of hospital care in an aged population. *Scand J Soc Med* 1992; **20**: 79–84.

287. van Tulder MW, Koes BW, Metsemakers JFM, Bauter LM. Chronic low back pain in primary care: a prospective study on the management and course. *Fam Pract* 1998; **15**: 126–132.

18 | Upper limb disorders

Gary J. Macfarlane

Pain is a common complaint in the general population. Approximately 60 per cent of the general population will report having experienced, during the previous month, pain which has lasted for 1 day or longer at one or more sites of the body [1]. The 1-month period-prevalence of pain (lasting at least 1 day) at individual regional sites, from a population-based survey of approximately 2000 subjects in the United Kingdom [1] is shown in Fig. 18.1. The most common sites for pain to be reported are the lower back (28 per cent), the hip and buttock area (28 per cent), the neck and shoulder (24 per cent), and the knee (21 per cent), all of which are reported by more than 1 in 5 of the population. Headache or facial pain (15 per cent), pain in the wrist or hand (15 per cent), elbow (11 per cent), and ankle or foot (13 per cent) are also common with more than 1 in 10 of the population reporting symptoms. These regional pain syndromes do not, however, occur in isolation. Considering the 15 regional sites shown in Fig. 18.1, the distribution of the number of sites at

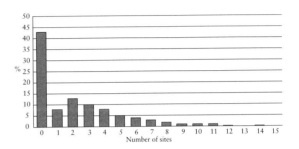

Fig. 18.2 The number of sites at which pain is reported in a population survey. Data from [1].

which subjects reported pain in this study is shown in Fig. 18.2. More than 12 per cent of the population report pain in at least six regional sites. An earlier survey of approximately 25 000 subjects, also in the United Kingdom, demonstrated that musculoskeletal pain syndromes were associated with important levels of disability: 8.2 per cent of the population reported disability arising from any rheumatic disorder, 2.5 per cent from a disorder of the back and neck, and 1.7 per cent from some other soft tissue disorder [2]. Of subjects with back/neck or other soft tissue disorder, respectively 81.6 per cent and 82 per cent had sought a consultation with a general practitioner in the past year, while 75.2 per cent and 59.8 per cent reported current use of medication for their symptoms. Disability from back, neck, and other soft tissue disorders (combined) increased markedly with age from 0.42 per cent of the population aged 16–34 years to 13.8 per cent at ages over 75 years, and overall was more common in females (5.8 per cent) than males (2.6 per cent). Regional musculoskeletal pain syndromes are therefore not only commonly reported in population surveys but a significant proportion result in disability. They are also associated with health-care seeking behaviour and time off work. Consequently the monetary costs associated with such symptoms both for the individual and society are enormous.

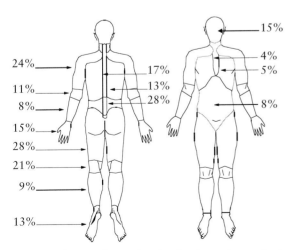

Fig. 18.1 The prevalence of regional pain syndromes in the general population. Data from [1].

This chapter will consider firstly the classification of upper limb disorders and thereafter the epidemiology of some of the most common disorders: shoulder and neck pain, forearm pain, carpal tunnel syndrome, and Dupuytren's disease.

Classification criteria of upper limb disorders

There are few agreed and validated classification criteria for upper limb disorders: one exception is carpal tunnel syndrome. It can be no coincidence that this syndrome has subsequently been a focus for research and consequently a greater amount of progress made in understanding the aetiology than for most other syndromes. Three principal methods have been used in classifying upper limb disorders:

1. The first is an anatomical/pathological classification based on a presumed pathological abnormality underlying symptoms. Examples of this include 'tenosynovitis' and 'medial epicondylitis'. This requires that the underlying cause of symptoms can be determined and that their classification is repeatable within and between observers. However, it has been demonstrated in several studies that the between-person repeatability of such diagnoses for upper limb disorders is poor [3–5]. In the study by Bamji *et al.* [3] three rheumatologists examined, separately, the same 44 patients with painful shoulders and agreed on the diagnosis in only 20. A further study in the

Netherlands of 120 patients with a new episode of shoulder pain, referred by general practitioners for physiotherapy, showed only moderate-poor agreement on diagnosis, using Dutch national guidelines, between the general practitioners and physiotherapists. For some conditions (e.g. acute bursitis) agreement was worse than could have been expected by chance [5].

2. The second method of classification used, particularly in population-based epidemiological studies, is according to anatomical site based on patient reporting of pain. This can be achieved by a simple question about having experienced pain in a particular area, for example 'During the past month, have you experienced shoulder pain lasting at least one day'. However, when dealing with regional sites such as shoulder or forearm, respondents may disagree as to precisely what area constitutes the shoulder or forearm. An alternative, to overcome this, can be to include a manikin with the particularly region under study shaded, and to ask subjects whether they have experienced pain in this area (Fig. 18.3a) [6]. To increase flexibility (i.e. to examine the effect of changes in the anatomical definitions of a regional pain site) subjects can be requested to shade on a blank body manikin the area where pain is felt (Fig. 18.3b), and the investigator can determine the effect of using different areas of definition for a particular regional pain syndrome. These methods have the advantage that they are simple and can be applied to large populations. However, differences in the precise question asked or

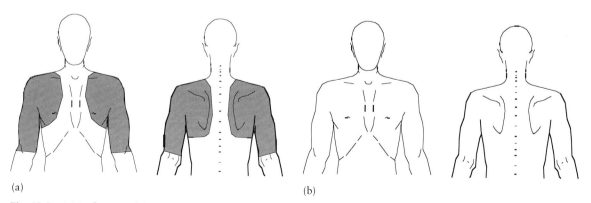

(a)   (b)

Fig. 18.3　(a) Definition of shoulder pain = pre-shaded manikin. Reproduced with permission of the BMJ Publishing Group from Pope DP, Croft PR, Pritchard CM, Silman AJ. *Ann Rheum Dis* 1997; 56: 308–312 [6]. (b) Definition of shoulder pain = blank manikin.

definition used, for example the reference period or the duration of pain, the definition of the region under study, can make substantial differences in prevalence estimates and make comparison between studies difficult. A study by Pope *et al.* [6] of shoulder pain used four different instruments to obtain information on the 1-month period prevalence, with prevalence estimates ranging from 31 per cent to 48 per cent depending on the definition used. The disadvantages of a system which does not consider underlying pathology is that pain experienced in, for example, the shoulder region may actually be arising from the neck. Conversely pain arising from the shoulder may only be felt outside the shoulder region, for example more distally in the forearm. There, therefore, may be some degree of misclassification. Further, a classification based only on experiencing pain currently, or within a specified period, may include many cases of relatively trivial pain. For this reason several studies

using this approach, in addition, make an assessment of severity or disability arising as a result of the pain.

3. The third method for classification of pain is by (presumed) aetiology. Examples of this are most common with respect to forearm pain and terms used include 'repetitive strain injury', 'overuse syndrome' and 'cumulative trauma disorder'. Such a scheme is unsatisfactory as a basis for diagnosis, classification, and for research studies, for several reasons. It classifies not only the condition but also implies that there is a single underlying cause and that this can be determined. It also implies that the syndrome is a distinct entity, which may not be true.

Instead of developing classification criteria by presumed aetiology a more logical sequence of scientific enquiry is to determine classification criteria for the condition which does not include presumed aetiology, and then, through epidemiological enquiry, determine

Table 18.1 Surveillance case definitions for major upper limb pain syndromes

Condition	Definition	Surveillance criteria
Carpal tunnel syndrome	A clinical syndrome caused by compression of the median nerve as it passes though the carpal tunnel.	Pain, or parathesia, or sensory loss in the median nerve distribution and one of: Tinel's test positive, Phalen's test positive, nocturnal exacerbation of symptoms, motor loss with wasting of abductor pollicis brevis, and abnormal nerve conduction
Tenosynovitis of the wrist	Inflammation of the extensor or flexor tendon sheaths at the wrist	Pain on movement localized to the affected tendon sheaths in the wrist and reproduction of pain of the affected tendons with the forearm stabilized
De Quervain's disease of the wrist	Painful swelling of the first extensor compartment containing extensor pollicis brevis and adductor pollicis longus	Pain which is centred over the radial styloid and tender swelling of first extensor compartment and either pain reproduced by resisted thumb extension or positive Finkelstein's test
Non-specific diffuse forearm pain	Pain in the forearm in the absence of a specific diagnosis or pathology	Pain in the forearm and failure to meet the diagnostic criteria for other specific diagnoses and diseases
Lateral epicondylitis	A lesion at the common extensor origin of the lateral epicondyle of the humerus causing the effects noted in the criteria	Lateral epicondylar pain and epicondylar tenderness and pain on restricted extension of the wrist.
Shoulder capsulitis (frozen shoulder)	A condition characterized by current or past pain in the upper arm, with global restriction of active or glenohumeral movement in a capsular pattern	History of unilateral pain in the deltoid area and equal restriction of active and passive glenohumeral movement in a capsular pattern (external rotation >abduction > internal rotation)
Shoulder tendonitis	Symptomatic inflammation or degeneration of the tendons of the rotator cuff or biceps	Rotator cuff: history of pain in the deltoid region and pain on or more resisted active movements (abduction of the supraspinatus; external rotation of the infraspinatus, teres minor; internal rotation of the subcapsularis); biceps: history of anterior shoulder pain and pain on resisted active flexion of elbow or supination of forearm

From [7]

the aetiology (or more commonly, aetiologies) of symptoms. This approach was adopted in a proposed set of surveillance case definitions for upper limb pain syndromes [7] and a criteria document for the evaluation of the work-relatedness of such disorders [8]. The definitions proposed by Harrington *et al.* [7] were developed using a Delphi process involving 29 experts from the United Kingdom in the following areas: rheumatology, surgery, occupational health, epidemiology, general practice, physiotherapy, ergonomics, psychiatry, psychology, and pain physiology. Thereafter there was a consensus conference. Definitions and surveillance criteria were agreed for carpal tunnel syndrome, tenosynovitis of the wrist, De Quervain's disease of the wrist, epicondylitis, shoulder capsulitis, and shoulder tendonitis. The consensus group also identified a condition which they called 'non-specific diffuse forearm pain'. The definitions and surveillance criteria for these are shown in Table 18.1 [7]. These have subsequently been developed into an examination schedule which has been validated in clinic attenders [9] and is currently being validated in the community. It will be noted that although the meeting had a particular interest in identifying case definitions for work-related syndromes, none of the conditions have such restrictions in the case definitions. This will allow researchers to use the definitions in a variety of settings and to determine the possible role of work-related exposures in their aetiology.

Shoulder and neck pain

Classification

Painful disorders of the shoulder and neck have been common subjects of enquiry in both population and occupational studies. Some have been conducted on 'shoulder disorders' or 'shoulder pain' while others have either concentrated on specific syndromes or made such diagnoses as part of multi-phase studies. These disorders have included bursitis, tendon related disorders, rotator cuff lesions, impingement syndrome, and 'frozen shoulder'. As discussed previously, clinical criteria are often poorly defined, and there has been a lack of validated classification criteria for these conditions suitable for use, particularly in epidemiological studies [10]. The conditions of shoulder and neck pain are considered together because of the difficulty of separating these two conditions in large-scale epidemiological enquiries. Even where a distinction has

been made they are often both considered in a single study.

Occurrence

Population studies which have examined the prevalence of shoulder or neck symptoms (predominantly pain) are summarized in Table 18.2. It will be noted that in almost all studies the measure of occurrence is point or period prevalence. Measures of episode incidence and first ever incidence are rarely reported. A large postal survey of 25 168 households, including 42 826 subjects aged 16 years and over, was conducted in the north of England [24]. Subjects were asked whether 'anyone in your household suffers from any pain, swelling or stiffness in their joints, neck or back?' For each subject with problem joints, the questionnaire asked for the site of the joints to be recorded on a chart. The prevalence of shoulder and neck problems was 6.9 per cent and 5.9 per cent respectively. A population study in Finland (The Mini-Finland Health Survey) recruited 7217 men and women representative of the whole Finnish population over 30 years of age [27]. Subjects completed a questionnaire that included enquiry about musculoskeletal symptoms and those who reported symptoms were invited for supplementary interview and a standardized physical examination. The prevalence of shoulder disorders and chronic neck pain was 1.9 per cent and 4.2 per cent aged 30–64 years, and 4.6 per cent and 4.9 per cent aged 65 years or more, respectively. Both disorders were frequently associated with a reduced working capacity and an occasional or regular need for help, but rates of disability were similar to those for musculoskeletal disorders overall (Table 18.3). The United States Health and Nutrition Examination Survey (HANES I) included a randomly selected group of 6913 adults aged 25–74 years from the general population, who were given both an interview about musculoskeletal symptoms and a thorough musculoskeletal evaluation [26]. The precise questions asked are not stated but physician-observed musculoskeletal abnormalities were defined as 'joint tenderness', 'joint swelling', 'limitation of motion' or 'pain on motion'. The estimated prevalence of shoulder symptoms in the United States population based on data from this study is 6.7 per cent, and 3 per cent for physician-observed abnormalities.

Other studies, mostly conducted in Northern Europe, have provided similar estimates of prevalence. The highest estimates of the prevalence of shoulder pain (~20–40 per cent) and neck pain (~15–25 per

Table 18.2 Population studies measuring the prevalence of shoulder and neck pain

Study location	Disease definition	Population	Sample size	Prevalence Shoulder	Prevalence Neck	Reference
Finland	Pain occurring fairly often, often or continuously during the year preceding investigation in: (S) shoulder-upper arm (N) neck, cervical spine, occiput	Sample of two rural communities 40–64 years	2268	17% (M) 17% (F)	18% (F) 16% (M)	[11]
Finland	'Shoulder disorder' and 'Chronic neck pain' determined by interview and examination	Representative sample of Finnish population ≥30 years	7217	1.9% <65 years 4.6% ≥65years	4.2% <65years 4.9% ≥65years	[12]
Netherlands	Current shoulder pain	A community survey of persons aged ≥85 years	95	19% (M) 29% (F)		[13]
Netherlands	Specific shoulder disorders—GP diagnosed	Incident cases from general practice	392	8.4 per 1000 person years (M)[a] 11.1 per 1000 person years (F)[a]		[14]
Norway	Persistent or regularly recurrent pain with a duration >3 months Site indicated on manikin	Random sample of subjects ages 25–74 from two primary health-care districts	1609	17.7% (M) 22.3% (F)	14.5% (M) 19.1% (F)	[15]
Norway	Experiencing neck or shoulder pain at least weekly	All persons 20–56 years in one municipality	17650	15.4% (M) 24.9% (F)		[16]
Sweden	(S) Restriction of shoulder movement with pain	Random sample of city residents 31–74 years	15268	10.3% (M)[b] 15.5% (F)		[17]
Sweden	(S) Have you had any joint trouble i.e. pain, tenderness, stiffness in the shoulders (N) Do you have any neck trouble i.e. pain, tenderness, stiffness	Sample of city residents 18–65 years	2537	8.0%	12.1%	[18]
Sweden	(S) Sub-acromial shoulder pain without neck pain (N) Neck pain—see reference for further details	Random samples of city residents who participated in previous health survey	445	6.7%	6.5%	[19]
Sweden	> 6 weeks during past year (S) Shoulder pain at some time during the previous month.	Follow-up subjects recruited from elementary school in 1938; 55 years of age	575	13% (M) 15% (F)		[20]
Sweden	Modified Nordic[c] Questionnaire	Random sample of semi-rural population who were working	637	35% (M) 40% (F)	33% (M) 53% (F)	[21]
Sweden	Symptoms (shoulder/neck) during the past month leading to medical consultation	Follow-up of a population sample resident in a city (mean age 48 years)	484	13% (M) 24% (F)	11% (M) 23% (F)	[22]

Table 18.2 Population studies measuring the prevalence of shoulder and neck pain (*continued*)

Study location	Disease definition	Population	Sample size	Prevalence Shoulder	Prevalence Neck	Reference
United Kingdom	Current shoulder symptoms (self-reported) and specific diagnosis on clinical examination	A random sample from the community of subjects ≥ 70 years	644	17% (M) 25% (F)		[23]
United Kingdom	'Does anyone in your household suffer from any pain, swelling or stiffness in their joints, neck or back ?' 18 joint sites included	Two-stage survey of randomly selected households of a town. Persons age ≥16 years	42826	6.9%	5.9%	[24]
United Kingdom	Shoulder pain on clinical history	Population sample of subjects >65 years	100	34% (9% severe pain)		[25]
United Kingdom	Pain in the shoulder (a manikin defined area) lasting at least 24 h during the past month	A random sample of community subjects aged 18–65 years	312	34%		[6]
United States	(S) Pain in shoulder on most days lasting at least 1 month OR shoulder swelling and pain or morning stiffness lasting at least 1 month	Sample representative of US population 25–74 years	6913	6.7%		[26]

[a] Cumulative incidence
[b] Calculated from data presented in the paper
[c] [116]

S = shoulder; N = neck

Table 18.3 Prevalence of disabilities associated with neck and shoulder disorders: a population-based study in Finland; modified from [27]

	N	Age 30–64		N	Age 65 or more	
		Reduced working capacity (%)	Need for help at least occasionally (%)		Need for help at least occasionally (%)	Need for help regularly (%)
All subjects	5673	24.2	15.3	1544	56.1	19.6
Any musculoskeletal disorder	1103	64.6	41.8	656	70.1	27.4
Chronic neck pain	239	64.9	36.8	76	72.4	18.4
Shoulder disorder	107	57.0	35.5	71	73.2	28.2

cent) are usually provided by population studies where classification is based only on self-reported symptoms [6,11,13,15,16,21]. High prevalence rates of shoulder and or neck pain have also been reported from specific population sub-groups such as the elderly [23,25] and those in employment [21]. In order to exclude relatively trivial pain episodes, some studies have supplemented information on pain, with an assessment of range of movement [17], disability [28], or health-seeking behaviour [22]. A variety of measures with demonstrated validity and repeatability [29] have been developed to measure shoulder disability including, the American Shoulder and Elbow Surgeons Evaluation Form [30], the Shoulder Pain and Disability Index [31], the Simple Shoulder Test [32], the Shoulder Severity Index [32,33], and the Manchester Shoulder Disability Questionnaire [34]. Two instruments to measure neck pain, the Neck Pain Disability Index [35] and the Northwick Park Neck Pain Questionnaire [36] have been developed, both based on the Oswestry Disability Questionnaire for Low Back Pain [37], but have not yet been used in population surveys. Lower rates of shoulder and neck pain are also reported when the population survey has relied on clinical examination with or without the use of standard criteria or presentation for medical care [14,19].

Overall, therefore, the population studies of neck and shoulder pain emphasize how common both are in the population, although prevalence rates are highly dependent on the classification scheme used and the method of collecting information.

Age and sex in relation to the occurrence of shoulder pain

Age

The prevalence of pain increases until around the fifth decade, with a slight decrease thereafter, and popu-

lation studies of neck pain have reported a similar relationship between age and prevalence. In a large study from the United Kingdom, prevalence of self-reported neck problems increased to a peak of 11.4 per cent at ages 55–64 years and decreased slightly to 9.3 per cent at ages over 85 years (Fig. 18.4) [24]. Andersson *et al.* [15] in a study from Sweden demonstrated a similar relationship: prevalence of pain in the neck/back of head increased to a peak of 24 per cent at ages 45–54 and decreased to 15 per cent by ages 65–74 years (Fig. 18.4).

A similar relationship between prevalence and age has been demonstrated in some studies for shoulder pain. Andersson *et al.* [15], in the study from Sweden, showed a very similar relationship to that found for neck pain in the same study. Prevalence increased to a peak of 28 per cent at ages 45–54 years and then decreased to around 20 per cent at ages 65–74 years (Fig. 18.5). Other population-based studies have found that shoulder pain becomes more common with increasing age, and that there is no decrease in pre-

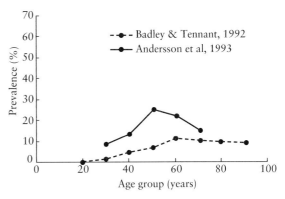

Fig. 18.4 The prevalence of neck pain with age in population-based studies. Data from [15,24].

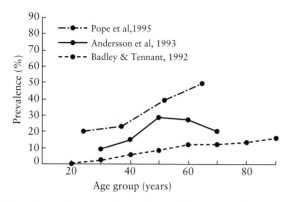

Fig. 18.5 The prevalence of shoulder pain with age in population-based studies. Data from [15,24,38].

valence at older ages [24,38]. In the large United Kingdom study of Badley and Tennant [24], prevalence of shoulder problems increased monotonically with age from 0.7 per cent at ages 16–24 years to 15.9 per cent over 85 years (Fig. 18.5). The difference in the pattern of prevalence at older ages may be due to varying definitions of the condition under study, the extent of exposure to risk factors for the disease, and the prevalence of co-morbidities in distinct populations.

Sex

The results in relation to the prevalence of shoulder and neck pain in males and females are consistent (Table 18.2). Females report higher rates than men. This is true whether the outcome of interest is pain or other symptoms and whether based on self-report, interview, or examination. Makela *et al.* [12], in a population study of neck pain amongst adults aged over 30 years in Finland, provided age and sex-specific estimates of the 1-month period prevalence. Females had higher rates at all ages. Similar conclusions were drawn from a population study of neck and shoulder pain among adults aged 20–56 years in a municipality of Norway [16].

Risk factors for shoulder and neck pain

Population studies which have examined risk factors for shoulder or neck symptoms (predominantly pain) are summarized in Table 18.4. The principal factors which have been examined are mechanical (injury), psychological, and psychosocial factors.

Social class

In the NHANES I study [26], both low income and having left formal education at an early age were associated with an increased likelihood of reporting musculoskeletal symptoms overall. In the study from Malmo [39], intelligence tests on men in elementary school predicted shoulder pain on follow-up, 45 years later. This remained an independent predictor even after adjustment for occupational workload and psychosocial factors [20]. In women, level of education attained rather than intelligence test score was associated with subsequent shoulder pain [39], although this was not an independent predictor of symptom onset [20].

In the population study of chronic neck syndrome in Finland [12], there was a strong association between the prevalence of symptoms and years of education (Fig. 18.6). Those with the longest years of education had the lowest prevalence of symptoms, irrespective of their current age. In the same study, there was a less clear association with occupational class. In men age 30–64 years the highest prevalence was in agricultural workers, while in older men the highest prevalence was in the 'clerical and services' category. In women the highest prevalence in age groups 30–64 years and ≥ 65 years was in the occupational groups 'industry' and 'clerical and services' respectively. However, it should be noted that the occupational category was an extremely broad classification system and, particularly in older subjects, may not even reflect the occupations which subjects held for most of their working life.

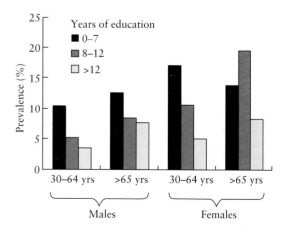

Fig. 18.6 Prevalence of chronic neck syndrome according to years of education: a population-based study in Finland. Data from [12].

Table 18.4 Population studies reporting risk factors for shoulder and neck pain

Country	Study method	Study sample	Disease definition	Sample size	Risk factors[a]		Reference
Finland	Cross-sectional	Sample of two rural communities 40–64 years	Pain occurring fairly often, often or continuously during the year preceding investigation in the shoulder–upper arm As above for symptoms in the neck, cervical spine or occiput	2268 (est. 396 with shoulder pain) (est. 390 with neck pain)	*Men:* Psychiatric symptoms *Women:* Psychiatric symptoms *Men:* Psychiatric symptoms *Women:* Psychiatric symptoms BMI ≥ 30	RR 2.4 95% CI (1.8, 3.1) RR 2.5 95% CI (2.0,3.2) RR 2.9 95% CI (2.2,3.8) RR 2.8 95% CI (2.2,3.6) RR 1.3 95% CI (1.0,1.7)	[11]
Finland	Cross-sectional	Representative sample of Finish population 30 years (results presented age 30–64 years	'Shoulder disorder' and 'chronic neck pain' determined by interview and examination	7217 (With symptoms)	*Men (30–64 years):* High physical stress at work High mental stress at work Neck/shoulder injury Current smoker Obese (BMI ≥ vs. <23) *Women (30–64 years)* High physical stress at work High mental stress at work Neck/shoulder injury Obese (BMI ≥35 vs. <23) Parity (≥ 7 vs. none)	RR 4.7 95% CI (3.0,7.4) RR 2.4 95% CI (1.7,3.4) RR 1.9 95% CI (1.5,2.4) RR 1.4 95% CI (1.0,2.0) RR 3.6 95% CI (1.8,7.5) RR 3.2 95% CI (2.4,4.3) RR 2.3 95% CI (1.8,2.9) RR 1.9 95% CI (1.6,2.4) RR 2.1 95% CI (1.3,3.5) RR 2.6 95% CI (1.7,3.8)	[12]
Sweden	Prospective cohort	Follow-up of subjects recruited from elementary school in 1938, 55 years of age	Shoulder pain at some time during previous month	574 subjects (79 with shoulder pain on follow-up)	*Men:* Lower intelligence (at recruitment) *Women:* Low job satisfaction (at follow-up)	P <0.05 P <0.05	[39]
Sweden	Cross-sectional	Random sample of city residents who participated in previous health survey	Sub-acromial shoulder pain without neck pain	445 (36 with shoulder pain) (35 with neck pain)	Self-rated heavy workload Low level of education Self-rated heavy workload Female sex	OR 5.4 95% CI (3.4,8.6) OR 2.4 95% CI (1.0,5.9) OR 8.0 95% CI (4.7,13.6) OR 4.8 95% CI (3.0,10.3)	[40]

Table 18.4 Population studies reporting risk factors for shoulder and neck pain(*continued*)

Country	Study method	Study sample	Disease definition	Sample size	Risk factors[a]		Reference
Sweden	Prospective cohort	Follow-up of population sample resident in a city	Neck symptoms during a 12-year period, leading to consultation	484 (132 with neck symptoms)	*Women:* Monotonous work Unsatisfactory leisure time	CIR 1.7 95% CI (1.0,2.9) CIR 1.9 95% CI (1.3,2.8)	[22]
			As above for shoulder symptoms		*Men:* Additional domestic load	CIR 2.3 95% CI (1.0,5.2)	
				(120 with shoulder symptoms)	*Women:* Unsatisfactory leisure time	CIR 2.3 95% CI (1.0,5.2)	[28]
					Men: Manual work Night or shift work	CIR 2.9 95% CI (1.4,6.1) CIR 3.1 95% CI (1.4,7.0)	
United Kingdom	Case–control	Random sample of community subjects aged 18–65 years	Pain in the shoulder (a manikin-defined area) lasting at least 24 h during past month and ⩾ 1 related disability	39 cases 178 controls	*Men:* Carried weights on one shoulder	RR 5.5 95% CI (1.8, 17)	
					Working conditions always damp Working conditions always cold	RR 5.4 95% CI (1.6,19) RR 6.4 95% CI (1.5, 27)	
					Women: No significant factors *Men and women:* Work was monotonous	RR 2.7 95% CI (1.3,5.4)	

[a] Only risk factors which were statistically significant are reported

RR = relative risk; OR = odds ratio; CIR = cumulative incidence ratio.

Social class or years of education *per se* obviously does not alter one's risk of future shoulder or neck symptoms. Instead they are likely to be a marker for future individual and environmental exposures experienced. In particular, a considerable amount of research interest has focused on mechanical factors (physical load, posture, and repetitive movements) and psychological and psychosocial factors. Population studies which have examined exposure to these factors, many of which have been measured with reference to occupation, will be reviewed. However, the sizeable literature pertaining to research studies conducted solely on specific occupational groups is outside the remit of this section and have recently been reviewed elsewhere [41,42].

Mechanical and psychosocial risk factors

These risk factors are considered together because individual studies have often considered both and it is important to consider the possible confounding effects of the other in examining any associations. A population-based study of shoulder pain conducted in north-west England involving 217 subjects compared work-place exposures amongst those subjects with and without disabling shoulder pain (Table 18.4) [28]. The exposures were those reported at the time of symptom onset (for cases) and at the same date for controls (who were matched by age and sex). Despite the small size of this study, strong associations, among men, were noted between disabling shoulder pain and mechanical factors (carrying weights on one shoulder) and work-place environment factors (conditions always damp or always cold) (Table 18.4). Increased risks of shoulder pain (although not statistically significant) were also noted for those who reported frequently working with hands above shoulder level (RR = 2.1), stretching to below knee level (RR = 2.0) and using arms (RR = 1.7) or wrists (RR = 2.0) in a repetitive way. There was no statistically significant associations found among women for exposure to mechanical factors, in whom many of the examined exposures were uncommon. However, working frequently with arms in a repetitive way was associated with a doubling of risk of shoulder pain, and frequently working in damp conditions with a three-fold increased risk. Men and women who reported work was monotonous had an almost three-fold increased risk of reporting shoulder pain, while those whose work caused stress and worry had a non-significant increased risk (RR = 1.9).

Bergenudd *et al.* [20] reported from Sweden a 45-year follow-up of elementary schoolchildren in third grade: 574 of 1542 participants in the original study were contacted and information on shoulder pain status collected (Table 18.4). Performing poorly in intelligence tests while a schoolchild was a predictor of shoulder pain on follow-up amongst men, while amongst women reporting poor job satisfaction was also associated with symptoms. There was a moderate, but not significant, increased risk of shoulder pain (RR = 1.4) associated with jobs that were evaluated as involving a moderate or heavy amount of physical workload. There was no investigation of psychological or psychosocial factors in this study.

A further survey (the 'Malmo Food Survey') in Sweden during 1984 involved 552 subjects out of 900 invited (Table 18.4). These subjects were then approached the following year, and 445 agreed to take part in a further survey which included enquiry about rheumatic complaints [40]. Both shoulder and neck pain were related to self-reports of a heavy physical workload, while in addition neck pain was related to a low level of education. While shoulder pain was not related to any of the specific occupational mechanical factors examined, neck pain was associated with reports of awkward working position for the neck and shoulders, for the back or legs, heavy work with the hands or forearms, and repetitive or static work tasks.

The third and most recent population survey in Sweden of risk factors for neck and upper limb disorders [22] involved 484 subjects aged 42–59 years (Table 18.4). Information was available on potential risk factors among the participating subjects from a study conducted 24 years previously. Shoulder symptoms were related, in men, to previous reports of manual work and night/shift work, and in women to low satisfaction with leisure time (i.e. insufficient or unsatisfactory leisure time). The authors also examined the combined effects of some of the exposures recorded. In men supra-additive effects were noted for the interactions of low family support with both high physical load and high mental load at work. Among women supra-additive interactions were noted for a high mental load at work in combination with additional domestic workload, and for manual work in combination with dissatisfactory leisure time. For neck pain, the single factor related to the onset in men was the reporting of an additional domestic workload, which was defined as being both gainfully employed and having responsibility for children and household. A greater than additive effect on risk was noted when this was combined with undertaking over-time work. Among women, two factors increased the risk of future neck pain—unsatisfactory leisure time and perceiving work as monotonous. When these were combined with a high physical workload and a low family support respectively, significant supra-additive interactive effects were noted.

A screening programme for musculoskeletal disorders was carried out in 1973–4 amongst residents aged 40–64 years of two rural municipalities in northwestern Finland (Table 18.4) [11]. As part of this study the authors examined the relationship between regional musculoskeletal disorders (including neck and shoulder) and obesity, psychiatric symptoms, and sector of employment. Only neck pain in women was associated with obesity (body mass index $\geq 30 \text{ kg/m}^2$), but there were strong relationships between neck and shoulder pain and the presence of multiple psychiatric symptoms [43] in both genders. Both neck and shoulder symptoms were most common in pensioners (most probably a reflection of their older age) and thereafter in agriculture/forestry and in industry/mining and construction. The lowest prevalence of both regional pain syndromes was observed in office-workers, managers, and service occupations.

Overall, these six population studies, conducted amongst different study populations and using different study methods, provide evidence for the role of both mechanical and psychosocial factors in the onset of neck and shoulder pain. Many of these exposures (particularly high exposures) occur in the work-place setting. However, the study by Fredriksson *et al.* [22] emphasizes the potential interaction of these two types of exposure and, further, of an interactive effect between exposures occurring at the workplace and at home. The majority of the data presented on risk factors in the population comes from cross-sectional studies and, as noted elsewhere, this provides problems in the measurement of relevant exposures and determining the temporal relationship between symptoms and the (perceived) exposure. Future work requires prospective studies on shoulder/neck-pain free populations with detailed assessment of potential risk factors and periodic follow-up to allow measurement of both changes in exposure and symptom occurrence.

Forearm pain

The problems, of a lack of classification criteria for upper limb syndromes in general, particularly relate to forearm pain, making review of the epidemiological literature problematic. Studies are usually based on diagnoses of specific soft tissue syndromes which have pain in the forearm (at rest and/or with specific movements) as one symptom. With the exception of carpal tunnel syndrome, which is considered separately in this chapter, there have been no validated criteria for these syndromes suitable for use in large-scale studies. Some 'diagnostic labels' use terms such as 'cumulative trauma disorder' or 'repetitive strain injury' which for reasons previously noted are particularly unsatisfactory and will not be considered further. Finally, there are a few studies based on the reporting of pain in a defined anatomical area. This approach not only aids comparison between studies but generally provides a suitable methodology for investigating the possible aetiology of forearm pain.

Occurrence

There have been relatively few epidemiological studies of forearm pain: four population-based studies which measured prevalence are listed in Table 18.5. In a population study in the United Kingdom in 1956 of subjects aged 18–65 years, the prevalence of elbow and forearm pain (experienced during the past month and lasting at least 1 day, and with the area indicated on a manikin) was 11 per cent and 8 per cent respectively (Fig. 18.1). At follow-up 2 years later, amongst subjects who were initially free of forearm pain, 105 subjects (8.3 per cent) had developed a new episode (using the same definition as previously) [45]. This is in close agreement with another United Kingdom based survey using a very similar definition, which found a prevalence of 9.4 per cent for elbow and forearm pain, and was reported by Helliwell [46].

During the 1980s an 'epidemic' of chronic upper limb pain syndrome (often labelled as repetitive strain injury) occurred in Australia, and subsequently in some other countries. Up to one-third of workers in some industries were away from work with such symptoms at the peak of the epidemic [47]. The role of mechanical, particularly workplace exposures, and the role of stress, personal susceptibility, and wider social and legal factors have all been proposed as having an influence on the 'epidemic'. Kivi [48], using reports on occupational disorders, submitted to a national board in Finland examined the trends in the number of cases of 'pain syndrome of the forearm' between 1975 and 1979. In contrast to the number of reports of shoulder pain, which remained constant during this period at

Table 18.5 Population and work place studies measuring the prevalence of elbow and/or forearm pain

Study location	Disease definition	Population	Sample size	Prevalence	Reference
General populations					
Finland	Pain (fairly often, often or continuously) in elbows or forearms during past year	Adults aged 40–64 years in two rural Finnish municipalities	2268	11% (M) 12% (F)	[11]
Norway	Persistent or regular recurrent pain with a duration >3 months. Site indicated on manikin	Random sample of subjects ages 25–74 years from two primary health care districts	1609	8.3% (M) 11.9% (F)	[15]
Sweden	Pain in elbow for at least 1 month and tenderness over lateral epicondyle and pain on pronation against resistance and report of pain when carrying	Random sample of city residents aged 31–74 years	15268	a	[17]
United Kingdom	Pain in (manikin-defined) forearm or elbow and lasting at least 24 h during past month	Adults aged 18–65 years in city suburb	1956	11% (elbow) 8% (forearm)	[44]
United Kingdom	New onset of forearm pain at 2 years follow-up in subjects initially forearm pain free	As above	1398	8%	[45]
United Kingdom	Pain in (manikin-defined) forearm and elbow lasting at least 24h during the past month	Community-based survey (age-range not reported)	Not reported	9% (elbow or forearm pain)	McCarney (unpublished data) reported in [46]

[a] Rates provided only in graphical form

approximately 50 cases per year, the number of cases of forearm pain increased from around 300 cases per year to more than 400.

Risk factors for the development of forearm pain

Age and sex

A population study in Norway found prevalence rates higher in females (8.3 per cent males vs. 11.9 per cent females). In a survey conducted in Finland of 2268 persons aged 40–64 years, pain in the elbows or forearm (occurring fairly often, often, or continuously) during the past year was reported by 11 per cent of men and 12 per cent of women. Prevalence rates in both sexes were higher over 50 years (men: 14 per cent, women: 15 per cent) than under 50 years (men 7 per cent, women 10 per cent) [11]. The United Kingdom population-based study, however, reported higher rates in males (8.9 per cent males vs. 7.9 per cent females) [45]. In the same study prevalence increased with age from 5.8 per cent at ages 18–39 years, to 9.0 per cent at ages 40–59 years, to 9.6 per cent at ages ≥ 60 years.

Mechanical and psychosocial factors

In examining associated features of symptoms, the Finnish population-based study discussed above found a two to three-fold increase in prevalence rates of elbow and forearm pain amongst subjects who reported multiple psychiatric symptoms (men 18 per cent, women 23 per cent) in comparison to those who did not (men 8 per cent, women 8 per cent) [11]. In comparison to some of the other regional pain syndromes considered in this study, the prevalence rates across agricultural, industrial, clerical, and housework showed little variation. However, this classification is likely to have been insufficiently precise to identify important mechanical factors in the aetiology of such symptoms.

In a study conducted across 12 workplaces amongst 1081 newly employed workers, the influence of short-term exposure to adverse psychosocial factors (job demands, support, and control) on the risk of regional pain syndromes was examined. Those who perceived their work as stressful always or most of the time were more likely to report forearm pain (OR 2.0, 95 per cent CI: 0.9–4.5) as well as other regional pain syndromes. Relationships with psychosocial factors were relatively modest; however, of all the regional sites

examined, the most consistent associations were with forearm pain: monotonous work (RR = 2.1), hectic work (RR = 1.4), and low job autonomy (RR = 1.7) [49]. Examining the role of short-term mechanical factors on regional pain syndromes, the only strong association with forearm pain in this study was with the reporting of frequent repetitive movement of the wrists (OR 1.8, 95 per cent CI: 1.04–3.1) [50].

The study in Finland of all reports of occupational disorders submitted to a national board between 1975 and 79 found that the upper limb was involved in 93 per cent of cases and specifically the forearm in 63 per cent [48]. Repetitive, monotonous tasks were considered to be a contributing factor by the reporting physician for forearm pain in 40 per cent of cases, and the occupations associated with highest risk were butchers and packers.

A study amongst 401 subjects employed in 11 factories in South Africa found that forearm, wrist, and hand pain (assessed by body manikin) was most common amongst workers involved in chicken processing, nylon spinners, and workers in a potato crisp factory and canning factory [51]. In comparison to the other occupations considered, these were assessed as having higher levels of repetitive upper limb movements. On regression analysis male sex and a composite factor assessing dynamic postures of the wrist and hand were the two factors predictive of forearm, wrist, or hand pain. In a United States study of soft tissue upper limb disorders in female garment workers, elbow and wrist pain were significantly more common in garment workers when compared with female hospital employees and rates were particularly high amongst those employed in 'stitching', 'finishing', or 'ironing' [52].

Although there has been considerable interest in this area, with substantial media coverage, there is a lack of large, population-based studies to allow an assessment of the range of possible aetiological factors. A recent population-based, prospective study of forearm pain attempted to evaluate the relative role of mechanical, psychosocial, and psychological factors in its onset. A total of 1398 subjects, who were initially free of forearm pain, provided information on their workplace mechanical and psychosocial factors and levels of psychological distress. At follow-up 2 years later, 105 subjects had developed a new episode of forearm pain (lasting at least 24 h in the past month and defined using a body manikin). It was uncommon for pain to be confined to the forearm (only 9 per cent of new cases). Shoulder pain and back pain were common co-morbidities while in 45 per cent of cases, subjects satisfied the ACR definition of chronic widespread pain used in the criteria for fibromyalgia [53]. An increased risk of developing forearm pain was identified for subjects who reported, at recruitment, high levels of psychological distress (RR 2.4, 95 per cent CI: 1.5–3.8) or other somatic symptoms (RR 1.7, 95 per cent CI: 0.95–3.0). The strongest workplace mechanical factors predicting onset were repetitive movements of the arm (RR 4.7, 95 per cent CI: 2.2–10) or wrists (RR 3.4, 95 per cent CI: 1.3–8.7) while the strongest workplace psychosocial factor was lack of support from colleagues and/or supervisors (RR 4.7, 95 per cent CI: 2.2–10) [45].

The review of the above data has concentrated, necessarily, on studies which have been based on symptom reporting. The results suggest that, in common with other regional pain syndromes, both psychosocial and specific mechanical factors are important in the onset of forearm pain. The ability to determine the epidemiology of specific clinical diagnoses with forearm pain as one feature will await similar studies using validated criteria for these conditions. Only then can it be determined whether any such clinical conditions have a distinct aetiology from the broad grouping of forearm pain syndromes.

There are, however, some studies which have examined the prevalence and aetiology of epicondylitis. Allander [17] examined the prevalence in random population samples of residents in the city of Stockholm aged 31–74 years. Although prevalence rates are not stated, graphical displays allow certain conclusions to be drawn—the prevalence in both sexes peaked in the fifth decade and with the exception of females in the fifth decade, amongst whom a prevalence rate of approximately 10 per cent was observed, all other rates were below 5 per cent. In the United States Health and Nutrition Examination Survey (HANES I), conducted on a random sample of 6913 adults aged 25–74 years, the estimated 'prevalence' (no further details reported) of self-reported elbow symptoms was 4.2 per cent and for physician-observed abnormalities was 1.2 per cent [26].

The aetiology of epicondylitis has been examined, principally in relation to employment, and generally conclude that those with upper limb physically demanding jobs have higher prevalence than 'control' populations. However, such 'control' populations may differ in a variety of additional aspects from the 'high risk' populations, and it remains to be elucidated the precise physical exposure(s) associated with risk. A study in Sweden amongst 2933 workers at an aircraft engine factory, which examined the role of the psychosocial work environment in upper limb symptoms, found that although neck and shoulder symptoms were more common amongst subjects in jobs considered stressful, there was no difference observed for epicondylitis [54]. The likelihood of symptoms increased with age, and with time spent in the job. Epicondylitis was more common in workers (rather than salaried staff) and those who used vibrating hand tools. Kivi [48] reported that in Finland between 1975 and 1979 the number of occupationally related cases of epicondylitis increased from around 100 to over 200 cases per year.

Hand and wrist syndromes

Two specific syndromes of the hand and wrist will be considered: Dupuytren's disease and carpal tunnel syndrome.

Dupuytren's disease

Dupuytren's disease was first described in the early 19th century by a French surgeon, Guillane Dupuytren [55]. The clinical deformity is a progressive flexion of the fingers arising from thickening and contracture of fibrous bands on the palmar surface of the hands and fingers. Although advanced cases present little problem in diagnosis, in the early stages differentiating from a normal hand with thick skin or prominent fascia can be difficult [56]. Given the lack of diagnostic tests, difficulties in ensuring repeatability of diagnosis between observers should be borne in mind when comparing prevalence rates across studies.

A study from Aberdeen in the United Kingdom involving 200 consecutive patients admitted to a geriatric ward assessed the interobserver repeatability of the diagnosis using two orthopaedic surgeons. Agreement was assessed using the Kappa (κ) statistic: where a κ value of 1 indicates perfect agreement and 0 a level of agreement that would be expected by chance. There was perfect agreement for measuring flexion contractures ($\kappa = 1.0$) and moderate agreement for observing skin tethering ($\kappa = 0.8$), palmar modules ($\kappa = 0.7$), and knuckle pads ($\kappa = 0.7$) [57].

Occurrence

Studies which have measured the prevalence of Dupuytren's disease in population samples are shown

Table 18.6   Studies measuring the prevalence of Dupuytren's disease

Study location	Population	Sample size	Prevalence	Reference
Australia	Medical institutions and work-place settings 30–80 years	3700	15.2% (F) 13.8% (M)	[58][a]
Canada	Hospital in-patients (all ages)	2705	9.9% (F) 15.4% (M)	[59]
Japan	Orthopaedic out-patient clinic	3852	0.9% (F) 2.9% (M)	[60]
Norway	General population ≥16 years	15950	2.8% (F) 9.4% (M)	[61]
Spain	General medical examinations >15 years	1455	4.4% (F) 12.1% (M)	[62]
Sweden	General population 55 years	574	2% (F) 10% (M)	[63]
United Kingdom	Hospital patients (general ward) >60 years	200	21% (F) 39% (M)	[57]
United Kingdom	Hospital patients (fracture ward)	555	16% (F) 16% (M)	[64]
United Kingdom	Exservicemen ≥65 years	400	14%	[65]
United Kingdom	Orthopaedic clinic 29–81 years	919	3.5% (F) 5.0% (M)	[66]
United Kingdom	Locomotive works (15–75 years)	5273	0.3% (F) 3.3% (M)	[67]
	Elderly care home (≥65 years)	466	9.2% (F) 17.2% (M)	
	General population (15–75 years)	1240	0.5% (F) 3.9% (M)	
United States	Hospital admissions ≥13 years	5062	1.8% (F) 4.3% (M)	[68]

[a] There was a marked difference in the age-distribution of male and female subjects in this study. Males had a higher prevalence within each of the age groups 30–39, 40–59 and 60–79 years.

in Table 18.6. Dupuytren's disease has traditionally been considered to be a disease of northern European populations and their descendants and to be more common in men than women. In the largest population study conducted Mikkelsen [61] took advantage of a mass screening programme in Hangasund in Norway, to examine approximately 16 000 adult participants using standardized diagnostic criteria for Dupuytren's disease. The overall prevalence rate found was 9.4 per cent in men and 2.8 per cent in women. In men, rates increased from 0.2 per cent at ages 20–24 years to a peak of 36.7 per cent at ages 70–74 with a slight decrease in rates thereafter to 30.8 per cent at ages 85–89 years. In women there were no diagnoses of Dupuytren's disease below aged 40, thereafter rates increased monotonically to 25.0 per cent at ages 85–89 years (Fig. 18.7). A smaller study from Sweden amongst 55-year-olds reported similar rates of disease amongst this age-group (males 10 per cent females 2 per cent) in comparison to the Norwegian study [63].

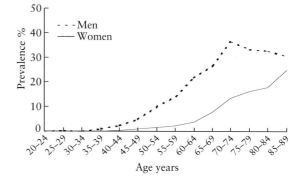

Fig. 18.7   Prevalence of Dupuytren's disease in Norway. Data from [61].

Results from other countries show great variability. In the United Kingdom, Lennox *et al.* [57] conducted a study amongst 200 patients, over 60 years, in geriatric wards in Aberdeen and reported higher rates in comparable age groups (male 39 per cent, female 21 per cent) than the study from Norway. A further study from London amongst ex-servicemen (aged 65 to 97 years), however, reported a much lower prevalence rate—14 per cent [65]. Although it has traditionally been considered uncommon outside Northern Europe, an epidemiological study from Spain reported high rates (male 12.1 per cent, female 4.4 per cent) suggesting that such generalizations may not hold [62]. Anecdotal evidence suggests that Dupuytren's disease is rare in Africa and much of Asia, and the latter is supported by a study from Japan amongst patients in an orthopaedic clinic which found low rates (male 2.9 per cent, female 0.9 per cent) [60].

Risk factors for Dupuytren's disease

Large variations in the prevalence of Dupuytren's disease between geographic areas and very high rates of disease in some populations, such as in Scandinavia, suggest that genetic factors may be important in disease onset. Further, it has been shown that Northern Europe populations maintain their high disease prevalence even on migration to warmer environments such as Australia. Hueston [69] hypothesized that such a genetic predisposition could have originated in Celtic or Viking populations, although subsequent studies have shown cases of disease to occur in populations outside areas of influence or migration of these populations. In many families there appears to be a dominant mode of inheritance of Dupuytren's disease although it is unclear whether many apparently sporadic cases also have a genetic basis [70].

The other factors consistently associated with Dupuytren's disease are diabetes mellitus, seizure disorders, alcohol intake, and manual occupations. Arkilla *et al.* [71] in a 5-year prospective study of 207 patients with type I diabetes (mean age 30 years) found an incidence rate for Dupuytren's disease of 2 per cent per annum (a very high rate for this age-group) and risk of onset was related to age and duration of diabetes. There was also an association between onset and complications of diabetes such as retinopathy or neuropathy after allowance for disease duration. However, the reason for an association between Dupuytren's disease and diabetes remains unknown.

A high prevalence of disease amongst those with a heavy consumption of alcohol has been reported by some although not all studies. Burge *et al.* [72], in a case–control study of patients operated on for Dupuytren's disease, and with both hospital and community control groups, found that alcoholics had approximately twice the risk of disease in comparison to non-alcoholics. Although the mechanism by which alcohol consumption may increase risk is unknown, it appears not to be through altered liver function since an association between hepatic pathology from other causes and Dupuytren's disease has not been demonstrated [73]. The same study also reported an independent increased risk associated with cigarette smoking, which the author's believed, as in the association with diabetes, may be as a result of microvascular impairment [74]. A link with seizure disorders has been demonstrated and the mechanism has been suggested as anticonvulsant drug treatment such as phenobarbitone [75], and improvement in signs has been noted after discontinuation of treatment [76].

Finally, whether mechanical factors have a role in onset has been a long-standing source of debate. The mechanism proposed for an association is through microtrauma to the palmar fascia resulting in fibrillar ruptures and microhaemorrhages. Two recent reviews [77,78] have addressed this topic but their conclusion is that evidence available to support an association with mechanical load is weak. Early [67] in a study from Manchester, United Kingdom of over 5000 employees in a locomotive works, found no difference in the prevalence of palmar contracture between office and manual workers. A previous study by Herzog [79], also from the United Kingdom, had reported similar rates of contracture amongst steelworkers, miners, and clerks. Evidence is stronger, however, to support a relationship between vibration and Dupuytren's disease, with three studies having reported such an association [80–82], and with some evidence of a dose–risk relationship.

Carpal tunnel syndrome

Carpal tunnel syndrome is a clinical disorder arising from compression of the median nerve at the wrist. Diagnosis is straightforward in patients with characteristic history, signs, and electrophysiological abnormalities—although this is likely to represent only one end of a clinical spectrum. To what extent, however, can those who present with deviations from this 'classical case' still be considered as part of this spectrum, that is what is an appropriate case definition? In the absence of a gold standard, studies have used various combinations of symptoms, signs, and electrophysiological abnormalities to define caseness and within these have used different definitions of abnormality. Apart from methodological issues, the practicality of using these measures may differ depending upon the size and the nature of the study sample selected, for example a small clinical sample may be investigated in greater detail than a large population sample, in whom either different criteria may need to be employed or use made of multistage sampling strategies.

Two recent studies have shown that agreement between single methods of identifying subjects with carpal tunnel syndrome can be relatively poor. A study of 824 workers across six companies in the United States found that only 5 per cent of subjects satisfying one criteria met all three criteria for carpal tunnel syndrome (symptoms, physical examination, electophysicological abnormalities) and that κ values, evaluating agreement between different definitions, showed agreement that was little better than chance [83]. A population study of 648 subjects conducted in the United Kingdom showed no relationship between symptom classification for carpal tunnel syndrome (classical/probable, possible, and unlikely) and delayed sensory or motor nerve conduction [84]. The presence of symptoms considered typical of carpal tunnel syndrome had a sensitivity of only around 20 per cent or less in detecting those with delayed nerve conduction. However, a population-based study of 2466 subjects in Sweden reported 'fair to moderate' agreement ($\kappa = 0.36$) between the clinical diagnosis of carpal tunnel syndrome and the identification of median neuropathy from electrophysiology [85].

A recent ad hoc working group in the United States have published criteria for the classification of carpal tunnel syndrome and reached consensus on the following conceptual issues. Firstly, that there is no perfect gold standard for carpal tunnel syndrome. Secondly, that the combination of symptoms and electrophysiological findings are the most accurate in making a diagnosis. If both these are available, physical examination findings add little diagnostic value, but in the absence of electrophysiological findings, physical examination findings in combination with symptoms provide the greatest diagnostic information [86]. Consequently, two sets of case definitions were proposed, those involving: (a) symptoms and electrophysiological findings (Table 18.7a; and (b) symptoms and physical examination findings (Table 18.7b). Each classifies symptoms as classic/probable, possible, or unlikely. 'Classic/probable' is defined as numbness, tingling, burning, or pain in at least two of digits 1–3 (palm pain, wrist pain, or radiation proximal to the wrist is allowed). 'Possible' is defined as tingling, numbness,

Table 18.7a Estimated likelihood of carpal tunnel syndrome for case definitions that include electrophysiological studies (EPS); reproduced with permission of the American Public Health Association from Rempel D, Evanoff B, Amadio PC *et al. Am J Public Health* 1998; 88: 1447–1451[86].

Symptom	EPS	Ordinal likelihood of CTS
Classic/probable	Positive	+++
Possible	Positive	++
Classic/probable	Negative	+/–[a]
Possible	Negative	–
Unlikely	Positive	–
Unlikely	Negative	—

[a] No consensus achieved on whether likelihood should be – or +

Table 18.7b Case definitions of Carpal Tunnel Syndrome that do not include electrophysiological studies; reproduced with permission of the American Public Health Association from Rempel D, Evanoff B, Amadio PC *et al. Am J Public Health* 1998; 88: 1447–1451[86]

Criteria evaluated in workplace studies	Sensitivity	Specificity	PPV
Classic/probable and PE and night symptoms[a]	0.07	0.99	0.44
Classic/probable and PE[a]	0.12	0.97	0.31
Classic/probable and night symptoms[a]	0.12	0.96	0.25
Classic/probable[a]	0.22	0.90	0.20
Possible[b]	0.34	0.84	0.19
PE[c]	0.41	0.76	0.16

Electrophysiological study findings alone were used as the gold standard. PPV was calculated assuming a disease prevalence of 0.10. PE = positive physical examination (Tinel's test, Phalen's test, 2-point discrimination, or carpal compression test).
[a] [83].
[b] [87].
[c] [88].

burning, or pain in at least one of digits 1–3, and 'unlikely' if there are no symptoms in digits 1–3 [89].

Occurrence

Prevalence and incidence studies are summarized in Table 18.8a and b, respectively. These studies, conducted in Europe and the United States, have all used different case definitions, and therefore comparison of results is difficult. The lowest prevalence rates were found in a United States population survey [92]. Amongst the 30 074 subjects who reported currently (or recently) being in employment 1.5 per cent self-reported that they had during the previous 12 months

357

Table 18.8a Population studies measuring the prevalence of carpal tunnel syndrome

Study location	Disease definition	Population	Sample size	Prevalence	Reference
Netherlands	BPN and ML >4.5 mn	Population sample from one city	504	0.6% (M) 6.8% (F)	[90]
Sweden	(a) pain/ numbness/ tingling in median nerve distribution (b) clinically certain CTS[a] (c) EP Median Neuropathy[a] (d) Definitions b and c	Population sample from single geographical area	2466	(a) 10.4% (M) 17.9% (F) (b) 2.8% (M) 4.6% (F) (c) 4.3% (M) 5.2% (F) (d) 2.1% (M) 3.0% (F)	[85]
United Kingdom	(a) SL >3.7 ms (b) SL >4.0 ms (c) ML >4.5 ms (d) Definitions a or c (e) Definitions b or c	Population sample registered with one general practice	648	(a) 11.7% (M) 11.1% (F) (b) 8.3% (M) 9.9% (F) (c) 8.2% (M) 6.4% (F) (d) 14.6% (M) 14.0% (F) (e) 18.0% (M) 12.9% (F)	[91]
United States	(a) 'During the past 12 months have you had a condition affecting the wrist and hand called carpal tunnel syndrome?' (b) Medically called CTS[a]	Workers amongst national survey participants	30074	(a) 1.2% (M) 1.8% (F) 1.6% (white) 0.7% (non-white) (b) 0.4% (M) 0.7% (F) 0.7% (white) 0.1% (non-white)	[92]

Table 18.8b Population studies measuring incidence of carpal tunnel syndrome

Study location	Disease definition	Population	Sample size	Incidence per 1000 person-years	Reference
United Kingdom	First referral to hospital for CTS	Sample from women in family planning clinics	17032 (154 cases)	1.0	[93]
United States	Physician diagnosis of CTS	Population in a defined geographical area	1016 cases	1.0	[94]
United States	Physician diagnosis of: (1) possible, probable or definite CTS (2) probable or definite CTS (3) possible, probable or definite CTS and at least 1/6 clinical signs	Population sample in defined geographical area	302 cases	(1) 4.03 (M) 4.90 (F) (2) 3.18 (M) 3.73 (F) (3) 3.16 (M) 3.62 (F)	[95]

[a] Refer to reference for details of definition
CTS = Carpal Tunnel Syndrome
EP = Electrophysiology
SL = Median Nerve Sensory Latency
BPN = Brachialgia Parasthetica Nocturna
ML = Medial Nerve Motor Latency

'a condition affecting the hand called carpal tunnel syndrome' while 0.5 per cent reported physician diagnosis. In population-cohort studies from defined geographical areas within the United States, incident rates of diagnosed carpal tunnel syndrome of 3.5 and 1.0 per 1000 person years of follow-up have been reported in two separate studies [94,95]. Both were based on retrospective review of case notes and the requirements for classification as a case differed between the two studies. Higher prevalence rates are found when definition is based on symptom reporting or electrophysiological studies. Atroshi *et al.* [85], in a population study from Sweden, found prevalence rates of 14 per cent when based on self-report of pain, numbness, and/or tingling in the median nerve distribution, during the previous 4 weeks. When based on electrophysiologically determined median neuropathy or 'clinically certain' carpal tunnel syndrome, prevalence fell to 4.8 per cent and 3.7 per cent respectively, and 2.6 per cent if both definitions required to be satisfied.

Time trends

The only study to provide information on time trends in occurrence is the population study in the United States from Rochester. These are based on clinical diagnoses, and over four quinquennia beginning with 1961–65, rates increased from 0.88, 1.00, 1.02, to 1.25 per 1000 person-years. These increases were observed in both males and females [94]. The authors conclude that such an increase could be due to increased exposure to risk factors (particularly exogenous hormones—discussed below) but may also be related to increased awareness of the condition, the changing nature of electrophysiological investigation, and the introduction of specialist hand clinics in the geographical area under study.

Aetiology

Gender

Studies based on symptom reporting and clinical diagnosis of carpal tunnel syndrome always report higher prevalence or incidence rates in females. In the population-based study from Sweden the prevalence of symptoms in the median nerve distribution was 17.9 per cent in females and 10.4 per cent in males (prevalence rate ratio (PRR) = 1.72). When based on 'clinically certain' carpal tunnel syndromes, the excess was maintained (4.6 per cent in females and 2.8 per cent in males, PRR = 1.64). Similar results were obtained from the national survey in the United States, where amongst those working the PRR (females vs. males) was 1.5 and 1.75 for symptom reporting and clinically certain CTS respectively [92]. In the population-based cohort study in Rochester (United States) incidence rates were three times higher in females (1.5 per 1000 person-years) than males (0.5 per 1000 person-years) [94]. Even where definition has been based on electrophysiology an excess amongst females has been reported. Atroshi *et al.* [85] report a PRR of 1.21 based on 'median neuropathy'. In contrast, however, a population-based study of 648 subjects in the United Kingdom did not find any difference in median nerve conduction between males and females, indeed the rates of combined sensory and motor delayed conduction were higher in males [91].

Age

In the population-based study of adults from the United States, Tanaka *et al.* [92] found that the prevalence of self-reported carpal tunnel syndrome increased from 18–24 years to a peak in the group 45–54 years, with thereafter a slight decrease in prevalence. A similar pattern was found with 'medically certain' cases, although the peak occurred slightly earlier—in the 35–44 years age-group. These results were confirmed by those of the Swedish study of Atroshi *et al.* [85]: prevalence of self-reported symptoms peaked between the ages of 55–64 years, with the prevalence of 'clinically certain' cases peaking earlier at 45–54 years. The incidence of diagnosed carpal tunnel syndrome increased with age in the cohort study of Nordstrom *et al.* [95]. The rate of physician diagnosis was very low in those under 18 years (0.30 per 1000 person years) and increased to a peak in the age group 50–64 years (7.81 per 1000 person-years), with only a slight decrease at older ages (7.54 per 1000 person-years). Indeed when only probable or definite diagnoses were included (or diagnosis and signs) the incidence rates increased monotonically with age. In the study of incidence from Rochester (United States), rates in females increased sharply to a peak of 4.2 per 1000 person-years at age 45–54 years and decreasing thereafter to 1.4 per 1000 person–years in the age group over 85 years [94]. In males, however, rates of new cases increased with age, the highest incidence rate (1.9 per 1000 person-years) being observed in those 85 years and over. Delayed nerve conduction increased with age in the study by Atroshi *et al.* [85] while it was found to be more common amongst subjects 55 years and above (in comparison to younger subjects) in the study by Ferry [91]: a difference particularly marked for motor latency.

Other demographic and socio-economic factors

Few studies have collected further information on the demographic or socio-economic factors associated with carpal tunnel syndrome. However, the study by Tanaka *et al.* [96] in the United States found that self-reported carpal tunnel syndrome was more than twice as common in whites than non-whites, and medically certain carpal tunnel syndrome six times as common. In addition self-reported carpal tunnel syndrome was found to be more common amongst those with more years of education (>12 years vs. ≤ 12 years; OR 1.4, 95 per cent CI: 1.1, 1.8) and higher levels of income (≥ $20000 vs. < $20000; OR 1.3, 95 per cent CI: 1.0, 1.7). Risk factors for the development of carpal tunnel syndrome were investigated in a nested case–control analysis from a prospective cohort study of the health effects of oral contraceptives in women on the United Kingdom. Cases were 1264 women who were diagnosed with carpal tunnel syndrome either in general practice or hospital, although no standardized criteria were used. Controls were age-matched women who did not have this diagnosis. This study found the diagnosis more common in subjects of low social class, even after adjustment for other risk factors [97].

Anthropometry

Several studies have reported a positive association between body mass and the risk of carpal tunnel syndrome. In the large UK study of women discussed above, the diagnosis of carpal tunnel syndrome was associated with previous consultation to general practice about obesity (OR 2.0, 95 per cent CI: 1.6, 2.6) [97]. In a cross-sectional study of 441 adult volunteers across six industries in the United States [98], a high body mass index (BMI) (i.e. weight (kg)/height (m^2)) was independently associated on multivariate analysis with median nerve sensory latency and with an increased likelihood of a diagnosis of carpal tunnel syndrome. On symptom analysis it was also associated with numbness but not tingling, pain, clumsiness, or nocturnal awakening. The Swedish population-based study of Atroshi *et al.* [85] found that a significantly higher proportion (70 per cent) of subjects with clinically and electrophysiologically confirmed carpal tunnel syndrome were obese (BMI > 25 kg/m^2) compared to those without carpal tunnel syndrome (47 per cent), a finding confirmed by Tanaka *et al.* [96] in the United States and de Krom *et al.* [99] in the

Netherlands. In the latter studies, with each unit increase in BMI the odds ratio of reporting medically confirmed carpal tunnel syndrome was 1.03 and 1.09 respectively. Studies by Werner *et al.* [100] and Nathan *et al.* [101] estimated that 8–9 per cent of the total risk of carpal tunnel syndrome could be explained by obesity. The prospective study of Vessey *et al.* [93] has further shown that subjects with a high BMI are at greater risk of developing carpal tunnel syndrome, after adjusting the analysis for the effects of cigarette smoking and the use of oral contraceptives (both possible confounding factors, discussed below).

The finding of a relationship between carpal tunnel syndrome and body mass is consistent across different study designs, different geographical locations, and using case-definitions. Where adjustment is made for confounding factors the relationship is still found to persist. The biological explanation of the relationship is thought to be an increased fatty tissue or oedema around the carpal tunnel.

Hormonal factors

One explanation of the sex differential in occurrence of carpal tunnel syndrome, which has been postulated, is hormonal factors. These have also been postulated to be implicated in other regional pain syndromes such as migraine and temporomandibular joint disorder. Both of these syndromes, more common in females, have been noted to be relatively uncommon in children with prevalence rates rising markedly after puberty—a feature also of carpal tunnel syndrome. Biological mechanisms linking hormonal factors with carpal tunnel syndrome have usually involved fluid retention or the observation that carpal tunnel syndrome appears to be common amongst pregnant women. The evidence that hormonal factors may be important in the aetiology is reviewed below.

The Oxford Family Planning Study involved prospective follow-up of 17 032 women attending family planning clinics in the United Kingdom [93]. At the time of recruitment women were aged 25–39 years, married, white, and either a user of oral contraceptives for at least 5 months or user of an alternative contraceptive (intrauterine device, diaphragm) without previous exposure to the pill. The outcome of interest was first referral rates for carpal tunnel syndrome (n = 154). There was no influence of parity or time since last pregnancy on outcome: only one women was pregnant at the time of referral. Referral rates, however, were related to duration of use of the oral contraceptive. Rates of referral amongst users for 10 years or more were more than double that of non-users: these associations remained even after adjusting for possible confounding factors including age and body mass.

The findings of a lack of association with pregnancy have been confirmed by other studies. In the United Kingdom study of 1264 women diagnosed with carpal tunnel syndrome, there was no effect of parity [97]. Dieck and Kelsey [102] in a case–control study of 44 women admitted to hospital for surgical treatment of carpal tunnel syndrome and 1043 admitted for other surgical procedures, found no relationship either with ever having been pregnant or the number of pregnancies. And a case–control study of 156 hospital and community-ascertained cases of carpal tunnel syndrome found no difference in parity status compared to 473 symptom-free community controls [99]. However, a prospective study from the United States, based in the Mayo clinic, has reported an effect with parity. The study involved hospital-diagnosed cases in the general population of Rochester and incident rates were estimated to be more than twice as high among pregnant in comparison to non-pregnant women aged 15–44 years [103]. The latter positive result, combined with anecdotal reports of carpal tunnel syndrome being common during pregnancy, and negative results from other case–control studies of referral for treatment may indicate that episodes are more common during pregnancy but relatively transient.

The observation by the Oxford Planning Study of an association with duration of use of oral contraceptives was partly confirmed by studies of Sabour and Fadel [104] and de Krom et al. [99]. In the former (uncontrolled) follow-up study of 62 clinical patients, symptoms were noted to resolve in all patients 1 month after discontinuation of the pill. In the latter study, although there was no overall association of the syndrome with use of oral contraceptives, subjects who used them for more than 5 years had a (non-significant) doubling of risk. The United Kingdom study of Ferry et al. [97] showed no association with current or previous oral contraceptive use. Although a United States case–control study of subjects (cases: 626, controls: 3618) undergoing carpal tunnel release within medical care programmes involved subjects too old to examine the influence of oral contraceptives, the use of oestrogen replacement therapy was associated with case status [105].

Several studies have examined the relationship between carpal tunnel syndrome and menstrual disorder and the menopause. The Oxford Planning Study [93] found rates of referral for carpal tunnel syndrome

were higher amongst women who had previously been referred for 'menstrual problems'—an association which the authors hypothesized to be a result of fluid retention. Such a hypothesis may also explain why the study of de Krom et al. [99] found that, amongst hospital cases, menopause (and hysterectomy) increased the immediate risk of the syndrome. Ferry et al. [97] reported that a diagnosis of carpal tunnel syndrome was associated with previous consultation for 'any menstrual disorder' (OR 1.4, 95 per cent CI: 1.1, 1.7) and in particular ammenorrhea, dysmenorrhoea, and heavy periods. Premenstrual tension and menopausal symptoms were also associated with the diagnosis for carpal tunnel syndrome. Hysterectomy has also been identified as a risk factor in other studies, including an occupational case–control study of 30 workers from one factory with clinically-confirmed carpal tunnel syndrome and 90 controls [106]. Risk was not significantly increased with hysterectomy alone, but increased in those with unilateral oophorectomy (OR = 3.4) and particularly those who had undergone bilateral oophorectromy (OR = 8.9). In a study of 53 healthy women who had undergone hysterectomy and bilateral oophorectomy 1–4 years previously and a group of 70 healthy age-matched women still menstruating, carpal tunnel symptoms (OR 4.3, 95 per cent CI: 1.5, 12.6) and abnormal nerve conduction studies were significantly more common in the former group [107].

Other hormone-related conditions have been associated with carpal tunnel syndrome. The study of Solomon et al. [105] found, using medical records, that diabetes mellitus, hypothyroidism, and inflammatory arthritis were all significantly more common in those undergoing carpal tunnel release. The latter association remained even after adjusting for the use of corticosteroids, a possible confounding factor. The population study of de Krom et al. [99] using both clinically diagnosed and population controls did not find a relationship with any of the aforementioned conditions, but with only 156 cases in total, the numbers of cases reporting these conditions was low, and the confidence intervals wide. In the large Swedish study of Atroshi et al. [85], based on participant self-reports, there was no difference in the prevalence of diabetes or hypothyroidism amongst clinically and electrophysiologically determined cases of carpal tunnel syndrome, but rheumatoid arthritis was more than twice as common. A study of 711 consecutive patients referred for electrophysiological testing to a private physical medicine practice in the United States, found that those subjects with confirmed carpal tunnel syndrome were more likely to have diabetes (significant), rheumatoid arthritis, and hypothyroidism (non-significant) [108].

Smoking

Smoking showed a strong positive relationship with carpal tunnel syndrome in the Oxford Family Planning Study [93]. Those smoking more than 25 cigarettes per day had a referral rate three times that of non- or ex-smokers (after adjustment for oral contraceptive use and body mass). At the time the study was published this was an isolated finding, with other studies reporting negative findings [102,109] and the authors could not provide a hypothesis for the mechanism of this association. Since that time, however, the relationship has been reported by other studies. Tanaka *et al.* [96] in the large population-based United States study found that carpal tunnel syndrome was significantly more common amongst current or ex-smokers. In a study within two groups of American industrial workers those with definite carpal tunnel syndrome were significantly more likely to be current smokers and had a higher lifetime consumption than those without carpal tunnel syndrome [110]. However, the large United Kingdom general practice based study failed to find an association between smoking status at the time of recruitment to the study and subsequent diagnosis [97].

Mechanical factors

The role of mechanical factors in the aetiology of carpal tunnel syndrome has been principally studied in occupational settings. A review of studies in occupational settings is outside the remit of this chapter, and is available elsewhere [111]. Instead, this section will discuss population studies which have examined the role of mechanical factors and highlight some studies in the work place which provide important information on their role. The factors which have been considered include repetitive upper limb movements, wrist flexion and extension, and upper limb vibration.

In the population-based study conducted with a sample of United States citizens, those subjects with self-reported carpal tunnel syndrome were significantly more likely to report bending or twisting of the wrist (OR 3.2, 95 per cent CI: 2.4, 4.1) or the use of hand-held vibrating tools (OR 1.7, 95 per cent CI: 1.3, 2.2) as part of their work [96]. The associations with medically confirmed cases was even stronger. Similarly, in the population-based study of de Krom *et al.* [99] in the Netherlands, reporting activities either with flexed or extended wrist was more common amongst those with carpal tunnel syndrome. Further, risk increased with increasing time of exposure to these tasks. The same study, however, reported no association with tasks involving pinch grasp nor was there a relationship with time spent typing [99]. A population study in Canada, on the island of Montreal, considered risk factors for first surgery for carpal tunnel syndrome. Overall, manual workers were observed to have an increased standardized incidence ratio (SIR) (men: SIR 180, 95 per cent CI: 140, 220; women: SIR 190, 95 per cent CI: 140, 250). Increased risks were also reported in six specific occupational groups: housekeepers/cleaners, data processing operators, material handlers, food and beverage service/processing, child-care workers (women), and lorry/bus drivers (men). Estimates of the attributable fraction in persons employed in these occupations varied from 75 per cent to 99 per cent. There was, however, no specific assessment of the mechanical exposures involved in subjects in this study. A study within an aircraft engine manufacturing plant, of 30 subjects diagnosed with carpal tunnel syndrome and 90 controls, found cases significantly more likely (OR = 14) to be employed in tasks which required the use of hand-held vibrating tools, but there was no difference regarding tasks involving repetitive motion [106]. In contrast, a study involving 1200 workers involved in repetitive work across 53 different companies in France found increasing risk (with caseness defined based on clinical examination or nerve conduction tests) with a decrease in the cycle time of the repetitive movement [112].

Psychological and psychosocial factors

In contrast to many regional pain syndromes, the role of psychosocial factors in the aetiology of carpal tunnel syndrome has received relatively little attention. The study considered above, conducted amongst workers in France whose tasks involved repetitive movement, considered aspects of job demand and control in addition to psychological well-being. In a multivariate model— including adjustment for mechanical factors—those workers with poor psychological well-being were at increased risk of carpal tunnel syndrome (OR 2.3, 95 per cent CI: 1.4, 3.9) as were those with low job control (OR 1.6, 95 per cent CI: 1.04, 2.4). Increased risk was also associated with a 'just in time' production system (OR 2.2, 95 per cent CI: 1.4, 3.6). Whether these associations hold with electrophysiological abnormalities or only with reporting of symptoms is unclear. Further, the large United Kingdom general practice-based study found an increased likelihood of a previous diagnosis of a psychotic (OR 1.4, 95 per cent CI: 0.9, 2.0) or non-psychotic (OR 1.3, 95 per cent CI: 1.1, 1.5) illness in those diagnosed with carpal tunnel syndrome.

The extensive literature on the aetiology of carpal tunnel syndrome provides some consistency in results. This is despite differences in study design, population studies, methods of classification, and exposure. Carpal tunnel syndrome is more common in women than men, and amongst women occurrence peaks in middle age. In women it appears to be related to hormonal factors—the use of exogenous oestrogens, the menopause, and hysterectomy (particularly with oophorectomy) all appear to increase the risk of symptoms in the short-term. A consistent relationship is also noted with obesity, and there is some evidence that smoking may be an independent risk factor. Both population and occupational studies suggest that mechanical factors may be important, in particular repetitive tasks, wrist flexion and extension, and the use of hand-held vibrating tools. Finally the study of Ferry *et al.* [97] show that carpal tunnel syndrome is not unrelated to other musculoskeletal disorders. In this study those with the diagnosis were significantly more likely to have been diagnosed with another musculoskeletal disorder (OR 2.4, 95 per cent CI: 2.0, 2.9). The particular disorders associated included arm fracture, osteoarthritis, arthritis (unspecified), fibrosis, neck pain, tennis elbow, limb pain, and joint pain.

Other upper limb conditions

Other conditions of the hand and wrist, such as tenosynovitis and De Quervain's disease of the wrist, are not considered separately within this chapter. There has been little consistency in the use of terminology. Proposed surveillance criteria are listed in Table 18.1, but at present information on their epidemiology comes from a few studies in the workplace, As an example, a cross-sectional study conducted amongst 2261 textile workers in four geographic areas of the United States [113] found a prevalence of tendinitis of 3.5 per cent. Prevalence was higher in the younger workers and amongst those categorized as having physically demanding job categories. Occupational and non-occupational upper limb physical tasks, particularly involving use of the thumbs, has certainly been noted clinically amongst individuals diagnosed with De Quervain's disease of the wrist [114], although again

there is a lack of epidemiological studies which have investigated this further. A prospective study at a meat packing plant in Canada measured the episode incidence of stenosing flexor tenosynovitis (trigger finger) amongst 454 workers initially symptom free [115]. The incidence rate was high and was particularly related to the use of hand tools (12.4 per cent hand-tool users vs. 2.6 per cent non-users). The particular aspect associated with increase risk (e.g. type of tool, force, duration) was not investigated.

Acknowledgements

Daniel Pope provided assistance with references on shoulder and neck pain, Isabelle Hunt provided assistance with reference on forearm pain, and helped in producing the figures for the chapter. Lesley Jordan typed the manuscript.

References

1. Hunt IM, Silman AJ, Benjamin S, McBeth J, Macfarlane GJ. The prevalence and associated features of chronic widespread pain in the community using the 'Manchester' definition of chronic widespread pain. *Rheumatology* 1999; 38: 275–279.
2. Badley EM, Tennant A. Impact of disablement due to rheumatic disorders in a British population: estimates of severity and prevalence from the Calderdale rheumatic disablement survey. *Ann Rheum Dis* 1993; 52: 6–13.
3. Bamji AN, Erhardt CC, Price TR, Williams PL. The painful shoulder: can consultants agree? *Br J Rheumatol* 1996; 35: 1172–1174.
4. Buchbinder R, Goel V, Bombardier C, Hogg Johnson S. Classification systems of soft tissue disorders of the neck and upper limb: do they satisfy methodological guidelines? *J Clin Epidemiol* 1996; 49: 141–149.
5. Liesdek C, van der Windt DA, Koes BW, Bouter LM. Soft-tissue disorders of the shoulder: a study of the inter-observer agreement between general practioners and pysiotherapists and an overview of physiotherapeutic treatment. *Physiotherapy* 1997; 83: 12–17.
6. Pope DP, Croft PR, Pritchard CM, Silman AJ. Prevalence of shoulder pain in the community: the influence of case definition. *Ann Rheum Dis* 1997; 56: 308–312.
7. Harrington JM, Carter JT, Birrell L, Gompertz D. Surveillance case definitions for work related upper limb pain syndromes. *Occup Environ Med* 1998; 55: 264–271.
8. Sluiter JS, Rest KM, Frings-Dresen MH. *Criteria document for the evaluation of work-relatedness of upper extremity musculoskeletal disorders.* University of Amsterdam: Coronel Institute for Occupational and Environmental Health, Academic Medical Center, 2000.

9. Palmer K, Walker Bone K, Linaker C *et al.* The Southampton examination schedule for the diagnosis of musculoskeletal disorders of the upper limb. *Ann Rheum Dis* 2000; **59**: 5–11.

10. Norregaard J, Jacobsen S, Kristensen JH. A narrative review on classification of pain conditions of the upper extremities. *Scand J Rehabil Med* 1999; **31**: 153–164.

11. Takala J, Sievers K, Klaukka T. Rheumatic symptoms in the middle-aged population in southwestern Finland. *Scand J Rheumatol Suppl* 1982; **47**: 15–29.

12. Makela M, Heliovaara M, Sievers K, Impivaara O, Knekt P, Aromaa A. Prevalence, determinants, and consequences of chronic neck pain in Finland. *Am J Epidemiol* 1991; **134**: 1356–1367.

13. van Schaardenburg D, Van den Brande KJ, Ligthart GJ, Breedveld FC, Hazes JM. Musculoskeletal disorders and disability in persons aged 85 and over: a community survey. *Ann Rheum Dis* 1994; **53**: 807–811.

14. van der Windt DA, Koes BW, de Jong BA, Bouter LM. Shoulder disorders in general practice: incidence, patient characteristics, and management. *Ann Rheum Dis* 1995; **54**: 959–964.

15. Andersson HI, Ejlertsson G, Leden I, Rosenberg C. Chronic pain in a geographically defined general population: studies of differences in age, gender, social class, and pain localization. *Clin J Pain* 1993; **9**: 174–182.

16. Hasvold T, Johnsen R. Headache and neck or shoulder pain—frequent and disabling complaints in the general population. *Scand J Prim Health Care* 1993; **11**: 219–224.

17. Allander E. Prevalence, incidence, and remission rates of some common rheumatic diseases or syndromes. *Scand J Rheumatol* 1974; **3**: 145–153.

18. Westerling D, Jonsson BG. Pain from the neck-shoulder region and sick leave. *Scand J Soc Med* 1980; **8**: 131–136.

19. Jacobsson L, Lindgarde F, Manthorpe R. The commonest rheumatic complaints of over six weeks' duration in a twelve-month period in a defined Swedish population. Prevalences and relationships. *Scand J Rheumatol* 1989; **18**: 353–360.

20. Bergenudd H, Nilsson B. The prevalence of locomotor complaints in middle age and their relationship to health and socioeconomic factors. *Clin Orthop* 1994; **308**: 264–270.

21. Ekberg K, Karlsson M, Axelson O, Malm P. Cross-sectional study of risk factors for symptoms in the neck and shoulder area. *Ergonomics* 1995; **38**: 971–980.

22. Fredriksson K, Alfredsson L, Koster M *et al.* Risk factors for neck and upper limb disorders: results from 24 years of follow up. *Occup Environ Med* 1999; **56**: 59–66.

23. Chard MD, Hazleman R, Hazleman BL, King RH, Reiss BB. Shoulder disorders in the elderly: a community survey. *Arthritis Rheum* 1991; **34**: 766–769.

24. Badley EM, Tennant A. Changing profile of joint disorders with age: findings from a postal survey of the population of Calderdale, West Yorkshire, United Kingdom. *Ann Rheum Dis* 1992; **51**: 366–371.

25. Chakravarty K, Webley M. Shoulder joint movement and its relationship to disability in the elderly. *J Rheumatol* 1993; **20**: 1359–1361.

26. Cunningham LS, Kelsey JL. Epidemiology of musculoskeletal impairments and associated disability. *Am J Public Health* 1984; **74**: 574–579.

27. Makela M, Heliovaara M, Sievers K, Knekt P, Maatela J, Aromaa A. Musculoskeletal disorders as determinants of disability in Finns aged 30 years or more. *J Clin Epidemiol* 1993; **46**: 549–559.

28. Pope DP, Croft PR, Pritchard CM, Silman AJ, Macfarlane GJ. Occupational factors related to shoulder pain and disability. *Occup Environ Med* 1997; **54**: 316–321.

29. Beaton D, Richards RR. Assessing the reliability and responsiveness of 5 shoulder questionnaires. *J Shoulder Elbow Surg* 1998; **7**: 565–572.

30. Richards RR, An KN, Bigliani LU *et al.* A standardised method for the assessment of shoulder function. *J Shoulder Elbow Surg* 1994; **3**: 347–352.

31. Roach KE, Budiman ME, Songsiridej N, Lertratanakul Y. Development of a shoulder pain and disability index. *Arthritis Care Res* 1991; **4**: 143–149.

32. Lippett SB, Harryman DT, Matsen FA. A practical tool for evaluating funstion: the simple shoulder test. In: Matsen FA, Fu FH, Hawkins RJ, editors. *The shoulder: a balance of mobility and stability*. Rosemont, Illinois: American Academy of Orthapaedic Surgeons Symposium, 1993: 501–518.

33. Patte D. Directions for the use of the index severity for painful and/or chronically disabled shoulders. *Abstracts of the First Open Congress of the European Society of Surgery of the Shoulder and Elbow (SECEC)*, 1987: 36–41.

34. Croft P, Pope D, Zonca M, O'Neill T, Silman A. Measurement of shoulder related disability: results of a validation study. *Ann Rheum Dis* 1994; **53**: 525–528.

35. Vernon H, Mior S. The Neck Disability Index: a study of reliability and validity. *J Manipulative Physiol Ther* 1991; **14**: 409–415.

36. Leak AM, Cooper J, Dyer S, Williams KA, Turner Stokes L, Frank AO. The Northwick Park neck pain questionnaire, devised to measure neck pain and disability. *Br J Rheumatol* 1994; **33**: 469–474.

37. Fairbank JC, Couper J, Davies JB, O'Brien JP. The Oswestry low back pain disability questionnaire. *Physiotherapy* 1980; **66**: 271–273.

38. Pope D. *A survey of shoulder pain in the community: issues of response, case definition and prevalence*. MSc Thesis, University of Manchester, 1995.

39. Bergenudd H, Lindgarde F, Nilsson B, Petersson CJ. Shoulder pain in middle age. A study of prevalence and relation to occupational work load and psychosocial factors. *Clin Orthop* 1988; **231**: 234–238.

40. Jacobsson L, Lindgarde F, Manthorpe R, Ohlsson K. Effect of education, occupation and some lifestyle factors on common rheumatic complaints in a Swedish group aged 50–70 years. *Ann Rheum Dis* 1992; **51**: 835–843.

41. Ariens GAM, Borghouts JAJ, Koes BW. Neck pain. In: Crombie IK, Croft PR, Linton SJ, LeResche L, von Korff M, editors. *Epidemiology of pain*. Seattle: IASP Press, 1999.

42. van der Windt DA, Thomas E, Pope DP *et al.* Occupational risk factors for shoulder pain: a systematic review. *Occup Environ Med* 2000; **57**: 433–442.

43. Goldberg DP. *The detection of psychiatric illness by questionnaire*. London: Oxford University Press, 1972.

44. Macfarlane GJ. Musculoskeletal pain in the community and workplace. In: McCaig R, Harrington M, editors. *The changing nature of occupational health*. UK: HSE books, 1998: 119–136.

45. Macfarlane GJ, Hunt IM, Silman AJ. The role of mechanical and psychosocial factors in the onset of forearm pain. *BMJ* 2000; **32**: 676–9.

46. Helliwell P. The elbow, forearm, wrist and hand. *Best Pract Res Cl Rh* 1999; **13**: 311–328.

47. Miller MH, Topliss DJ. Chronic upper limb pain syndrome (repetitive strain injury) in the Australian workforce: a systematic cross sectional rheumatological study of 229 patients. *J Rheumatol* 1988; **15**: 1705–1712.

48. Kivi P. Rheumatic disorders of the upper limbs associated with repetitive occupational tasks in Finland in 1975–1979. *Scand J Rheumatol* 1984; **13**: 101–107.

49. Nahit ES, Pritchard CM, Cherry NM, Silman AJ, Macfarlane GJ. The influence of work-related psychosocial factors and psychological distress on regional musculoskeletal pain. *J Rheumatol* 2001; **28**: 1378–1384.

50. Nahit ES, Macfarlane GJ, Pritchard C, Cherry NM, Silman AJ. The short term influence of mechanical factors on regional musculoskeletal pain: a study of new workers from twelve occupational groups. *Occup Environ Med* 2001; **58**: 374–381.

51. Schierhout GH, Meyers JE, Bridger RS. Work related musculoskeletal disorders and ergonomic stressors in the South African workforce. *Occup Environ Med* 1995; **52**: 46–50.

52. Punnett L, Robins JM, Wegman DH, Keyserling WM. Soft tissue disorders in the upper limbs of female garment workers. *Scand J Work Environ Health* 1985; **11**: 417–425.

53. Wolfe F, Smythe HA, Yunus MB *et al*. The American College of Rheumatology 1990 criteria for the classification of fibromyalgia. Report of the multicenter criteria committee. *Arthritis Rheum* 1990; **33**: 160–172.

54. Dimberg L, Olafsson A, Stefansson E *et al*. The correlation between work environment and the occurrence of cervicobrachial symptoms. *J Occup Med* 1989; **31**: 447–453.

55. Dupuytren G. *Lecons orale de clinique chirurgicale*. Paris: Germer-Bailliere, 1832.

56. McGrouther DA. The clinical diagnosis. In: McFarlane RM, McGrouther DA, Flint MH, editors. *Dupuytren's disease: biology and treatment*. New York: Churchill Livingstone, 1990: 191–200.

57. Lennox IA, Murali SR, Porter R. A study of the repeatability of the diagnosis of Dupuytren's contracture and its prevalence in the Grampian region. *J Hand Surg Br* 1993; **18**: 258–261.

58. Hueston JT. The incidence of Dupuytren's contracture. *Med J Aust* 1960; **2**: 999–1007.

59. Gordon S. Dupuytren's contracture: the significance of various factors in its etiology. *Ann Surg* 1954; **140**: 683–686.

60. Egawa T. Dupuytren's contracture in the hand: incidental study on outpatients in a private practice of general orthopaedics. *J Japanese Soc Surg* 1985; **2**: 536–539.

61. Mikkelsen OA. The prevalence of Dupuytren's disease in Norway. A study in a representative population sample of the municipality of Haugesund. *Acta Chir Scand* 1972; **138**: 695–700.

62. Guitain AQ. Quelques aspects epidemiologiques de la maladie de Dupuytren. *Ann Chir Main* 1988; **7**: 256–262.

63. Bergenudd H, Lindgarde F, Nilsson BE. Prevalence of Dupuytren's contracture and its correlation with degenerative changes of the hands and feet and with criteria of general health. *J Hand Surg Br* 1993; **18B**: 254–257.

64. Arafa M, Noble J, Royle SG, Trail IA, Allen J. Dupuytren's and epilepsy revisited. *J Hand Surg Br* 1992; **17**: 221–224.

65. Carson J, Clarke C. Dupuytren's contracture in pensioners at the Royal Hospital Chelsea. *J R Coll Physicians Lond* 1993; **27**: 25–27.

66. Mackenney RP. A population study of Dupuytren's contracture. *Hand* 1983; **15**: 155–161.

67. Early PF. Population studies in Dupuytren's contracture. *J Bone Joint Surg Br* 1962; **44**: 602–613.

68. Yost J, Winters T, Fett HC. Dupuytren's contracture. A statistical study. *Am J Surg* 1955; **99**: 568–571.

69. Hueston JT. Overview of aetiology and pathology. In: Hueston JT, Tubiana R, editors. *Dupuytren's disease*. Edinburgh: Churchill Livingstone, 1985: 75–81.

70. Burge P. Genetics of Dupuytren's disease. *Hand Clin* 1999; **15**: 63–71.

71. Arkkila PET, Kantola IM, Viikari JSA, Ronnemaa T, Vahatalo MA. Dupuytren's disease in type 1 diabetic patients: a five-year prospective study. *Clin Exp Rheumatol* 1996; **14**: 59–65.

72. Burge P, Hoy G, Regan P, Milne R. Smoking, alcohol and the risk of Dupuytren's contracture. *J Bone Joint Surg Br* 1997; **79**: 206–210.

73. Noble J, Arafa M, Royle SG, McGeorge G, Crank S. The association between alcohol, hepatic pathology and Dupuytren's disease. *J Hand Surg Br* 1992; **17**: 71–74.

74. van Adrichem LN, Hovius SE, van Strik R, van der Meulen JC. Acute effects of cigarette smoking on microcirculation of the thumb. *Br J Plast Surg* 1992; **45**: 9–11.

75. Critchley EM, Vakil SD, Hayward HW, Owen VM. Dupuytren's disease in epilepsy: result of prolonged administration of anticonvulsants. *J Neurol Neurosurg Psychiatry* 1976; **39**: 498–503.

76. Froscher W, Hoffman F. Dupuytren's contracture in patients with epilepsy: follow-up study. In: Oxley J, Janz D, Meinardi H, editors. *Chronic toxicity of antiepileptic drugs*. New York: Raven Press, 1983: 147.

77. Ross DC. Epidemiology of Dupuytren's disease. *Hand Clin* 1999; **15**: 53–62.

78. Liss GM, Stock SR. Can Dupuytren's contracture be work-related?: review of the evidence. *Am J Ind Med* 1996; **29**: 521–532.

79. Herzog EG. The aetiology of Dupuytren's contracture. *Lancet* 1951; **i**: 305.

80. Cocco PL, Frau P, Rapallo M, Casula D. Occupational exposure to vibration and Dupuytren's disease: a case-controlled study. *Med Lav* 1987; **78**: 386–392.

81. Thomas PR, Clarke D. Vibration white finger and Dupuytren's contracture: are they related? *Occup Med Lond* 1992; **42**: 155–158.

82. Bovenzi M. Hand-arm vibration syndrome and dose-response relation for vibration induced white finger among quarry drillers and stonecarvers. Italian study group on physical hazards in the stone industry. *Occup Environ Med* 1994; **51**: 603–611.

83. Homan MM, Franzblau A, Werner RA, Albers JW, Armstrong TJ, Bromberg MB. Agreement between symptom surveys, physical examination procedures and electrodiagnostic findings for the carpal tunnel syndrome. *Scand J Work Environ Health* 1999; **25**: 115–124.

84. Ferry S, Silman AJ, Pritchard T, Keenan J, Croft P. The association between different patterns of hand symptoms and objective evidence of median nerve compression: a community-based survey. *Arthritis Rheum* 1998; **41**: 720–724.

85. Atroshi I, Gummesson C, Johnsson R, Ornstein E, Ranstam J, Rosen I. Prevalence of carpal tunnel syndrome in a general population. *JAMA* 1999; **282**: 153–158.

86. Rempel D, Evanoff B, Amadio PC *et al.* Consensus criteria for the classification of carpal tunnel syndrome in epidemiologic studies. *Am J Public Health* 1998; **88**: 1447–1451.

87. Franzblau A, Werner RA, Albers JW, Grant CL, Olinskis D, Johnston E. Workplace surveillance for carpal-tunnel syndrome using hand-diagrams. *J Occup Rehabil* 1994; **4**: 185–198.

88. Franzblau A, Werner R, Valle J, Johnston E. Workplace surveillance for carpal tunnel syndrome: a comparison of methods. *J Occup Rehabil* 1993; **3**: 1–14.

89. Katz JN, Stirrat CR. A self-administered hand diagram for the diagnosis of carpal-tunnel syndrome. *J Hand Surg Am* 1990; **15A**: 360–363.

90. de Krom MC, Knipschild PG, Kester AD, Thijs CT, Boekkooi PF, Spaans F. Carpal tunnel syndrome: prevalence in the general population. *J Clin Epidemiol* 1992; **45**: 373–376.

91. Ferry S, Pritchard T, Keenan J, Croft P, Silman AJ. Estimating the prevalence of delayed median nerve conduction in the general population. *Br J Rheumatol* 1998; **37**: 630–635.

92. Tanaka S, Wild DK, Seligman PJ, Behrens V, Cameron L, Putz Anderson V. The US prevalence of self-reported carpal tunnel syndrome: 1988 National Health Interview Survey data. *Am J Public Health* 1994; **84**: 1846–1848.

93. Vessey MP, Villard Mackintosh L, Yeates D. Epidemiology of carpal tunnel syndrome in women of childbearing age. Findings in a large cohort study. *Int J Epidemiol* 1990; **19**: 655–659.

94. Stevens JC, Sun S, Beard CM, O'Fallon WM, Kurland LT. Carpal tunnel syndrome in Rochester, Minnesota, 1961 to 1980. *Neurology* 1988; **38**: 134–138.

95. Nordstrom DL, DeStefano F, Vierkant RA, Layde PM. Incidence of diagnosed carpal tunnel syndrome in a general population. *Epidemiology* 1998; **9**: 342–345.

96. Tanaka S, Wild DK, Cameron LL, Freund E. Association of occupational and non-occupational risk factors with the prevalence of self-reported carpal tunnel syndrome in a national survey of the working population. *Am J Ind Med* 1997; **32**: 550–556.

97. Ferry S, Hannaford P, Warskyj M, Lewis M, Croft P. Carpal tunnel syndrome: a nested case-control study of risk factors in women. *Am J Epidemiol* 2000; **151**: 566–574.

98. Keniston RC, Nathan PA, Leklem JE, Lockwood RS. Vitamin B6, vitamin C, and carpal tunnel syndrome. A cross-sectional study of 441 adults. *J Occup Environ Med* 1997; **39**: 949–959.

99. de Krom MC, Kester AD, Knipschild PG, Spaans F. Risk factors for carpal tunnel syndrome. *Am J Epidemiol* 1990; **132**: 1102–1110.

100. Werner RA, Albers JW, Franzblau A, Armstrong TJ. The relationship between body mass index and the diagnosis of carpal tunnel syndrome. *Muscle Nerve* 1994; **17**: 632–636.

101. Nathan PA, Keniston RC, Meadows KD, Lockwood RS. The relationship between body mass index and the diagnosis of carpal tunnel syndrome. *Muscle Nerve* 1994; **17**: 1491–1493.

102. Dieck GS, Kelsey JL. An epidemiologic study of the carpal tunnel syndrome in an adult female population. *Prev Med* 1985; **14**: 63–69.

103. Stevens JC, Beard CM, O'Fallon WM, Kurland LT. Conditions associated with carpal tunnel syndrome. *Mayo Clin Proc* 1992; **67**: 541–548.

104. Sabour MS, Fadel HE. The carpal tunnel syndrome—a new complication ascribed to the 'pill'. *Am J Obstet Gynecol* 1970; **107**: 1265–1267.

105. Solomon DH, Katz JN, Bohn R, Mogun H, Avorn J. Nonoccupational risk factors for carpal tunnel syndrome. *J Gen Intern Med* 1999; **14**: 310–314.

106. Cannon LJ, Bernacki EJ, Walter SD. Personal and occupational factors associated with carpal tunnel syndrome. *J Occup Med* 1981; **23**: 255–258.

107. Pascual E, Giner V, Arostegui A, Conill J, Ruiz MT, Pico A. Higher incidence of carpal tunnel syndrome in oophorectomized women. *Br J Rheumatol* 1991; **30**: 60–62.

108. Radecki P. The familial occurrence of carpal tunnel syndrome. *Muscle Nerve* 1994; **17**: 325–330.

109. Wieslander G, Norback D, Gothe CJ, Juhlin L. Carpal tunnel syndrome (CTS) and exposure to vibration, repetitive wrist movements, and heavy manual work: a case-referent study. *Br J Ind Med* 1989; **46**: 43–47.

110. Nathan PA, Keniston RC, Lockwood RS, Meadows KD. Tobacco, caffeine, alcohol, and carpal tunnel syndrome in American industry. A cross-sectional study of 1464 workers. *J Occup Environ Med* 1996; **38**: 290–298.

111. Abbas MA, Afifi AA, Zhang ZW, Kraus JF. Meta-analysis of published studies of work-related carpal tunnel syndrome. *Int J Occup Environ Health* 1998; **4**: 160–167.

112. Leclerc A, Franchi P, Cristofari MF *et al.* Carpal tunnel syndrome and work organisation in repetitive work: a cross sectional study in France. Study group on repetitive work. *Occup Environ Med* 1998; **55**: 180–187.

113. McCormack RR Jr, Inman RD, Wells A, Berntsen C, Imbus HR. Prevalence of tendinitis and related disorders of the upper extremity in a manufacturing workforce. *J Rheumatol* 1990; **17**: 958–964.

114. Moore JS. De Quervain's tenosynovitis. Stenosing teno-synovitis of the first dorsal compartment. *J Occup Environ Med* 1997; **39**: 990–1002.

115. Gorsche R, Wiley JP, Renger R, Brant R, Gemer TY, Sasyniuk TM. Prevalence and incidence of stenosing flexor tenosynovitis (trigger finger) in a meat-packing plant. *J Occup Environ Med* 1998; **40**: 556–560.

116. Kourinka I, Jonsson B, Kilbom A *et al*. Standardised Nordic questionnaires for the analysis of musculo-skeletal symptoms. *Appl Ergon* 1987; **18**: 233–237.

19 | *Chronic widespread pain and fibromyalgia*

Gary J. Macfarlane

Pain is a common complaint in the general population. Approximately 60 per cent of individuals will report having experienced pain, which has lasted for one day or longer, during the past month [1]. Some of these reports will be about relatively trivial pain, limited to one region of the body, with little or no impact on subjects' daily activities and which does not result in consultation to medical services. However, more than one-fifth of subjects with pain (13 per cent of the general population) will report pain that it is both chronic and widespread throughout the body. Chronic widespread pain, one of the core features of the fibromyalgia syndrome, is commonly associated with significant morbidity, frequent health service utilization, and indeed is estimated to be one of the most common reasons for referral to rheumatologists in Western Europe and North America [2].

Definition and classification

The concept of a syndrome encompassing pain, stiffness, tenderness, and fatigue has been recognized since the time of Hippocrates. It has been classified in diverse ways and known by a variety of names, the most modern of which include 'muscular rheumatism', 'fibrositis', and, latterly, 'fibromyalgia'. The groups of symptoms and signs which together are recognized clinically as fibromyalgia also overlap to a considerable extent with several other 'syndromes', particularly chronic fatigue syndrome, but also multiple chemical sensitivities, chronic candidiasis, silicone-associated atypical rheumatic disease, and what has been labelled as 'Gulf war syndrome' [3]. One of the major problems in studying conditions such as fibromyalgia is the lack of a gold standard against which classification criteria can be developed and evaluated. In 1977 Smythe and Moldofsky [4], in describing patients with the 'fibrositis' syndrome, noted that reports of pain and generalized tenderness on examination were often accompanied by a cycle of disturbed sleep, fatigue, and emotional distress. Subsequently, Yunus *et al.* [5] derived criteria for the syndrome by comparing a group of clinically diagnosed subjects with 'primary' fibromyalgia against both normal controls and subjects with other types of pain (mild rheumatoid arthritis and local fibromyalgia secondary to trauma). The criteria proposed were pain and/or stiffness at four or more anatomic sites for 3 months or longer (with bilateral involvement of a site counting as one site) and exclusion of an underlying condition. In addition, subjects were required either to have (a) at least two from six historical variables plus four or more specific anatomical sites which were painful on palpation (so called tender points) or (b) at least three from six historical variables plus two or more tender points. The historical variables were general fatigue, poor sleep, anxiety/tension, irritable bowel syndrome, and pain in seven or more areas. These criteria (incorporating some minor modifications) were subsequently used in population surveys, while studies based in clinics used a wide array of similar, but not identical, criteria.

Yunus's classification for fibromyalgia was one of several commonly in use until, in 1990, the American College of Rheumatology (ACR) published classification criteria [6]. Lacking a gold standard for the syndrome, individual rheumatologists, with an interest in fibromyalgia, identified a group of their own clinic patients who they considered to have fibromyalgia (using whatever criteria they considered suitable), and a comparison group of age- and sex-matched clinic patients with other painful rheumatic conditions. The subjects selected included both those with primary fibromyalgia (occurring in the absence of another rheumatic disorder) and those with secondary fibromyalgia (occurring as part of an underlying disease process such as osteoarthritis or rheumatoid arthritis). Information collected from each subject related to both

Table 19.1   The American College of Rheumatology 1990 criteria for the classification of fibromyalgia[a]; reproduced from [6] by permission of Lippincott, Williams and Wilkins

---

1. **History of widespread pain**
   Definition. Pain is considered widespread when all of the following are present: pain in the left side of the body, pain in the right side of the body, pain above the waist, and pain below the waist. In addition, axial skeletal pain (cervical spine or anterior chest or thoracic spine or low back) must be present. In this definition, shoulder and buttock pain is considered as pain for each involved side. 'Low back' pain is considered lower segment pain.
2. Pain in 11 of 18 tender point sites on digital palpation
   Definition. Pain, on digital palpation, must be present in at least 11 of the following 18 tender points sites:
   Occiput: bilateral, at the suboccipital muscle insertions.
   Low cervical: bilateral, at the anterior aspects of the intertransverse spaces at C5-C7.
   Trapezius: bilateral, at the midpoint of the upper border.
   Supraspinatus: bilateral, at origins, above the scapula spine near the medial border.
   Second rib: bilateral, at the second costochondral junctions, just lateral to the junctions on upper surfaces.
   Lateral epicondyle: bilateral, 2 cm distal to the epicondyles.
   Gluteal: bilateral, in upper outer quadrants of buttocks in anterior fold of muscle.
   Greater trochanter: bilateral, posterior to the trochanteric prominence.
   Knee: bilateral, at the medial fat pad proximal to the joint line.

   Digital palpation should be performed with an approximate force of 4 kg.
   For a tender point to be considered 'positive' the subject must state that the palpation was painful. 'Tender' is not to be considered 'painful'.

---

[a] For classification purposes, patients will be said to have fibromyalgia if both criteria are satisfied. Widespread pain must have been present for at least 3 months. The presence of a second clinical disorder does not exclude the diagnosis of fibromyalgia.

pain and other symptoms, modulating factors, and included an examination for tenderness. The combination of factors which best discriminated between those with and without fibromyalgia was a history of widespread pain and tenderness on examination (Table 19.1). Overall, the criteria correctly classified 85 per cent of patients in the fibromyalgia and non-fibromyalgia pain groups and discriminated better than any previous criteria. These criteria worked equally well for patients with 'primary' and 'secondary' fibromyalgia, and therefore it was suggested that the distinction be abolished. Fibromyalgia was a valid construct irrespective of other diagnoses. The general use of such criteria in both clinical and epidemiological studies has aided their interpretation and comparison. However, the necessity to examine subjects makes their use difficult in large-scale population surveys. More recently, two questionnaire-only screening instruments for fibromyalgia have been proposed: the first, the London Fibromyalgia Epidemiology Study Screening Questionnaire (LFESSQ) (Table 19.2), includes four questions on pain and two on fatigue, and has shown a positive predictive value (against the ACR criteria) of 71 per cent [7], while the second criteria (Manchester criteria) use only the distribution of pain reported on body manikins, but require genuinely more diffuse pain than in the ACR criteria [8].

Table 19.2   The London Fibromyalgia Epidemiology Study Screening Questionnaire (LFESSQ); reproduced by permission of the Journal of Rheumatology from [7]

Pain criteria

In the past 3 months:
1. Have you had pain in the muscles, bones, or joints, lasting at least 1 week?
2. Have you had pain in your shoulders, arms, or hands? On which side? Right, left, or both?
3. Have you had pain in your legs or feet? On which side? Right, left, or both?
4. Have you had pain in your neck, chest, or back?

Fatigue criteria

---

1. Over the past 3 months, have you often felt tired or fatigued?
2. Does tiredness or fatigue significantly limit your activities?

Meeting the pain criteria requires 'yes' responses to all four pain items, and either
1. Both a right and left side positive response, or
2. A both sides positive response
Screening positive for chronic, debilitating fatigue requires a 'yes' response to both fatigue items.

The publication and acceptance of standard classification criteria has given rise to a common view that subjects or patients satisfying such criteria have a

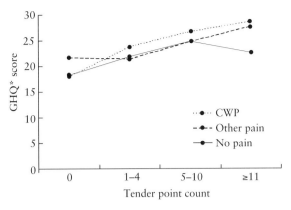

Fig. 19.1 The relationship between psychological distress and tenderness on examination: a population-based study in (Cheshire/United Kingdom). Source: [9].

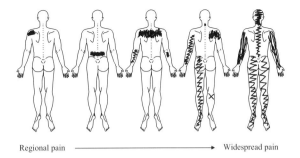

Regional pain ⟶ Widespread pain

Fig. 19.2 A pain spectrum. Reprinted from Macfarlane GJ. *Baillieres Best Pract Res Clin Rheumatol* 1999; 13: 403–414 [12] by permission of the publisher Baillière Tindall.

distinct syndrome in comparison, for example, to others with less widespread pain or less tenderness on examination. In fact, rather than uniquely occurring with widespread pain or causing an enhancement of pain, tender points appear to be a general measure of distress which are also independently associated with fatigue and depression [9–11]. Data from a population survey in the United Kingdom demonstrate that amongst subjects with chronic widespread pain, greater numbers of tender points on examination are associated with higher levels of distress (Fig. 19.1). However, this relationship holds true also amongst subjects with regional pain and even those with no pain—it is therefore not unique to subjects with chronic widespread pain [9]. This provides a rationale, when considering the epidemiology, to consider individual features of the syndrome, for example pain, rather than necessarily their co-occurrence in a syndrome such as fibromyalgia. In support of this, a review of the descriptive and analytical epidemiology reveals many similarities in patterns of occurrence, co-morbidities, and risk factors between chronic widespread pain (and fibromyalgia) and regional pain syndromes, such as low back pain

and shoulder pain [12]. This argues in favour of considering a 'pain spectrum' ranging from acute regional pain to chronic widespread pain syndromes, rather than distinct entities (Fig. 19.2). Acknowledging, therefore, that from an epidemiological viewpoint it represents an artificial division, this chapter will consider chronic widespread pain while regional pain syndromes will be considered in other chapters.

Prevalence of chronic widespread pain and fibromyalgia

Chronic widespread pain

Three population-based questionnaire surveys in the United Kingdom, United States, and Sweden have all provided remarkably similar prevalence estimates of chronic widespread pain: 11.2 per cent, 10.6 per cent, and 10.7 per cent respectively [13–15] (Table 19.3). Information on pain and its location is typically collected, in such surveys, by means of a body manikin, which is then coded according to the definition of chronic widespread pain used in the ACR definition for fibromyalgia. A further survey, conducted in Canada

Table 19.3 Population estimates of the prevalence of chronic widespread pain

Study location	Disease definition	Population (years)	Sample size	Prevalence (%)	Reference
United Kingdom	ACR[a]	18–85	1340	11.2	[13]
United States	ACR[a]	≥18	3006	10.6	[14]
Sweden	Chronic pain with multiple localization	25–74	1609	10.7	[15]
Canada	LFESSQ[b]/ACR[a]	≥18	3395	7.3	[16]

[a] American College of Rheumatology definition in the 1990 fibromyalgia classification criteria: [6].
[b] London Fibromyalgia Epidemiology Study Screening Questionnaire: [7].

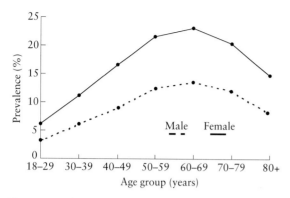

Fig. 19.3 The prevalence of chronic widespread pain by age in Wichita (United States). Reproduced from [14] by permission of Lippincott, Williams and Wilkins.

by telephone, using the LFESSQ to screen for chronic widespread pain, provided a slightly lower prevalence estimate at 7.3 per cent [16]. Clearly, therefore, this is a commonly reported symptom in populations. It is also a consistent finding that prevalence estimates are almost double in females in comparison to males. For example in Canada rates for males and females were 4.7 per cent and 9.0 per cent [16] while in the United Kingdom rates were 9.4 per cent and 15.6 per cent respectively [13]. The prevalence pattern by age in both sexes is typically of an increasing prevalence until around the seventh decade with decreases thereafter (Fig. 19.3) [14]. In this respect it mirrors the pattern found in common regional pain syndromes such as back and shoulder pain [17,18]. Why this pattern of a decrease in point and period prevalence rates at older ages should be observed, is unclear. Firstly, subjects with such pain syndromes may die at earlier ages,

although there is at present no evidence for this. Alternatively, pain reporting may be affected both by subjects' expectations of pain and other experienced symptoms. If subjects at older ages have a higher expectation of pain and are experiencing a variety of other symptoms, this may lead to lower relative awareness and reporting of pain in epidemiological surveys.

Fibromyalgia

Most studies conducted in Scandinavia and North and Central America have reported population prevalence rates of between 0.5 and 2.0 per cent (Table 19.4). At the bottom end of the range two studies in Denmark and Finland reported prevalence rates of 0.66 per cent and 0.75 per cent respectively [20,23], while at the upper end of the range a population study in Wichita (United States) reported prevalence rates of 2.0 per cent [14]. Higher prevalence rates have been reported in Canada (3.3 per cent), from a study which paradoxically had reported lower than average rates of chronic widespread pain [15], from a study of women only in Norway (10.5 per cent) [21], and a study of schoolchildren in Israel (6.2 per cent) [22]. There may be a variety of reasons for such variation in estimates. Firstly, there may be a real difference between populations, although the consistency of the majority of studies would argue against this. Secondly it may relate to methodological aspects of individual studies: there may be a biased sample of responders or biases in the responses given, or there may be variation particularly in the examination of tender points between individual studies. While reliability within centres has been shown to be good for tender point examination [25,26], there

Table 19.4 Population estimates of the prevalence of fibromyalgia

Study location	Disease definition	Population (years)	Sample size	Prevalence (%)	Reference
Sweden	Yunus[a]	50–70	876	1.0	[19]
Finland	Yunus[a]	≥30	7217	0.75	[20]
Norway	ACR[b]	20–49 (females only)	2038	10.5	[21]
Israel	ACR[b]	9–15	338	6.2	[22]
Denmark	ACR[b]	18–79	1219	0.66	[23]
United States	ACR[b]	≥18	3006	2.0	[14]
Mexico	ACR[b]	9–15	548	1.2	[24]
Canada	LFESSQ[c]/ACR[b]	≥18	3395	3.3	[16]

[a] Source: [5]
[b] American College of Rheumatology definition in the 1990 fibromyalgia classification criteria: [6].
[c] London Fibromyalgia Epidemiology Study Screening Questionnaire: [7].

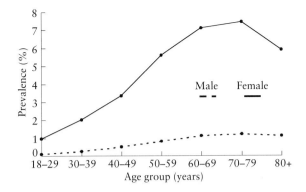

(a)

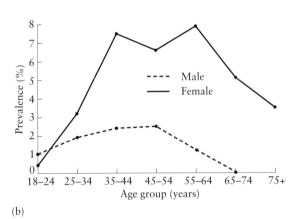

(b)

Fig. 19.4 (a) The prevalence of fibromyalgia by age in Wichita (United States). Reproduced from [14] by permission of Lippincott, Williams and Wilkins. (b) The prevalence of fibromyalgia by age in Ontario (Canada), source: [16].

is considerable scope for variation in examination between centres. Dolorimetry has the advantage of being more objective with a standard stimulus, but both the surface area of the dolorimeter and the rate of force can still influence the results [27,28].

There appears to be an even greater female: male prevalence ratio for fibromyalgia in comparison to chronic widespread pain. The United States study found a prevalence in females of 3.4 per cent compared to 0.5 per cent in males [14], while the study in Canada found prevalence rates of 4.9 per cent and 1.6 per cent respectively [16]. The shape of the age–prevalence curve remains the same, however, with increases observed until the sixth or seventh decades, when the Canadian study found a peak prevalence of 7.9 per cent, but with a decrease in prevalence at older ages (Fig. 19.4).

In contrast to population studies, studies relying on clinics for ascertainment and recruitment of subjects rarely provide useful information on the prevalence of fibromyalgia. This is because they are conducted on selected populations: selected on the basis of the decision to consult and on the further referral process. Given the differences that exist between countries in consultation and referral processes there is little to be gained from comparisons. Such studies can, however, give indications of population groups in which fibromyalgia is particularly common. In a primary care study from the United States, of 692 patients evaluated in a 1-month period, 4.6 per cent of subjects had symptoms of unexplained, chronic diffuse muscular pain [29]. The authors of this study note, however, that only a minority of these groups formally satisfied various sets of criteria for fibromyalgia, and emphasize, as has been discussed above, that such criteria merely define one end of a spectrum. Moving from primary care to specialist referral centres for pain or rheumatic conditions, fibromyalgia becomes relatively more common. In a United States study of 125 patients referred to a spine centre for back pain, 12 per cent were diagnosed with fibromyalgia on the basis of tenderness and pain intensity and distribution [30]. Fibromyalgia has also been reported as having a high prevalence in patients with other conditions, for example rheumatoid arthritis (13.6 per cent; n = 280) [31], systemic lupus erythematosus (22.0 per cent; n = 102) [32], and Behçet's syndrome (9.2 per cent; n = 108) [33]. Overall, of 285 new patients seen at rheumatology clinic in the United States over a period of 1 year, 20 per cent were referred with 'primary' fibromyalgia, and, in patients under 50, this was the most common reason for referral [34].

Wolfe and Cathey [35] specifically examined 1520 consecutive patients at a rheumatic disease clinic for tenderness at 14 anatomical locations. Forty percent of patients reported at least one tender point, 23 per cent had four or more, 14 per cent had seven or more, and 14 per cent had 12 or more tender points. The count of number of tender points generally increased with age and was higher in females. A high number of tender points was associated with high levels of anxiety, disability, fatigue, and disturbed sleep. Although they were also associated with regional pain syndromes such as neck and low back pain, the sites of tender points did not generally correspond to the site of joint pathology. In a population study of 177 subjects from the United Kingdom (including subjects with and without pain) the median number of tender points, using the eighteen sites defined in the

ACR criteria for fibromyalgia [6], increased from three (in subjects with no pain) to eight (in subjects with widespread pain) [10]. The recording of a tender point as positive was associated with an increased odds of reporting pain in the same anatomical site of between two to three-fold, depending on the specific anatomical site.

Time trends in occurrence

There is little direct evidence available to determine whether chronic widespread pain or fibromyalgia is becoming more common. Although the term fibrositis (subsequently called fibromyalgia) seems first to have been used at the beginning of the 20th century [36], only in the past 20 years has there been an explosion of research interest, amongst rheumatologists, in this syndrome. This may be due to a true increase in the occurrence of such symptoms. However, the levels of reporting and likelihood of seeking treatment for a condition and the type of diagnosis made can be influenced by a host of factors other than a true change in occurrence: social forces (e.g. financial, legal, the popular media) can determine the 'acceptability' of certain conditions and the likelihood of subjects reporting or presenting for medical care. Further, the diagnosis and treatment of ailments by health-care professionals is affected by a variety of social factors and political considerations in addition to current medical views on the aetiology of disease [37]. It may be, for example, that chronic widespread pain has always been common but that health-care systems through time have changed patterns of referral for such patients within health-care systems. From a rheumatologists viewpoint, Wolfe [38] suggests that in the United States fibromyalgia is currently 'out of control', with a logarithmic increase in the number of cases diagnosed and in medicolegal claims for disability entitlement. While acknowledging that 'fibromyalgia' (or whatever name one gives to the constellation of symptoms) will always be with us because patients suffer with these symptoms, he proposes that the trend towards labelling fibromyalgia patients as disabled must be halted and that a societal trend towards encouragement of such a disability concept should be discouraged [38].

Data above have shown that amongst developed countries there is little evidence for variation in the prevalence of chronic widespread pain and fibromyalgia. The only available data on time trends within a country come from the United Kingdom. Within the Greater Manchester area several population-based pain surveys have been undertaken using a similar methodology. In 1991, amongst a sample of 1340 subjects the prevalence of chronic widespread pain (using the definition in the ACR criteria for fibromyalgia) was 13 per cent [13]. Data obtained from a 2-year follow-up study of 141 participants in this study suggested that while some subjects had developed chronic widespread pain, the symptoms of others had resolved; the overall effect of these changes in status would be an unchanged population prevalence [39]. Further, in 1995, amongst a different population of 3004 subjects from the same area, the prevalence of chronic widespread pain was still found to be 13 per cent [1]. There is, therefore, no evidence to support the view that in population terms such a condition has recently become more frequent although presentation for health care may be more common.

Risk factors for chronic widespread pain and fibromyalgia

Genetic factors

There is relatively little research work examining the possible role of genetic factors in chronic widespread pain and fibromyalgia. Buskila *et al.* [40] examined 58 offspring of 20 female clinic patients with fibromyalgia in Israel. Sixteen offspring (28 per cent) were found to satisfy criteria for the fibromyalgia syndrome according to the ACR criteria. Age-specific prevalence rates were compared with those from a population-based study in the United States [14] and found to be higher, particularly in the youngest and oldest age groups (although numbers of subjects were small and the comparison group was not ideal) [40]. An excess could come about not only as a result of genetic factors, but due to common environmental factors such as anxiety, depression, and illness behaviour. A further study from the same research group reported that the mean tender point count amongst relatives of female fibromyalgia patients was higher than an unmatched control population [41]. The few association studies which have been conducted of fibromyalgia with HLA have provided conflicting results. Hørven *et al.* [42] found no association with HLA in a study of 60 fibromyalgia and 159 healthy controls, while a another study of 52 fibromyalgia patients and 869 healthy controls found a significant association with HLA-B58,

DR8, and DR5 [43]. A recent linkage analysis of 40 multicase families with fibromyalgia suggested that there may be some linkage to the HLA region although the effect noticed was modest [44]. In summary, the studies to date in this area are few, generally involving small groups of subjects, and using unmatched and selected control groups.

Further work is required before one can draw conclusions about the role of genetic and family environment factors in chronic widespread pain and fibromyalgia. However, a study on pain perception, using dolorimeter measurements of pressure pain threshold (PPT), on 269 and 340 pairs of monozygotic (MZ) and dizygotic (DZ) healthy female–female twin pairs found a strong and approximately equal correlation of PPT in MZ (correlation coefficient r = 0.57, 95 per cent CI: 0.49, 0.65) and DZ (r = 0.51, 95 per cent CI: 0.42, 0.59) twins [45]. These results would suggest that learned behaviour within families rather than genetic factors are important with respect to pain sensitivity.

Non-genetic host factors

Comorbidities are the rule amongst patients in the clinic with fibromyalgia. Indeed early criteria sets, such as those of Yunus *et al.* [5], required that some of these co-morbidities (e.g. general fatigue, poor sleep, anxiety/tension, or irritable bowel syndrome) be present. There is therefore some circularity in an argument that then describes these features as more common in patients. The increased prevalence of fibromyalgia and chronic widespread pain with age (at least until older ages) has previously been discussed as has the excess in females compared to males. Population studies have shown that the prevalence of fibromyalgia is inversely associated with level of education [14]. In the population study of Mäkelä and Heliövaara [20], prevalence increased from 0 per cent amongst 806 subjects with at least high school education to 2.7 per cent amongst 736 subjects with less than an elementary level of education. Further, amongst subjects with fibromyalgia low education has been associated with a greater impact of symptoms, likelihood of disability, and persistence of symptoms [39,46,47].

Although the observation has been made of differing prevalence rates between males and females both of regional and widespread chronic pain syndromes, the role of sex hormones on the occurrence and severity of symptoms is largely unknown. One retrospective study of a small group of 26 women with fibromyalgia found that they reported a worsening of symptoms during pregnancy and a further worsening of symptoms in the post-partum period. However, the hormonal changes associated with abortion or oral contraceptive use were not associated with changes in self-reported symptoms [48].

Most clinic and population studies have, to date, been of cross-sectional design. It is has thus been difficult to determine whether some of the features that are commonly associated with chronic widespread pain are risk factors for the onset of widespread pain, and/or are consequences of having such symptoms or whether they merely share common aetiological factors.

Population studies have demonstrated that chronic widespread pain and fibromyalgia are associated with fatigue, psychological distress, and have shown that subjects score highly on scales of anxiety and depression [1,13,14]. Subjects with regional or widespread pain also commonly report other somatic symptoms [13,49]. A problem in interpreting clinical studies is disentangling the extent to which observed associations are with the symptoms themselves and to what extent they reflect factors associated with seeking consultation. A population-based study in the United Kingdom demonstrated a stronger cross-sectional association between chronic widespread pain and psychological distress amongst those who had consulted in comparison to those with symptoms but who had not consulted their general practitioner [50]. A study of patients and population volunteers with fibromyalgia in the United States suggested that an association between psychiatric disorder and fibromyalgia was confined to clinic patients [51].

An evaluation of the temporal relationship between depression and chronic musculoskeletal pain was possible within The National Health and Nutrition Survey (NHANES) in the United States which collected information on chronic pain and depression firstly between 1974 and 5 and again between 1981 and 4 [52]. Chronic pain was defined as pain present on most days for 1 of the 12 months preceding baseline evaluation (not necessarily widespread) while depression was assessed using the Centre for Epidemiologic Studies Depression Scale [53]. Amongst subjects without chronic pain at baseline, depressive symptoms at baseline were associated with a doubling in risk of chronic pain at follow-up. Similarly however, amongst subjects without depressive symptoms at baseline, chronic pain at baseline was associated with a doubling in risk of depressive symptoms at follow-up. This would suggest that the relationship between pain and psychological factors operates in both directions, an observation which has also been made for regional pain syndromes [54]. In identifying subjects without symptoms but who are at high risk to develop chronic widespread pain the factors conferring the highest risk, in addition to high levels of psychological distress, appear to be female gender, older age, somatic symptoms, and aspects of illness behaviour [55]. This gives weight to the opinion that chronic widespread pain may be one manifestation of somatization, even though subjects rarely meet formal criteria for the diagnosis of somatoform disorder [50].

Environmental factors

Several studies have examined the relationship between abuse in childhood (particularly sexual abuse) and chronic widespread pain and fibromyalgia in adults. Boisset-Pioro *et al.* [56] compared 83 female fibromyalgia clinic patients with 161 clinic subjects with other rheumatic disease. Overall, there was no statistical difference in the rates of reporting of abuse (at any time) between the two groups, although childhood physical and sexual abuse were more common amongst fibromyalgia patients. Another clinic study comparing 104 patients with fibromyalgia with 44 patients with rheumatoid arthritis also found an association between fibromyalgia and childhood physical and sexual abuse [57] while a study amongst patients with fibromyalgia found that those reporting a past history of abuse were characterized by having greater pain, disability, and levels of stress [58]. Not all studies, however, have found a difference in reported rates of sexual abuse [59]. In interpreting these (and other) studies it is important to consider that they are conducted in selected populations, almost all have low participation rates in the fibromyalgia and/or 'control' groups, and are clearly open to the potential of differential recall of past events between subjects with and without current symptoms. A population study in the United Kingdom found that subjects with chronic widespread pain reported greater levels of five adverse childhood factors: illness in family members, parental loss, hospitalization, operations, and abuse. When self-reports of hospitalization and operation were compared with available medical notes there was evidence of differential recall of past events between subjects with and without chronic widespread pain which could explain some of the observed relationship [60]. Determining whether there is an association between

adverse childhood factors and chronic pain in adulthood will rely on future studies. Such studies, in this methodologically difficult area, will require to be of high quality design, if advances in knowledge are to be made.

The role of physical (mechanical) factors in the aetiology of chronic widespread pain and fibromyalgia has received relatively little attention. Although there appears to be acknowledgment in the literature that previous trauma can be related to symptoms, there is a lack of well-designed studies to evaluate this. Mäkelä and Heliövaara [20], in a population survey, reported that the prevalence of fibromyalgia was more than twice as common in those reporting high physical work stress in comparison to those reporting low levels. A further retrospective study of 161 cases of traumatic injury found different subsequent rates of development of fibromyalgia according to site and type of injury: it was 13 times more common in those with a neck injury in comparison to those with an injury of the lower extremity [41]. As noted previously, differential recall and attribution may affect cross-sectional or retrospective studies relying on self-reports by those with and without chronic widespread pain. The role of mechanical factors in the aetiology of symptoms can therefore best be addressed by prospective studies which assess exposure prior to the onset of symptoms. A variety of other factors have been investigated, although mainly in cross-sectional and retrospective studies. Foremost amongst these has been the role of infection. However, one prospective study of 150 subjects with acute infectious mononucleosis (AIM) which enrolled them around the time of diagnosis, found that while 19 per cent of subjects satisfied ACR criteria for fibromyalgia at enrolment, prevalence rates subsequently fell to 3 per cent and 1 per cent at 2 and 6 months follow-up [61]. The authors concluded that a tender point count and fibromyalgia were infrequent sequelae of AIM. Indeed, at follow-up a high tender point count was predicted by older age, female sex, less family social support, and baseline tender point count, rather than any baseline laboratory tests.

Finally, fibromyalgia has been reported as common in persons with other environmental exposures. Widespread body pain has been a common symptom reported by armed forces personnel who served in the Gulf war. They report fibromyalgia (based on questionnaires), in addition to a variety of other conditions, more commonly than personnel who were not deployed [62]. Those deployed were exposed to a variety of environmental and physical exposures including smoke from oil-well fires, pesticides, nerve agent prophylaxis, and multiple inoculations. Adverse psychological experiences, including seeing maimed soldiers and dismembered bodies, were also commonly reported. However, to date, no specific associations with fibromyalgia have been elucidated. The symptoms reported by patients with fibromyalgia are shared with a variety of other 'unexplained syndromes'. They include chronic fatigue syndrome, repetitive strain injury, sick building syndrome, and irritable bowel syndrome. Some are defined by symptoms alone while others require, in addition, specific exposure. An exposure-defined syndrome, which has been closely associated with the symptoms of fibromyalgia, is the side-effects of silicone breast implants. Studies of women with breast implants have failed to demonstrate a subsequent increase in risk either of connective tissue disease overall or of fibromyalgia in particular [63,64]. However, it has been suggested that such syndromes may frequently co-occur because common psycho-social characteristics of those who have fibromyalgia and those who choose to have silicone breast implants.

In summary therefore, the research studies discussed above have shown that chronic widespread pain and fibromyalgia are common in the population as well as in rheumatology clinics. However, they do not represent specific disease entities, but rather should be considered at one end of a pain spectrum from acute regional pain to chronic widespread pain. Similarly, tender points are a general measure of distress rather than specifically associated with widespread pain. In terms of aetiology, adverse psychological factors are associated with and predict symptoms onset. The view that fibromyalgia is one manifestation of somatization seems likely in view of its co-occurrence with, and that it is predicted by, other somatic symptoms. Whether adverse childhood factors are a possible early part of this aetiological pathway is at present unclear. It is outside the remit of this chapter to review the interesting results emerging from clinical and laboratory studies on the pathophysiology associated with chronic pain syndromes (e.g. alterations in central neurochemical transmission, pain processing pathways). However, advances in our understanding of these painful and disabling conditions is most likely to follow from unravelling these mechanisms in combination with a greater understanding of the epidemiology of symptom onset.

References

1. Hunt IM, Silman AJ, Benjamin S, McBeth J, Macfarlane GJ. The prevalence and associated features of chronic widespread pain in the community using the 'Manchester' definition of chronic widespread pain. *Rheumatol* 1999; **38**: 275–279.
2. White KP, Speechley M, Harth M, Østbye T. Fibromyalgia in rheumatology practice: a survey of Canadian rheumatologists. *J Rheumatol* 1995; **22**: 722–726.
3. Hyams KC. Developing case definitions for symptom-based conditions: the problem of specificity. *Epidemiol Rev* 1998; **20**: 148–156.
4. Smythe HA, Moldofsky H. Two contributions to understanding of the 'fibrositis' syndrome. *Bull Rheum Dis* 1977; **28**: 928–931.
5. Yunus MB, Masi AT, Aldag JC. Preliminary criteria for primary fibromyalgia syndrome (PFS): multivariate analysis of a consecutive series of PFS, other pain patients, and normal subjects. *Clin Exp Rheumatol* 1989; **7**: 63–69.
6. Wolfe F, Smythe HA, Yunus MB *et al.* The American College of Rheumatology 1990 Criteria for the Classification of Fibromyalgia. Report of the Multicenter Criteria Committee. *Arthritis Rheum* 1990; **33**: 160–172.
7. White KP, Harth M, Speechley M, Østbye T. Testing an instrument to screen for fibromyalgia syndrome in general population studies: the London Fibromyalgia Epidemiology Study Screening Questionnaire. *J Rheumatol* 1999; **26**: 880–884.
8. Macfarlane GJ, Croft PR, Schollum J, Silman AJ. Widespread pain: is an improved classification possible? *J Rheumatol* 1996; **23**: 1628–1632.
9. Croft P, Schollum J, Silman A. Population study of tender point counts and pain as evidence of fibromyalgia. *BMJ* 1994; **309**: 696–699.
10. Croft P, Burt J, Schollum J, Thomas E, Macfarlane G, Silman A. More pain, more tender points: is fibromyalgia just one end of a continuous spectrum? *Ann Rheum Dis* 1996; **55**: 482–485.
11. Wolfe F. The relation between tender points and fibromyalgia symptom variables: evidence that fibromyalgia is not a discrete disorder in the clinic. *Ann Rheum Dis* 1997; **56**: 268–271.
12. Macfarlane GJ. Generalized pain, fibromyalgia and regional pain: an epidemiological view. *Baillieres Best Pract Res Clin Rheumatol* 1999; **13**: 403–414.
13. Croft P, Rigby AS, Boswell R, Schollum J, Silman A. The prevalence of chronic widespread pain in the general population. *J Rheumatol* 1993; **20**: 710–713.
14. Wolfe F, Ross K, Anderson J, Russell IJ, Hebert L. The prevalence and characteristics of fibromyalgia in the general population. *Arthritis Rheum* 1995; **38**: 19–28.
15. Andersson HI, Ejlertsson G, Leden I, Rosenberg C. Characteristics of subjects with chronic pain, in relation to local and widespread pain report. A prospective study of symptoms, clinical findings and blood tests in subgroups of a geographically defined population. *Scand J Rheumatol* 1996; **25**: 146–154.

16. White KP, Speechley M, Harth M, Østbye T. The London fibromyalgia epidemiology study: The prevalence of fibromyalgia syndrome in London, Ontario. *J Rheumatol* 1999; **26**: 1570–1576.

17. Andersson HI, Ejlertsson G, Leden I, Rosenberg C. Chronic pain in a geographically defined general population: studies of differences in age, gender, social class, and pain localization. *Clin J Pain* 1993; **9**: 174–182.

18. Papageorgiou AC, Croft PR, Ferry S, Jayson MI, Silman AJ. Estimating the prevalence of low back pain in the general population. Evidence from the South Manchester Back Pain Survey. *Spine* 1995; **20**: 1889–1894.

19. Jacobsson L, Lindgarde F, Manthorpe R. The commonest rheumatic complaints of over six weeks' duration in a twelve-month period in a defined Swedish population. Prevalences and relationships. *Scand J Rheumatol* 1989; **18**: 353–360.

20. Mäkelä M, Heliövaara M. Prevalence of primary fibromyalgia in the Finnish population. *BMJ* 1991; **303**: 216–219.

21. Forseth KO, Gran JT. The prevalence of fibromyalgia among women aged 20–49 years in Arendal, Norway. *Scand J Rheumatol* 1992; **21**: 74–78.

22. Buskila D, Press J, Gedalia A *et al.* Assessment of nonarticular tenderness and prevalence of fibromyalgia in children. *J Rheumatol* 1993; **20**: 368–370.

23. Prescott E, Kjoller M, Jacobsen S, Bulow PM, Danneskiold-Samsoe B, Kamper-Jorgensen F. Fibromyalgia in the adult Danish population: I. A prevalence study. *Scand J Rheumatol* 1993; **22**: 233–237.

24. Clark P, Burgos-Vargas R, Medina-Palma C, Lavielle P, Marina FF. Prevalence of fibromyalgia in children: a clinical study of Mexican children. *J Rheumatol* 1998; **25**: 2009–2014.

25. Jacobs JWG, Geenen R, Van Der Heide A, Rasker JJ, Bijlsma JWJ. Are tender point scores assessed by manual palpation in fibromyalgia reliable? An investigation into the variance of tender point scores. *Scand J Rheumatol* 1995; **24**: 243–247.

26. Tunks E, McCain GA, Hart LE *et al.* The reliability of examination for tenderness in patients with myofascial pain, chronic fibromyalgia and controls. *J Rheumatol* 1995; **22**: 944–952.

27. Smythe HA, Buskila D, Urowitz S, Langevitz P. Control and 'fibrositic' tenderness: comparison of two dolorimeters. *J Rheumatol* 1992; **19**: 768–771.

28. White KP, McCain GA, Tunks E. The effects of changing the painful stimulus upon dolorimetry scores in patients with fibromyalgia. *J Musculoskelet Pain* 1993; **1**: 43–58.

29. Hartz A, Kirchdoerfer E. Undetected fibrositis in primary care practice. *J Fam Pract* 1987; **25**: 365–369.

30. Borenstein D. Prevalence and treatment outcome of primary and secondary fibromyalgia in patients with spinal pain. *Spine* 1995; **20**: 796–800.

31. Wolfe F, Cathey MA, Kleinheksel SM. Fibrositis (fibromyalgia) in rheumatoid arthritis. *J Rheumatol* 1984; **11**: 814–818.

32. Middleton GD, McFarlin JE, Lipsky PE. The prevalence and clinical impact of fibromyalgia in systemic lupus erythematosus. *Arthritis Rheum* 1994; **37**: 1181–1188.

33. Yavuz S, Fresko I, Hamuryudan V, Yurdakul S, Yazici H. Fibromyalgia in Behc[,]et's syndrome. *J Rheumatol* 1998; **25**: 2219–2220.

34. Yunus M, Masi AT, Calabro JJ, Miller KA, Feigenbaum SL. Primary fibromyalgia (fibrositis): Clinical study of 50 patients with matched normal controls. *Semin Arthritis Rheum* 1981; **11**: 151–171.

35. Wolfe F, Cathey MA. The epidemiology of tender points: a prospective study of 1520 patients. *J Rheumatol* 1985; **12**: 1164–1168.

36. Gowers WR. Lumbago: its lessons and analogues. *BMJ* 1904; **1**: 117–121.

37. Cockerham WC. *Medical sociology.* Englewood Cliffs, New Jersey: Prentice Hall, 1986.

38. Wolfe F. The fibromyalgia problem. *J Rheumatol* 1997; **24**: 1247–1249.

39. Macfarlane GJ, Thomas E, Papageorgiou AC, Schollum J, Croft PR, Silman AJ. The natural history of chronic pain in the community: a better prognosis than in the clinic? *J Rheumatol* 1996; **23**: 1617–1620.

40. Buskila D, Neumann L, Hazanov I, Carmi R. Familial aggregation in the fibromyalgia syndrome. *Semin Arthritis Rheum* 1996; **26**: 605–611.

41. Buskila D, Neumann L, Vaisberg G, Alkalay D, Wolfe F. Increased rates of fibromyalgia following cervical spine injury. A controlled study of 161 cases of traumatic injury. *Arthritis Rheum* 1997; **40**: 446–452.

42. Hørven S, Stiles TC, Holst A, Moen T. HLA antigens in primary fibromyalgia syndrome. *J Rheumatol* 1992; **19**: 1269–1270.

43. Branco JC, Tavares V, Abreu I, Correia MM, Caetano JAM. HLA studies in fibromyalgia. *J Musculoskelet Pain* 1996; **4**: 21–27.

44. Yunus MB, Khan MA, Rawlings KK, Green JR, Olson JM, Shah S. Genetic linkage analysis of multicase families with fibromyalgia syndrome. *J Rheumatol* 1999; **26**: 408–412.

45. MacGregor AJ, Griffiths GO, Baker J, Spector TD. Determinants of pressure pain threshold in adult twins: evidence that shared environmental influences predominate. *Pain* 1997; **73**: 253–257.

46. Neumann L, Buskila D. Ethnocultural and educational differences in Israeli women correlate with pain perception in fibromyalgia. *J Rheumatol* 1998; **25**: 1369–1373.

47. White KP, Speechley M, Harth M, Østbye T. Comparing self-reported function and work disability in 100 community cases of fibromyalgia syndrome versus controls in London, Ontario: the London Fibromyalgia Epidemiology Study. *Arthritis Rheum* 1999; **42**: 76–83.

48. Ostensen M, Rugelsjoen A, Wigers SH. The effect of reproductive events and alterations of sex hormone levels on the symptoms of fibromyalgia. *Scand J Rheumatol* 1997; **26**: 355–360.

49. Von Korff M, Dworkin SF, Le Resche L, Kruger A. An epidemiologic comparison of pain complaints. *Pain* 1988; **32**: 173–183.

50. Macfarlane GJ, Morris S, Hunt IM *et al.* Chronic widespread pain in the community: the influence of psychological symptoms and mental disorder on healthcare seeking behavior. *J Rheumatol* 1999; **26**: 413–419.

51. Aaron LA, Bradley LA, Alarcon GS *et al.* Psychiatric diagnoses in patients with fibromyalgia are related to health care-seeking behavior rather than to illness. *Arthritis Rheum* 1996; **39**: 436–445.

52. Magni G, Moreschi C, Rigatti-Luchini S, Merskey H. Prospective study on the relationship between depressive symptoms and chronic musculoskeletal pain. *Pain* 1994; **56**: 289–297.

53. Radloff L. The CES-D scale: a self-report depression scale for research in the general population. *J Appl Psychol Meas* 1977; **1**: 385–401.

54. Hotopf M, Mayou R, Wadsworth M, Wessely S. Temporal relationships between physical symptoms and psychiatric disorder. Results from a national birth cohort. *Br J Psychiatry* 1998; **173**: 255–261.

55. Silman AJ, McBeth J, Papageorgiou AC, Hunt IM, Benjamin S, Macfarlane GJ. Features of somatisation predict onset of chronic widespread pain: Results from a large prospective population study. *Arthritis Rheum* 1998; **41**: S358.

56. Boisset-Pioro MH, Esdaile JM, Fitzcharles MA. Sexual and physical abuse in women with fibromyalgia syndrome. *Arthritis Rheum* 1995; **38**: 235–241.

57. Carpenter MT, Hugler R, Enzenauer RJ, Rosier KFD, Kirk JM, Brehm WT. Physical and sexual abuse in female patients with fibromyalgia. *J Clin Rheumatol* 1998; **4**: 301–306.

58. Alexander RW, Bradley LA, Alarcon GS *et al.* Sexual and physical abuse in women with fibromyalgia: association with outpatient health care utilization and pain medication usage. *Arthritis Care Res* 1998; **11**: 102–115.

59. Taylor ML, Trotter DR, Csuka ME. The prevalence of sexual abuse in women with fibromyalgia. *Arthritis Rheum* 1995; **38**: 229–234.

60. McBeth J, Morris S, Papageorgiou AC, Benjamin S, Silman AJ, Macfarlane GJ. Psychiatric morbidity, adverse childhood experiences and chronic widespread pain. *Arthritis Rheum* 1997; **40**: S304.

61. Rea T, Russo J, Katon W, Ashley RL, Buchwald D. A prospective study of tender points and fibromyalgia during and after an acute viral infection. *Arch Intern Med* 1999; **159**: 865–870.

62. The Iowa Persian Gulf Study Group. Self-reported illness and health status among Gulf War veterans. A population-based study. *JAMA* 1997; **277**: 238–245.

63. Nyren O, Yin L, Josefsson S *et al.* Risk of connective tissue disease and related disorders among women with breast implants: a nation-wide retrospective cohort study in Sweden. *BMJ* 1998; **316**: 417–422.

64. Wolfe F, Anderson J. Silicone filled breast implants and the risk of fibromyalgia and rheumatoid arthritis. *J Rheumatol* 1999; **26**: 2025–2028.

Index